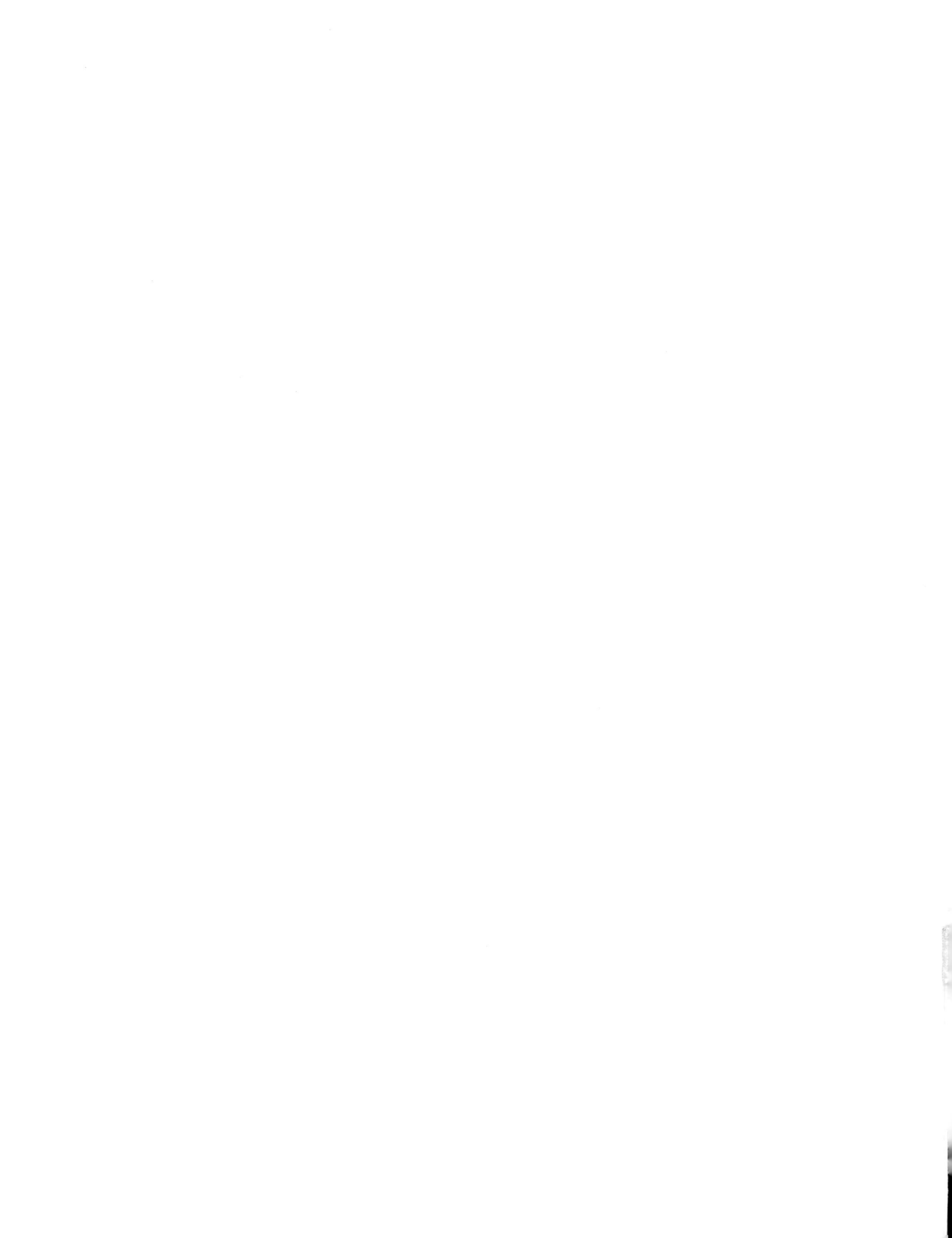

Advances in Genome Medicine

Advances in Genome Medicine

Editor: Stuart Gates

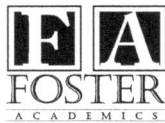

FA
FOSTER
ACADEMICS

www.fosteracademics.com

www.fosteracademics.com

FA
FOSTER
ACADEMICS

Cataloging-in-Publication Data

Advances in genome medicine / edited by Stuart Gates.
    p. cm.
Includes bibliographical references and index.
ISBN 978-1-63242-698-7
1. Medical genetics. 2. Genomics. 3. Genomes. 4. Human genome. I. Gates, Stuart.
RB155 .A38 2019
616.042--dc23

Foster Academics,
118-35 Queens Blvd., Suite 400,
Forest Hills, NY 11375, USA

ISBN 978-1-63242-698-7 (Hardback)

Contents

Preface

The diagnosis and management of hereditary disorders and conditions, such as birth defects and dysmorphology, autism, mental retardation, connective tissue disorders, mitochondrial disorders, skeletal dysplasia, etc. is encompassed under genome medicine. It incorporates diverse areas within its domain such as personalized medicine, gene therapy and predictive medicine. A diagnostic examination customized according to an understanding of existing signs and symptoms is used for establishing a differential diagnosis and developing an appropriate treatment. Such diagnostic tests help in determining whether the condition is an inborn error of metabolism, a chromosomal disorder or a single gene disorder. There is no cure for genetic disorders. However, there is a potential for the dietary and medical management of the conditions to reduce or prevent long-term complications. This book is a compilation of chapters that discuss the most vital concepts and emerging trends in the field of genome medicine. It aims to shed light on some of the unexplored aspects of genome medicine and the recent researches in this field. For all those who are interested in this field, this book can prove to be an essential guide.

After months of intensive research and writing, this book is the end result of all who devoted their time and efforts in the initiation and progress of this book. It will surely be a source of reference in enhancing the required knowledge of the new developments in the area. During the course of developing this book, certain measures such as accuracy, authenticity and research focused analytical studies were given preference in order to produce a comprehensive book in the area of study.

This book would not have been possible without the efforts of the authors and the publisher. I extend my sincere thanks to them. Secondly, I express my gratitude to my family and well-wishers. And most importantly, I thank my students for constantly expressing their willingness and curiosity in enhancing their knowledge in the field, which encourages me to take up further research projects for the advancement of the area.

Editor

Elevated polygenic burden for autism is associated with differential DNA methylation at birth

Eilis Hannon[1], Diana Schendel[2], Christine Ladd-Acosta[3,4], Jakob Grove[5,6,7,8], iPSYCH-Broad ASD Group, Christine Søholm Hansen[6,9,10], Shan V. Andrews[3,4], David Michael Hougaard[6,9], Michaeline Bresnahan[11], Ole Mors[6,13], Mads Vilhelm Hollegaard[6,9^], Marie Bækvad-Hansen[6,9], Mady Hornig[11,12], Preben Bo Mortensen[6,14,15,16], Anders D. Børglum[5,6,7], Thomas Werge[6,10,17], Marianne Giørtz Pedersen[6,13,16], Merete Nordentoft[6,18], Joseph Buxbaum[19], M. Daniele Fallin[4,11,20,21], Jonas Bybjerg-Grauholm[6,9], Abraham Reichenberg[19] and Jonathan Mill[1]*

Abstract

Background: Autism spectrum disorder (ASD) is a severe neurodevelopmental disorder characterized by deficits in social communication and restricted, repetitive behaviors, interests, or activities. The etiology of ASD involves both inherited and environmental risk factors, with epigenetic processes hypothesized as one mechanism by which both genetic and non-genetic variation influence gene regulation and pathogenesis. The aim of this study was to identify DNA methylation biomarkers of ASD detectable at birth.

Methods: We quantified neonatal methylomic variation in 1263 infants—of whom ~ 50% went on to subsequently develop ASD—using DNA isolated from archived blood spots taken shortly after birth. We used matched genotype data from the same individuals to examine the molecular consequences of ASD-associated genetic risk variants, identifying methylomic variation associated with elevated polygenic burden for ASD. In addition, we performed DNA methylation quantitative trait loci (mQTL) mapping to prioritize target genes from ASD GWAS findings.

Results: We identified robust epigenetic signatures of gestational age and prenatal tobacco exposure, confirming the utility of DNA methylation data generated from neonatal blood spots. Although we did not identify specific loci showing robust differences in neonatal DNA methylation associated with later ASD, there was a significant association between increased polygenic burden for autism and methylomic variation at specific loci. Each unit of elevated ASD polygenic risk score was associated with a mean increase in DNA methylation of − 0.14% at two CpG sites located proximal to a robust GWAS signal for ASD on chromosome 8.

Conclusions: This study is the largest analysis of DNA methylation in ASD undertaken and the first to integrate genetic and epigenetic variation at birth. We demonstrate the utility of using a polygenic risk score to identify molecular variation associated with disease, and of using mQTL to refine the functional and regulatory variation associated with ASD risk variants.

Keywords: Autism, DNA methylation, Genetics, Neonatal, Genome-wide association study (GWAS), Epigenome-wide association study (EWAS), Birth, DNA methylation quantitative trait loci (mQTL), Polygenic risk score, Prenatal smoking

* Correspondence: J.Mill@exeter.ac.uk
^Deceased
[1]University of Exeter Medical School, University of Exeter, RILD Building, Level 4, Barrack Rd, Exeter EX2 5DW, UK
Full list of author information is available at the end of the article

Background

Autism spectrum disorder (ASD) defines a group of complex neurodevelopmental disorders marked by deficits in social communication and restricted, repetitive behaviors, interests, or activities [1]. ASD affects ~ 1–2% of the population, and confers severe lifelong disability [2–4]. Quantitative genetic studies indicate that ASD is highly heritable [5, 6], although population-based epidemiologic studies of environmental risks and ASD liability modeling using family designs also indicate environmental factors as important [7]. Genetic studies have shown that autism risk is strongly associated with both rare inherited and *de novo* DNA sequence variants [8–11]. In contrast, the identification of common genetic variants associated with ASD using genome-wide association studies (GWAS) has proven harder than for other complex neuropsychiatric traits such as schizophrenia [12], at least in part due to a lack of large sample datasets. Recent collaboration between the Psychiatrics Genomics Consortium autism workgroup (PGC-AUT) and the Lundbeck Foundation Initiative for Integrative Psychiatric Research (iPSYCH) has greatly expanded the number of ASD cases with GWAS data, enabling the identification of three genome-wide significant associations for ASD and evidence for a substantial polygenic component in signals falling below the stringent genome-wide significance threshold [13]. None of the three ASD-associated loci are predicted to result in coding changes or altered protein structure; instead they are hypothesized to influence gene regulation. Previous studies of other neurodevelopmental disorders have reported an enrichment of disease-associated variation in regulatory domains, including enhancers and regions of open chromatin [14].

Epigenetic variation induced by non-genetic exposures has been hypothesized to be one mechanism by which environmental factors can affect risk for ASD [15, 16]. Recent studies have provided initial evidence for autism-associated epigenetic variation in both brain and peripheral tissues [17–22], although these analyses have been undertaken on relatively small numbers of samples with limited statistical power. Existing analyses have assessed epigenetic variation in samples collected after a diagnosis of ASD has been assigned and are likely to be confounded by factors such as smoking [23–25], medication [26, 27], other environmental toxins [28], and reverse causation [29]. Furthermore, they have not investigated the role of genetic variation in mediating associations between epigenetic variation and ASD. The integration of genetic and epigenetic data will facilitate a better understanding of the molecular mechanisms involved in autism, especially given the high heritability of ASD and recent data showing how the epigenome can be directly influenced by genetic variation [30–33]. For example, we have previously demonstrated the potential for using polygenic risk scores (PRS)—defined as the sum of trait-associated alleles across many genetic loci, weighted by GWAS effect sizes—as disease biomarkers with utility for exploring the molecular genomic mechanisms involved in disease pathogenesis [34]. Of note, PRS-associated epigenetic variation is potentially less affected by factors associated with the disease itself, which can confound case–control analyses.

In this study, we quantified DNA methylation for ~ 1316 individuals (comprising equal numbers of ASD cases and matched controls, 50% male/female) using DNA samples isolated from neonatal blood spots collected proximal to birth (mean = 6.08 days; standard deviation (sd) = 3.24 days; Additional file 1: Figure S1). Known epigenetic signatures for gestational and chronological age [35, 36], and exposure to maternal smoking during pregnancy [24], were used to confirm the robust nature of genome-wide DNA methylation data generated from neonatal blood spots. Matched genome-wide single nucleotide polymorphism (SNP) genotyping data from the same individuals enabled us to undertake an integrated genetic–epigenetic analysis of ASD, exploring the extent to which neonatal methylomic variation at birth is associated with elevated polygenic burden for ASD. Finally, we generated an extensive database of DNA methylation quantitative trait loci (mQTL) in neonatal blood samples, which were used to characterize the molecular consequences of genetic variants associated with ASD.

Methods

Overview of the MINERvA cohort

Denmark has a comprehensive neonatal screening program which is used to test for innate errors of metabolism, hypothyroidism, and other treatable disorders. Neonatal blood is collected on standard Guthrie cards and residual material is stored within the Danish Neonatal Screening Biobank. The reason for storing the samples in prioritized order is: (1) diagnosis and treatment of congenital disorders, (2) diagnostic use later in infancy after informed consent, (3) legal use after court order, (4) research projects pending approval by the Scientific Ethical Committee System in Denmark, The Danish Data Protection Agency, and the NBS-Biobank Steering Committee. Thus, research is possible assuming sufficient material remains for the proceeding priorities [37]. Cases and controls were selected from the iPSYCH case–control sample, which has been recently described [38]. Briefly, the iPSYCH study population comprises all singletons born in Denmark between May 1st 1981 and December 31st 2005, who are still alive and residing in Denmark at their first birthday and with a known mother. iPSYCH ASD cases comprise all children in the study population with an ASD diagnosis reported before December 31st 2012. iPSYCH controls comprise 30,000 persons randomly selected from the study population (about 2% of the total study population).

The MINERvA study profiled a subsample of 1316 iPSYCH samples, including an equal number of ASD cases and controls that were selected using the following criteria. Cases were born between 1998 and 2002, with both parents born in Denmark themselves. We selected a 1:1 male to female ratio (i.e., by "oversampling" ASD females). Cases and controls were excluded if they had a reported diagnosis (before December 31st 2012) of select known genetic disorders: Down syndrome, Fragile X, Angelman, Prader Willi, Zellweger, William, tuberous sclerosis, Rett, Tourette, neurofibromatosis, Duchennes, Cornelia de Lange, DiGeorge, Smith-Lemli-Opitz, Klinfelter. In addition, controls were excluded if they had died or emigrated from Denmark before December 31st 2012, or had any reported psychiatric diagnosis. Eligible controls were individually matched to cases on sex, month of birth (month before, same month, or month after case month), and year of birth. Among the controls fulfilling these criteria, additional matching criteria were applied as closely as possible with regard to gestational age (in weeks) and the same urbanicity level of maternal residence at time of birth as cases. All perinatal data used for case–control matching, plus additional information on birth weight and maternal smoking were obtained from the Danish Medical Birth Register or the Central Person Register. Detailed maternal smoking data were used to generate a binary variable indicating whether the mother smoked during pregnancy or not. All diagnoses used for ASD case identification and case/control exclusions were obtained from the Danish Psychiatric Central Research Register (DPCRR) and Danish National Patient Register (DNPR). In Denmark, children and adolescents suspected of ASD or other mental or behavioral disorders are referred by general practitioners or school psychologists to a child and adolescent psychiatric department for a multidisciplinary evaluation, and their conditions are diagnosed by a child and adolescent psychiatrist. Registry reporting is done only by psychiatrists following mandatory training in the use of the World Health Organization International Classification of Diseases (ICD) [39]. The following ICD-10 diagnosis codes were used: ASD, F84.0, F84.1, F84.5, F84.8, F84.9; any psychiatric disorder, F00–F99. Reported diagnoses for the conditions used as exclusions were obtained from the DNPR, which holds all data on in- and out-patient diagnoses given at discharge from somatic wards in all hospitals and clinics since 1995 [40]. Additional file 2: Table S1 gives a full overview of relevant diagnosis codes. The MINERvA study was approved by the Regional Scientific Ethics Committee in Denmark and the Danish Data Protection Agency.

DNA methylation profiling in MINERvA
Neonatal dried blood spot samples were retrieved from the Danish Neonatal Screening Biobank, within the Danish National Biobank, as part of the iPSYCH study. Neonatal DNA extractions and DNA methylation quantification were performed at the Statens Serum Institut (SSI, Copenhagen, Capital Region, Denmark), building on a previously described protocol [41]. Briefly, from each dried blood spot sample two disks of 3.2 mm were used with the Extract-N-Amp Blood PCR kit (Sigma-Aldrich, St. Louis, USA) and eluted in 200 μL buffer. The isolated genomic DNA (160 μL) was converted with sodium bisulfite using the EZ-96 DNA Methylation Kit (Zymo Research, California, USA). DNA methylation was quantified across the genome using the Infinium HumanMethylation450k array ("450 K array"; Illumina, California, USA) and a modified protocol as previously described [40]. Fully methylated and unmethylated control samples were included on each plate throughout each stage of processing.

MINERvA Illumina 450 K array data pre-processing and quality control
Signal intensities for 1316 neonatal blood samples, 14 fully methylated control samples, and 14 fully unmethylated control samples were imported into the R programming environment using the *methylumIDAT()* function in the *methylumi* package [42]. Our stringent quality control (QC) pipeline included the following steps: 1) checking methylated and unmethylated signal intensities and excluding samples where either the median methylated or unmethylated intensity values were < 2500; 2) using the ten control probes to ensure the sodium bisulfite conversion was successful, excluding any samples with a median score < 80; 3) identifying the fully methylated and fully unmethylated control samples were in the correct location on each plate; 4) using the 65 SNP genotyping probes on the array to confirm no duplicate samples; 5) multidimensional scaling of data from probes on the X and Y chromosomes separately to confirm reported gender; 6) comparing genotype data for up to 65 SNP probes on the 450 K array with SNP array data; 7) using the *pfilter()* function in *wateRmelon* [43] to exclude samples with more than 1% of probes characterized by a detection P value > 0.05, in addition to probes characterized by > 1% of samples having a detection P value > 0.05. In total, 1263 samples (96.0%) passed all QC steps and were included in subsequent analyses. Normalization of the DNA methylation data was performed used the *dasen()* function in the *wateRmelon* package [43].

SNP genotyping and derivation of ASD polygenic risk scores
DNA was extracted at SSI as above and whole genome amplified in triplicate using the REPLI-g kit (Qiagen, Hilten, Germany). The triplicates were pooled and then quantified using Quant-iT picogreen (Invitrogen, California, USA). Samples were genotyped at the Broad Institute (Boston, Massachusetts, USA) using the Infinium

PsychChip v1.0 array (Illumina, San Diego, California, USA) using a standard protocol. Phasing and imputation was done using SHAPEIT [44] and IMPUTE2 with haplotypes from the 1000 Genomes Project, phase 3 [45, 46] as described previously [38]. ASD polygenic risk scores (PRSs) were generated as a weighted sum of associated variants as previously described [47]. Briefly, results from the largest autism GWAS available from a combined effort by the Psychiatric Genomics Consortium (PGC) and iPSYCH [13] was used to select genetic variants and provide weights. As the MINERvA cohort is a subset of the broader iPSYCH cohort we used GWAS results excluding MINERvA samples, so that there was no overlap between the training cohort and the test cohort. Ten different significance thresholds (p_T) from 5×10^{-8} to 1 were used to select sets of genetic variants, which were linkage disequilibrium (LD) clumped using *plink* with setting *–clump-p1 1 –clump-p2 1 –cump-r2 0.1 –clump-kb 500* to generate PRSs.

Statistical analysis

All statistical analyses were performed using the R statistical environment version 3.2.2 [48]. To test the validity and robustness of our blood spot DNA methylation measures, we implemented two DNA methylation clock algorithms to derive estimates for both age in years [36] and gestational age in weeks [35] for each sample. In addition, for each sample, we computed a score for prenatal exposure to maternal smoking using DNA methylation data as previously described by Elliott et al. [23]. To identify DNA methylation sites associated with ASD status in the MINERvA discovery dataset, a linear model was fitted for each DNA methylation site with DNA methylation as the dependent variable, case/control status as an independent variable, and a set of possible confounders as covariates—sex, experimental array number, urbanicity level, birth month, birth year, gestational age, smoking, and cell composition variables estimated using the Houseman algorithm with a reference dataset for whole blood [49, 50]. Regional analysis to identify differentially methylated regions (DMRs) spanning multiple DNA methylation sites was performed using a sliding-window approach as previously described [34]. Subsequent replication and meta-analysis was performed using summary statistics available from two US-based studies: the Study to Explore Early Development (SEED) [51] and the Simons Simplex Collection (SSC) [52]. Meta-analysis to combine the epigenome-wide association study (EWAS) results from MINERvA, SEED, and SSC studies was performed for DNA methylation loci present in at least two of the three studies. Data quality control, normalization, and ASD EWAS analysis was performed separately for each of the replication cohorts. A complete description of the SEED and SSC datasets can be found elsewhere [53]. The *P* values from the three independent EWAS analyses were combined using Fisher's method, focusing on DMPs where the

direction of effect was consistent across all studies. To identify DNA methylation sites associated with elevated autism polygenic risk burden, a linear model was used with DNA methylation as the dependent variable and ASD PRS, the number of non-missing genotypes contributing to the PRS, the first five genetic principal components, sex, experimental array number, six cell composition variables, smoking score, gestational age, and birth weight included as independent variables as described above. DNA methylation sites significantly associated with either ASD case control status or ASD PRS were identified at an experiment-wide significant threshold of $P < 1 \times 10^{-7}$, which is corrected for the number of DNA methylation sites profiled on the 450 K array.

DNA mQTL and co-localization analyses

All DNA methylation sites located within 250 kb of the three genome-wide significant genetic variants identified in the PGC-AUT GWAS [13] were identified and *cis* (defined as a 500-kb window) mQTL analysis was performed using the 1257 samples within MINERvA that had both DNA methylation and imputed genotype data. mQTL were identified using an additive linear model to test if the number of alleles (coded 0, 1, or 2) predicted DNA methylation at each site, including covariates for sex, and the first five principal components from the genotype data fitted using the MatrixEQTL package [54]. Co-localization analysis was performed for each DNA methylation site as previously described [55] using the R coloc package (http://cran.r-project.org/web/packages/coloc). From both the PGC-AUT GWAS data and our mQTL results we inputted the regression coefficients, their variances and SNP minor allele frequencies, and the prior probabilities were left as their default values. This methodology quantifies the support across the results of each GWAS for five hypotheses by calculating the posterior probabilities, denoted as *PPi* for hypothesis *Hi*.

H_0: there exist no causal variants for either trait;

H_1: there exists a causal variant for one trait only, ASD;

H_2: there exists a causal variant for one trait only, DNA methylation;

H_3: there exist two distinct causal variants, one for each trait;

H_4: there exists a single causal variant common to both traits.

Results

Robust epigenetic signatures of gestational age and prenatal tobacco exposure validate DNA methylation data generated from neonatal blood spots

Following our stringent QC pipeline (see "Methods") our final MINERvA DNA methylation dataset included 1263 samples comprising 629 ASD cases and 634 controls. The characteristics of this sample are displayed in

Table 1; of note, due to oversampling female cases, we had a near equal ratio of males and females (632:631). There were no significant differences between ASD cases and controls for maternal or paternal age, days to blood spot sampling, or birth weight ($P > 0.05$). There was a significantly higher rate of maternal smoking for the ASD cases ($P = 0.003$) and evidence of higher smoking quantity ($P = 0.006$). We used DNA methylation data to derive estimates of gestational age [35] and chronological age [36] for each sample. The mean predicted gestational age was 37.7 weeks (sd = 1.35 weeks; Additional file 1: Figure S2) compared to the actual mean of 39.6 weeks (sd = 1.77 weeks), with a strong positive correlation between estimated and actual gestational age (r = 0.602; Fig. 1a). The mean predicted

chronological age was 0.495 years (sd = 0.298; Additional file 1: Figure S3) and this was less strongly correlated with actual age (r = 0.139; Fig. 1b), consistent with data from Knight et al. [35]. Of note, "days to sampling"—i.e., the time between birth and blood draw—was not correlated with either predicted gestational age or chronological age, and controlling for this did not improve the strength of the correlation with gestational age (Additional file 1: Figure S4). We next tested robust markers of smoking exposure during pregnancy [24] and adulthood, using an established algorithm [23] to calculate a DNA methylation derived "smoking score" which we compared to reported *in utero* exposure. We identified a highly significant association between this smoking score and actual exposure, with offspring exposed to

Table 1 Characteristics of samples included in the MINERvA cohort

Characteristic	Unit/category	ASD	Controls	P value
Sex[a] (%)	Male	52.0	49.8	0.933
Birth year[a] (%)	1998	31.8	30.6	
	1999	28.3	29	
	2000	7	6.78	0.991
	2001	13.7	14.2	
	2002	19.2	19.4	
Gestational age[b] (mean (sd))	Weeks	39.6 (1.82)	39.6 (1.72)	0.96
Urbanicity[b] (%)	1: Capital	18.1	17	
	2: Suburb of the capital	14.9	13.4	
	3: Municipalities having a town with more than 100,000 inhabitants	8.27	8.68	0.879
	4: Municipalities having a town with between 10,000 and 100,000 inhabitants	27.3	29.2	
	5: Other municipalities in Denmark (largest town has less than 10,000 inhabitants)	31.3	31.7	
Time to sampling (mean (sd))	Days	6.01 (3.15)	6.15 (3.33)	0.46
Maternal age (mean (sd))	Years	29.2 (4.94)	29.7 (4.57)	0.07
Paternal age (mean (sd))	Years	32.1 (6.04)	31.9 (5.40)	0.476
Maternal smoking during pregnancy (%)	Smoke at any time	29.0	21.2	0.00256
	Non-smoker	71.0	78.8	
Maternal smoking amount during pregnancy (%)	5 or less cigarettes per day	6.46	7.25	
	6–10 cigarettes per day	11.2	7.59	0.00573
	11–20 cigarettes per day	9.6	5.06	
	21 or more cigarettes per day	1.05	1.18	
Birth weight (mean (sd))	Grams	3512 (581)	3541 (542)	0.355

[a]Primary characteristics used to match ASD cases and controls
[b]Secondary characteristics used to match ASD cases and controls as closely as possible. There was a significant difference in maternal smoking rates between ASD cases and controls

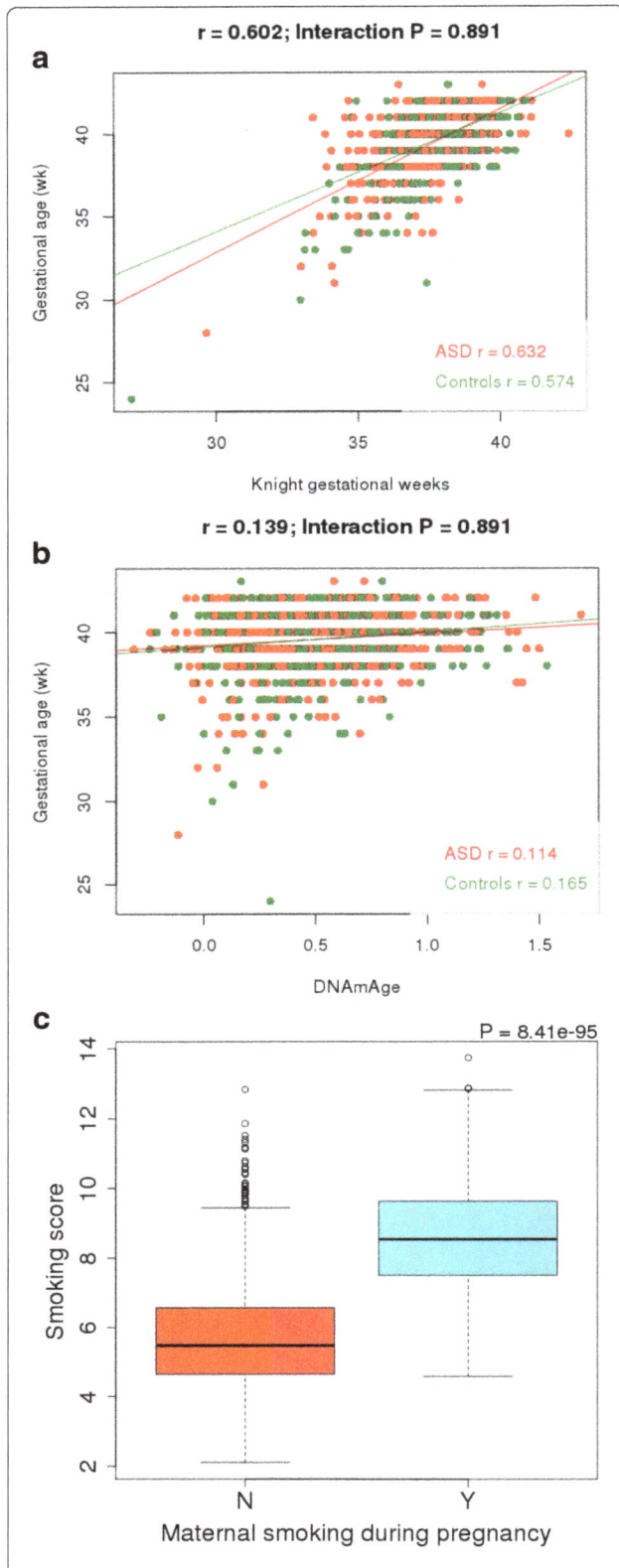

a r = 0.602; Interaction P = 0.891

ASD r = 0.632
Controls r = 0.574

Gestational age (wk)

Knight gestational weeks

b r = 0.139; Interaction P = 0.891

ASD r = 0.114
Controls r = 0.165

Gestational age (wk)

DNAmAge

c P = 8.41e-95

Smoking score

N   Y

Maternal smoking during pregnancy

Fig. 1 DNA methylation data from neonatal blood spots can be used to accurately predict age and maternal smoking status. **a** Scatterplot of gestational age predicted from DNA methylation data (using an algorithm generated by Knight et al. [35]) against actual gestational age. Autism cases are in red and controls are in green. **b** Scatterplot of chronological age predicted from DNA methylation data (using the online Epigenetic Clock software [36]) against actual gestational age. Autism cases are in *red* and controls are in *green*. **c** Boxplot of a smoking score derived from DNA methylation data [23] stratified by maternal smoking status during pregnancy

tobacco smoking in utero having higher smoking scores compared to offspring who were not exposed ($P = 8.41 \times 10^{-95}$; Fig. 1c) [23, 34]. Taken together these analyses highlight the utility of using DNA isolated from neonatal blood spots to generate reliable DNA methylation data that can robustly identify exposure/trait-associated variation.

Methylomic variation in perinatal blood is not significantly associated with childhood autism

Our initial analysis focused on identifying neonatal blood DNA methylation differences among MINERvA neonates who went on to later develop a childhood diagnosis of ASD. No global differences in DNA methylation—estimated by averaging across all probes on the array included in our analysis—were identified between ASD patients ($N = 629$) and controls ($N = 634$) (ASD mean = 50.0%, ASD sd = 0.0811%; controls mean = 50.0%, controls sd = 0.0917%; *t*-test $P = 0.695$). Using a linear model to identify DNA methylation differences in ASD cases compared to controls we did not identify any differentially methylated positions (DMPs) passing an experiment-wide significance threshold adjusted for multiple testing ($P < 1 \times 10^{-7}$). Twenty ASD-associated DMPs were identified at a "discovery" threshold of $P < 5 \times 10^{-5}$ (Additional file 1: Figures S5 and S6; Additional file 2: Table S2); the most significant association was at cg12699865, which is located the 5′ UTR of *RALY* where the mean level of DNA methylation was 0.647% lower ($P = 7.63 \times 10^{-7}$) in ASD cases compared to controls (Additional file 1: Figure S7). Regional analysis combining the EWAS *P* values for DNA methylation sites within a sliding window across the genome (see "Methods") did not identify any significant ASD-associated DMRs after correcting for multiple testing. Given the higher prevalence of ASD diagnosis in males, we also tested for an interaction between autism status and sex but identified no significant associations ($P < 1 \times 10^{-7}$) and only seven DMPs at our discovery threshold of $P < 5 \times 10^{-5}$ (Additional file 2: Table S3).

We next meta-analyzed these findings with summary statistics from 450K array measurements for two US-based studies of autism—the Study to Explore Early Development (SEED) [51] and Simons Simplex Collection (SSC) [52]. Although neither of these datasets was generated on

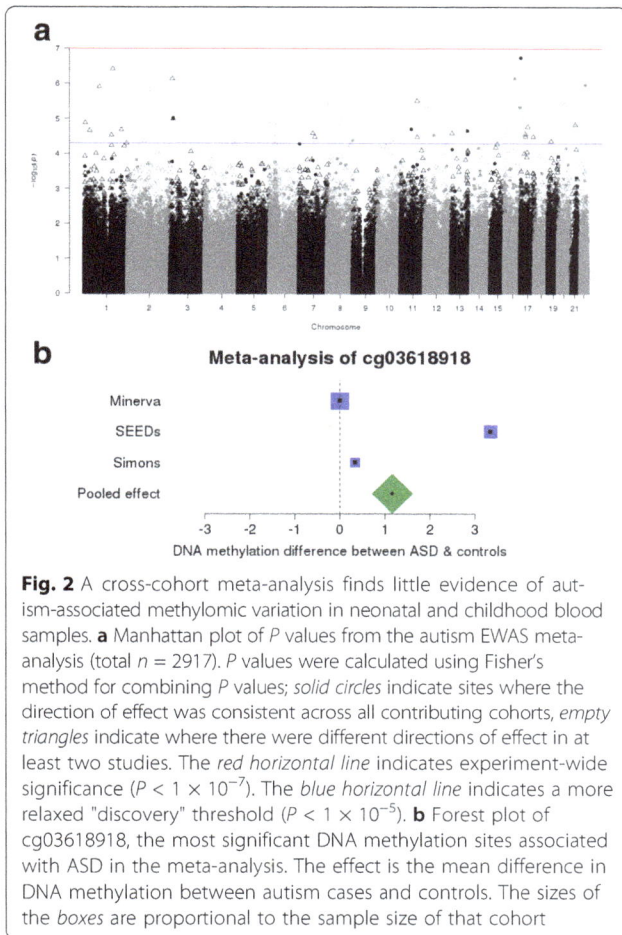

Fig. 2 A cross-cohort meta-analysis finds little evidence of autism-associated methylomic variation in neonatal and childhood blood samples. **a** Manhattan plot of P values from the autism EWAS meta-analysis (total $n = 2917$). P values were calculated using Fisher's method for combining P values; *solid circles* indicate sites where the direction of effect was consistent across all contributing cohorts, *empty triangles* indicate where there were different directions of effect in at least two studies. The *red horizontal line* indicates experiment-wide significance ($P < 1 \times 10^{-7}$). The *blue horizontal line* indicates a more relaxed "discovery" threshold ($P < 1 \times 10^{-5}$). **b** Forest plot of cg03618918, the most significant DNA methylation sites associated with ASD in the meta-analysis. The effect is the mean difference in DNA methylation between autism cases and controls. The sizes of the *boxes* are proportional to the sample size of that cohort

blood samples collected immediately after birth, they enabled us to assess a combined sample size of 1425 ASD cases and 1492 controls (Additional file 2: Table S4). We first took the top ranked loci identified in each independent study and compared the directions of effect (i.e., difference between autism and controls); we did not find any excess of consistent associations (all sign test $P > 0.05$; Additional file 1: Figure S8; Additional file 2: Table S5). Second, we combined the P values from the EWAS results of the three samples using Fisher's method (Fig. 2a; Additional file 1: Figure S9). There were no sites where the combined P value survived correction for multiple testing ($P < 1 \times 10^{-7}$), although 45 ASD-associated DMPs were identified at the discovery P value threshold ($P < 5 \times 10^{-5}$) (Additional file 2: Table S6). The most significant DNA methylation site, based on a consistent direction of effect across all three studies, was cg03618918 (combined $P = 3.85 \times 10^{-7}$; pooled mean = 1.17%; Fig. 2b), located ~ 10 kb from *ITLN1*. In general, the estimated effects of ASD-associated DMPs ($P < 5 \times 10^{-5}$) was very small (Additional file 1: Figure S10), typically ~ 1% difference between ASD and controls. Taken together, these data suggest that, based

on the sites assayed by the 450K array, ASD is not associated with robust methylomic signatures in blood obtained during early childhood.

Increased polygenic burden for autism is associated with methylomic variation in blood at birth

Like many complex diseases, individual genetic variants associated with autism explain only a small proportion of an individual's risk [6, 56]. Polygenic risk scores (PRSs), which essentially count the number of risk alleles across multiple associated loci, have been used successfully to capture the polygenic architecture of complex traits, including autism [47]. PRS have been used to establish genetic correlations between traits [6] and there has been recent interest in using PRS as a quantitative variable to identify molecular biomarkers of high genetic burden [34, 57, 58]. PRS-associated epigenetic variation is potentially less affected by non-genetic risk factors for the disease itself, which can confound case–control analyses, although pleiotropic effects of these genetic variants, which may themselves influence DNA methylation, cannot be excluded. We generated autism PRSs for individuals in the iPSYCH-MINERvA sample using recent results from a meta-analysis of samples in the PGC-AUT GWAS [13] excluding the subset of individuals included the MINERvA cohort ($n = 45,162$; 39.4% autism cases). Individual PRSs were calculated using a range of different GWAS P value thresholds ($p_T = 5 \times 10^{-8}$, ..., 1) to identify the optimal set of SNPs with the largest difference between ASD cases and controls in MINERvA. All scores based on P values < 1 significantly predicted autism status ($P < 0.05$; Additional file 2: Table S7; Additional file 1: Figure S11), with a PRS based on $p_T = 0.1$ having the most significant difference ($P = 9.49 \times 10^{-13}$) between ASD cases and controls (Fig. 3a). There was a strong positive correlation between scores based on SNPs selected at relatively relaxed significance thresholds (i.e., $p_T > 0.001$; Additional file 1: Figure S12), with weaker correlations between scores based on more limited (but more strongly associated) sets of variants, potentially reflecting the more dramatic effect a single SNP has on the PRS when the total number of SNPs is small. We next performed an EWAS of ASD PRS (Additional file 1: Figure S13; Additional file 1: Figure S14), observing strong correlations (r > 0.5) between the results of analyses of scores based on $p_T > 0.01$ (Additional file 1: Figure S15). Examples of PRS-associated DMPs identified using the most predictive ASD PRS ($p_T < 0.1$) are shown in Additional file 1: Figure S16; in total, we identified two DMPs significantly associated ($P < 1 \times 10^{-7}$) with elevated polygenic burden (cg02771117, $P = 3.14 \times 10^{-8}$; cg27411982, $P = 8.38 \times 10^{-8}$), with 49 DMPs associated at a more relaxed "discovery" P value threshold ($P < 5 \times 10^{-5}$) (Fig. 3; Additional file 3: Table S8). Both cg02771117 and cg27411982 are located on chromosome 8, but are ~ 5 kb

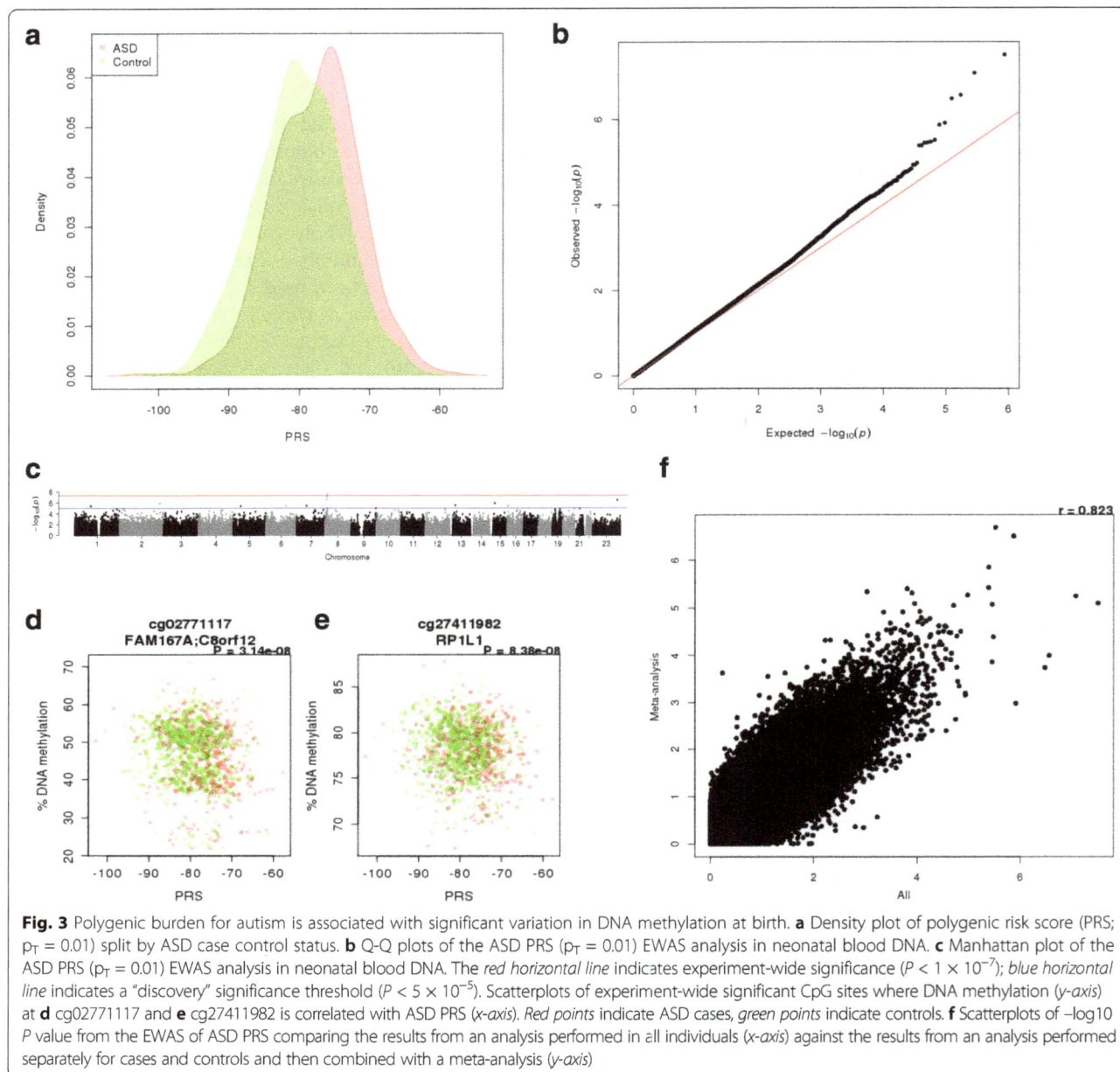

Fig. 3 Polygenic burden for autism is associated with significant variation in DNA methylation at birth. **a** Density plot of polygenic risk score (PRS; $p_T = 0.01$) split by ASD case control status. **b** Q-Q plots of the ASD PRS ($p_T = 0.01$) EWAS analysis in neonatal blood DNA. **c** Manhattan plot of the ASD PRS ($p_T = 0.01$) EWAS analysis in neonatal blood DNA. The *red horizontal line* indicates experiment-wide significance ($P < 1 \times 10^{-7}$); *blue horizontal line* indicates a "discovery" significance threshold ($P < 5 \times 10^{-5}$). Scatterplots of experiment-wide significant CpG sites where DNA methylation (*y-axis*) at **d** cg02771117 and **e** cg27411982 is correlated with ASD PRS (*x-axis*). *Red points* indicate ASD cases, *green points* indicate controls. **f** Scatterplots of –log10 P value from the EWAS of ASD PRS comparing the results from an analysis performed in all individuals (*x-axis*) against the results from an analysis performed separately for cases and controls and then combined with a meta-analysis (*y-axis*)

apart and annotated to two different genes (*FAM167A* and *RP1L1*, respectively). Differential DNA methylation at these sites on chromosome 8 is identified in each of the eight most inclusive ASD PRS EWAS analyses (i.e., those using the most relaxed GWAS *P* value threshold; Additional file 1: Figure S14). Of note, both DMPs flank a significant genetic association signal identified in the latest ASD GWAS (Additional file 1: Figure S17). We used ChromHMM classifications [59, 60] based on regulatory data from the Roadmap Epigenomics Project (http://www.roadmapepigenomics.org) [61] to characterize chromatin states across this region (Additional file 1: Figure S18). The index SNP for the GWAS signal is in a

region predicted to be characterized by a repressed polycomb state in blood and a quiescent/low state in brain. One of the ASD PRS-associated DNA methylation sites (cg02771117) is located in a predicted enhancer region, and the other (cg27411982) is in a region of predicted quiescent/low chromatin state. To establish whether the PRS-associated methylation signal in this region reflected direct effects of the GWAS signal itself, we iteratively added PRS variants within 100 kb of these two sites as covariates in our EWAS in order of significance (see "Methods"). After the addition of the four most significant genetic variants, which were independently associated with cg02771117 (Additional file 1: Figure S19), the ASD PRS term was no longer significant ($P = 0.0518$; Additional file 2: Table S9). In contrast cg27411982 was still nominally significant even after the addition of 12 ASD-associated SNPs, four of which were independently associated and largely explained the association between the ASD PRS and DNA methylation (Additional file 1: Figure S20; Additional file 2: Table S10). These data suggest that the PRS-associated variation in DNA methylation at both cg02771117 and cg27411982 results from the combined effects of multiple genetic variants associated with ASD in this region. In order to demonstrate that the PRS EWAS results are not simply a consequence of the ASD cases within the full MINERvA sample, we repeated the analysis separately for cases and controls. P values from this approach were strongly correlated with those for the analysis across all samples (Additional file 1: Figure S21), indicating that the methylomic consequences of high genetic burden are largely consistent across both groups.

Alignment of DNA methylation quantitative trait loci and ASD genetic signals

None of the GWAS-AUT identified genetic variants tag known nonsynonymous mutations; consistent with other complex phenotypes it is likely that disease-associated variants instead influence the regulation of gene expression [14, 62]. Building on our previous work showing how DNA methylation quantitative trait loci (mQTLs) can be used to refine GWAS loci through the identification of discrete sites of variable methylation associated with disease risk variants [30, 34], we used the matched MINERvA DNA methylation and genetic data (see "Methods") to identify mQTL located in the vicinity of ASD-associated GWAS variants (Fig. 4; Additional file 1: Figure S22). Simply aligning mQTL data with GWAS results is not sufficient to infer that there is a relationship between ASD and DNA methylation in these regions; instead it may reflect two distinct causal variants—one associated with ASD and the other with DNA methylation—in strong linkage disequilibrium. To establish whether there was evidence of a single causal variant influencing both DNA methylation and ASD in the regions nominated by the GWAS we performed a Bayesian co-localization analysis [55]. Briefly, this approach compares the pattern of association results from two independent GWAS (i.e., of ASD and DNA methylation) to see if associations colocalize to the same causal variant. We considered mQTL data for 457 unique DNA methylation sites located within 250 kb of three independent autosomal ASD GWAS variants. The posterior probabilities involving 91 of these sites were supportive of a co-localized association signal for both ASD and DNA methylation ($PP_3 + PP_4 > 0.99$; Additional file 3: Table S11). Four of these sites located on chromosome 20 had a higher posterior probability for both ASD and DNA methylation being associated with the same causal variant compared to them being associated with different causal variants ($PP_4/PP_3 > 1$; Additional file 1: Figure S23). The genes annotated to

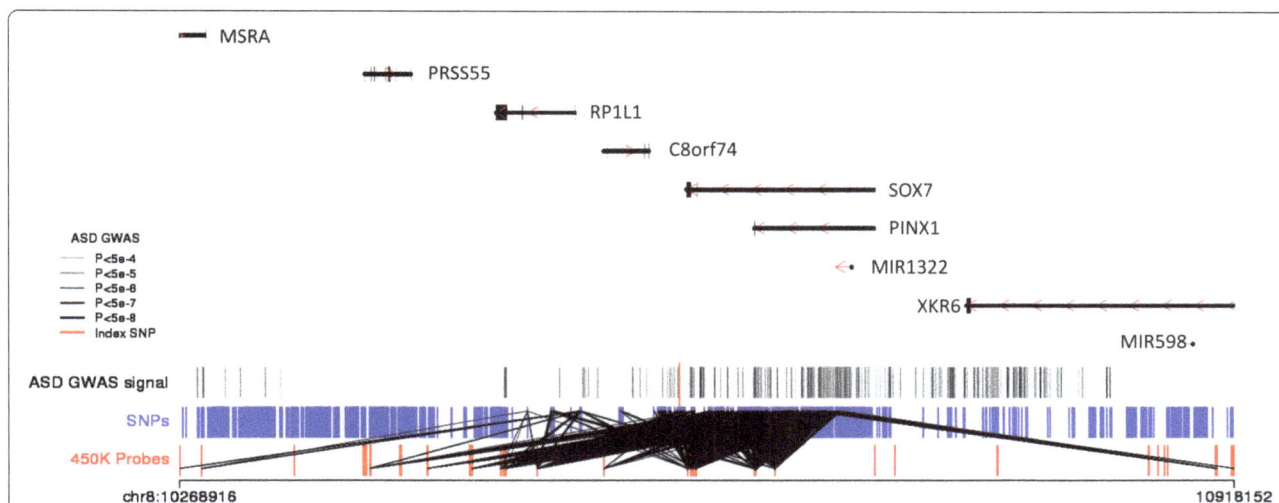

Fig. 4 DNA methylation quantitative trait loci (mQTL) mapping can localize putative causal loci associated with ASD. Presented here is a genomic region (chr8:10268916–10,918,152) identified in a recent GWAS analysis of ASD [13]. At the top of the figure is a schematic detailing the genes located in this region which are identified by their Entrez ID number. All genetic variants identified in the ASD GWAS ($P < 1 \times 10^{-4}$) are represented by *vertical solid lines* where the color reflects the strength of the association ranging from *gray* (less significant P values) to *black* (more significant P values). A *red vertical line* indicates the most significant genetic variant in this region. All DNA methylation sites tested for neonatal blood mQTL in the MINERvA dataset are indicated by *red vertical lines* and genetic variants by *blue vertical lines*. Significant neonatal blood mQTLs ($P < 1 \times 10^{-13}$) are indicated by *black diagonal lines* between the respective genetic variant and DNA methylation site. Genomic locations are based on hg19. Additional examples of mQTLs in genomic regions showing genome-wide significant association with ASD are given in Additional file 1: Figure S22

these sites (KIZ, XRN2, and NKX2–4) represent putative candidates for a potential functional role in ASD and warrant further investigation.

Discussion

In this study, we quantified neonatal methylomic variation in 1263 infants selected from the iPSYCH cohort [38] including samples from individuals who went on to develop ASD and carefully matched control samples. It represents the first attempt to integrate analyses of both genetic and epigenetic variation at birth in ASD, demonstrating the utility of using a polygenic risk score to identify molecular variation associated with disease, and of using DNA methylation quantitative trait loci to refine the functional and regulatory variation associated with ASD risk variants. While ASD itself was not associated with significant differences in neonatal DNA methylation, at an experiment-wide significance threshold, increased polygenic burden for autism was found to be associated with methylomic variation at specific loci in blood at birth. Our analysis of ASD PRS and DNA methylation supplements an increasing body of literature investigating the effects of high genetic burden for other complex traits on molecular variation [34, 57, 58]. We find that two CpGs located on chromosome 8 are associated with genetic risk for ASD, and are proximal to a robust GWAS signal for ASD. Furthermore, multiple associated SNPs on chromosome 8 have a polygenic effect on DNA methylation at these two CpG sites, demonstrating how a complex genetic architecture can converge on a common molecular consequence.

This study has several advantages over previous analyses of DNA methylation in ASD. We assessed a relatively large set of samples that is balanced with regard to both disease status and numbers of males and females. This contrasts with previous studies that have been undertaken on much smaller numbers of samples and focused primarily on ASD in males. Our control samples were stringently matched to cases on the basis of a number of criteria (see "Methods") to minimize the effects of confounding variables that often lead to false positives in molecular epidemiology. Furthermore, our use of neonatal DNA samples—collected before diagnosis and the manifestation of any ASD symptoms—means that we are uniquely positioned to identify epigenetic variation associated with later disease or elevated polygenic burden for later ASD, avoiding the confounding exposures often associated with disease (for example, medication, stress, and reverse causation) [63]. Finally, our study profiled whole blood from neonatal infants rather than cord blood; this minimizes confounding by maternal blood DNA and means our data can be more easily compared to blood datasets derived from later in life. A limitation of our sampling strategy, however, is that no blood cell reference DNA datasets

specifically for use on neonatal blood are yet available, likely reflecting the difficulties of obtaining sufficient volumes of neonatal blood for cell sorting and methylomic profiling. Instead, we corrected for blood cell-type composition using algorithms developed using adult datasets which may not fully represent the cellular diversity observed in neonatal blood.

We find little evidence to support an association between DNA methylation at birth and ASD, confirming this finding in a meta-analysis of three studies with a total sample of 2917. Power calculations show that we have > 90% power in our meta-analysis to identify an ASD-associated difference of 0.3% and a difference of 0.7% in the MINERvA cohort alone. While this suggests the lack of association was not due to sample size, we cannot fully conclude that DNA methylation is not associated with the onset of ASD. First, our analyses were constrained by the technical limitations of the Illumina 450K array, which only assays ~ 3% of CpG sites in the genome. Second, this work necessitated the use of a peripheral tissue that may provide limited information about variation in the presumed tissue of interest, i.e., the brain [64]. Although this is a salient point for understanding the role DNA methylation plays in the disease process, biomarkers—by definition—need to be measured in an accessible tissue and therefore justify the use of blood from neonates in this study. Third, given the chronology of sample collection prior to ASD diagnosis, it is plausible that we were looking too early on in the disease process. Another limitation of our study is the possibility of diagnostic misclassification; however, validation of select diagnoses (e.g., schizophrenia, single-episode depression, dementia, and childhood autism) has been previously performed with good results [39, 65].

In contrast, we find that polygenic burden for ASD is robustly associated with DNA methylation at two CpG sites on chromosome 8, with 49 DMPs associated with ASD polygenic burden at a more relaxed "discovery" P value threshold. Of note, both sites flank a significant genetic association signal identified in the latest ASD GWAS and our data suggest that the PRS-associated variation at these sites results from the combined effects of multiple genetic variants associated with ASD in this region. Finally, we have used mQTL analyses to annotate this extended genomic region nominated by GWAS analyses of ASD, using co-localization analyses to highlight potential regulatory variation causally involved in disease. Of interest, we found evidence that several SNPs on chromosome 20 were associated with both ASD and DNA methylation and the genes annotated to these sites (KIZ, XRN2, and NKX2–4) represent putative candidates for a potential functional role in ASD. The mechanisms linking DNA sequence variation to alterations in DNA methylation and other epigenetic modifications are not yet well understood; further exploration of these processes is warranted to provide insight into the functional consequences of disease-associated genetic variation.

Conclusions

Our data provide evidence for differences in DNA methylation at birth associated with an elevated polygenic burden for ASD. Our study represents the first analysis of epigenetic variation at birth associated with autism and highlights the utility of polygenic risk scores for identifying molecular pathways associated with etiological variation.

Acknowledgements
The iPSYCH-Broad ASD Group contains the following participants:
Esben Agerbo
Thomas D. Als
Rich Belliveau
Jonas Bybjerg-Grauholm
Marie Bækved-Hansen
Anders Børglum
Felecia Cerrato
Jane Christensen
Kimberly Chambert
Claire Churchhouse
Mark Daly
Ditte Demontis
Ashley Dumont
Jacqueline Goldstein
Jakob Grove
Christine Hansen
Mads Hauberg
David Hougaard
Daniel Howrigan
Hailiang Huang
Julian Maller
Alicia Martin
Joanna Martin
Manuel Mattheisen
Jennifer Moran
Ole Mors
Preben Mortensen
Benjamin Neale
Merete Nordentoft
Mette Nyegaard
Jonatan Pallsen
Duncan Palmer
Carsten Pedersen
Marianne Pedersen
Timothy Poterba
Jesper Poulsen
Per Qvist
Stephan Ripke
Elise Robinson
Kyle Satterstrom
Christine Stevens
Patrick Turley
Raymond Walters
Thomas Werge
(see Additional file 4 for full listing of e-mail addresses and affiliations).

Funding
This study was supported by grant HD073978 from the Eunice Kennedy Shriver National Institute of Child Health and Human Development, National Institute of Environmental Health Sciences, and National Institute of Neurological Disorders and Stroke; and by the Beatrice and Samuel A. Seaver Foundation. We acknowledge iPSYCH and The Lundbeck Foundation for providing samples and funding. The iPSYCH (The Lundbeck Foundation Initiative for Integrative Psychiatric Research) team acknowledges funding from The Lundbeck Foundation (grant numbers R102-A9118 and R155–2014-1724), the Stanley Medical Research Institute, the European Research Council (project number 294838), the Novo Nordisk Foundation for supporting the Danish National Biobank resource, and grants from Aarhus and Copenhagen Universities and University Hospitals, including support to the iSEQ Center, the GenomeDK HPC facility, and the CIRRAU Center. This research has been conducted using the Danish National Biobank resource, supported by the Novo Nordisk Foundation. JM is supported by funding from the UK Medical Research Council (MR/K013807/1) and a Distinguished Investigator Award from the Brain & Behavior Research Foundation. The SEED study was supported by Centers for Disease Control and Prevention (CDC) Cooperative Agreements announced under the RFAs 01086, 02199, DD11–002, DD06–003, DD04–001, and DD09–002 and the SEED DNA methylation measurements were supported by Autism Speaks Award #7659 to MDF. SA was supported by the Burroughs-Wellcome Trust training grant: Maryland, Genetics, Epidemiology and Medicine (MD-GEM). The SSC was supported by Simons Foundation (SFARI) award and NIH grant MH089606, both awarded to STW.

Authors' contributions
AR, DS, and JM designed and coordinated the study. GB-G, DMH, MVH, M-BH, and CSH led generation of DNA methylation data from dried neonatal bloodspots. AR, DS, JM, EH, JB-G, CL-A, and MDF oversaw implementation of the data analyses. EH led data analysis. CL-A and SVA analyzed data from replication datasets. JG provided autism polygenic risk scores. DMH, OM, PBM, ADB, TW, and MN are principal investigators of the iPSYCH study and obtained funding for genetic data. EH and JM drafted the manuscript, with input from AR, DS, CL-A, JG, SVA, MDF, MB, MH, JB, and JB-G. All coauthors read and approved the final manuscript.

Ethics approval and consent to participate
The MINERvA study has been approved by the Regional Scientific Ethics Committee in Denmark, the Danish Data Protection Agency and the NBS-Biobank Steering Committee. iPSYCH is a register-based cohort study solely using data from national health registries. The study was approved by the Scientific Ethics Committees of the Central Denmark Region (www.komite.rm.dk; J.nr. 1–10–72-287-12) and executed according to guidelines from the Danish Data Protection Agency (www.datatilsynet.dk; J.nr.: 2012–41-0110). Passive consent was obtained, in accordance with Danish Law nr. 593 of June 14, 2011, para 10, on the scientific ethics administration of projects within health research. Permission to use the dried blood spot samples stored in the Danish Neonatal Screening Biobank (DNSB) was granted by the steering committee of DNSB (SEP 2012/BNP). Research was conducted in accordance with the principles of the Declaration of Helsinki.

Competing interests
TW has acted as advisor and lecturer to H. Lundbeck A/S. The remaining authors declare that they have no competing interests.

Author details
[1]University of Exeter Medical School, University of Exeter, RILD Building, Level 4, Barrack Rd, Exeter EX2 5DW, UK. [2]Department of Public Health, Aarhus University, Aarhus, Denmark. [3]Department of Epidemiology, Johns Hopkins Bloomberg School of Public Health, Baltimore, MD, USA. [4]Wendy Klag Center for Autism and Developmental Disabilities, Johns Hopkins Bloomberg School of Public Health, Baltimore, MD, USA. [5]Department of Biomedicine, Aarhus University, Aarhus, Denmark. [6]iPSYCH, The Lundbeck Foundation Initiative for Integrative Psychiatric Research, Aarhus, Denmark. [7]Centre for Integrative Sequencing, iSEQ, Aarhus University, Aarhus, Denmark. [8]Bioinformatics

Research Centre, Aarhus University, Aarhus, Denmark. [9]Center for Neonatal Screening, Department for Congenital Disorders, Statens Serum Institut, Copenhagen, Denmark. [10]Institute of Biological Psychiatry, MHC Sct. Hans, Mental Health Services Copenhagen, Roskilde, Denmark. [11]Center for Infection and Immunity, Columbia University Mailman School of Public Health, New York, USA. [12]Department of Epidemiology, Columbia University Mailman School of Public Health, New York, USA. [13]Psychosis Research Unit, Aarhus University Hospital, Risskov, Denmark. [14]Department of Clinical Medicine, Aarhus University; Aarhus University Hospital, Risskov, Denmark. [15]National Centre for Register-Based Research, Aarhus University, Aarhus, Denmark. [16]Centre for Integrated Register-based Research, Aarhus University, Aarhus, Denmark. [17]Department of Clinical Medicine, University of Copenhagen, Copenhagen, Denmark. [18]Mental Health Services in the Capital Region of Denmark, Mental Health Center Copenhagen, University of Copenhagen, Copenhagen, Denmark. [19]Department of Psychiatry, Mount Sinai School of Medicine, New York City, USA. [20]Department of Psychiatry, Columbia University, New York, USA. [21]Department of Mental Health, Johns Hopkins Bloomberg School of Public Health, Baltimore, MD, USA.

References

1. American Psychiatric Association. Diagnostic and statistical manual of mental disorders. 4th ed. Washington, DC: The American Psychiatric Association; 2000.
2. Baron-Cohen S, Scott FJ, Allison C, Williams J, Bolton P, Matthews FE, Brayne C. Prevalence of autism-spectrum conditions: UK school-based population study. Br J Psychiatry. 2009;194:500–9.
3. Investigators ADDMNSYP, CfDCa P. Prevalence of autism spectrum disorders–Autism and Developmental Disabilities Monitoring Network, 14 sites, United States, 2008. MMWR Surveill Summ. 2012;61:1–19.
4. Christensen DL, Baio J, Van Naarden BK, Bilder D, Charles J, Constantino JN, Daniels A, Durkin MS, Fitzgerald RT, Kurzius-Spencer M, et al. Prevalence and characteristics of autism spectrum disorder among children aged 8 years–Autism and Developmental Disabilities Monitoring Network, 11 Sites, United States, 2012. MMWR Surveill Summ. 2016;65:1–23.
5. Robinson EB, St Pourcain B, Anttila V, Kosmicki JA, Bulik-Sullivan B, Grove J, Maller J, Samocha KE, Sanders SJ, Ripke S, et al. Genetic risk for autism spectrum disorders and neuropsychiatric variation in the general population. Nat Genet. 2016;48:552–5.
6. Consortium C-DGPG. Identification of risk loci with shared effects on five major psychiatric disorders: a genome-wide analysis. Lancet. 2013;381:1371–9.
7. Hallmayer J, Cleveland S, Torres A, Phillips J, Cohen B, Torigoe T, Miller J, Fedele A, Collins J, Smith K, et al. Genetic heritability and shared environmental factors among twin pairs with autism. Arch Gen Psychiatry. 2011;68:1095–102.
8. Iossifov I, O'Roak BJ, Sanders SJ, Ronemus M, Krumm N, Levy D, Stessman HA, Witherspoon KT, Vives L, Patterson KE, et al. The contribution of de novo coding mutations to autism spectrum disorder. Nature. 2014;515:216–21.
9. Sanders SJ, Ercan-Sencicek AG, Hus V, Luo R, Murtha MT, Moreno-De-Luca D, Chu SH, Moreau MP, Gupta AR, Thomson SA, et al. Multiple recurrent de novo CNVs, including duplications of the 7q11.23 Williams syndrome region, are strongly associated with autism. Neuron. 2011;70:863–85.
10. Sanders SJ, Murtha MT, Gupta AR, Murdoch JD, Raubeson MJ, Willsey AJ, Ercan-Sencicek AG, DiLullo NM, Parikshak NN, Stein JL, et al. De novo mutations revealed by whole-exome sequencing are strongly associated with autism. Nature. 2012;485:237–41.
11. Sebat J, Lakshmi B, Malhotra D, Troge J, Lese-Martin C, Walsh T, Yamrom B, Yoon S, Krasnitz A, Kendall J, et al. Strong association of de novo copy number mutations with autism. Science. 2007;316:445–9.
12. Schizophrenia Working Group of the PGC, Ripke S, Neale B, Corvin A, Walters J, Farh K, Holmans P, Lee P, Bulik-Sullivan B, Collier D, et al. Biological insights from 108 schizophrenia-associated genetic loci. Nature. 2014;511:421.
13. Grove J, Ripke S, Als TD, Mattheisen M, Walters R, Won H, Pallesen J, Agerbo E, Andreassen OA, Anney R, et al. Common risk variants identified in autism spectrum disorder. bioRxiv. 2017. https://www.biorxiv.org/content/early/2017/11/25/224774.

14. Schaub MA, Boyle AP, Kundaje A, Batzoglou S, Snyder M. Linking disease associations with regulatory information in the human genome. Genome Res. 2012;22:1748–59.
15. Siu MT, Weksberg R. Epigenetics of autism spectrum disorder. Adv Exp Med Biol. 2017;978:63–90.
16. Vogel Ciernia A, LaSalle J. The landscape of DNA methylation amid a perfect storm of autism aetiologies. Nat Rev Neurosci. 2016;17:411–23.
17. Wong CC, Meaburn EL, Ronald A, Price TS, Jeffries AR, Schalkwyk LC, Plomin R, Mill J. Methylomic analysis of monozygotic twins discordant for autism spectrum disorder and related behavioural traits. Mol Psychiatry. 2014;19:495–503.
18. Ladd-Acosta C, Hansen KD, Briem E, Fallin MD, Kaufmann WE, Feinberg AP. Common DNA methylation alterations in multiple brain regions in autism. Mol Psychiatry. 2014;19:862–71.
19. Nardone S, Sams DS, Reuveni E, Getselter D, Oron O, Karpuj M, Elliott E. DNA methylation analysis of the autistic brain reveals multiple dysregulated biological pathways. Transl Psychiatry. 2014;4:e433.
20. Nguyen A, Rauch TA, Pfeifer GP, Hu VW. Global methylation profiling of lymphoblastoid cell lines reveals epigenetic contributions to autism spectrum disorders and a novel autism candidate gene, RORA, whose protein product is reduced in autistic brain. FASEB J. 2010;24:3036–51.
21. Homs A, Codina-Solà M, Rodríguez-Santiago B, Villanueva CM, Monk D, Cuscó I, Pérez-Jurado LA. Genetic and epigenetic methylation defects and implication of the ERMN gene in autism spectrum disorders. Transl Psychiatry. 2016;6:e855.
22. Sun W, Poschmann J, Cruz-Herrera Del Rosario R, Parikshak NN, Hajan HS, Kumar V, Ramasamy R, Belgard TG, Elanggovan B, Wong CC, et al. Histone acetylome-wide association study of autism spectrum disorder. Cell. 2016; 167:1385–97.
23. Elliott HR, Tillin T, McArdle WL, Ho K, Duggirala A, Frayling TM, Davey Smith G, Hughes AD, Chaturvedi N, Relton CL. Differences in smoking associated DNA methylation patterns in South Asians and Europeans. Clin Epigenetics. 2014;6:4.
24. Joubert BR, Felix JF, Yousefi P, Bakulski KM, Just AC, Breton C, Reese SE, Markunas CA, Richmond RC, Xu CJ, et al. DNA Methylation in newborns and maternal smoking in pregnancy: genome-wide consortium meta-analysis. Am J Hum Genet. 2016;98:680–96.
25. Shenker NS, Polidoro S, van Veldhoven K, Sacerdote C, Ricceri F, Birrell MA, Belvisi MG, Brown R, Vineis P, Flanagan JM. Epigenome-wide association study in the European Prospective Investigation into Cancer and Nutrition (EPIC-Turin) identifies novel genetic loci associated with smoking. Hum Mol Genet. 2013;22:843–51.
26. Non AL, Binder AM, Kubzansky LD, Michels KB. Genome-wide DNA methylation in neonates exposed to maternal depression, anxiety, or SSRI medication during pregnancy. Epigenetics. 2014;9:964–72.
27. Gurnot C, Martin-Subero I, Mah SM, Weikum W, Goodman SJ, Brain U, Werker JF, Kobor MS, Esteller M, Oberlander TF, Hensch TK. Prenatal antidepressant exposure associated with CYP2E1 DNA methylation change in neonates. Epigenetics. 2015;10:361–72.
28. Panni T, Mehta AJ, Schwartz JD, Baccarelli AA, Just AC, Wolf K, Wahl S, Cyrys J, Kunze S, Strauch K, et al. A genome-wide analysis of DNA methylation and fine particulate matter air pollution in three study populations: KORA F3, KORA F4, and the normative aging study. Environ Health Perspect. 2016; 124(7):983–90.
29. Mill J, Heijmans BT. From promises to practical strategies in epigenetic epidemiology. Nat Rev Genet. 2013;14:585–94.
30. Hannon E, Spiers H, Viana J, Pidsley R, Burrage J, Murphy TM, Troakes C, Turecki G, O'Donovan MC, Schalkwyk LC, et al. Methylation QTLs in the developing brain and their enrichment in schizophrenia risk loci. Nat Neurosci. 2016;19(1):48–54.
31. Gaunt TR, Shihab HA, Hemani G, Min JL, Woodward G, Lyttleton O, Zheng J, Duggirala A, McArdle WL, Ho K, et al. Systematic identification of genetic influences on methylation across the human life course. Genome Biol. 2016;17:61.
32. Heyn H, Moran S, Hernando-Herraez I, Sayols S, Gomez A, Sandoval J, Monk D, Hata K, Marques-Bonet T, Wang L, Esteller M. DNA methylation contributes to natural human variation. Genome Res. 2013;23:1363–72.
33. Smith AK, Kilaru V, Kocak M, Almli LM, Mercer KB, Ressler KJ, Tylavsky FA, Conneely KN. Methylation quantitative trait loci (meQTLs) are consistently detected across ancestry, developmental stage, and tissue type. BMC Genomics. 2014;15:145.

34. Hannon E, Dempster E, Viana J, Burrage J, Smith AR, Macdonald R, St Clair D, Mustard C, Breen G, Therman S, et al. An integrated genetic-epigenetic analysis of schizophrenia: evidence for co-localization of genetic associations and differential DNA methylation. Genome Biol. 2016;17:176.

35. Knight AK, Craig JM, Theda C, Bækvad-Hansen M, Bybjerg-Grauholm J, Hansen CS, Hollegaard MV, Hougaard DM, Mortensen PB, Weinsheimer SM, et al. An epigenetic clock for gestational age at birth based on blood methylation data. Genome Biol. 2016;17:206.

36. Horvath S. DNA methylation age of human tissues and cell types. Genome Biol. 2013;14:R115.

37. Nørgaard-Pedersen B, Hougaard DM. Storage policies and use of the Danish Newborn Screening Biobank. J Inherit Metab Dis. 2007;30:530–6.

38. Pedersen CB, Bybjerg-Grauholm J, Pedersen MG, Grove J, Agerbo E, Bækvad-Hansen M, Poulsen JB, Hansen CS, McGrath JJ, Als TD, et al. The iPSYCH2012 case-cohort sample: new directions for unravelling genetic and environmental architectures of severe mental disorders. Mol Psychiatry. 2018;23(1):6–14.

39. Mors O, Perto GP, Mortensen PB. The Danish Psychiatric Central Research Register. Scand J Public Health. 2011;39:54–7.

40. Lynge E, Sandegaard JL, Rebolj M. The Danish National Patient Register. Scand J Public Health. 2011;39:30–3.

41. Hollegaard MV, Grauholm J, Nørgaard-Pedersen B, Hougaard DM. DNA methylome profiling using neonatal dried blood spot samples: a proof-of-principle study. Mol Genet Metab. 2013;108:225–31.

42. Davis S, Du P, Bilke S, Triche J, Bootwalla M. methylumi: Handle Illumina methylation data. R package version 2.14.0.; 2015. https://www.bioconductor.org/packages/release/bioc/html/methylumi.html.

43. Pidsley R, Wong CC, Volta M, Lunnon K, Mill J, Schalkwyk LC. A data-driven approach to preprocessing Illumina 450K methylation array data. BMC Genomics. 2013;14:293.

44. Delaneau O, Marchini J, Zagury JF. A linear complexity phasing method for thousands of genomes. Nat Methods. 2012;9:179–81.

45. Abecasis GR, Auton A, Brooks LD, DePristo MA, Durbin RM, Handsaker RE, Kang HM, Marth GT, McVean GA, Consortium GP. An integrated map of genetic variation from 1,092 human genomes. Nature. 2012;491:56–65.

46. Sudmant PH, Rausch T, Gardner EJ, Handsaker RE, Abyzov A, Huddleston J, Zhang Y, Ye K, Jun G, Fritz MH, et al. An integrated map of structural variation in 2,504 human genomes. Nature. 2015;526:75–81.

47. Purcell SM, Wray NR, Stone JL, Visscher PM, O'Donovan MC, Sullivan PF, Sklar P, Consortium IS. Common polygenic variation contributes to risk of schizophrenia and bipolar disorder. Nature. 2009;460:748–52.

48. R Core Team (2014). R: A language and environment for statistical computing. R Foundation for Statistical Computing, Vienna, Austria. http://www.R-project.org/.

49. Houseman EA, Accomando WP, Koestler DC, Christensen BC, Marsit CJ, Nelson HH, Wiencke JK, Kelsey KT. DNA methylation arrays as surrogate measures of cell mixture distribution. BMC Bioinformatics. 2012;13:86.

50. Koestler DC, Christensen B, Karagas MR, Marsit CJ, Langevin SM, Kelsey KT, Wiencke JK, Houseman EA. Blood-based profiles of DNA methylation predict the underlying distribution of cell types: a validation analysis. Epigenetics. 2013;8:816–26.

51. Schendel DE, Diguiseppi C, Croen LA, Fallin MD, Reed PL, Schieve LA, Wiggins LD, Daniels J, Grether J, Levy SE, et al. The Study to Explore Early Development (SEED): a multisite epidemiologic study of autism by the Centers for Autism and Developmental Disabilities Research and Epidemiology (CADDRE) network. J Autism Dev Disord. 2012;42:2121–40.

52. Fischbach GD, Lord C. The Simons Simplex Collection: a resource for identification of autism genetic risk factors. Neuron. 2010;68:192–5.

53. Andrews SV, Ellis SE, Bakulski KM, Sheppard B, Croen LA, Hertz-Picciotto I, Newschaffer CJ, Feinberg AP, Arking DE, Ladd-Acosta C, Fallin MD. Cross-tissue integration of genetic and epigenetic data offers insight into autism spectrum disorder. Nat Commun. 2017;8(1):1011.

54. Shabalin AA. Matrix eQTL: ultra fast eQTL analysis via large matrix operations. Bioinformatics. 2012;28:1353–8.

55. Giambartolomei C, Vukcevic D, Schadt EE, Franke L, Hingorani AD, Wallace C, Plagnol V. Bayesian test for colocalisation between pairs of genetic association studies using summary statistics. PLoS Genet. 2014;10:e1004383.

56. Gaugler T, Klei L, Sanders SJ, Bodea CA, Goldberg AP, Lee AB, Mahajan M, Manaa D, Pawitan Y, Reichert J, et al. Most genetic risk for autism resides with common variation. Nat Genet. 2014;46:881–5.

57. Viana J, Hannon E, Dempster E, Pidsley R, Macdonald R, Knox O, Spiers H, Troakes C, Al-Saraj S, Turecki G, et al. Schizophrenia-associated methylomic variation: molecular signatures of disease and polygenic risk burden across multiple brain regions. Hum Mol Genet. 2017;26(1):210–25.

58. Fromer M, Roussos P, Sieberts SK, Johnson JS, Kavanagh DH, Perumal TM, Ruderfer DM, Oh EC, Topol A, Shah HR, et al. Gene expression elucidates functional impact of polygenic risk for schizophrenia. Nat Neurosci. 2016;19:1442–53.

59. Ernst J, Kellis M. Chromatin-state discovery and genome annotation with ChromHMM. Nat Protoc. 2017;12:2478–92.

60. Ernst J, Kellis M. ChromHMM: automating chromatin-state discovery and characterization. Nat Methods. 2012;9:215–6.

61. Consortium RE, Kundaje A, Meuleman W, Ernst J, Bilenky M, Yen A, Heravi-Moussavi A, Kheradpour P, Zhang Z, Wang J, et al. Integrative analysis of 111 reference human epigenomes. Nature. 2015;518:317–30.

62. Maurano MT, Humbert R, Rynes E, Thurman RE, Haugen E, Wang H, Reynolds AP, Sandstrom R, Qu H, Brody J, et al. Systematic localization of common disease-associated variation in regulatory DNA. Science. 2012;337:1190–5.

63. Heijmans BT, Mill J. The seven plagues of epigenetic epidemiology. Int J Epidemiol. 2012;41:74–8.

64. Hannon E, Lunnon K, Schalkwyk L, Mill J. Interindividual methylomic variation across blood, cortex, and cerebellum: implications for epigenetic studies of neurological and neuropsychiatric phenotypes. Epigenetics. 2015; 10:1024–32.

65. Lauritsen MB, Jørgensen M, Madsen KM, Lemcke S, Toft S, Grove J, Schendel DE, Thorsen P. Validity of childhood autism in the Danish Psychiatric Central Register: findings from a cohort sample born 1990-1999. J Autism Dev Disord. 2010;40:139–48.

2

Human genetic variants and age are the strongest predictors of humoral immune responses to common pathogens and vaccines

Petar Scepanovic[1,2†], Cécile Alanio[3,4,5†], Christian Hammer[1,2,6], Flavia Hodel[1,2], Jacob Bergstedt[7], Etienne Patin[8,9,10], Christian W. Thorball[1,2], Nimisha Chaturvedi[1,2], Bruno Charbit[4], Laurent Abel[11,12,13], Lluis Quintana-Murci[8,9,10], Darragh Duffy[3,4,5], Matthew L. Albert[6*], Jacques Fellay[1,2,14*] [iD] and for The Milieu Intérieur Consortium

Abstract

Background: Humoral immune responses to infectious agents or vaccination vary substantially among individuals, and many of the factors responsible for this variability remain to be defined. Current evidence suggests that human genetic variation influences (i) serum immunoglobulin levels, (ii) seroconversion rates, and (iii) intensity of antigen-specific immune responses. Here, we evaluated the impact of intrinsic (age and sex), environmental, and genetic factors on the variability of humoral response to common pathogens and vaccines.

Methods: We characterized the serological response to 15 antigens from common human pathogens or vaccines, in an age- and sex-stratified cohort of 1000 healthy individuals (*Milieu Intérieur* cohort). Using clinical-grade serological assays, we measured total IgA, IgE, IgG, and IgM levels, as well as qualitative (serostatus) and quantitative IgG responses to cytomegalovirus, Epstein-Barr virus, herpes simplex virus 1 and 2, varicella zoster virus, *Helicobacter pylori*, *Toxoplasma gondii*, influenza A virus, measles, mumps, rubella, and hepatitis B virus. Following genome-wide genotyping of single nucleotide polymorphisms and imputation, we examined associations between ~ 5 million genetic variants and antibody responses using single marker and gene burden tests.

Results: We identified age and sex as important determinants of humoral immunity, with older individuals and women having higher rates of seropositivity for most antigens. Genome-wide association studies revealed significant associations between variants in the human leukocyte antigen (HLA) class II region on chromosome 6 and anti-EBV and anti-rubella IgG levels. We used HLA imputation to fine map these associations to amino acid variants in the peptide-binding groove of HLA-DRβ1 and HLA-DPβ1, respectively. We also observed significant associations for total IgA levels with two loci on chromosome 2 and with specific KIR-HLA combinations.

Conclusions: Using extensive serological testing and genome-wide association analyses in a well-characterized cohort of healthy individuals, we demonstrated that age, sex, and specific human genetic variants contribute to inter-individual variability in humoral immunity. By highlighting genes and pathways implicated in the normal antibody response to frequently encountered antigens, these findings provide a basis to better understand disease pathogenesis.

(Continued on next page)

* Correspondence: albert.matthew@gene.com; jacques.fellay@epfl.ch
†Petar Scepanovic and Cécile Alanio contributed equally to this work.
[6]Department of Cancer Immunology, Genentech, South San Francisco, CA, USA
[1]School of Life Sciences, École Polytechnique Fédérale de Lausanne, Lausanne, Switzerland
Full list of author information is available at the end of the article

(Continued from previous page)

Keywords: Infection, Vaccination, GWAS, Serology, Human genomics, HLA, Age, Sex, Humoral immunity, Immunoglobulins

Background

Humans are regularly exposed to infectious agents, including common viruses such as cytomegalovirus (CMV), Epstein-Barr virus (EBV), or herpes simplex virus-1 (HSV-1) that have the ability to persist as latent infections throughout life—with possible reactivation events depending on extrinsic and intrinsic factors [1]. Humans also receive multiple vaccinations, which in many cases are expected to achieve lifelong immunity in the form of neutralizing antibodies. In response to each of these stimulations, the immune system mounts a humoral response, triggering the production of specific antibodies that play an essential role in limiting infection and providing long-term protection. Although the intensity of the humoral response to a given stimulation has been shown to be highly variable [2–4], the genetic and non-genetic determinants of this variability are still largely unknown. The identification of such factors may lead to improved vaccination strategies by optimizing vaccine-induced immunoglobulin G (IgG) protection, or to new understanding of autoimmune diseases, where immunoglobulin levels can correlate with disease severity [5].

Several genetic variants have been identified that account for inter-individual differences in susceptibility to pathogens [6–9] and in infectious [10] or therapeutic [11] phenotypes. By contrast, relatively few studies have investigated the variability of humoral responses in healthy humans [12–14]. In particular, Hammer et al. examined the contribution of genetics to variability in human antibody responses to common viral antigens, and fine-mapped variants at the HLA class II locus that associated with IgG responses. To replicate and extend these findings, we measured IgG responses to 15 antigens from common infectious agents or vaccines as well as total IgG, IgM, IgE, and IgA levels in 1000 well-characterized healthy donors. We used an integrative approach to study the impact of age, sex, non-genetic, and genetic factors on humoral immunity in healthy humans.

Methods

Study participants

The *Milieu Intérieur* cohort consists of 1000 healthy individuals that were recruited by BioTrial (Rennes, France). The cohort is stratified by sex (500 men, 500 women) and age (200 individuals from each decade of life, between 20 and 70 years of age). Donors were selected based on stringent inclusion and exclusion criteria, previously described [15]. Briefly, recruited individuals had no evidence of any severe/chronic/recurrent medical conditions. The main exclusion criteria were seropositivity for human immunodeficiency virus (HIV) or hepatitis C virus (HCV); ongoing infection with the hepatitis B virus (HBV)—as evidenced by detectable HBs antigen levels; travel to (sub-) tropical countries within the previous 6 months; recent vaccine administration; and alcohol abuse. To avoid the influence of hormonal fluctuations in women during the peri-menopausal phase, only pre- or post-menopausal women were included. To minimize the importance of population substructure on genomic analyses, the study was restricted to self-reported Metropolitan French origin for three generations (i.e., with parents and grandparents born in continental France). Whole blood samples were collected from the 1000 fasting healthy donors on lithium heparin tubes, from September 2012 to August 2013. The clinical study was approved by the Comité de Protection des Personnes - Ouest 6 on June 13, 2012, and by the French Agence Nationale de Sécurité du Médicament on June 22nd, 2012. The study is sponsored by Institut Pasteur (Pasteur ID-RCB Number: 2012-A00238-35) and was conducted as a single-center study without any investigational product. The protocol is registered under ClinicalTrials.gov (study# NCT01699893).

Serologies

Total IgG, IgM, IgE, and IgA levels were measured using clinical grade turbidimetric test on AU 400 Olympus at the BioTrial (Rennes, France). Antigen-specific serological tests were performed using clinical-grade assays measuring IgG levels, according to the manufacturer's instructions. A list and description of the assays is provided in Additional file 1: Table S1. Briefly, anti-HBs and anti-HBc IgGs were measured on the Architect automate (CMIA assay, Abbott). Anti-CMV IgGs were measured by CMIA using the CMV IgG kit from Beckman Coulter on the Unicel Dxl 800 Access automate (Beckman Coulter). Anti-measles, anti-mumps, and anti-rubella IgGs were measured using the BioPlex 2200 MMRV IgG kit on the BioPlex 2200 analyzer (Bio-Rad). Anti-*Toxoplasma gondi*, and anti-CMV IgGs were measured using the BioPlex 2200 ToRC IgG kit on the BioPlex 2200 analyzer (Bio-Rad). Anti-HSV1 and anti-HSV2 IgGs were measured using the BioPlex 2200 HSV-1 and

HSV-2 IgG kit on the BioPlex 2200 analyzer (Bio-Rad). IgGs against *Helicobacter Pylori* were measured by EIA using the PLATELIA *H. pylori* IgG kit (BioRad) on the VIDAS automate (Biomérieux). Anti-influenza A IgGs were measured by ELISA using the NovaLisa IgG kit from NovaTec (Biomérieux) that explores responses to grade 2 H3N2 Texas 1/77 strain. In all cases, the criteria for serostatus definition (positive, negative, or indeterminate) were established by the manufacturer and are indicated in Additional file 1: Table S2. Donors with an unclear result were retested and assigned a negative result if borderline levels were confirmed with repeat testing.

Non-genetic variables

A large number of demographical and clinical variables are available in the Milieu Intérieur cohort as a description of the environment of the healthy donors [15]. These include infection and vaccination history, childhood diseases, health-related habits, and socio-demographical variables. Of these, 53 where chosen for subsequent analysis of their impact on serostatus. This selection is based on the one done in [16], with a few variables added, such as measures of lipids and C-reactive protein (CRP).

Testing of non-genetic variables

Using serostatus variables as the response, and non-genetic variables as treatment variables, we fitted a logistic regression model for each response and treatment variable pair. A total of $14 \times 52 = 742$ models where therefore fitted. Age and sex where included as controls for all models, except if that variable was the treatment variable. We tested the impact of the clinical and demographical variables using a likelihood ratio test. All 742 tests where considered a multiple testing family with the false discovery rate (FDR) as error rate.

Age and sex testing

To examine the impact of age and sex, we performed logistic and linear regression analyses for serostatus and IgG levels, respectively. For logistic regression, we included both scaled linear and quadratic terms for the age variable (model = glm($y \sim$ Age + I(Age^2) + Sex, family = binomial)). Scaling was achieved by centering age variable at the mean age. When indicated, we used a second model that includes age, sex as well as an interaction term for age and sex (model = glm($y \sim$ Age + Sex + Age $\times$ Sex, family = binomial)). All continuous traits (i.e., quantitative measurements of antibody levels) were log10-transformed in donors assigned as positive using the clinical cutoff suggested by the manufacturer. We used false discovery rate (FDR) correction for the number of serologies tested (associations with $P < 0.05$ were considered significant).

DNA genotyping

Blood was collected in 5-mL sodium EDTA tubes and was kept at room temperature (18°–25°) until processing. DNA was extracted from human whole blood and genotyped at 719,665 single nucleotide polymorphisms (SNPs) using the HumanOmniExpress-24 BeadChip (Illumina). The SNP call rate was higher than 97% in all donors. To increase coverage of rare and potentially functional variation, 966 of the 1000 donors were also genotyped at 245,766 exonic variants using the HumanExome-12 BeadChip. The HumanExome variant call rate was lower than 97% in 11 donors, which were thus removed from this dataset. We filtered out from both datasets genetic variants that (i) were unmapped on dbSNP138, (ii) were duplicated, (iii) had a low genotype clustering quality (GenTrain score < 0.35), (iv) had a call rate < 99%, (v) were monomorphic, (vi) were on sex chromosomes, or (vii) diverged significantly from Hardy-Weinberg equilibrium (HWE $P < 10^{-7}$). These quality-control filters yielded a total of 661,332 and 87,960 variants for the HumanOmniExpress and HumanExome BeadChips, respectively. Average concordance rate for the 16,753 SNPs shared between the two genotyping platforms was 99.9925%, and individual concordance rates ranged from 99.8 to 100%.

Genetic relatedness and structure

As detailed elsewhere [16], relatedness was detected using KING [17]. Six pairs of related participants (parent-child, first and second-degree siblings) were detected, and one individual from each pair, randomly selected, was removed from the genetic analyses. The genetic structure of the study population was estimated using principal component analysis (PCA), implemented in EIGENSTRAT (v6.1.3) [18]. The PCA plot of the study population is shown in Additional file 2: Figure S1.

Genotype imputation

We used positional Burrows-Wheeler transform for genotype imputation, starting with the 661,332 quality-controlled SNPs genotyped on the HumanOmniExpress array. Phasing was performed using EAGLE2 (v2.0.5) [19]. As reference panel, we used the haplotypes from the Haplotype Reference Consortium (release 1.1) [20]. After removing SNPs that had an imputation info score < 0.8, we obtained 22,235,661 variants. We then merged the imputed dataset with 87,960 variants directly genotyped on the HumanExome BeadChips array and removed variants that were monomorphic or diverged significantly from Hardy-Weinberg equilibrium ($P < 10^{-7}$). We obtained a total of 12,058,650 genetic variants to be used in association analyses.

We used SNP2HLA (v1.03) [21] to impute 104 four-digit HLA alleles and 738 amino acid residues (at

315 variable amino acid positions of the HLA class I and II proteins) with a minor allele frequency (MAF) of > 1%.

We used KIR*IMP [22] to impute KIR alleles, after haplotype inference on chromosome 19 with SHAPEIT2 (v2.r790) [23]. A total of 19 KIR types were imputed: 17 loci plus two extended haplotype classifications (A vs. B and KIR haplotype). A MAF threshold of 1% was applied, leaving 16 KIR alleles for association analysis.

Genetic association analyses

For single-variant association analyses, we only considered SNPs with a MAF of > 5% ($N = 5,699,237$). We used PLINK (v1.9) [24] to perform logistic regression for binary phenotypes (serostatus: antibody positive versus negative) and linear regression for continuous traits (log10-transformed quantitative measurements of antibody levels in seropositive donors). The first two principal components of a PCA based on genetic data, age and sex, were used as covariates in all tests. In order to correct for baseline difference in IgG production in individuals, total IgG levels were included as covariates when examining associations with antigen-specific antibody levels, total IgM, IgE, and IgA levels. From a total of 53 additional variables additional co-variates, selected by using elastic net [25] and stability selection [26] as detailed elsewhere [16], were included in some analyses (Additional file 1: Table S3). For all genome-wide association studies, we used a genome-wide significant threshold ($P_{\text{threshold}} < 2.6 \times 10^{-9}$) corrected for the number of antigens and immunoglobulin classes tested ($N = 19$). For specific HLA analyses, we used PLINK (v1.07) [27] to perform conditional haplotype-based association tests and multivariate omnibus tests at multi-allelic amino acid positions.

Variant annotation and gene burden testing

We used SnpEff (v4.3g) [28] to annotate all 12,058,650 variants. A total of 84,748 variants were annotated as having (potentially) moderate (e.g., missense variant, inframe deletion) or high impact (e.g., stop gained, frameshift variant) and were included in the analysis. We used bedtools v2.26.0 [29] to intersect variant genomic location with gene boundaries, thus obtaining sets of variants per gene. By performing kernel-regression-based association tests with SKAT_Common-Rare (testing the combined effect of common and rare variants) and SKATBinary implemented in the SKAT v1.2.1 [30], we tested 16,628 gene sets for association with continuous and binary phenotypes, respectively. By SKAT default parameters, variants with MAF $\leq \frac{1}{\sqrt{2n}}$ are considered rare, whereas variants with MAF $\geq \frac{1}{\sqrt{2n}}$ were considered common, where N is the sample size. We used genome-wide Bonferroni correction for multiple testing, accounting for the number of phenotypes tested ($P_{\text{threshold}} < 2.6 \times 10^{-9}$).

Results

Characterization of humoral immune responses in the 1000 study participants

To characterize the variability in humoral immune responses between healthy individuals, we measured total IgG, IgM, IgA, and IgE levels in the plasma of the 1000 donors of the *Milieu Interieur* (MI) cohort. After log10 transformation, total IgG, IgM, IgA, and IgE levels showed normal distributions, with a median ± sd of 1.02 ± 0.08 g/l, 0.01 ± 0.2 g/l, 0.31 ± 0.18 g/l, and 1.51 ± 0.62 UI/ml, respectively (Additional file 2: Figure S2A).

We then evaluated specific IgG responses to multiple antigens from the following infections and vaccines: (i) seven common persistent pathogens, including five viruses: CMV, EBV (EA, EBNA, and VCA antigens), herpes simplex virus 1 and 2 (HSV-1 & 2), varicella zoster virus (VZV), one bacterium: *Helicobacter pylori* (*H. pylori*), and one parasite: *Toxoplasma gondii* (*T. gondii*); (ii) one recurrent virus: influenza A virus (IAV); and (iii) four viruses for which most donors received vaccination: measles, mumps, rubella, and HBV (HBs and HBc antigens). The distributions of log10-transformed antigen-specific IgG levels in the 1000 donors for the 15 serologies are shown in Additional file 2: Figure S2B. Donors were classified as seropositive or seronegative using the thresholds recommended by the manufacturer (Additional file 1: Table S2).

The vast majority of the 1000 healthy donors were chronically infected with EBV (seropositivity rates of 96% for EBV VCA, 91% for EBV EBNA, and 9% for EBV EA) and VZV (93%). Many also showed high-titer antibodies specific for IAV (77%), HSV-1 (65%), and *T. gondii* (56%). By contrast, fewer individuals were seropositive for CMV (35%), HSV-2 (21%), and *H. pylori* (18%) (Additional file 2: Figure S3A). The majority of healthy donors carried antibodies against five or more persistent/recurrent infections of the eight infectious agents tested (Additional file 2: Figure S3B). Fifty-one percent of *MI* donors were positive for anti-HBs IgG—a large majority of them as a result of vaccination, as only 15 study participants (3% of the anti-HBs-positive group) were positive for anti-HBc IgG, indicative of previous HBV infection (spontaneously cured, as all donors were negative for HBs antigen, criteria for inclusion in the study). For rubella, measles, and mumps, seropositivity rates were 94, 91, and 89%, respectively. For the majority of the donors, this likely reflects vaccination with a trivalent vaccine, which was integrated in 1984 as part of national recommendations in France, but for some, in particular the > 40-year-old individuals of the cohort, it may reflect acquired immunity due to natural infection.

Associations of age, sex, and non-genetic variables with serostatus

Subjects included in the *Milieu Interieur* cohort were surveyed for a large number of variables related to infection and vaccination history, childhood diseases, health-related habits, and socio-demographical variables (http://www.milieuinterieur.fr/en/research-activities/cohort/crf-data). Of these, 53 where chosen for subsequent analysis of their impact on serostatus. This selection is based on the one done in [16], with a few variables added, such as measures of lipids and CRP. Applying a mixed model analysis that controls for potential confounders and batch effects, we found expected associations of HBs seropositivity with previous administration of HBV vaccine, as well as of influenza seropositivity with previous administration of flu vaccine. We also found associations of HBs seropositivity with previous administration of typhoid and hepatitis A vaccines—which likely reflects co-immunization, as well as with income, employment, and owning a house—which likely reflects confounding epidemiological factors (Additional file 2: Figure S4). Full results of the association of non-genetic variables with serostatus are available in Additional file 1: Table S4.

We observed a significant impact of age on the probability of being seropositive for antigens from persistent or recurrent infectious agents and/or vaccines. For 14 out of the 15 examined serologies, older people (> 45 years old) were more likely to have detectable specific IgG, with a mean beta estimate of 0.04 for linear associations (Fig. 1a). Additionally, we found a significant quadratic term for five out of the 15 serologies, highlighting that the rate of change in probability of seropositivity with respect to age is higher for rubella and lower for HSV-1, HP, HBs, and EBV EBNA in older people as compared to younger donors (Additional file 2: Figure S5A). We identified four different profiles of age-dependent evolution of seropositivity rates (Fig. 1b). Profile 1 is typical of childhood-acquired infection, i.e., microbes that most donors had encountered by age 20 (EBV, VZV, and influenza). We observed in this case either (i) a limited increase in seropositivity rate after age 20 for EBV; (ii) stability for VZV; or (iii) a small decrease in seropositivity rate with age for IAV (Additional file 2: Figure S5B-F). Profile 2 concerns prevalent infectious agents that are acquired throughout life, with steadily increasing prevalence (observed for CMV, HSV-1, and *T. gondii*). We observed in this case either (i) a linear increase in seropositivity rates over the five decades of age for CMV (seropositivity rate 24% in 20-29 years old, 44% in 60-69 years old, slope = 0.02) and *T. gondii* (seropositivity rate 21% in

20-29 years old, 88% in 60-69, slope = 0.08); or (ii) a non-linear increase in seropositivity rates for HSV-1, with a steeper slope before age 40 (seropositivity rate 36% in 20-29 years old, 85% in 60-69, slope = 0.05) (Additional file 2: Figure S5G-I). Profile 3 showed microbial agents with limited seroprevalence—in our cohort, HSV-2, HBV (anti-HBs and anti-HBc positive individuals, indicating prior infection rather than vaccination), and *H. pylori*. We observed a modest increase of seropositivity rates throughout life, likely reflecting continuous low-grade exposure (Additional file 2: Figure S5J-L). Profile 4 is negatively correlated with increasing age and is unique to HBV anti-HBs serology (Additional file 2: Figure S5M). This reflects the introduction of the HBV vaccine in 1982 and the higher vaccination coverage of younger populations. Profiles for measles, mumps and rubella are provided in Additional file 2: Figure S5N-P.

We also observed a significant association between sex and serostatus for 8 of the 15 antigens, with a mean beta estimate of 0.07 (Fig. 1c). For six serological phenotypes, women had a higher rate of positivity, IAV being the notable exception. These associations were confirmed when considering "Sharing house with partner" and "Sharing house with children" as covariates. Full results of associations of age and sex with serostatus are present in Additional file 1: Table S5. Finally, we found a significant interaction of age and sex for odds of being seropositive for EBV EBNA, reflecting a decrease in seropositivity rate in older women (beta − 0.0414814; $P = 0.02$, Additional file 2 Figure S5Q).

Impact of age and sex on total and antigen-specific antibody levels

We further examined the impact of age and sex on the levels of total IgG, IgM, IgA, and IgE detected in the serum of the patients, as well as on the levels of antigen-specific IgGs in seropositive individuals. We observed a low impact of age and sex with total immunoglobulin levels (Fig. 2a). Age also had a strong impact on specific IgG levels in seropositive individuals, affecting 9 out of the 15 examined serologies (Fig. 2b). Correlations between age and pathogen-specific IgG levels were mostly positive, i.e., older donors had more specific IgG than younger donors, as for example in the case of rubella (Additional file 2: Figure S6A). The notable exception was *T. gondii*, where we observed lower amounts of specific IgG in older individuals ($b = − 0.013(− 0.019, − 0.007)$, $P = 3.7 × 10^{-6}$, Additional file 2: Figure S6B). On the other hand, sex was significantly correlated with IgG levels specific to mumps and VZV (Fig. 2c). Full results of associations of age and sex with total immunoglobulin and antigen-specific antibody levels are presented in Additional file 1: Table S5.

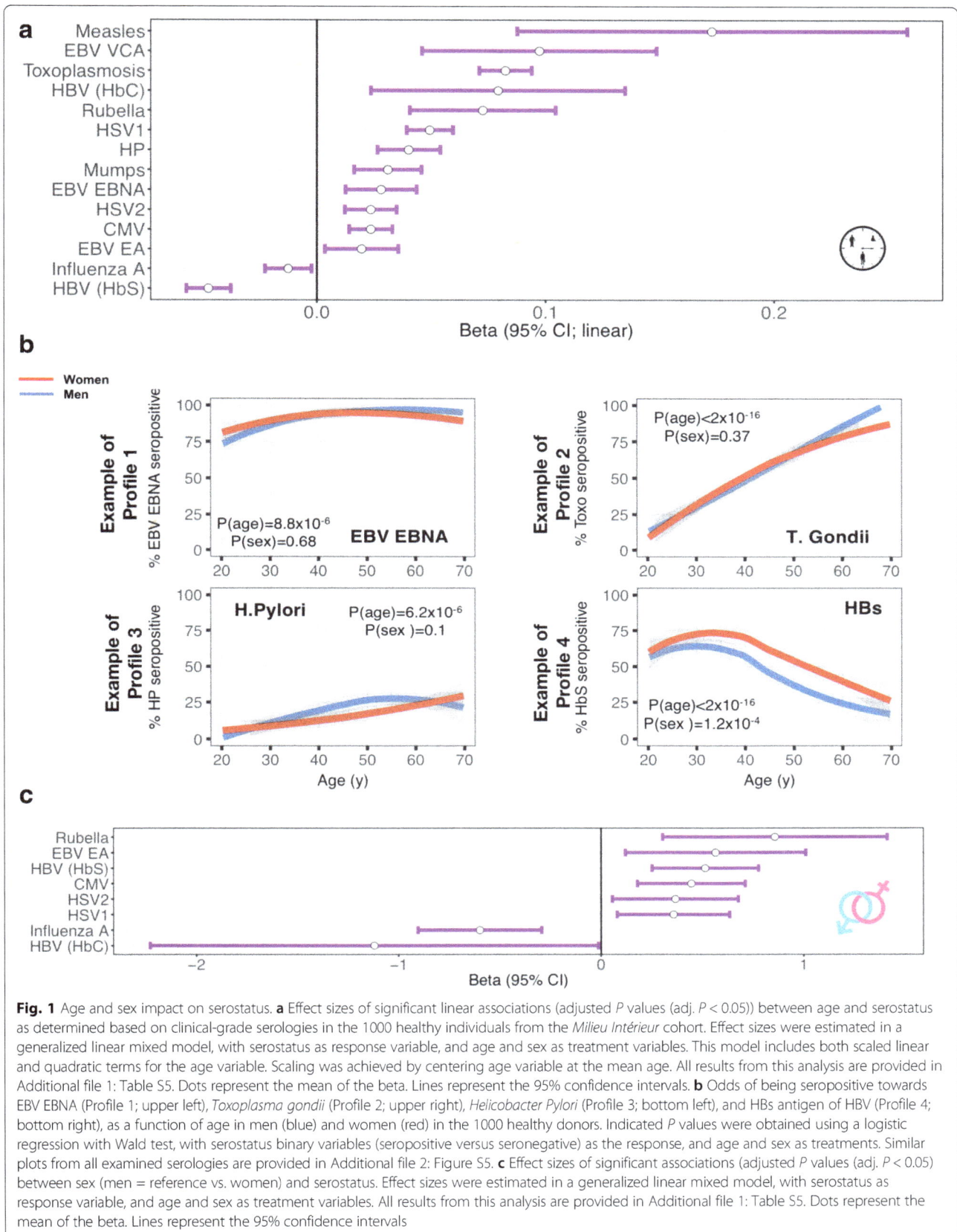

Fig. 1 Age and sex impact on serostatus. **a** Effect sizes of significant linear associations (adjusted *P* values (adj. *P* < 0.05)) between age and serostatus as determined based on clinical-grade serologies in the 1000 healthy individuals from the *Milieu Intérieur* cohort. Effect sizes were estimated in a generalized linear mixed model, with serostatus as response variable, and age and sex as treatment variables. This model includes both scaled linear and quadratic terms for the age variable. Scaling was achieved by centering age variable at the mean age. All results from this analysis are provided in Additional file 1: Table S5. Dots represent the mean of the beta. Lines represent the 95% confidence intervals. **b** Odds of being seropositive towards EBV EBNA (Profile 1; upper left), *Toxoplasma gondii* (Profile 2; upper right), *Helicobacter Pylori* (Profile 3; bottom left), and HBs antigen of HBV (Profile 4; bottom right), as a function of age in men (blue) and women (red) in the 1000 healthy donors. Indicated *P* values were obtained using a logistic regression with Wald test, with serostatus binary variables (seropositive versus seronegative) as the response, and age and sex as treatments. Similar plots from all examined serologies are provided in Additional file 2: Figure S5. **c** Effect sizes of significant associations (adjusted *P* values (adj. *P* < 0.05)) between sex (men = reference vs. women) and serostatus. Effect sizes were estimated in a generalized linear mixed model, with serostatus as response variable, and age and sex as treatment variables. All results from this analysis are provided in Additional file 1: Table S5. Dots represent the mean of the beta. Lines represent the 95% confidence intervals

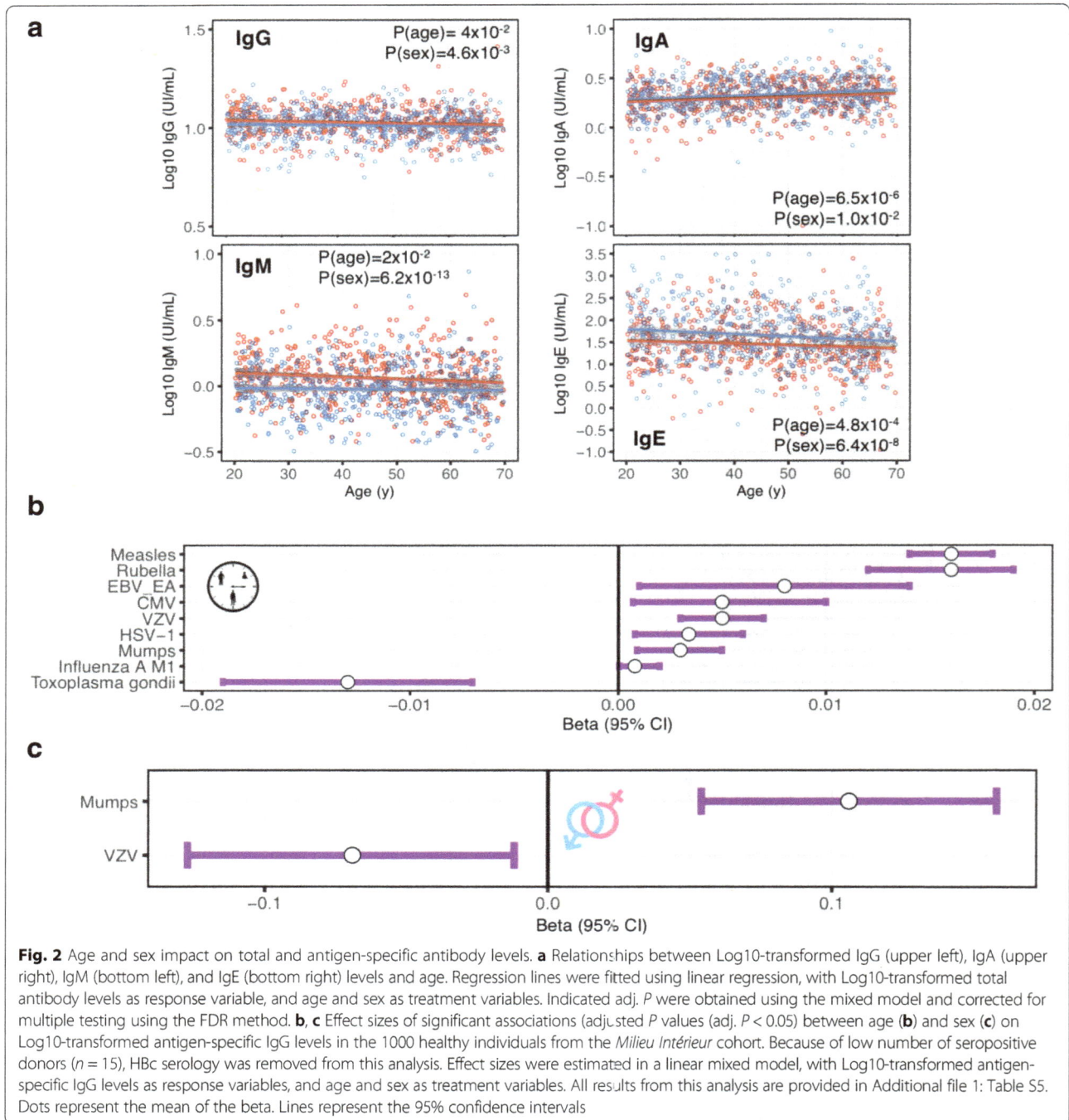

Fig. 2 Age and sex impact on total and antigen-specific antibody levels. **a** Relationships between Log10-transformed IgG (upper left), IgA (upper right), IgM (bottom left), and IgE (bottom right) levels and age. Regression lines were fitted using linear regression, with Log10-transformed total antibody levels as response variable, and age and sex as treatment variables. Indicated adj. *P* were obtained using the mixed model and corrected for multiple testing using the FDR method. **b**, **c** Effect sizes of significant associations (adjusted *P* values (adj. *P* < 0.05) between age (**b**) and sex (**c**) on Log10-transformed antigen-specific IgG levels in the 1000 healthy individuals from the *Milieu Intérieur* cohort. Because of low number of seropositive donors (*n* = 15), HBc serology was removed from this analysis. Effect sizes were estimated in a linear mixed model, with Log10-transformed antigen-specific IgG levels as response variables, and age and sex as treatment variables. All results from this analysis are provided in Additional file 1: Table S5. Dots represent the mean of the beta. Lines represent the 95% confidence intervals

Genome-wide association study of serostatus

To test if human genetic factors influence the rate of seroconversion upon exposure, we performed genome-wide association studies. Specifically, we searched for associations between 5.7 million common polymorphisms (MAF > 5%) and the 15 serostatus in the 1000 healthy donors. Based on our results regarding age and sex, we included both as covariates in all models. After correcting for the number of antibodies considered, the threshold for genome-wide significance was $P_{\text{threshold}} = 2.6 \times 10^{-9}$, for which we did not observe any significant association. In particular, we did not replicate the previously reported associations with *H. pylori* serostatus on chromosomes 1 (rs368433, *P* = 0.56, OR = 1.08) and 4 (rs10004195, *P* = 0.83, OD = 0.97) [31]. We verified this result by performing an additional analysis that matched the design of the previous study, i.e., a case-control association study comparing individuals in the upper quartile of the anti-*H.*

pylori antibody distribution to the rest of the study population: no association was found ($P = 0.42$ and $P = 0.48$ for rs368433 and rs10004195, respectively). The quantile-quantile (QQ) plots and lambda values of all genome-wide logistic regressions are available in Additional file 2: Figure S7.

We then focused on the HLA region and confirmed the previously published association of influenza A serostatus with specific amino acid variants of HLA class II molecules [12]. The strongest association in the *MI* cohort was found with residues at position 31 of the HLA-DRβ1 subunit (omnibus $P = 0.009$, Additional file 1: Table S6). Residues found at that position, isoleucine ($P = 0.2$, OD (95% CI) = 0.8 (0.56, 1.13)) and phenylalanine ($P = 0.2$, OR (95% CI) = 0.81 (0.56, 1.13)), are consistent in direction and in almost perfect linkage disequilibrium (LD) with the glutamic acid residue at position 96 in HLA-DRβ1 that was identified in the previous study (Additional file 1: Table S7). As such, our result independently validates the previous observation.

Genome-wide association study of total and antigen-specific antibody levels

To test whether human genetic factors also influence the intensity of antigen-specific immune response, we performed genome-wide association studies of total IgG, IgM, IgA and IgE levels, as well as antigen-specific IgG levels.

We found no SNPs associated with total IgG, IgM, IgE, and IgA levels. Additional file 2: Figure S8 shows QQ plots and lambda values of these studies. However, we observed nominal significance and the same direction of the effect for 3 out of 11 loci previously

published for total IgA [13, 32–35], 1 out of 6 loci for total IgG [13, 32, 36], and 4 out of 11 loci for total IgM [13, 37] (Additional file 1: Table S8). Finally, we also report a suggestive association (genome-wide significant, $P < 5.0 \times 10^{-8}$, but not significant when correcting for the number of antibody levels tested in the study) of a SNP rs11186609 on chromosome 10 with total IgA levels ($P = 2.0 \times 10^{-8}$, beta = -0.07 for the C allele). The closest gene for this signal is *SH2D4B*.

We next explored associations between human genetic variants and antigen-specific IgG levels in seropositive donors. Information on possible inflation of false positive rates of these linear regressions is available in Additional file 2: Figure S9. We detected significant associations for anti-EBV (EBNA antigen) and anti-rubella IgGs. Associated variants were in both cases located in the HLA region on chromosome 6. For EBV, the top SNP was rs74951723 ($P = 3 \times 10^{-14}$, beta = 0.29 for the A allele) (Fig. 3a). For rubella, the top SNP was rs115118356 ($P = 7.7 \times 10^{-10}$, beta = -0.11 for the G allele) (Fig. 3b). rs115118356 is in LD with rs2064479, which has been previously reported as associated with titers of anti-rubella IgGs ($r^2 = 0.53$ and $D' = 0.76$) [38].

To fine map the associations observed in the HLA region, we tested four-digit HLA alleles and variable amino positions in HLA proteins. At the level of HLA alleles, *HLA-DQB1*03:01* showed the lowest P value for association with EBV EBNA ($P = 1.3 \times 10^{-7}$), and *HLA-DPB1*03:01* was the top signal for rubella ($P = 3.8 \times 10^{-6}$). At the level of amino acid positions, position 58 of the HLA-DRβ1 protein associated with anti-EBV (EBNA antigen) IgG levels ($P = 2.5 \times 10^{-11}$). This is consistent with the results of previous studies linking

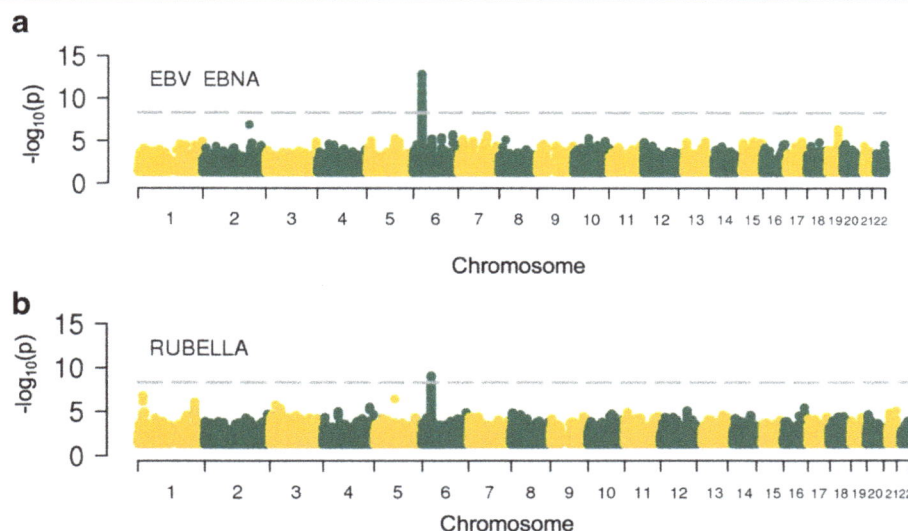

Fig. 3 Association between host genetic variants and serological phenotypes. Manhattan plots of association results for **a** EBV anti-EBNA IgG and **b** rubella IgG levels. The dashed horizontal line denotes genome-wide significance ($P = 2.6 \times 10^{-9}$)

genetic variations in HLA-DRβ1 with levels of anti-EBV EBNA-specific IgGs [12, 39, 40] (Additional file 1: Table S9). In addition, position 8 of the HLA-DPβ1 protein associated with anti-rubella IgG levels ($P = 1.1 \times 10^{-9}$, Table 1). Conditional analyses on these amino-acid positions did not reveal any additional independent signals.

KIR associations

To test whether specific KIR genotypes, and their interaction with HLA molecules, are associated with humoral immune responses, we imputed KIR alleles from SNP genotypes using KIR*IMP [22]. First, we searched for potential associations with serostatus or IgG levels for 16 KIR alleles that had a MAF > 1%. We did not find any significant association after Bonferroni correction for multiple testing. Second, we tested specific KIR-HLA combinations. We filtered out rare combinations by removing pairs that were observed less than four times in the cohort. After correction for the number of tests performed and phenotypes considered ($P_{\text{threshold}} < 5.4 \times 10^{-7}$), we observed significant associations between total IgA levels and the two following HLA-KIR combinations: HLA-B*14:02/KIR3DL1 and HLA-C*08:02/KIR2DS4 ($P = 3.9 \times 10^{-9}$ and $P = 4.9 \times 10^{-9}$ respectively, Table 2).

Burden testing for rare variants

Finally, to search for potential associations between the burden of low-frequency variants and the serological phenotypes, we conducted a rare variant association study. This analysis only included variants annotated as missense or putative loss-of-function (nonsense, essential splice-site, and frame-shift, $N = 84,748$), which we collapsed by gene and tested together using the kernel-regression-based association test SKAT [30]. We restricted our analysis to genes that contained at least

Table 1 Associations of EBV EBNA and rubella antigens with HLA (SNP, allele, and amino acid position)

	Phenotype	
	EBV EBNA IgG levels	Rubella IgG levels
SNP		
ID (Allele)	rs74951723 (A)	rs115118356 (G)
P-value	3×10^{-14}	7.68×10^{-10}
Beta (95% CI)	0.29 (0.21, 0.36)	−0.11 (−0.15, −0.08)
Classical HLA allele		
Allele	HLA-DQB1*03:01	HLA-DPB1*03:01
P value	1.26×10^{-7}	3.8×10^{-6}
Beta (95% CI)	0.17 (0.11, 0.23)	−0.12 (−0.18, −0.07)
Amino acid		
Protein (position)	HLA-DRβ1 (56)	HLA-DPβ1 (8)
Omnibus P value	2.53×10^{-11}	1.12×10^{-9}

Table 2 Association testing between KIR-HLA interactions and serology phenotypes

Phenotype	KIR	HLA	Estimate	Std. error	P value
IgA levels	KIR3DL1	HLA-B*14:02	0.456	0.077	3.9×10^{-09}
IgA levels	KIR2DS4	HLA-B*14:02	0.454	0.077	4.5×10^{-09}
IgA levels	KIR3DL1	HLA-C*08:02	0.449	0.076	4.9×10^{-09}
IgA levels	KIR2DS4	HLA-C*08:02	0.448	0.076	5.7×10^{-09}

five variants. Two genes were identified as significantly associated with total IgA levels using this approach: *ACADL* ($P = 3.4 \times 10^{-11}$) and *TMEM131* ($P = 7.8 \times 10^{-11}$) (Table 3). By contrast, we did not observe any significant associations between rare variant burden and antigen-specific IgG levels or serostatus. All the QQ plots and lambda values of analysis of binary, total Ig levels, and pathogen-specific quantitative phenotypes are shown in Additional file 2: Figure S10, S11, and S12.

Discussion

We performed genome-wide association studies for a number of serological phenotypes in a well-characterized age- and sex-stratified cohort and included a unique examination of genetic variation at HLA and KIR loci, as well as KIR-HLA associations. As such, our study provides a broad resource for exploring the variability in humoral immune responses across different isotypes and different antigens in humans.

Using a fine-mapping approach, we replicated the previously reported associations of variation in the HLA-DRβ1 protein with influenza A serostatus and anti-EBV IgG titers [4, 12], implicating amino acid residues in strong LD with the ones previously reported by Hammer et al. In accordance with the same study, we did not observe any significant association with another measure of EBV serostatus, the presence of anti-EBNA antibodies, suggesting that a larger sample size will be required to uncover potentially associated variants. We replicated an association between HLA class II variation and anti-rubella IgG titers [38] and further fine-mapped it to position 8 of the HLA-DPβ1 protein. Interestingly, position 8 of HLA-DPβ1 and positions 58 and 31 of HLA-DRβ1 are all part of the extracellular domain of the respective proteins. Our findings confirm these proteins as critical elements for the presentation of processed peptide to CD4+ T cells and as such may reveal important clues in the fine regulation of class II antigen presentation. We also identified specific HLA/KIR combinations, namely HLA-B*14:02/KIR3DL1 and HLA-C*08:02/KIR2DS4, which associate with higher levels of circulating IgA. Combinations of HLA and killer cell immunoglobulin-like receptor (KIR) genes have been associated with diseases as diverse as autoimmunity, viral infections, reproductive failure, and

Table 3 Significant associations of rare variants collapsed per gene set with IgA levels

Phenotype	Chromosome	Gene	P value	Q	No. of rare markers	No. of Common Markers
IgA levels	2	ACADL	3.42×10^{-11}	18.09	5	2
	2	TMEM131	7.83×10^{-11}	17.89	13	2

cancer [41]. To date, the molecular basis for these associations is mostly unknown. One could speculate that the association identified between IgA levels and specific KIR-HLA combinations may reflect different levels of tolerance to commensal microbes. However, formal testing of this hypothesis will require additional studies. Also, given the novelty of KIR imputation method and the lack of possibility of benchmarking its reliability in the *MI* cohort, further replication of these results will be needed. Yet these findings support the concept that variations in the sequence of HLA class II molecules, or specific KIRs/HLA class I interactions play a critical role in shaping humoral immune responses in humans. In particular, our findings confirm that small differences in the capacity of HLA class II molecules to bind specific viral peptides can have a measurable impact on downstream antibody production. As such, our study emphasizes the importance of considering HLA diversity in disease association studies where associations between IgG levels and autoimmune diseases are being explored.

We identified nominal significance for some but not all of the previously reported associations with levels of total IgG, IgM, and IgA, as well as a suggestive association of total IgA levels with an intergenic region on chromosome 10—closest gene being *SH2D4B*. By collapsing the rare variants present in our dataset into gene sets and testing them for association with the immunoglobulin phenotypes, we identified two additional loci that participate to natural variation in IgA levels. These associations mapped to the genes *ACADL* and *TMEM131*. *ACADL* encodes an enzyme with long-chain acyl-CoA dehydrogenase activity, and polymorphisms have been associated with pulmonary surfactant dysfunction [42]. As the same gene is associated with levels of circulating IgA in our cohort, we speculate that *ACADL* could play a role in regulating the balance between mucosal and circulating IgA. Further studies will be needed to test this hypothesis, as well as the potential impact of our findings in other IgA-related diseases.

We were not able to replicate previous associations of *TLR1* and *FCGR2A* locus with serostatus for *H. pylori* [31]. We believe this may be a result of (i) different analytical methods or (ii) notable differences in previous exposure among the different cohorts as illustrated by the different levels of seropositivity—17% in the *Milieu Interieur* cohort, versus 56% in the previous ones, reducing the likelihood of replication due to decreased statistical power.

In addition to genetics findings, our study re-examined the impact of age and sex, as well as non-genetic variables, on humoral immune responses. Although this question has been previously addressed, our well-stratified cohort brings interesting additional insights. One interesting finding is the high rate of seroconversion for CMV, HSV-1, and *T. gondii* during adulthood. In our cohort, the likelihood of being seropositive for one of these infections is comparable at age 20 and 40. This observation raises interesting questions about the factors that could prevent some individuals from becoming seropositive upon late-life exposure, considering the high likelihood of being in contact with the pathogens because of their high prevalence in humans (CMV and HSV-1) or because of frequent interactions with an animal reservoir (toxoplasmosis). Second, both age and sex have a strong correlation with serostatus, i.e., older and female donors were more likely to be seropositive. Although increased seropositivity with age probably reflects continuous exposure, the sex effect is intriguing. Indeed, our study considered humoral immunity to microbial agents that differ significantly in terms of physiopathology and that do not necessarily have a childhood reservoir. Also, our analysis shows that associations persist after removal of potential confounding factors such as marital status and/or number of kids. As such, we believe that our results may highlight a general impact of sex on humoral immune response variability, i.e., a tendency for women to be more likely to seroconvert after exposure, as compared to men of same age. Gender-specific differences in humoral responses have been previously observed for a large number of viral and bacterial vaccines including influenza, hepatitis A and B, rubella, measles, rabies, yellow fever, meningococcus, pneumococcus, diphtheria, tetanus, and Brucella [43, 44]. Along the same line, women often respond to lower vaccine doses than men [43, 45], and higher levels of antibodies have been found in female schoolchildren after rubella and mumps vaccination [46] as well as in adult women after smallpox vaccination [47]. This could be explained, at least partially, by a shift towards Th2 immunity in women as compared to men [48]. Finally, we observed an age-related increase in antigen-specific IgG levels in seropositive individuals for most serologies, with the notable exception of toxoplasmosis. This may indicate that aging plays a general role in IgG production. An alternative explanation that requires further study is that this could be the consequence of reactivation or recurrent exposure.

Conclusions

In sum, our study provides evidence that age, sex, and host genetics contribute to natural variation in humoral immunity in humans. The identified associations have the potential to help improve vaccination strategies and/or dissect pathogenic mechanisms implicated in human diseases related to immunoglobulin production such as autoimmunity.

Additional files

Additional file 1: Table S1. Assay details for serologies. Table S2. Cutoffs and seroprevalence for serologies. Table S3. List of covariates used for each phenotype. Table S4. Associations of environmental variables with serostatus. Table S5. Association of serologies with age and sex. Table S6. Associations of amino acid positions in HLA proteins with Influenza A serology. Table S7. LD between residues in HLA-DRβ1 at position 13 and 96. Table S8. Replication of SNPs associated with levels of total IgM, IgA and IgG. Table S9. LD between residues in HLA-DRβ1 at position 15 and 11.

Additional file 2: Figure S1. Principal Component Analysis. Figure S2. Distribution of serological variables, and clinical thresholds. Figure S3. Seroprevalence data. Figure S4. Impact of non-genetic factors on serostatus. Figure S5. Evolution of serostatus with age and sex. Figure S6. Correlations between age and IgG specific to Rubella and T. gondii. Figure S7. QQ plots for logistic regressions preformed in the study. Figure S8. QQ plots for linear regressions preformed on total Ig levels. Figure S9. QQ plots for linear regressions preformed for pathogen-specific IgG levels. Figure S10. QQ plots for burden testing analyses preformed for all binary phenotypes. Figure S11. QQ plots for burden testing analyses preformed for total Ig levels. Figure S12. QQ plots for burden testing analyses preformed for pathogen-specific IgG levels.

Abbreviations

CMV: Cytomegalovirus; CRP: C-reactive protein; EBV: Epstein-Barr virus; FDR: False discovery rate; H. pylori: Helicobacter pylori; HBV: Hepatitis B virus; HCV: Hepatitis C virus; HLA: Human leukocyte antigen; HSV1: Herpes simplex virus 1; HSV2: Herpes simplex virus 2; IAV: Influenza A virus; Ig: Immunoglobulin; LD: Linkage disequilibrium; MAF: Minor allele frequency; MI: Milieu Interieur; QQ: Quantile-quantile; SNP: Single nucleotide polymorphism; T. gondii: Toxoplasma gondii; VZV: Varicella zoster virus

Acknowledgements

We would like to thank all the donors for their contribution to the study. We also thank the members of the The Milieu Intérieur Consortium for their insightful comments. The Milieu Intérieur Consortium is composed of the following team leaders: Laurent Abel (Hôpital Necker, Paris, France), Andres Alcover (Institut Pasteur, Paris, France), Hugues Aschard (Institut Pasteur, Paris, France), Kalla Astrom (Lund University, Lund, Sweden), Philippe Bousso (Institut Pasteur, Paris, France), Pierre Bruhns (Institut Pasteur, Paris, France), Ana Cumano (Institut Pasteur, Paris, France), Caroline Demangel (Institut Pasteur, Paris, France), Ludovic Deriano (Institut Pasteur, Paris, France), James Di Santo (Institut Pasteur, Paris, France), Françoise Dromer (Institut Pasteur, Paris, France), Darragh Duffy (Institut Pasteur, Paris, France), Gérard Eberl (Institut Pasteur, Paris, France), Jost Enninga (Institut Pasteur, Paris, France), Jacques Fellay (EPFL, Lausanne, Switzerland) Odile Gelpi (Institut Pasteur, Paris, France), Ivo Gomperts-Boneca (Institut Pasteur, Paris, France), Milena Hasan (Institut Pasteur, Paris, France), Serge Hercberg (Université Paris 13, Paris, France), Olivier Lantz (Institut Curie, Paris, France), Claude Leclerc (Institut Pasteur, Paris, France), Hugo Mouquet (Institut Pasteur, Paris, France), Sandra Pellegrini (Institut Pasteur, Paris, France), Stanislas Pol (Hôpital Côchin, Paris, France), Antonio Rausell (INSERM UMR 1163 – Institut Imagine, Paris, France), Lars Rogge (Institut Pasteur, Paris, France), Anavaj Sakuntabhai (Institut Pasteur, Paris, France), Olivier Schwartz (Institut Pasteur, Paris, France), Benno Schwikowski (Institut Pasteur, Paris, France), Spencer Shorte (Institut Pasteur, Paris, France), Vassili Soumelis (Institut Curie, Paris, France), Frédéric Tangy (Institut Pasteur, Paris, France), Eric Tartour (Hôpital Européen George Pompidou, Paris, France), Antoine Toubert (Hôpital Saint-Louis, Paris, France), Mathilce Touvier (Université Paris 13, Paris, France), Marie-Noëlle Ungeheuer (Institut Pasteur, Paris, France), Matthew L. Albert (Roche Genentech, South San Francisco, CA, USA), Lluis Quintana-Murci (Institut Pasteur, Paris, France).

Funding

This work benefited from support of the French government's Invest in the Future Program, managed by the Agence Nationale de la Recherche (ANR, reference 10-LABX-69-01). It was also supported by a grant from the Swiss National Science Foundation (31003A_175603, to JF). C.A. received a PostDoctoral Fellowship from Institut National de la Recherche Médicale.

Authors' contributions

CA, LA, LQ-M, DD, MLA, and JF contributed to the conception of the study. PS, CA, CH, DD, MLA, and JF contributed to the design of the study. PS, CA, CH, FH, EP, and BC contributed to the acquisition of the data. PS, CA, CH, FH, JB, CWT, and NC contributed to the analysis of the data. PS, CA, CH, DD, MLA, anc JF contributed to the drafting of the manuscript. PS, CA, CH, FH, JB, EP, CWT, LA, DD, MLA, and JF contributed to the revising of the manuscript. All authors read and approved the final manuscript.

Competing interests

C.H. and M.L.A. are employees of Genentech Inc., a member of The Roche Group. The remaining authors declare that they have no competing interests.

Author details

[1]School of Life Sciences, École Polytechnique Fédérale de Lausanne, Lausanne, Switzerland. [2]Swiss Institute of Bioinformatics, Lausanne, Switzerland. [3]Immunobiology of Dendritic Cell Unit, Institut Pasteur, Paris, France. [4]Center for Translational Research, Institut Pasteur, Paris, France. [5]Inserm U1223, Institut Pasteur, Paris, France. [6]Department of Cancer Immunology, Genentech, South San Francisco, CA, USA. [7]Department of Automatic Control, Lund University, Lund, Sweden. [8]Unit of Human Evolutionary Genetics, Department of Genomes and Genetics, Institut Pasteur, Paris, France. [9]Centre National de la Recherche Scientifique, URA 3012, Paris, France. [10]Center of Bioinformatics, Biostatistics and Integrative Biology, Institut Pasteur, 75015 Paris, France. [11]Laboratory of Human Genetics of Infectious Diseases, Necker branch, Inserm U1163, Paris, France. [12]Imagine Institute, Paris Descartes University, Paris, France. [13]St Giles laboratory of Human Genetics of Infectious Diseases, Rockefeller Branch, The Rockefeller University, New York, NY, USA. [14]Precision Medicine Unit, Lausanne University Hospital, Lausanne, Switzerland.

References

1. Traylen CM, Patel HR, Fondaw W, Mahatme S, Williams JF, Walker LR, Dyson OF, Arce S, Akula SM. Virus reactivation: a panoramic view in human infections. Future Virol. 2011;6:451–63.
2. Grundbacher FJ. Heritability estimates and genetic and environmental correlations for the human immunoglobulins G, M, and A. Am J Hum Genet. 1974;26:1–12.
3. Tsang JS. Schwartzberg PL, Kotliarov Y, Biancotto A, Xie Z, Germain RN, Wang E, Olnes MJ, Narayanan M, Golding H, Moir S, Dickler HB, Perl S, Cheung F, Baylor HIPC Center; CHI Consortium. Global analyses of human immune variation reveal baseline predictors of postvaccination responses. Cell. 2014;157:499–513.
4. Rubicz R, Leach CT, Kraig E, Dhurandhar NV, Duggirala R, Blangero J, Yolken R, Göring HH. Genetic factors influence serological measures of common infections. Hum Hered. 2011;72:133–41.
5. Almohmeed YH, Avenell A, Aucott L, Vickers MA. Systematic review and meta-analysis of the sero-epidemiological association between Epstein Barr virus and multiple sclerosis. PLoS One. 2013;8:e61110.

6. Timmann C, Thye T, Vens M, Evans J, May J, Ehmen C, Sievertsen J, Muntau B, Ruge G, Loag W, Ansong D, Antwi S, Asafo-Adjei E, Nguah SB, Kwakye KO, Akoto AO, Sylverken J, Brendel M, Schuldt K, Loley C, Franke A, Meyer CG, Agbenyega T, Ziegler A, Horstmann RD. Genome-wide association study indicates two novel resistance loci for severe malaria. Nature. 2012;489:443–6.

7. McLaren PJ, Coulonges C, Ripke S, van den Berg L, Buchbinder S, Carrington M, Cossarizza A, Dalmau J, Deeks SG, Delaneau O, De Luca A, Goedert JJ, Haas D, Herbeck JT, Kathiresan S, Kirk GD, Lambotte O, Luo M, Mallal S, van Manen D, Martinez-Picado J, Meyer L, Miro JM, Mullins JI, Obel N, O'Brien SJ, Pereyra F, Plummer FA, Poli G, Qi Y, Rucart P, Sandhu MS, Shea PR, Schuitemaker H, Theodorou I, Vannberg F, Veldink J, Walker BD, Weintrob A, Winkler CA, Wolinsky S, Telenti A, Goldstein DB, de Bakker PI, Zagury JF, Fellay J. Association study of common genetic variants and HIV-1 acquisition in 6,300 infected cases and 7,200 controls. PLoS Pathog. 2013;9:e1003515.

8. Casanova JL, Abel L. The genetic theory of infectious diseases: a brief history and selected illustrations. Annu Rev Genomics Hum Genet. 2013;14:215–43.

9. Tian C, Hromatka BS, Kiefer AK, Eriksson N, Noble SM, Tung JY, Hinds DA. Genome-wide association and HLA region fine-mapping studies identify susceptibility loci for multiple common infections. Nat Commun. 2017;8:599.

10. McLaren PJ, Coulonges C, Bartha I, Lenz TL, Deutsch AJ, Bashirova A, Buchbinder S, Carrington MN, Cossarizza A, Dalmau J, De Luca A, Goedert JJ, Gurdasani D, Haas DW, Herbeck JT, Johnson EO, Kirk GD, Lambotte O, Luo M, Mallal S, van Manen D, Martinez-Picado J, Meyer L, Miro JM, Mullins JI, Obel N, Poli G, Sandhu MS, Schuitemaker H, Shea PR, Theodorou I, Walker BD, Weintrob AC, Winkler CA, Wolinsky SM, Raychaudhuri S, Goldstein DB, Telenti A, de Bakker PI, Zagury JF, Fellay J. Polymorphisms of large effect explain the majority of the host genetic contribution to variation of HIV-1 virus load. Proc Natl Acad Sci U S A. 2015;112:14658–63.

11. Ge D, Fellay J, Thompson AJ, Simon JS, Shianna KV, Urban TJ, Heinzen EL, Qiu P, Bertelsen AH, Muir AJ, Sulkowski M, McHutchison JG, Goldstein DB. Genetic variation in IL28B predicts hepatitis C treatment-induced viral clearance. Nature. 2009;461:399–401.

12. Hammer C, Begemann M, McLaren PJ, Bartha I, Michel A, Klose B, Schmitt C, Waterboer T, Pawlita M, Schulz TF, Ehrenreich H, Fellay J. Amino acid variation in HLA class II proteins is a major determinant of humoral response to common viruses. Am J Hum Genet. 2015;97:738–43.

13. Jonsson S, Sveinbjornsson G, de Lapuente Portilla AL, Swaminathan B, Plomp R, Dekkers G, Ajore R, Ali M, Bentlage AEH, Elmér E, Eyjolfsson GI, Gudjonsson SA, Gullberg U, Gylfason A, Halldorsson BV, Hansson M, Holm H, Johansson Å, Johnsson E, Jonasdottir A, Ludviksson BR, Oddsson A, Olafsson I, Olafsson S, Sigurdardottir O, Sigurdsson A, Stefansdottir L, Masson G, Sulem P, Wuhrer M, Wihlborg AK, Thorleifsson G, Gudbjartsson DF, Thorsteinsdottir U, Vidarsson G, Jonsdottir I, Nilsson B, Stefansson K. Identification of sequence variants influencing immunoglobulin levels. Nat Genet. 2017;49:1182–91.

14. Rubicz R, Yolken R, Drigalenko E, Carless MA, Dyer TD, Kent J Jr, Curran JE, Johnson MP, Cole SA, Fowler SP, Arya R, Puppala S, Almasy L, Moses EK, Kraig E, Duggirala R, Blangero J, Leach CT, Göring HH. Genome-wide genetic investigation of serological measures of common infections. Eur J Hum Genet. 2015;23:1544–8.

15. Thomas S, Rouilly V, Patin E, Alanio C, Dubois A, Delval C, Marquier LG, Fauchoux N, Sayegrih S, Vray M, Duffy D, Quintana-Murci L, Albert ML. Milieu Intérieur Consortium. The Milieu Intérieur study—an integrative approach for study of human immunological variance. Clin Immunol. 2015;157:277–93.

16. Patin E, Hasan M, Bergstedt J, Rouilly V, Libri V, Urrutia A, Alanio C, Scepanovic P, Hammer C, Jönsson F, Beitz B, Quach H, Lim YW, Hunkapiller J, Zepeda M, Green C, Piasecka B, Leloup L, Rogge L, Huetz F, Peguillet I, Lantz O, Fontes M, Di Santo JP, Thomas S, Fellay J, Duffy D, Quintana-Murci L, Albert ML, for The Milieu Intérieur Consortium. Natural variation in innate immune cell parameters is preferentially driven by genetic factors. Nat Immunol 2018;19:302–314.

17. Manichaikul A, Mychaleckyj JC, Rich SS, Daly K, Sale M, Chen WM. Robust relationship inference in genome-wide association studies. Bioinformatics. 2010;26:2867–73.

18. Patterson N, Price AL, Reich D. Population structure and eigenanalysis. PLoS Genet. 2006;2:e190.

19. Loh PR, Danecek P, Palamara PF, Fuchsberger C, A Reshef Y, K Finucane H, Schoenherr S, Forer L, McCarthy S, Abecasis GR, Durbin R, L Price A. Reference-based phasing using the Haplotype Reference Consortium panel. Nat Genet. 2016;48:1443–8.

20. McCarthy S, et al. A reference panel of 64,976 haplotypes for genotype imputation. Nat Genet. 2016;48:1279–83.

21. Jia X, Han B, Onengut-Gumuscu S, Chen WM, Concannon PJ, Rich SS, Raychaudhuri S, de Bakker PI. Imputing amino acid polymorphisms in human leukocyte antigens. PLoS One. 2013;8:e64683.

22. Vukcevic D, Traherne JA, Næss S, Ellinghaus E, Kamatani Y, Dilthey A, Lathrop M, Karlsen TH, Franke A, Moffatt M, Cookson W, Trowsdale J, McVean G, Sawcer S, Leslie S. Imputation of KIR types from SNP variation data. Am J Hum Genet. 2015;97:593–607.

23. O'Connell J, Gurdasani D, Delaneau O, Pirastu N, Ulivi S, Cocca M, Traglia M, Huang J, Huffman JE, Rudan I, McQuillan R, Fraser RM, Campbell H, Polasek O, Asiki G, Ekoru K, Hayward C, Wright AF, Vitart V, Navarro P, Zagury JF, Wilson JF, Toniolo D, Gasparini P, Soranzo N, Sandhu MS, Marchini J. A general approach for haplotype phasing across the full spectrum of relatedness. PLoS Genet. 2014;10:e1004234.

24. Chang CC, Chow CC, Tellier LC, Vattikuti S, Purcell SM, Lee JJ. Second-generation PLINK: rising to the challenge of larger and richer datasets. Gigascience. 2015;4:7.

25. Zhou X, Stephens M. Efficient multivariate linear mixed model algorithms for genome-wide association studies. Nat Methods. 2014;11:407–9.

26. Meinshausen N, Bühlmann P. Stability selection. J R Stat Soc Ser B: Stat Methodol. 2010;72:417–73.

27. Purcell S, Neale B, Todd-Brown K, Thomas L, Ferreira MA, Bender D, Maller J, Sklar P, de Bakker PI, Daly MJ, Sham PC. PLINK: a tool set for whole-genome association and population-based linkage analyses. Am J Hum Genet. 2007;81:559–75.

28. Cingolani P, Platts A, Wang le L, Coon M, Nguyen T, Wang L, Land SJ, Lu X, Ruden DM. A program for annotating and predicting the effects of single nucleotide polymorphisms, SnpEff: SNPs in the genome of Drosophila melanogaster strain w1118; iso-2; iso-3. Fly (Austin). 2012;6:80–92.

29. Quinlan AR, Hall IM. BEDTools: a flexible suite of utilities for comparing genomic features. Bioinformatics. 2010;26:841–2.

30. Ionita-Laza I, Lee S, Makarov V, Buxbaum JD, Lin X. Sequence kernel association tests for the combined effect of rare and common variants. Am J Hum Genet. 2013;92:841–53.

31. Mayerle J, den Hoed CM, Schurmann C, Stolk L, Homuth G, Peters MJ, Capelle LG, Zimmermann K, Rivadeneira F, Gruska S, Völzke H, de Vries AC, Völker U, Teumer A, van Meurs JB, Steinmetz I, Nauck M, Ernst F, Weiss FU, Hofman A, Zenker M, Kroemer HK, Prokisch H, Uitterlinden AG, Lerch MM, Kuipers EJ. Identification of genetic loci associated with Helicobacter pylori serologic status. JAMA. 2013;309:1912–20.

32. Swaminathan B, Thorleifsson G, Jöud M, Ali M, Johnsson E, Ajore R, Sulem P, Halvarsson BM, Eyjolfsson G, Haraldsdottir V, Hultman C, Ingelsson E, Kristinsson SY, Kähler AK, Lenhoff S, Masson G, Mellqvist UH, Månsson R, Nelander S, Olafsson I, Sigurðardottir O, Steingrimsdóttir H, Vangsted A, Vogel U, Waage A, Nahi H, Gudbjartsson DF, Rafnar T, Turesson I, Gullberg U, Stefánsson K, Hansson M, Thorsteinsdóttir U, Nilsson B. Variants in ELL2 influencing immunoglobulin levels associate with multiple myeloma. Nat Commun. 2015;6:7213.

33. Viktorin A, Frankowiack M, Padyukov L, Chang Z, Melén E, Sääf A, Kull I, Klareskog L, Hammarström L, Magnusson PK. IgA measurements in over 12 000 Swedish twins reveal sex differential heritability and regulatory locus near CD30L. Hum Mol Genet. 2014;23:4177–84.

34. Frankowiack M, Kovanen RM, Repasky GA, Lim CK, Song C, Pedersen NL, Hammarström L. The higher frequency of IgA deficiency among Swedish twins is not explained by HLA haplotypes. Genes Immun. 2015;16:199–205.

35. Yang C, Jie W, Yanlong Y, Xuefeng G, Aihua T, Yong G, Zheng L, Youjie Z, Haiying Z, Xue Q, Min Q, Linjian M, Xiaobo Y, Yanling H, Zengnan M. Genome-wide association study identifies TNFSF13 as a susceptibility gene for IgA in a South Chinese population in smokers. Immunogenetics. 2012;64:747–53.

36. Liao M, Ye F, Zhang B, Huang L, Xiao Q, Qin M, Mo L, Tan A, Gao Y, Lu Z, Wu C, Zhang Y, Zhang H, Qin X, Hu Y, Yang X, Mo Z. Genome-wide association study identifies common variants at TNFRSF13B associated with IgG level in a healthy Chinese male population. Genes Immun. 2012;13:509–13.

37. Yang M, Wu Y, Lu Y, Liu C, Sun J, Liao M, Qin M, Mo L, Gao Y, Lu Z, Wu C, Zhang Y, Zhang H, Qin X, Hu Y, Zhang S, Li J, Dong M, Zheng SL, Xu J, Yang X, Tan A, Mo Z. Genome-wide scan identifies variant in TNFSF13 associated with serum IgM in a healthy Chinese male population. PLoS One. 2012;7:e47990.

38. Lambert ND, Haralambieva IH, Kennedy RB, Ovsyannikova IG, Pankratz VS, Poland GA. Polymorphisms in HLA-DPB1 are associated with differences in rubella virus-specific humoral immunity after vaccination. J Infect Dis. 2015; 211:898–905.

39. Rubicz R, Yolken R, Drigalenko E, Carless MA, Dyer TD, Bauman L, Melton PE, Kent JW, Jr HJB, Curran JE, Johnson MP, Cole SA, Almasy L, Moses EK, Dhurandhar NV, Kraig E, Blangero J, Leach CT, Göring HH. A genome-wide integrative genomic study localizes genetic factors influencing antibodies against Epstein-Barr virus nuclear antigen 1 (EBNA-1). PLoS Genet. 2013;9: e1003147.

40. Pedergnana V, Syx L, Cobat A, Guergnon J, Brice P, Fermé C, Carde P, Hermine O, Le-Pendeven C, Amiel C, Taoufik Y, Alcaïs A, Theodorou I, Besson C, Abel L. Combined linkage and association studies show that HLA class II variants control levels of antibodies against Epstein-Barr virus antigens. PLoS One. 2014;9:e102501.

41. Rajagopalan S, Long EO. Understanding how combinations of HLA and KIR genes influence disease. J Exp Med. 2005;201:1025–9.

42. Goetzman ES, Alcorn JF, Bharathi SS, Uppala R, McHugh KJ, Kosmider B, Chen R, Zuo YY, Beck ME, McKinney RW, Skilling H, Suhrie KR, Karunanidhi A, Yeasted R, Otsubo C, Ellis B, Tyurina YY, Kagan VE, Mallampalli RK, Vockley J. Long-chain acyl-CoA dehydrogenase deficiency as a cause of pulmonary surfactant dysfunction. J Biol Chem. 2014;289:10668–79.

43. Giefing-Kröll C, Berger P, Lepperdinger G, Grubeck-Loebenstein B. How sex and age affect immune responses, susceptibility to infections, and response to vaccination. Aging Cell. 2015;14:309–21.

44. Cook IF. Sexual dimorphism of humoral immunity with human vaccines. Vaccine. 2008;26:3551–5.

45. Klein SL, Jedlicka A, Pekosz A. The Xs and Y of immune responses to viral vaccines. Lancet Infect Dis. 2010;10:338–49.

46. Ovsyannikova IG, Jacobson RM, Dhiman N, Vierkant RA, Pankratz VS, Poland GA. Human leukocyte antigen and cytokine receptor gene polymorphisms associated with heterogeneous immune responses to mumps viral vaccine. Pediatrics. 2008;121:e1091–9.

47. Kennedy RB, Ovsyannikova IG, Pankratz VS, Vierkant RA, Jacobson RM, Ryan MA, Poland GA. Gender effects on humoral immune responses to smallpox vaccine. Vaccine. 2009;27:3319–23.

48. Girón-González JA, Moral FJ, Elvira J, García-Gil D, Guerrero F, Gavilán I, Escobar L. Consistent production of a higher TH1:TH2 cytokine ratio by stimulated T cells in men compared with women. Eur J Endocrinol. 2000;143:31–6.

3

Sensitivity to sequencing depth in single-cell cancer genomics

João M. Alves[1,2,3]* and David Posada[1,2,3]*

Abstract

Background: Querying cancer genomes at single-cell resolution is expected to provide a powerful framework to understand in detail the dynamics of cancer evolution. However, given the high costs currently associated with single-cell sequencing, together with the inevitable technical noise arising from single-cell genome amplification, cost-effective strategies that maximize the quality of single-cell data are critically needed. Taking advantage of previously published single-cell whole-genome and whole-exome cancer datasets, we studied the impact of sequencing depth and sampling effort towards single-cell variant detection.

Methods: Five single-cell whole-genome and whole-exome cancer datasets were independently downscaled to 25, 10, 5, and 1× sequencing depth. For each depth level, ten technical replicates were generated, resulting in a total of 6280 single-cell BAM files. The sensitivity of variant detection, including structural and driver mutations, genotyping, clonal inference, and phylogenetic reconstruction to sequencing depth was evaluated using recent tools specifically designed for single-cell data.

Results: Altogether, our results suggest that for relatively large sample sizes (25 or more cells) sequencing single tumor cells at depths > 5× does not drastically improve somatic variant discovery, characterization of clonal genotypes, or estimation of single-cell phylogenies.

Conclusions: We suggest that sequencing multiple individual tumor cells at a modest depth represents an effective alternative to explore the mutational landscape and clonal evolutionary patterns of cancer genomes.

Keywords: Single-cell sequencing, Intratumor genetic heterogeneity, Variant calling, Clonal inference, Tumor phylogenies

Background

Recent advances in next-generation sequencing (NGS) technologies revealed that the large majority of cancer genomes are heterogeneous despite their monoclonal origin, with the continuous expansion of the tumor mass contributing to the accumulation of somatic mutations within malignant cells, hence promoting the proliferation of distinct genetic lineages (i.e., clones) through time [1]. While quantifying this intratumor heterogeneity (ITH) remains a difficult task, as standard methods in cancer genomics generally rely on population-level analysis from bulk experiments, single-cell sequencing (SC-Seq) approaches are now widely viewed as a promising alternative to explore tumor evolution [2]. Indeed, a collection of recent studies have successfully applied SC-Seq to determine the mutational load in individual tumors [3], estimate the frequency of subclones [4], infer evolutionary relationships [5], or explore the role of ITH in metastatic dissemination [6].

Nevertheless, several technical challenges surrounding current SC-Seq methodologies greatly limit our ability to obtain reliable genomic information from single cells. For instance, the multiple rounds of whole genome amplification (WGA) usually required prior to SC-Seq are known to introduce a high number of sequence artifacts that can be confounded with genuine biological variation (see [7] for a detailed review). Other technical errors, such as insufficient physical coverage, uneven genome amplification, and allelic dropout, may also generate substantial artificial variability in cancer genomes, compromising the ability to detect real somatic heterogeneity

* Correspondence: jalves@uvigo.es; dposada@uvigo.es
[1]Department of Biochemistry, Genetics and Immunology, University of Vigo, Vigo, Spain
Full list of author information is available at the end of the article

from SC-Seq data [8]. As a consequence, alternative strategies are needed in order to eliminate the noise generated during WGA while effectively allowing the quantification of ITH from single cells.

Zhang et al. [9] started addressing some of these issues and demonstrated the efficiency of a census-based strategy for accurate variant detection in single cells. By using multiple cells and trusting only variants detected in at least two single-cell libraries, they detected up to 80% of germline SNPs in the human chromosome 5 with 59 cells sequenced at 0.3× or 22 cells at 1×. Their results suggest that for detecting clonal and subclonal variants in single cells, and given a fixed sequencing effort, it is best to sequence multiple cells (in their case a minimum of 20) at a modest depth ($\sim 1\times$).

Here, we further explore the sensitivity of SC-seq to sequencing depth using five publicly available single-cell whole-genome (scWGS) and whole-exome (scWXS) cancer datasets. We expand not only on the scale of the datasets, but also on the scope of the inferences, including copy-number variant detection, clonal inference, and phylogenetic estimation. Altogether, our results suggest that even though sequencing depth does indeed contribute to a better refinement of somatic variant characterization from tumor single cells, sample size plays a more determinant role for a reliable assessment of the general patterns of somatic variation in cancer genomes. For relatively large sample sizes (e. g., ≥ 25 samples), sequencing single cells at modest depths (i.e., 5×) enables a similar description of somatic variation, clonal composition, and evolutionary history compared to sequencing depths one order of magnitude higher.

Methods

Five publicly available sequencing datasets from four single-cell studies were retrieved from the Sequence Read Archive (SRA) in FASTQ format, including four single-cell genomes from a breast cancer patient [5] (we will call this dataset "W4" to indicate the authors and the number of cells), eight single-cell exomes from circulating tumor cells from one lung adenocarcinoma patient [10] ("N8" dataset), 25 single-cell exomes derived from a kidney tumor patient [11] ("X25" dataset), 55 single-cell exomes from a breast cancer patient [5] ("W55" dataset), and 65 single-cell exomes from a single JAK-2 negative neoplasm myeloproliferative patient [12] ("H65" dataset). Normal and tumor bulk WGS/WXS data from the same patients were also retrieved. Normal single cells were only available for the three largest datasets. A list of the individual samples and corresponding accession codes is available in Additional file 1: Table S1.

All the analyses enumerated below are described in detail in the accompanying Additional file 1: Note, including command lines. Both single-cell and bulk reads were aligned to human reference GRCh37 using the *MEM* algorithm in the BWA software [13]. Following a standardized best-practices pipeline [14], mapped reads from all datasets were independently processed by filtering reads displaying low mapping-quality, performing local realignment around indels, and removing PCR duplicates. Raw single-nucleotide variant (SNV) calls for the bulk datasets were obtained using the paired-sample variant-calling approach implemented in the VarDict software [15]. For the N8 dataset, since samples from both primary tumor and metastasis were available, VarDict was run twice, independently for both samples, and the resulting SNVs subsequently merged using the *CombineVariants* tool from the Genome Analysis Toolkit (GATK) [16]. Low-quality SNV calls were removed using the *SelectVariants* tool from GATK. The remaining SNVs were further subdivided into two distinct categories: "germline" SNVs if present in both tumor and normal bulk samples, and "somatic" SNVs if found solely in the tumor bulk samples. Small indels and other complex structural rearrangements were ignored in order to generate a final list of "gold-standard" bulk SNVs. All analyses presented here were based on this set of variants.

The single-cell BAM files were independently downscaled to 25, 10, 5, and 1× sequencing depth using Picard [17]. For each depth level, ten technical replicates were generated for statistical validation, resulting in a total of 6280 BAM files. Single-cell SNV calls were obtained from the original and down-sampled single-cell BAM files using Monovar [18], a variant caller specifically designed for single-cell data, under default settings. Single-cell variant-calling performance was evaluated by estimating the proportion of "gold-standard" germline and somatic bulk SNVs identified in the down-sampled single-cell datasets (germline and somatic recall, respectively). To further characterize the effect of sequencing depth on single-cell variant calling, we determined the fraction of somatic SNVs found in the down-sampled single-cell replicates that were also identified in the original single-cell datasets ("somatic precision"). In addition, we repeated the recall analysis focusing only on the somatic SNVs already described in the Catalogue Of Somatic Mutations In Cancer (COSMIC) database [19] and on the non-synonymous SNVs previously detected (Additional file 1: Table S2).

Single-cell copy-number variants (CNVs) were identified with Ginkgo [20] using variable-length bins of around 500 kb. After binning, data for each cell was normalized and segmented using default parameters. Sensitivity was evaluated by assessing the recall of the CNVs and segment breakpoints at the different sequencing depths.

Clonal genotypes were estimated from the somatic SNVs using the Single-Cell Genotyper (SCG) [21] (Additional file 1: Note), and their recall across sequencing depth was measured with the adjusted Rand Index [22], a version of the Rand Index corrected for chance [23]. The Rand-Index is a popular statistical measure of the similarity between two data clusterings (corresponding here to groups of mutations, or clones). In addition, clonal trees were also inferred from the somatic SNVs with OncoNEM [24]. Using a similar approach to Ross and Markowetz [24], the pairwise cell shortest-path distance was used to measure the consistency in tree reconstruction across the different sequencing depths. Furthermore, maximum-likelihood single-cell phylogenies were estimated from the SNVs using SiFit [25]. In this case, phylogenetic recall across sequencing depth was measured using the standard Robinson-Foulds tree distance [26]. In addition, we also calculated the homoplasy index (HI), a measure of the

amount of homoplasy on a tree, using the phangorn R package [27]. The HI is one minus the ratio between the minimum number of changes required and the actual number observed [28].

Statistical significance for the differences in recall or HI for the experiments described above were assessed using Tukey's HSD test with a family-wise error rate of 0.05 in R. See the Additional file 1: Note for a detailed description.

Results

Genome coverage

Genome coverage (percentage of the reference genome covered by ≥ 1 read) for the single-cell down-sampled datasets decreased non-linearly with lower sequencing depths, in particular when moving from 5× to 1× (Fig. 1).

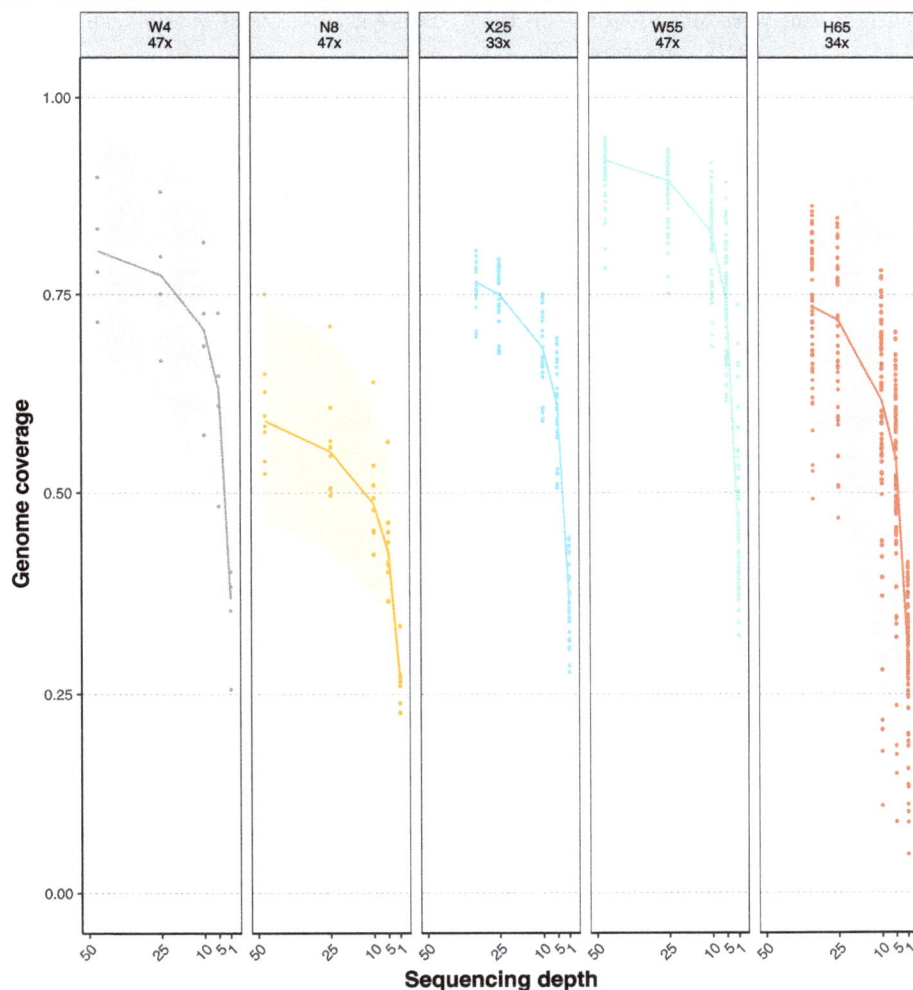

Fig. 1 Genome coverage and sequencing depth in the down-sampled single-cell datasets. Each panel depicts a single-cell dataset (e.g., W4) where the number in the header indicates its original sequencing depth (e.g., 47×). *Solid lines* represent the average genome coverage (proportion of bases covered by at least one read, measured per nucleotide) obtained for the different replicates at the different down-sampled depths. *Dots* correspond to single cells. *Shaded areas* indicate the standard deviation from the mean

Single-nucleotide variants

SNV detection

The observed decline in genome coverage was logically reflected in the proportion of bulk germline and somatic SNVs found in the single-cell down-sampled datasets ("germline and somatic recall"), which decreased significantly (Tukey HSD p value < 0.05) at lower sequencing depths (Fig. 2). The germline recall decrease was much less pronounced when the number of cells was large (≥25). Thus, for the X25, W55, and H65 datasets the germline recall was at 1× as high as 70–80%, and at 5× close to 100% (Fig. 2a). On the other hand, when only four or eight cells were available (W4, N8 datasets), the germline recall at 1× decreased dramatically to 5–13%. The somatic recall rate was, as expected, much more modest than for the germline variants (Fig. 2b). The effect of sequencing depth was significant in practically every case. Notably, the fraction of SNVs found in the down-sampled replicates that were also identified in the original single-cell datasets ("somatic precision"; Fig. 2c) was much less affected by sequencing depth, with many non-significant variations between "contiguous" levels of coverage (i.e., 1–5, 5–10, 10–25×).

Interestingly, a significant amount of somatic variants was detected exclusively in the single-cells (i.e., absent in the bulk), particularly at higher sequencing depths (Additional file 1: Figure S1A). However, the overall variant quality scores for these calls were much lower than for those shared with the bulk dataset (Additional file 1: Figure S1B), suggesting that most might be untrustworthy.

COSMIC and non-synonymous SNV detection

Moreover, the somatic recall specific for COSMIC somatic variants (Fig. 3a, b) decreased very rapidly and significantly (p value < 0.05) with lower sequencing depths for the smallest datasets (W4 and N8), but not as abruptly for the larger ones, in particular for the X25 and W55 datasets. For example, for the latter the recall was already around 70% at only 5×. A statistically significant trend was also observed for non-synonymous SNVs, which were very difficult to detect at 5× or 1× only for the smaller datasets (Fig. 3c, d). For larger sample sizes, the non-synonymous SNV recall rate was already above 70% at 1×.

SNV genotyping

The recall for single-cell SNV genotyping also dropped significantly at lower sequencing depth for all datasets (Fig. 4). Nevertheless, at 5×, 60–90% of the genotypes identified in the original single-cell datasets were already recovered without error. Importantly, discordant SNV genotype calls were relatively infrequent, and differences between depth levels and datasets were usually due to different amounts of missing calls.

Copy-number variants

Single-cell copy-number profiles were remarkably consistent across sequencing depth (Fig. 5). Breakpoint detection was slightly better for higher sequencing depths, but always quite accurate. For example, more than 70% of the CNV breakpoints inferred from the original dataset were already detected at 1× in all datasets. Moreover, CNV genotype calls were not affected by sequencing depth. Indeed, at 1× the CNV genotype recall was already > 99% for all datasets.

Clonal genotypes

Clonal inference recall by SCG [21], as measured by the adjusted Rand Index, was not affected by sequencing depth

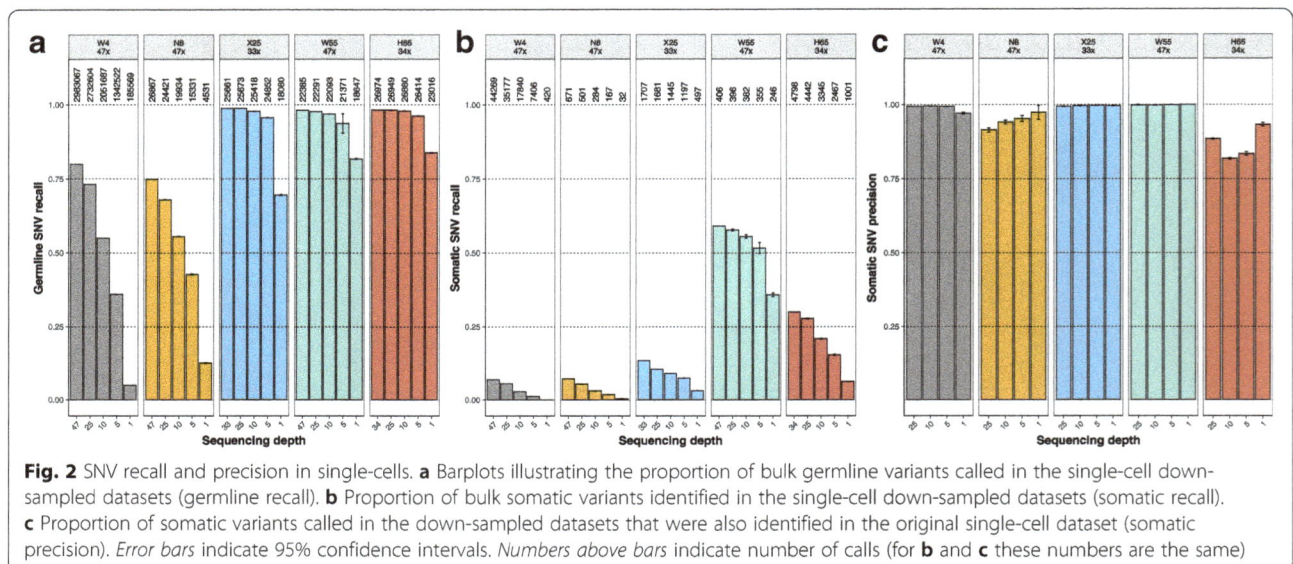

Fig. 2 SNV recall and precision in single-cells. **a** Barplots illustrating the proportion of bulk germline variants called in the single-cell down-sampled datasets (germline recall). **b** Proportion of bulk somatic variants identified in the single-cell down-sampled datasets (somatic recall). **c** Proportion of somatic variants called in the down-sampled datasets that were also identified in the original single-cell dataset (somatic precision). *Error bars* indicate 95% confidence intervals. *Numbers above bars* indicate number of calls (for **b** and **c** these numbers are the same)

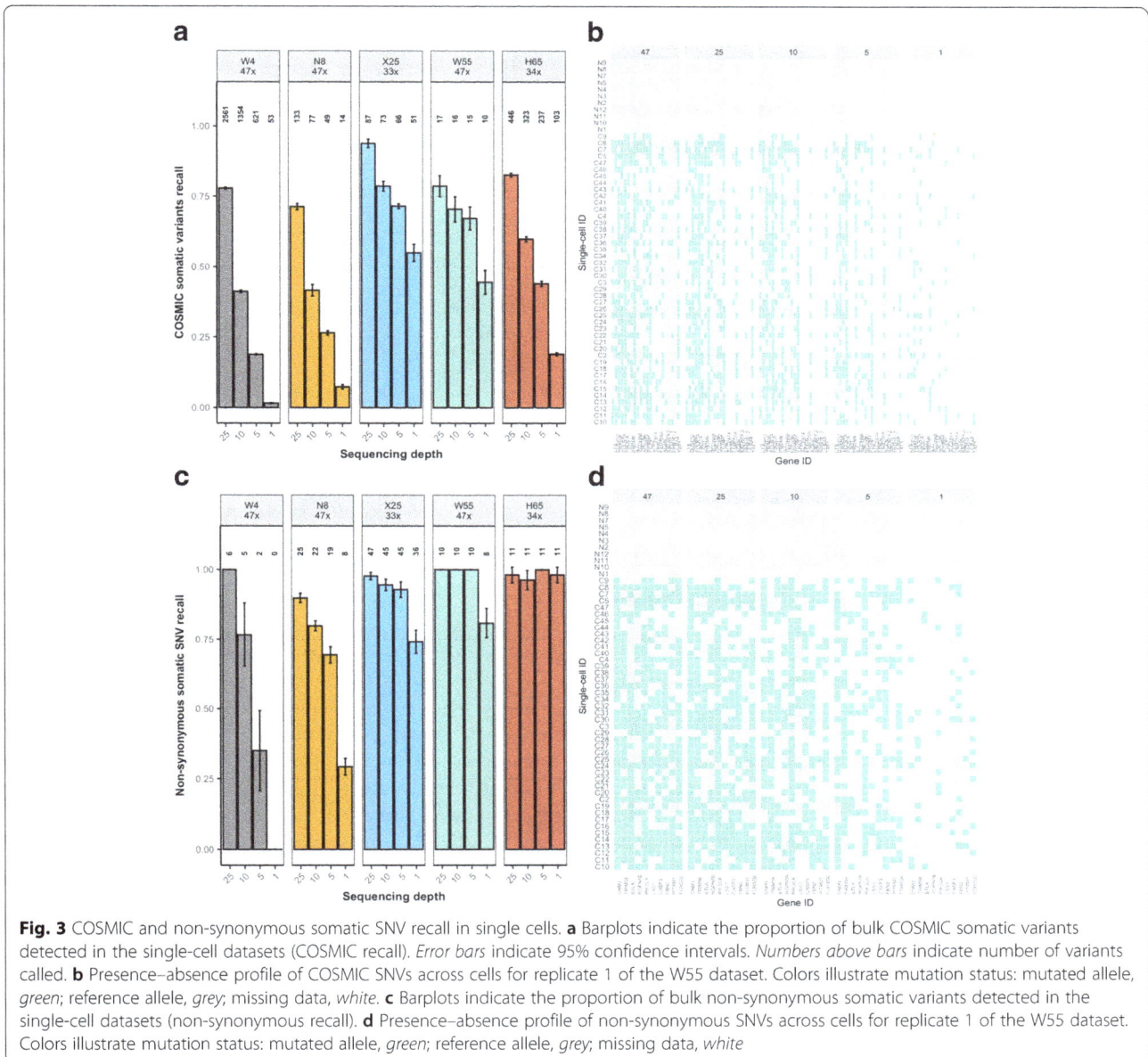

Fig. 3 COSMIC and non-synonymous somatic SNV recall in single cells. **a** Barplots indicate the proportion of bulk COSMIC somatic variants detected in the single-cell datasets (COSMIC recall). *Error bars* indicate 95% confidence intervals. *Numbers above bars* indicate number of variants called. **b** Presence–absence profile of COSMIC SNVs across cells for replicate 1 of the W55 dataset. Colors illustrate mutation status: mutated allele, *green*; reference allele, *grey*; missing data, *white*. **c** Barplots indicate the proportion of bulk non-synonymous somatic variants detected in the single-cell datasets (non-synonymous recall). **d** Presence–absence profile of non-synonymous SNVs across cells for replicate 1 of the W55 dataset. Colors illustrate mutation status: mutated allele, *green*; reference allele, *grey*; missing data, *white*

in the smallest and largest datasets (W4, N8, and H65) where the number of inferred clones was always one (data not shown), but decreased to a different extent at lower depths in the X25 and W55 datasets (Fig. 6a, b). Indeed, despite the improvements observed at sequencing depths beyond 5× for the X25 dataset, the distinct clonal clusters of the W55 dataset were only distinguishable at 25×.

Clonal trees

In contrast to the smallest datasets, the recall of the clonal trees inferred by OncoNEM [24] (Fig. 7a, b) was maintained or decreased slightly—not significantly in multiple occasions—at lower sequencing depths for the

larger datasets (X25, N55, and H65) where the number of potential phylogenetic solutions is much bigger.

Single-cell phylogenies

SiFit [25] single-cell phylogenies were also very stable at sequencing depths equal to or larger than 5× (Fig. 8a, b). In most instances the differences due to depth were not statistically significant. At 1×, in some cases the inferred phylogeny displayed healthy cells intermixed with tumor cells, likely due to poor resolution. Nevertheless, this effect disappeared at 5× and beyond, when all tumor cells always clustered together in a single clade, as expected. Despite the observed stability in tree topology, variants present in all cells in the original single-cell datasets

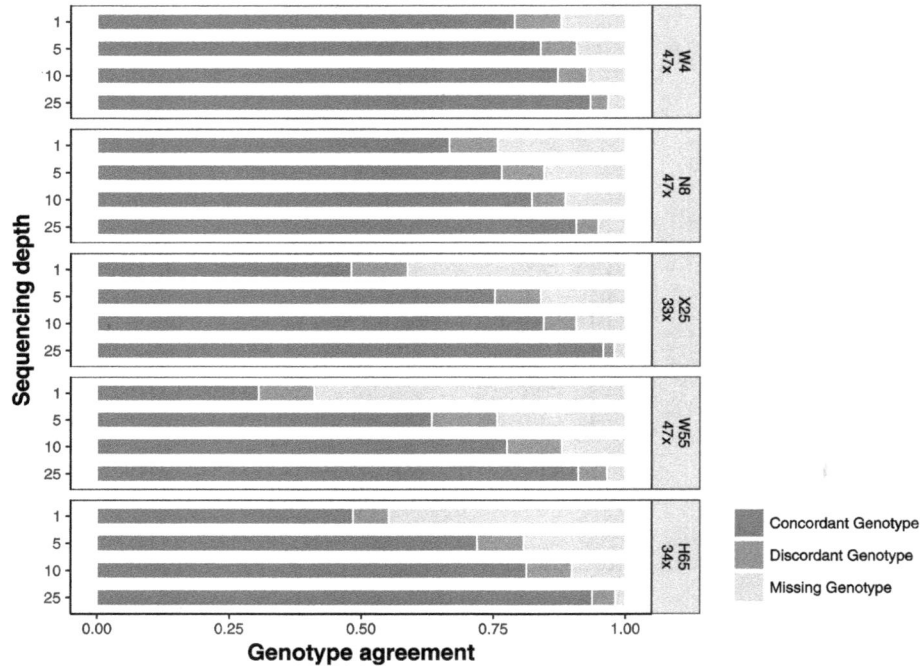

Fig. 4 SNV genotype recall in single cells. *Horizontal bars* represent the proportion of concordant (*dark blue*), discordant (*dark gray*), and missing (*light gray*) SNV genotype calls (homozygous for the reference allele, heterozygous or homozygous for the alternative allele) for the down-sampled datasets

increasingly became subclonal at lower depths (Additional file 1: Figure S2). The amount of homoplasy was, however, generally constant across sequencing depths with the exception of 1×, where for the larger datasets (X25, W55, H65) there was a significant decrease of the HI scores (Additional file 1: Figure S3).

Discussion

In this study we aimed to characterize the impact of sequencing depth in single-cell cancer genomics studies. Undeniably, here we have used five datasets with specific characteristics like number of mutations, number of clones, tissue of origin, genomic target, sequencing depth, or amplification bias. In consequence, although some general patterns seem to be more or less clear, care must be taken in generalizing our findings as particular trends may vary for other cancer datasets.

With this caveat in mind, our downsampling experiments suggest that, overall, larger sequencing depths for small numbers of cells (eight or less) might lead to relevant improvements. In contrast, for relatively large datasets (25 or more cells), our results indicate that sequencing single cells at moderate depths (i.e., 5×) should represent a reasonable approach to characterize the genomic diversity and evolution of tumors, including the identification of putative driver alterations. This is in line with the results of Zhang et al. [9], who showed that for

variant detection it is better to have multiple cells sequenced at low depth, given a fixed sequencing effort.

Unsurprisingly, all recalls (SNVs, CNVs, clones, phylogenies) showed some kind of decrease at smaller sequencing depths. In many cases the drop was statistically significant despite being of small magnitude. Notably, for the larger datasets (and by large here we mean—only—dozens of cells), the impact of sequencing depth was much smaller, with the exception of the H65 dataset. This particular dataset, albeit being the largest, displays a very heterogeneous genome coverage for the single cells sampled which may have mislead some of the analyses. Indeed, genome coverage bias has been shown to contribute to a lower sensitivity to detect variants [9], hence potentially explaining some of the somewhat discordant results of the H65 dataset.

In any case, bulk germline SNVs were relatively easy to identify for the three largest datasets even at low sequencing depth. This was indeed expected since germline variants should be present in the vast majority, if not all, of tumor cells. Nevertheless, when the number of single cells was small, the effect of sequencing depth on germline SNV recall was much more pronounced and reached a limit of ~ 75% at the highest sequencing depth (i.e., 47×) reinforcing the idea that, due to the inherent bias in single-cell genome amplification, broader sampling effort should be favored over increased sequencing depth in variant detection analysis [9].

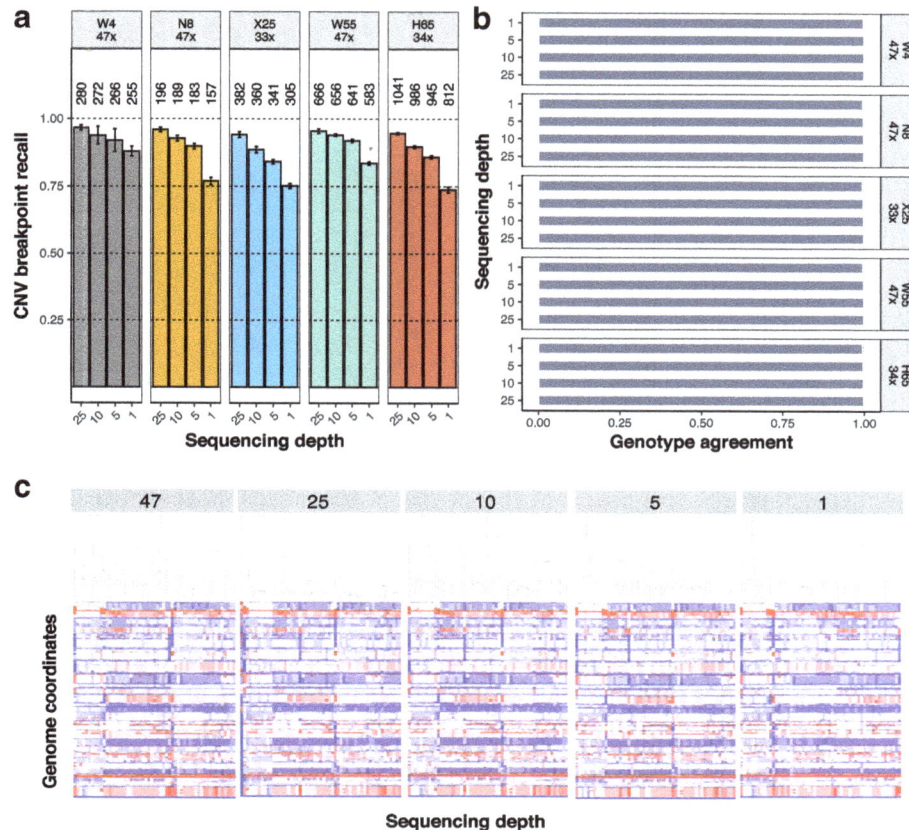

Fig. 5 CNV recall in single cells. **a** Barplots indicate the proportion of CNV breakpoints detected in the down-sampled datasets that were also called in the original single-cell dataset (recall). *Numbers above bars* indicate number of breakpoints detected. *Error bars* indicate 95% confidence intervals. **b** *Horizontal bars* represent the proportion of concordant (*dark blue*), discordant (*dark gray*), and missing (*light gray*) CNV genotype calls. **c** Copy-number profiles at different depths for replicate 1 of the W55 dataset. Distinct colors represent the CN configuration: CN gain, *red*; CN loss, *blue*

While somatic SNVs were much more difficult to detect, it should be highlighted that the number of somatic mutations detected at 5× were usually at the same order of magnitude as the number of mutations detected at higher sequencing depths, except for the smaller datasets. Still, for the smallest dataset analyzed (W4), the high number of somatic SNVs detected at 5× (7406) seem plenty enough to conduct many subsequent analyses, like clonal inference or phylogeny reconstruction.

In relation to this, it is important to highlight that, aside from sample size and sequencing depth, somatic variant detection can additionally be affected by the choice of thresholds during variant calling. Indeed, conservative thresholds may prevent the discovery of true mutations due to excessive filtering, whereas relaxed thresholds may cause an increase of false-positive calls. Determining the best parameters for filtering variants is, therefore, difficult. Most studies analyzing SC-Seq data have relied on "hard" filtering thresholds for a minimum depth of coverage (e.g., > 10 reads; e.g., [5]). Here, a similar filtering strategy would prove too stringent for most down-sampled datasets. To allow proper comparisons among the different depth levels we decided not to use a minimum depth threshold. Instead, we required each variant to be detected in at least two single cells. Such a consensus strategy has already been shown to be quite efficient [9, 18].

Remarkably, the somatic single-cell SNV precision was, in general, very robust to sequencing depth, suggesting that lower depths do not result in new calls that would not have been made at higher depths. Intuitively, this observation makes perfect sense since at lower sequencing depths the variants detected tend to be the clonal ones (i.e., variants shared by the majority of the single cells sampled) whereas the detection of low-frequency mutations required higher read depths (data not shown).

One might be worried, however, about missing putative driver mutations, but our results suggest that, as far as the number of single cells is reasonably large (here 25 or more), most COSMIC somatic variants can be detected at modest sequencing depths (here 5× or more).

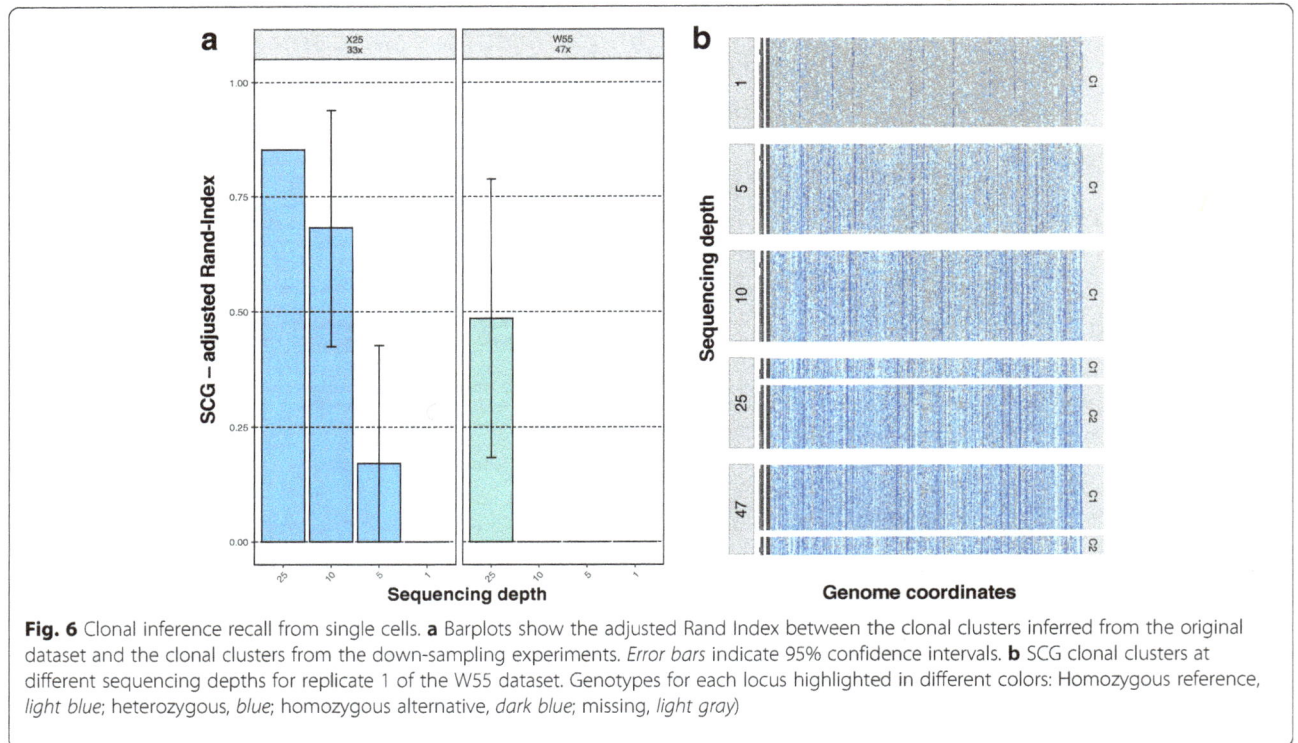

Fig. 6 Clonal inference recall from single cells. **a** Barplots show the adjusted Rand Index between the clonal clusters inferred from the original dataset and the clonal clusters from the down-sampling experiments. *Error bars* indicate 95% confidence intervals. **b** SCG clonal clusters at different sequencing depths for replicate 1 of the W55 dataset. Genotypes for each locus highlighted in different colors: Homozygous reference, *light blue*; heterozygous, *blue*; homozygous alternative, *dark blue*; missing, *light gray*)

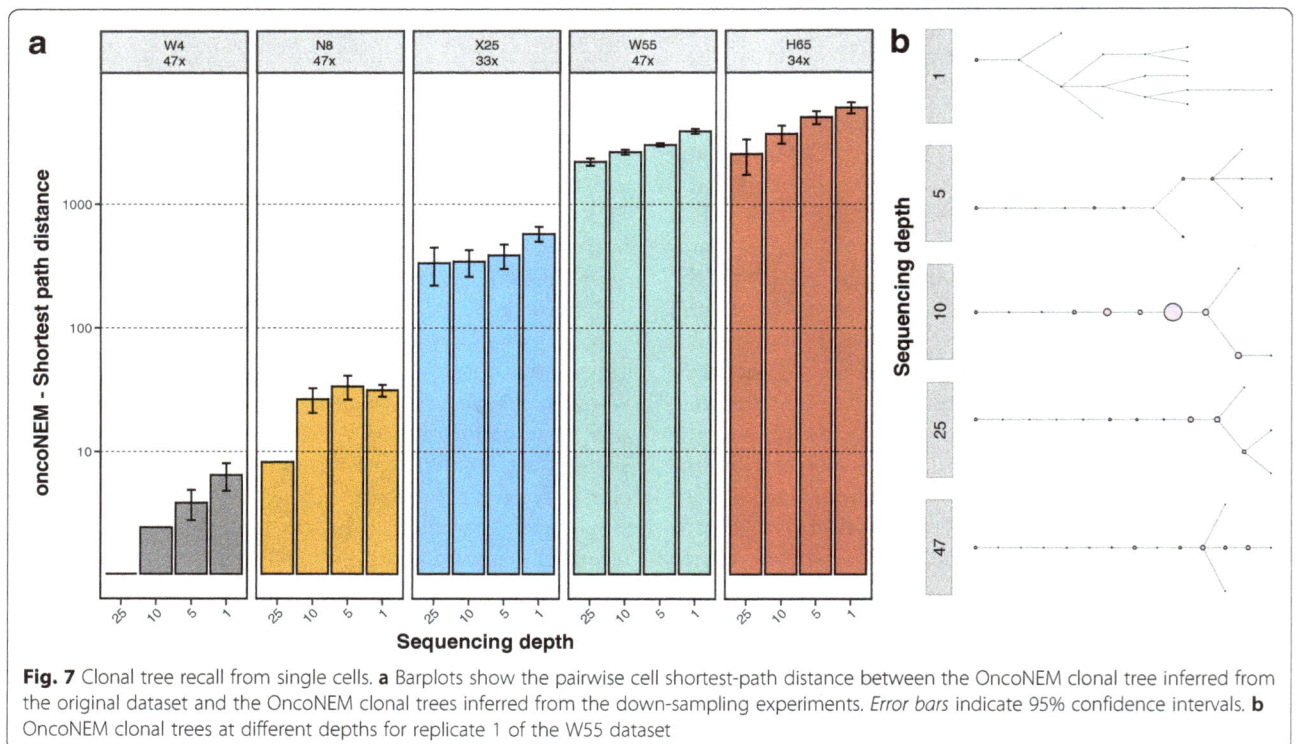

Fig. 7 Clonal tree recall from single cells. **a** Barplots show the pairwise cell shortest-path distance between the OncoNEM clonal tree inferred from the original dataset and the OncoNEM clonal trees inferred from the down-sampling experiments. *Error bars* indicate 95% confidence intervals. **b** OncoNEM clonal trees at different depths for replicate 1 of the W55 dataset

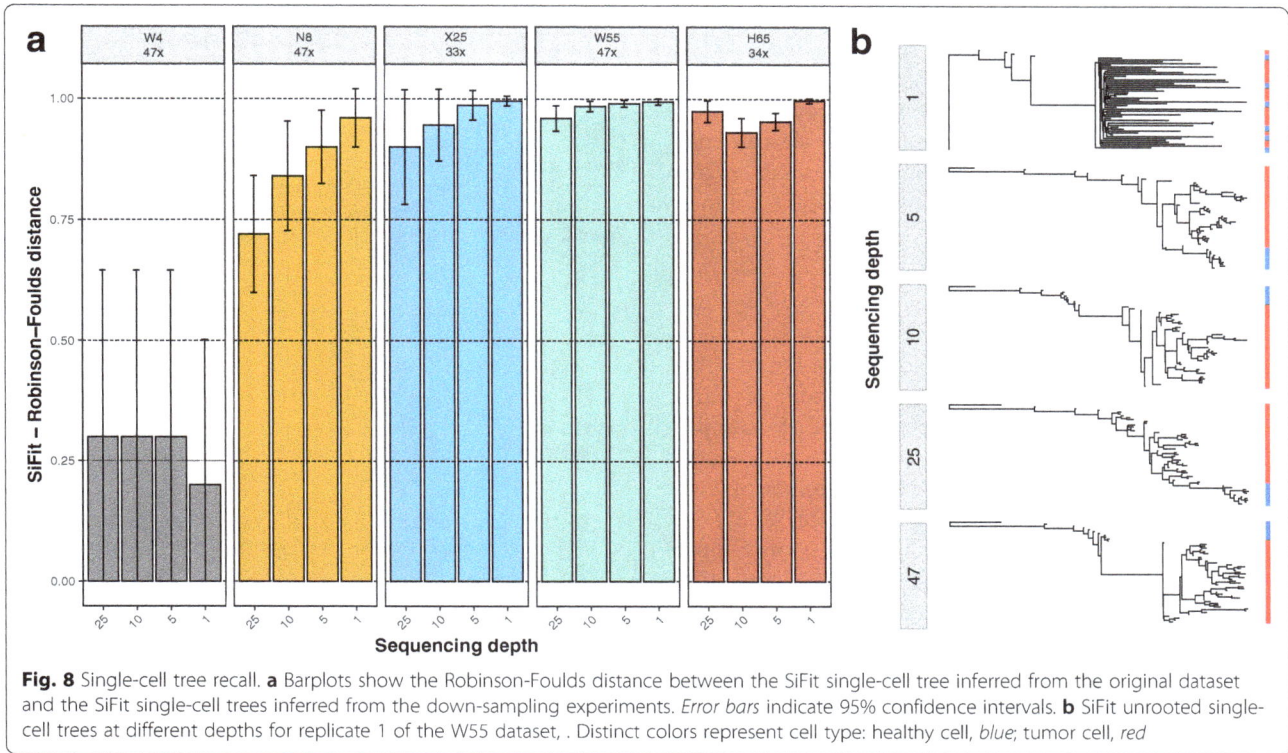

Fig. 8 Single-cell tree recall. **a** Barplots show the Robinson-Foulds distance between the SiFit single-cell tree inferred from the original dataset and the SiFit single-cell trees inferred from the down-sampling experiments. *Error bars* indicate 95% confidence intervals. **b** SiFit unrooted single-cell trees at different depths for replicate 1 of the W55 dataset, . Distinct colors represent cell type: healthy cell, *blue*; tumor cell, *red*

Similar results were also observed for the somatic non-synonymous variants, suggesting that, in principle, many relevant variants in single-cell genomes are likely to be detected at modest sequencing depths.

Obviously, assigning particular genotypes to the individual cells is a much more involved task than just detecting variants. Importantly, for SNV genotyping, reducing sequencing depth generally resulted in an increased amount of missing data in the single-cell genotype matrix, rather than different genotype calls.

Moreover, and in agreement with previous studies [20, 29], CNV characterization from single cells was also very robust to sequencing depth, with all down-sampled datasets showing remarkable preservation of CNV breakpoints. Furthermore, CNV genotype assignment was insensitive to the variation in the sequencing depths explored. In general, the copy-number analysis of single-cell libraries can be confounded by amplification bias. However, previous studies suggest that amplification biases are randomly distributed and sufficiently separated throughout the genome [30] as to not affect CNV calling at the level of resolution chosen here (500-kb bins). Popular single-cell amplification methods like multiple displacement amplification (MDA) and multiple annealing and looping-based amplification cycles (MALBAC) usually generate amplicons of around 10–100 kb and 1–5 kb, respectively; therefore, we do not expect many false positive CNV calls [31]. Yet, we acknowledge that

our choice of bin size may have prevented the identification of small CNVs [20].

It is relatively well established that an accurate identification of clonal genotypes can be very important to understand tumor dynamics and genomic architecture [32–34]. For the datasets analyzed here, our results suggest that SC-Seq depth does not affect the identification of tumor clones when the genomic variability between malignant cells is small (i.e., displaying limited clonal population genetic diversification). However, the same was not true for tumors comprising a larger number of subclones, where the different clonal genotypes were only distinguishable at higher sequencing depths. While these results are not necessarily surprising, as clonal identification remains a complex problem even for bulk sequencing data [35, 36], they seem to suggest that higher sequencing coverage is ultimately required to resolve fine-scale clonal structure in more heterogeneous tumors.

Finally, in our evolutionary analyses, we observed a moderate impact of sequencing depth with respect to the estimated phylogenetic relationships of the inferred clones and single cells. Perhaps due to the uncertainty stemming from significant amounts of missing data, datasets down-sampled to 1× resulted in phylogenetic trees with healthy cells intermingled with tumor cells, which can be safely considered as artifacts. While the amount of homoplasy was lower at 1×, this was likely an effect of the smaller amount of variant calls per cell at such a low depth. Otherwise, tree topologies at 5× seemed quite similar to those inferred at higher depths, suggesting that relatively few clonal variants might be enough to resolve the topology of the single-cell trees. Note that the topology does not include branch lengths, whose accurate estimation might require higher sequencing depths.

Conclusions

Single-cell DNA sequencing is expected to be key to obtain accurate inferences of the clonal architecture of tumor samples, which shall ultimately prove crucial to compare models of cancer evolution, trace cell lineages, measure mutation rates, and decipher cell clones responsible for metastatic dissemination and drug resistance [2, 37, 38]. While recent experimental and analytical improvements have improved the quality of single-cell DNA sequencing data [9, 18, 20, 21, 25, 39–41], the costs associated with sequencing multiple single-cell genomes or exomes at high depths are still largely prohibitive. Our results support the idea that sequencing multiple individual tumor cells at a modest depth, such as 5×, may help circumvent this limitation at least for the type of analyses implemented here. Finally, the results obtained here might be extrapolatable to some extent to non-tumor single-cell genomes.

Abbreviations

CNV: Copy-number variant; COSMIC: Catalogue of somatic mutations in cancer; GATK: Genome analysis toolkit; HI: Homoplasy index; ITH: Intratumor genomic heterogeneity; MALBAC: Multiple annealing and looping-based amplification cycles; MDA: Multiple displacement amplification; NGS: Next-generation sequencing; SC-Seq: Single-cell sequencing; SNV: Single-nucleotide variant; WGA: Whole-genome amplification; WGS: Whole-genome sequencing; WXS: Whole-exome sequencing

Acknowledgements

We would like to thank Sereina Rutschmann, Harald Detering, Laura Tomás, and Sara Rocha for their comments on earlier versions of the manuscript. We also thank the anonymous reviewers for their useful suggestions.

Funding

This work was supported by the European Research Council (ERC-617457-PHYLOCANCER awarded to D.P.) and by the Ministry of Economy and Competitiveness—MINECO (BFU2015-63774-P awarded to D.P.) D.P. receives further support from the Galician government.

Authors' contributions

DP conceived the project. DP designed and JMA performed the analyses. JMA and DP wrote the manuscript. Both authors read and approved the final manuscript.

Competing interests

The authors declare that they have no competing interests.

Author details

[1]Department of Biochemistry, Genetics and Immunology, University of Vigo, Vigo, Spain. [2]Biomedical Research Center (CINBIO), University of Vigo, Vigo, Spain. [3]Galicia Sur Health Research Institute, Vigo, Spain.

References

1. Gerlinger M, Swanton C. How Darwinian models inform therapeutic failure initiated by clonal heterogeneity in cancer medicine. Br J Cancer. 2010;103: 1139–43.
2. Navin NE. Cancer genomics: one cell at a time. Genome Biol. 2014;15:452.
3. Potter NE, Ermini L, Papaemmanuil E, Cazzaniga G, Vijayaraghavan G, Titley I, et al. Single-cell mutational profiling and clonal phylogeny in cancer. Genome Res. 2013;23:2115–25.
4. Hughes AEO, Magrini V, Demeter R, Miller CA, Fulton R, Fulton LL, et al. Clonal architecture of secondary acute myeloid leukemia defined by single-cell sequencing. PLoS Genet. 2014;10:e1004462.
5. Wang Y, Waters J, Leung ML, Unruh A, Roh W, Shi X, et al. Clonal evolution in breast cancer revealed by single nucleus genome sequencing. Nature. 2014;512:155–60.
6. Lawson DA, Bhakta NR, Kessenbrock K, Prummel KD, Yu Y, Takai K, et al. Single-cell analysis reveals a stem-cell program in human metastatic breast cancer cells. Nature. 2015;526:131–5.
7. Van Loo P, Voet T. Single cell analysis of cancer genomes. Curr Opin Genet Dev. 2014;24:82–91.
8. Wang Y, Navin NE. Advances and applications of single-cell sequencing technologies. Mol Cell. 2015;58:598–609.
9. Zhang C-Z, Adalsteinsson VA, Francis J, Cornils H, Jung J, Maire C, et al. Calibrating genomic and allelic coverage bias in single-cell sequencing. Nat Commun. 2015;6:6822.
10. Ni X, Zhuo M, Su Z, Duan J, Gao Y, Wang Z, et al. Reproducible copy number variation patterns among single circulating tumor cells of lung cancer patients. Proc Natl Acad Sci U S A. 2013;110:21083–8.
11. Xu X, Hou Y, Yin X, Bao L, Tang A, Song L, et al. Single-cell exome sequencing reveals single-nucleotide mutation characteristics of a kidney tumor. Cell. 2012;148:886–95.
12. Hou Y, Song L, Zhu P, Zhang B, Tao Y, Xu X, et al. Single-cell exome sequencing and monoclonal evolution of a JAK2-negative myeloproliferative neoplasm. Cell. 2012;148:873–85.
13. Li H. Aligning sequence reads, clone sequences and assembly contigs with BWA-MEM. arXiv. 2013;1303:3997v1.
14. Van der Auwera GA, Carneiro MO, Hartl C, Poplin R, Del Angel G, Levy-Moonshine A, et al. From FastQ data to high confidence variant calls: the Genome Analysis Toolkit best practices pipeline. Curr Protoc Bioinformatics. 2013;43:11.10.1–33.
15. Lai Z, Markovets A, Ahdesmaki M, Chapman B, Hofmann O, McEwen R, et al. VarDict: a novel and versatile variant caller for next-generation sequencing in cancer research. Nucleic Acids Res. 2016;44:e108.
16. McKenna A, Hanna M, Banks E, Sivachenko A, Cibulskis K, Kernytsky A, et al. The Genome Analysis Toolkit: a MapReduce framework for analyzing next-generation DNA sequencing data. Genome Res. 2010;20:1297–303.
17. Picard software. http://broadinstitute.github.io/picard.Accessed 12 Apr 2018.
18. Zafar H, Wang Y, Nakhleh L, Navin N, Chen K. Monovar: single-nucleotide variant detection in single cells. Nat Methods. 2016;13:505–7.
19. Forbes SA, Beare D, Boutselakis H, Bamford S, Bindal N, Tate J, et al. COSMIC: somatic cancer genetics at high-resolution. Nucleic Acids Res. 2017;45: D777–D83.
20. Garvin T, Aboukhalil R, Kendall J, Baslan T, Atwal GS, Hicks J, et al. Interactive analysis and assessment of single-cell copy-number variations. Nat Methods. 2015;12:1058–60.

21. Roth A, McPherson A, Laks E, Biele J, Yap D, Wan A, et al. Clonal genotype and population structure inference from single-cell tumor sequencing. Nat Methods. 2016;13:573–6.
22. Hubert L, Arabie P. Comparing partitions. J Classification. 1985;2:193–218.
23. Rand WM. Objective criteria for the evaluation of clustering methods. J Am Stat Assoc. 1971;66:846.
24. Ross EM, Markowetz F. OncoNEM: inferring tumor evolution from single-cell sequencing data. Genome Biol. 2016;17:69.
25. Zafar H, Tzen A, Navin N, Chen K, Nakhleh L. SiFit: inferring tumor trees from single-cell sequencing data under finite-sites models. Genome Biol. 2017;18:178.
26. Robinson DF, Foulds LR. Comparison of phylogenetic trees. Math Biosci. 1981;53:131–47.
27. Schliep KP. phangorn: phylogenetic analysis in R. Bioinformatics. 2010;27: 592–3.
28. Kluge AG, Farris JS. Quantitative phyletics and the evolution of anurans. Syst Zool. 1969;18:1.
29. Zahn H, Steif A, Laks E, Eirew P, VanInsberghe M, Shah SP, et al. Scalable whole-genome single-cell library preparation without preamplification. Nat Methods. 2017;14:167–73.
30. Navin N, Kendall J, Troge J, Andrews P, Rodgers L, McIndoo J, et al. Tumour evolution inferred by single-cell sequencing. Nature. 2011;472:90–4.
31. Sherman MA, Barton AR, Lodato MA, Vitzthum C, Coulter ME, Walsh CA, et al. PaSD-qc: quality control for single cell whole-genome sequencing data using power spectral density estimation. Nucleic Acids Res. 2017; https://doi.org/10.1093/nar/gkx1195.
32. Alves JM, Prieto T, Posada D. Multiregional tumor trees are not phylogenies. Trends Cancer Res. 2017;3:546–50.
33. Kuipers J, Jahn K, Beerenwinkel N. Advances in understanding tumour evolution through single-cell sequencing. Biochim Biophys Acta. 1867;2017: 127–38.
34. Beerenwinkel N, Schwarz RF, Gerstung M, Markowetz F. Cancer evolution: mathematical models and computational inference. Syst Biol. 2015;64:e1–25.
35. Turajlic S, McGranahan N, Swanton C. Inferring mutational timing and reconstructing tumour evolutionary histories. Biochim Biophys Acta. 1855; 2015:264–75.
36. Beerenwinkel N, Greenman CD, Lagergren J. Computational cancer biology: an evolutionary perspective. PLoS Comput Biol. 2016;12:e1004717.
37. Tsoucas D, Yuan G-C. Recent progress in single-cell cancer genomics. Curr Opin Genet Dev. 2017;42:22–32.
38. Casasent AK, Schalck A, Gao R, Sei E, Long A, Pangburn W, et al. Multiclonal invasion in breast tumors identified by topographic single cell sequencing. Cell. 2018;172:205–17. e12
39. Chen C, Xing D, Tan L, Li H, Zhou G, Huang L, et al. Single-cell whole-genome analyses by Linear Amplification via Transposon Insertion (LIANTI). Science. 2017;356:189–94.
40. Borgström E, Paterlini M, Mold JE, Frisen J, Lundeberg J. Comparison of whole genome amplification techniques for human single cell exome sequencing. PLoS One. 2017;12:e0171566.
41. Dong X, Zhang L, Milholland B, Lee M, Maslov AY, Wang T, et al. Accurate identification of single-nucleotide variants in whole-genome-amplified single cells. Nat Methods. 2017;14:491–3.

4

Genetic variants associated with Alzheimer's disease confer different cerebral cortex cell-type population structure

Zeran Li[1], Jorge L. Del-Aguila[1], Umber Dube[1,2], John Budde[1], Rita Martinez[1], Kathleen Black[1], Qingli Xiao[3], Nigel J. Cairns[3,4,5], The Dominantly Inherited Alzheimer Network (DIAN), Joseph D. Dougherty[1,7], Jin-Moo Lee[3], John C. Morris[3,5,6], Randall J. Bateman[3,5,6], Celeste M. Karch[1], Carlos Cruchaga[1,5,6*] and Oscar Harari[1*]

Abstract

Background: Alzheimer's disease (AD) is characterized by neuronal loss and astrocytosis in the cerebral cortex. However, the specific effects that pathological mutations and coding variants associated with AD have on the cellular composition of the brain are often ignored.

Methods: We developed and optimized a cell-type-specific expression reference panel and employed digital deconvolution methods to determine brain cellular distribution in three independent transcriptomic studies.

Results: We found that neuronal and astrocyte relative proportions differ between healthy and diseased brains and also among AD cases that carry specific genetic risk variants. Brain carriers of pathogenic mutations in APP, PSEN1, or PSEN2 presented lower neuron and higher astrocyte relative proportions compared to sporadic AD. Similarly, the APOE ε4 allele also showed decreased neuronal and increased astrocyte relative proportions compared to AD non-carriers. In contrast, carriers of variants in TREM2 risk showed a lower degree of neuronal loss compared to matched AD cases in multiple independent studies.

Conclusions: These findings suggest that genetic risk factors associated with AD etiology have a specific imprinting in the cellular composition of AD brains. Our digital deconvolution reference panel provides an enhanced understanding of the fundamental molecular mechanisms underlying neurodegeneration, enabling the analysis of large bulk RNA-sequencing studies for cell composition and suggests that correcting for the cellular structure when performing transcriptomic analysis will lead to novel insights of AD.

Keywords: Digital deconvolution, Alzheimer's disease, Brain cellular composition, Bulk RNA-sequencing, Autosomal dominant AD, TREM2

Background

Alzheimer's disease (AD) is a neurodegenerative disorder characterized clinically by gradual and progressive memory loss and pathologically by the presence of senile plaques (Aβ deposits) and neurofibrillary tangles (NFTs, Tau deposits) in the brain [1]. AD has a substantial but heterogeneous genetic component. Mutations in the amyloid-beta

* Correspondence: ccruchaga@wustl.edu; harario@wustl.edu
[1]Department of Psychiatry, Washington University School of Medicine, 660 S. Euclid Ave. B8134, St. Louis, MO 63110, USA
Full list of author information is available at the end of the article

precursor protein (APP) and Presenilin genes (PSEN1 and PSEN2) [2, 3] cause autosomal dominant AD (ADAD) which is typically associated with early-onset (< 65 years). In contrast, the most common manifestation of AD presents late-onset (LOAD) and accounts for the majority of the cases (90–95%). Despite appearing sporadic in nature, a complex genetic architecture underlies LOAD risk. APOE ε4 is the most common genetic risk factor, increasing the risk in three- to eightfold [4]. In addition, recent whole genome and whole exome analyses have identified rare coding variants in TREM2 [5, 6], PLD3 [7],

ABCA7 [8, 9], and SORL1 [10, 11] that are associated with AD and confer risk comparable to that of carrying one APOE ε4 allele. Besides age at onset, the clinical presentations of LOAD and ADAD are remarkably similar with an amnestic and cognitive impairment phenotype [12, 13]. A minor fraction of cases of ADAD have additional neurological findings, sometimes also seen in LOAD [12, 13].

Altered cellular composition is associated with AD progression and decline in cognition. Neuronal loss in the hippocampus is characteristic in the initial stages of AD, which could explain early memory disturbances [14, 15]. As the disease progresses, neuronal death is observed throughout the cerebral cortex. Furthermore, ~ 25% of cognitively normal individuals who die by the age of ~ 75 years also presented substantial cerebral lesions that resemble AD pathology, including amyloid plaque, NFTs, and neuronal loss [16]. Thus, the identification of the brain cellular population structure is essential for understanding neurodegenerative disease progression [17]. However, stereology protocols for counting neurons can be tedious, require extensive training, and are susceptible to technical artifacts which may lead to biased quantification of cell-type distributions [17].

Recently there has been a growing interest in understanding the transcriptomic changes attributed to AD [18–25], as these may point to underlying molecular mechanisms of disease. These studies are typically designed to analyze the expression profiles of large cohorts ascertained from homogenized regions of the brain (e.g. bulk RNA-sequencing [RNA-seq]) of affected and control donors. However, as bulk RNA-seq captures the gene expression of all the constituent cells in the sampled tissue; the altered cellular composition associated with AD has been reported to confound downstream analyses [20].

Digital deconvolution approaches enhance the interrogation of expression profiles to identify the cellular population structure of individual samples, alleviating the requirement of additional neurostereology procedures. These approaches have been developed, tested, and applied to ascertain cellular composition altered in many traits [26–29]. However, digital deconvolution has not been applied to identify the cellular population structure from RNA-seq from human brain of AD cases and controls. Technical constraints restrict the dissociation of cells from the brains for very specific conditions [30–32]. Nevertheless, a limited number of RNA-seq from isolated cell populations from the brain have been generated [30–32]. Using these resources, we are now able to generate a reference panel for digital deconvolution of human brain bulk RNA-seq data.

We sought to investigate the cellular population structure in AD by analyzing RNA-seq from multiple brain regions of LOAD participants. To do so, we assembled a novel brain reference panel and evaluated the accuracy of digital deconvolution methods by analyzing additional cell-type-specific RNA-seq samples and by creating synthetic admixtures with defined cellular distributions. Then we analyzed large cohorts of pathologically confirmed AD cases and controls (n = 613) and verified that our model predicts cellular distribution patterns consistent with neurodegeneration. Finally, we generated RNA-seq from the parietal lobe of participants from the Charles F. and Joanne Knight Alzheimer's Disease Research Center (Knight-ADRC) [33], including non-demented controls, LOAD cases, with enriched proportions of carriers of high-risk coding variants associated with AD, and also ADAD from The Dominantly Inherited Alzheimer Network [34] (DIAN). We compared the cell composition in ADAD and LOAD; and also evaluated differences among carriers of coding high-risk variants in PLD3, TREM2, and APOE ε4. Our findings indicate that cell-type composition differs among carriers of specific genetic risk factors, which might be revealing distinct pathogenic mechanisms contributing to disease etiology.

Methods
Subjects and samples
DIAN and Knight-ADRC
Parietal lobe tissue of post-mortem brain was obtained with informed consent for research use and was approved by the review board of Washington University in St. Louis. RNA was extracted from frozen brain using Tissue Lyser LT and RNeasy Mini Kit (Qiagen, Hilden, Germany). RNA-seq paired-end reads with read lengths of 2 × 150 bp were generated using Illumina HiSeq 4000 with a mean coverage of 80 million reads per sample (Table 1; Additional file 1: Table S1). RNA-seq was generated for 19 brains from DIAN, 84 brains with LOAD and 16 non-demented controls from Knight-ADRC [33]. The AD brains selected from Knight-ADRC are enriched for carrier of variants in TREM2 (n = 20; Additional file 1: Table S1) and PLD3 (n = 33; Additional file 1: Table S1). The clinical status of participants was neuropathologically confirmed [35]. We identified three additional participants from the Knight-ADRC study with PSEN1 (A79V, I143T, S170F) mutations. Clinical Dementia Rating (CDR) scores were obtained during regular visits throughout the study before the subject's decease [36]. A range of other pathological measurements were collected during autopsy including Braak staging, as previously described [37].

RNA was extracted from frozen brain tissues using Tissue Lyser LT and RNeasy Mini Kit (Qiagen, Hilden, Germany) following the manufacturer's instruction. RIN (RNA integrity) and DV200 were measured with RNA 6000 Pico Assay using Bioanalyzer 2100 (Agilent

Table 1 Demographics and disease status of cohorts from four brain bank resources

	Mayo	MSBB	DIAN	Knight-ADRC
Sample size	191	300	19	103
Age (years)	83 ± 7.77	83.3 ± 7.55	50.6 ± 7.06	85.1 ± 9.78
Male (%)	45.5	36	68.4	38.8
APOE ε4+ (%)	33.2	31.7	14.3	45.6
Brain weight	–	–	1187.7 ± 184.5	1138.1 ± 142.5
AD	82	135	19	87
PA	29	0	0	0
Control	80	85	0	16
CDR = 0	–	40	0	13
CDR = 0.5	–	40	0	9
CDR = 1	–	30	2	11
CDR = 2	–	44	4	14
CDR = 3	–	146	1	56

Mayo Mayo Clinic, *MSBB* Mount Sinai Brain Bank, *AD* Alzheimer's disease, *PA* pathological aging, *CDR* Clinical Dementia Rating for available samples

Technologies). The RIN is determined by the software on the Bioanalyzer taking into account the entire electrophoretic trace of the RNA including the presence or absence of degradation products. The DV200 value is defined as the percentage of nucleotides > 200 nt. RIN and DV200 for all the samples can be found on Additional file 1: Table S1. The yield of each sample is determined by the Quant-iT RNA Assay (Life Technologies) on the Qubit Fluorometer (Fisher Scientific). The complementary DNA (cDNA) library was prepared with the TruSeq Stranded Total RNA Sample Prep with Ribo-Zero Gold kit (Illumina) and then sequenced by HiSeq 4000 (Illumina) using 2 × 150 paired-end reads at McDonnell Genome Institute, Washington University in St. Louis with a mean of 58.14 ± 8.62 million reads. Number of reads and other quality control (QC) metrics can be found in Additional file 1: Table S1.

Mayo Clinic Brain Bank

Mayo Clinic Brain Bank RNA-seq was accessed from the Advanced Medicines Partnership – Alzheimer's Disease (AMP-AD) portal (synapse ID = 5,550,404; accessed January 2017) (Table 1). Paired end reads of 2 × 101 base pairs were generated by Illumina HiSeq 2000 sequencers for an average of 134.9 million reads per sample. Neuropathology criteria, quality control procedures, RNA extraction, and sequencing details are explained elsewhere [18].

RNA-seq based transcriptome data were generated from post-mortem brain tissue collected from cerebellum (CB; 189 samples) and temporal cortex (TC; 191 samples) of Caucasian subjects [18, 38]. RNA was extracted using Trizol® reagent and cleaned with Qiagen

RNeasy. RIN measurement was performed with Agilent Technologies 2100 Bioanalyzer. Samples with RIN > 5 were included. Library was prepared by Mayo Clinic Medical Genome Facility Gene Expression and Sequencing Cores with TruSeq RNA Sample Prep Kit (Illumina).

Mount Sinai Brain Bank

The Mount Sinai Brain Bank (MSBB) RNA-seq study was downloaded from the AMP-AD portal (synapse ID = 3,157,743; accessed January 2017) (Table 1). Single-end reads of 100 nt were generated by Illumina HiSeq 2500 System (Illumina, San Diego, CA, USA) for an average of 38.7 million reads per sample [39].

This dataset contains 1030 samples collected from four post-mortem brain regions of 300 subjects: anterior prefrontal cortex (APC; BA10); superior temporal gyrus (STG; BA22); parahippocampal gyrus (PHG; BA36); and inferior frontal gyrus (IFG; BA44). RNA-seq was generated using the TruSeq RNA Sample Preparation Kit v2 and Ribo-Zero rRNA removal kit (Illumina, San Diego, CA, USA) [39].

Induced pluripotent stem cell (iPSC)-derived neurons

Dermal fibroblasts were obtained from skin biopsies from research participants in the Knight-ADRC (Fibroblast lines: F11362, F12455, and F13504). Human fibroblasts were reprogrammed into iPSCs using non-integrating Sendai virus carrying OCT3/4, SOX2, KLF4, and cMYC [40, 41]. iPSCs were manually selected and expanded on Matrigel in mTesR1 (StemCell Techologies). iPSCs were characterized for expression of pluripotency markers by immunocytochemistry and quantitative polymerase chain reaction (qPCR). qPCR with probes specific to the Sendai virus were used to confirm the absence of virus in the isolated clones. All cell lines were confirmed to have a normal karyotype based on G-band karyotyping. To generate cortical neurons, iPSCs were plated in a v-bottom plate in neural induction media (StemCell Technologies; 65,000 per well) to form highly uniform neural aggregates. After five days, neural aggregates were transferred onto PLO/laminin-coated tissue culture plates. Neural rosettes formed over 5–7 days. The resulting neural rosettes were then isolated by enzymatic selection (StemCell Technologies) and cultured as neural progenitor cells (NPCs). NPCs were then differentiated by culturing in neural maturation medium (neurobasal medium supplemented with B27, GDNF, BDNF, cAMP). RNA was collected from the cells and sequenced following the same protocol and processing pipeline as the DIAN and Knight-ADRC dataset.

In addition, we accessed RNA-seq data generated for iPSC-derived neurons from the Broad iPSC study [42] (synapse ID: syn3607401). Forebrain neurons from wild-type background were generated using an embryoid body-based protocol to produce neural progenitor cells (day 17) and mature neurons (days 57 and 100). RNA was purified using a PureLink RNA mini-kit (Life Technologies). RNA-seq libraries were prepared using Illumina Strand Specific TruSeq protocol and sequenced to obtain an average of 75 M reads in paired reads per sample.

Translating ribosome affinity purification (TRAP)-seq mice

All animal procedures were performed in accordance with the guidelines of Washington University's Institutional Animal Care and Use Committee. The Rosa26^{fsTRAP} mice (Gt(ROSA)26Sor$^{tm1(CAG-EGFP/Rpl10a,-birA)Wtp}$) [43] (The Jackson Laboratory) were crossed with PV^{Cre} mice (Pvalb$^{tm1(cre)Arbr}$) [44] (The Jackson Laboratory) to produce PV-TRAP mice directing expression of EGFP-L10a ribosomal fusion protein in parvalbumin (PV) expressing cells.

Purification of cell-type-specific messenger RNA (mRNA) by TRAP was described previously [45] with modifications. Briefly, PV-TRAP mouse brain was removed and quickly washed in ice-cold dissection buffer (1× HBSS, 2.5 mM HEPES-KOH (pH 7.3), 35 mM glucose, and 4 mM NaHCO$_3$ in RNase-free water). Barrel cortex was rapidly dissected and flash-frozen in liquid nitrogen, and then stored at − 80 °C until use. Affinity matrix was prepared with 150 µL of Streptavidin MyOne T1 Dynabeads, 60 µg of Biotinylated Protein L, and 25 µg of each of GFP antibodies 19C8 and 19F7. The tissue was homogenized on ice in 1 mL of tissue-lysis buffer (20 mM HEPES KOH (pH 7.4), 150 mM KCl, 10 mM MgCl$_2$, EDTA-free protease inhibitors, 0.5 mM DTT, 100 µg/mL cycloheximide, and 10 µL/mL rRNasin and Superasin). Homogenates were centrifuged for 10 min at 2000×g, 4 °C, and 1/9 sample volume of 10% NP-40 and 300 mM DHPC were added to the supernatant at final concentration of 1% (vol/vol). After incubation on ice for 5 min, the lysate was centrifuged for 10 min at 20,000×g to pellet insolubilized material. Then 200 µL of freshly resuspended affinity matrix was added to the supernatant and incubated at 4 °C for 16–18 h with gentle end-over-end mixing in a tube rotator. After incubation, the beads were collected with a magnet and resuspended in 1000 µL of high-salt buffer (20 mM HEPES KOH (pH 7.3), 350 mM KCl, 10 mM MgCl$_2$, 1% NP-40, 0.5 mM DTT, and 100 µg/mL cycloheximide) and collected with magnets as above. After four times of washing with high-salt buffer, RNA was extracted using Absolutely RNA Nanoprep Kit (Agilent Technologies) following the manufacturer's instructions. RNA quantification was measured using Qubit RNA HS Assay Kit (Life Technologies) and the integrity was determined by Bioanalyzer 2100 using an RNA Pico chip (Agilent Technologies). The cDNA library was prepared with Clontech SMARTer and then sequenced by HiSeq3000. Single-end reads of 50 base pairs were generated for an average of 29.2 million reads per sample (24 samples).

iPSC-derived microglia

The data were accessed from the AMP-AD portal (synapse ID: syn7203233). This dataset comprises iPSC-derived microglia (n = 10) from human primitive streak-like cells [46]. Within 30 days of differentiation, myeloid progenitors co-expressing CD14 and CX3CR1 were generated. These iPSC-derived microglia were able to perform phagocytosis and elicit ADP-induced intracellular Ca^{2+} transients that asserted their microglia identity as opposed to macrophage. Single-ended RNA-seq data were generated with the Illumina HiSeq 2500 platform following the Illumina protocol.

RNA-seq QC and alignment

FastQC was applied to DIAN and Knight-ADRC RNA-seq data to perform quality checks on various aspects of sequencing quality [47]. The DIAN and Knight-ADRC dataset was aligned to human GRCh37 primary assembly using Star (ver 2.5.2b) [48]. We used the primary assembly and aligned reads to the assembled chromosomes, un-localized and unplaced scaffolds, and discarded alternative haploid sequences. Sequencing metrics, including coverage, distribution of reads in the genome [49], ribosomal and mitochondrial contents, and alignment quality, were further obtained by applying Picard CollectRnaSeqMetrics (ver 2.8.2) to detect sample deviation. Additional QC metrics can be found in Additional file 1: Table S1.

Aligned and sorted bam files were loaded into IGV [50] to perform visual inspection of target variants. Samples carrying unexpected variants or missing expected variants were labeled as potential swapped samples. In addition, variants were called from RNA-seq following BWA/GATK pipeline [51, 52]. The identity of the samples was later verified by performing IBD analysis against genomic typing from genome-wide association study chipsets.

Expression quantification

We applied Salmon transcript expression quantification (ver 0.7.2) [53] to infer the gene expression for all samples included in the reference panel and participants in the Mayo, MSBB, DIAN, and Knight-ADRC. We quantified the coding transcripts of *Homo sapiens* included in the GENCODE reference genome (GRCh37.75). Similarly, we quantified the expression of the mice samples included in the reference panel using the *Mus musculus* reference genome (mm10).

Reference panel
Reference samples

We assembled a cell-type-specific reference panel from publicly available RNA-seq datasets comprising both immunopanning collected or iPSC-derived neurons, astrocytes, oligodendrocytes, and microglial cells from human and murine samples. For immunopanning collected cells, antibodies for cell-type-specific antigens were utilized to bind and immobilize their targeted cell types in order to immunoprecipitate and purify each cell type from the suspensions [30]. cDNA synthesis was accomplished using Ovation RNA-seq system V2 (Nugen 7102) and library prepared with Next Ultra RNA-seq library prep kit from Illumina (NEB E7530) and NEB-Next® multiplex oligos from Illumina (NEB E7335 E7500). TruSeq RNA Sample Prep Kit (Illumina) was used to prepare library for paired-end sequence on 100 ng of total RNA extracted from each sample. Illumina HiSeq 2000 Sequencer was used to sequence all libraries [30].

Both human adult TC tissue, collected from patients receiving neurological surgeries, and mice cells were disassociated, sorted and sequenced as described elsewhere [31], and deposited in the Gene Expression Omnibus GSE73721 and GSE52564. We also accessed neural progenitor cells (day 17) and mature human neurons (days 57 and 100) from Broad iPSC deposited in the AMP-AD portal [42] and neural progenitor cells and iPSC-derived neurons from [54]. Broad iPSC-derived neurons accessed from the AMP-AD portal were generated using an embryoid body-based protocol to differentiate into forebrain neurons. Wild-type cells used in the protocol were obtained from UConn StemCell Core. RNA was purified using PureLink RNA mini-kit (Life Technologies) and libraries were prepared by Broad Institute's Genomics Platform using TruSeq protocol. Please refer to Additional file 1: Table S2 for additional information.

Marker genes
The reference panel was assembled with samples from four distinct cell types. A redundant set of well-known cell-type markers was selected from the literature [31, 55, 56] (Additional file 1: Table S3). Principal component analysis (PCA) was performed on the reference panel using R function *prcomp* (version 3.3.3) to verify that the expressions of these gene were clustering samples by their cell types (Additional file 1: Figure S1b; Additional file 1: Figure S2a).

Inference of the cellular population structure
We ascertained alternative computation deconvolution algorithms implemented in the CellMix package (ver 1.6). Based on accuracy and robustness evaluation results, we compared and reported the following three algorithms that outperformed the others: Digital Sorting Algorithm (named "DSA") [27], which employs linear modeling to infer cell distributions; the method population-specific expression analysis (PSEA, also named meanProfile in CellMix implementation) [29] that calculates estimated expression profiles relative to the average of the marker

gene list for each cell type [29]; and a semi-supervised learning method that employs non-negative matrix factorization (ssNMF in CellMix implementation) [57]. We employed a leave-one-out cross-validation (LOOCV) procedure to evaluate the accuracy provided by each method. The best performing algorithm ssNMF integrates cell-type marker genes to resolve the drawbacks of completely unsupervised standard non-negative matrix factorization. We followed the standard procedure described in the CellMix package, which included the extraction of marker genes from the reference samples (function extractMarkers from the CellMix package), and the posterior invocation of the function *ged* to infer cellular population from the gene expression of bulk RNA-seq data. Besides, we tested additional methods which provided considerably lower accuracy (least-squares fit [58], quadratic programing [59]) or no significant difference (support vector regression [26] or latent variable analysis [60]) to the methods presented.

We selected the reference samples that provide the most faithful transcriptomic profile for their respective cell types by following a LOOCV approach. We trained iteratively deconvolution models using all but one of the samples that was tested. Only samples predicted with a composition > 80% were kept for the reference panel (Additional file 1: Table S2; Additional file 1: Figure S2b).

Accuracy and robustness evaluation
Chimeric validation
To emulate heterogeneous tissue with known and controlled cellular composition, we generated chimeric libraries pooling reads (to a total of 400,000) contributed from the human reference samples (see Additional file 1: Table S2). This process was repeated 720 times, using alternative reference samples to model each cell type. The proportion of reads that the libraries of neurons, astrocytes, oligodendrocytes, and microglia provided to the chimeric libraries varied in predefined ranges (Additional file 1: Figure S3). As a result, each of the chimeric libraries contained reads that followed 32 different distributions (neuronal reads contributed 2–36% of reads, astrocytes 22–76%, oligodendrocytes 6–62%, and microglia 1–5%). Refer to Additional file 1: Table S4 for detailed description of the 32 different distributions. We quantified the chimeric reads using Salmon (v0.7.2) [53] and employed the reference samples that did not contribute reads to the chimeric library as reference panel for the deconvolution methods.

Overall, we quantified the expression of 23,040 (720 × 32) chimeric libraries. We evaluated the accuracy using the root-mean-square error (RMSE, Eq. 1 to compare the digital deconvolution cellular proportion estimates (method ssNMF) vs the defined proportion of reads specific to each of the chimeric libraries:

$$RMSE = \sqrt{\frac{\sum_{i=1}^{n}(\hat{y}i - yi)^2}{n}} \qquad (1)$$

$\hat{y}i$–estimated value, yi–observed value

We also tested whether the deconvolution results were dominated by the expression of any specific marker gene and ascertained the robustness of the inferred cellular population structure to any possibly altered expression of marker genes. To do so, we performed the deconvolution analysis discarding each of the marker genes one at a time and evaluated how these distributions differed in comparison to the full gene reference panel.

Statistical analysis

We employed linear regression models to test the association between cell-type proportions and disease status (R Foundation for Statistical Computing, ver.3.3.3). We used stepwise discriminant analysis (stepAIC function of R package MASS, version 7.3–45) to determine significant covariates and to correct for confounding effects. We included RIN, batch, age at death, and post-mortem interval (PMI) as covariates for the Mayo Clinic analyses. For MSBB analyses, we corrected for RIN, PMI, race, batch, and age at death. We also used linear-mixed models to perform multiple-region association analysis, employing random slopes and random intercepts grouping by observations and by donors [61], and correcting for the same covariates previously described.

To analyze the DIAN and Knight-ADRC studies, we applied linear-mixed models (function lmer and Anova, R packages lme4 ver.1.1 and car ver.2.1, respectively), clustering at family level to ascertain the effect of the neuropathological status in the cell proportion and corrected for RIN and PMI. For late-onset specific analyses we also corrected for age at death.

Cellular composition shown as proportions were plotted using R package ggplot2 (ver 2.2.1).

Results

Study design

To infer cellular composition from RNA-seq, we first assembled a reference panel to model the transcriptomic signature of neurons, astrocytes, oligodendrocytes, and microglia. The panel was created by analyzing expression data from purified cell lines. We evaluated alternative digital deconvolution methods and selected the best performing for our primary analyses. We tested the digital deconvolution accuracy on iPSC-derived neurons/microglia cells and neuronal TRAP-seq (Fig. 1).

Finally, we verified its accuracy by creating artificial admixture with pre-defined cellular proportions.

Once the deconvolution approach was optimized, we calculated the cell proportion in AD cases and controls from the different brain regions of Mayo and MSBB datasets. The RNA-seq data for the Mayo Clinic study (n = 191) [18] and MSBB (n = 300) [39] are deposited in the AMP-AD knowledge portal (synapse ID: syn5550404 and syn3157743; Table 1). The Mayo study includes RNA-seq from the TC and CB for AD affected and non-demented controls, in addition to pathological aging (PA) participants (Fig. 1). The MSBB also profiled four additional cerebral cortex areas: APC; STG; PGH; and IFG; Table 1 and Fig. 1). We restricted the case-control analysis to subjects with definite AD and autopsy-confirmed controls. In addition, we generated RNA-seq from parietal lobe for participants of the Knight-ADRC (84 late-onset cases, carriers of genetic risk factors and 16 controls; Additional file 1: Table S1) and The Dominantly Inherited Alzheimer Network (DIAN; 19 carriers of mutations in *APP, PSEN1, PSEN2*) (Table 1; Fig. 1). We employed the same pipeline to process all of the samples in order to avoid any bias. Furthermore, RNA-seq from the Knight-ADRC and DIAN studies allowed us to compare the cell composition from ADAD vs LOAD brains, and similarly to test for differences in brains of controls, sporadic AD who do not carry any known high-risk variant, carriers of high-risk variants in *TREM2* (n = 20), *PLD3* (n = 33), and *APOE* ε4 allele.

Development of a reference panel to estimate brain cellular population structure

Due to limited availability of brain cell-type-specific transcriptomic data, we compiled reference samples from different sources, including single-population RNA-seq from mice and human (immunopan-purified oligodendrocytes, neurons, astrocytes and microglia, and iPSC-derived neurons and astrocytes).

We first tried to create a transcriptome-wide reference panel by selecting the genes that are differentially expressed among cell types [26, 60, 62]. However, the species heterogeneity of the reference samples we compiled ruled out this attempt, as the PCA showed that differences between the human and mice donor samples dominated the transcriptome-wide profiles (Additional file 1: Figure S1a). For this reason, we curated a list of marker genes that have been described to tag these distinct cell types [31, 55, 56] (Additional file 1: Table S3). A visual inspection of the expression of these marker genes in the samples we compiled suggested a divergent transcriptomic profile among the cell types (Additional file 1: Figure S2a). The PCA showed that their expression was sufficient to cluster samples of neurons, astrocytes, oligodendrocytes, and microglia with their respective cell types, regardless of

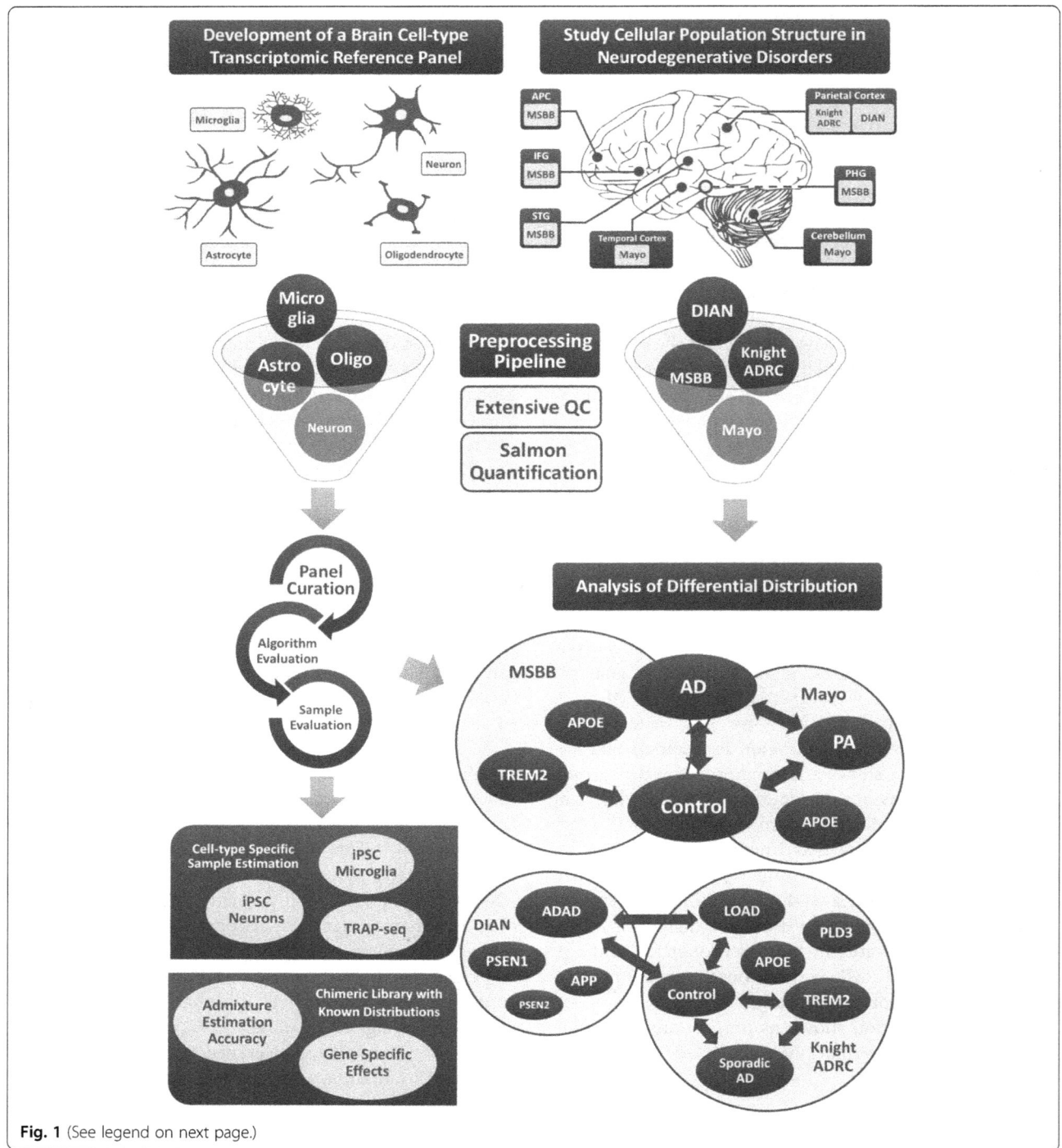

Fig. 1 (See legend on next page.)

Fig. 1 Study design development of the brain cell-type transcriptomic reference panel (*left column*): the expression signatures of key cell types of the brain were curated by compiling publicly available RNA-seq data from neurons, astrocytes, oligodendrocytes, and microglia. The panel was curated iteratively to retain only those samples that showed the most faithful expression signature, while evaluating alternative digital deconvolution methods. The accuracy of digital deconvolution to estimate brain cellular proportion was validated using additional cell-type-specific samples and also by generating chimeric libraries. To study cellular population structure in AD (*right column*), we accessed publicly available data from the AMP-AD, including Mayo Clinic and MSBB datasets. In addition, we generated RNA-seq from participants of the Knight-ADRC and DIAN studies. These three studies generated RNA-seq data from PA brains, AD cases, and neuropath-free controls in a total of six cerebral cortex regions and cerebellum. We quantified the gene expression for all of the samples included in these studies using the same RNA-seq processing pipeline. Using digital deconvolution methods, we estimated the brain cellular proportions of the samples and compared the proportion between AD cases and controls. We studied the cell structure of brain carriers of Mendelian pathological mutations and variants that confer high-risk to AD. APC anterior prefrontal cortex, STG superior temporal gyrus, PHG parahippocampal gyrus, IFG inferior frontal gyrus, MSBB Mount Sinai Brain Bank, AD Alzheimer's disease, PA pathological aging

the species of the reference samples (Additional file 1: Figure S1b; Additional file 1: Table S2). We observed that some samples did not cluster with their expected cell types and coincidently the LOOCV indicated that these samples had an expression signatures that differed from the other samples of the same cell type. However, we found that all of these outliers correspond to samples not correctly purified or that were sequenced in early stages of differentiation (Additional file 1: Supplementary Results). After discarding these samples, we assessed six digital deconvolution algorithms implemented in the CellMix package [62] and found that the ssNMF [57] calculated the most accurate estimates (see "Methods"). Our final reference panel (Additional file 1: Table S2; Additional file 1: Table S3) had a very high confidence to predict cell types with a mean predicted accuracy = 95.2%, s.d. = 4.3 (Additional file 1: Figure S2b), and a RMSE = 0.06 (Additional file 1: Table S5).

Optimization, validation, and accuracy estimation of the reference panel and digital deconvolution method

Once we identified the optimal approach to perform digital deconvolution from brain RNA-seq, we benchmarked it by using three sets of independent pure cell populations and simulated chimeric libraries.

We first validated the accuracy to predict neuronal composition by generating RNA-seq for eight iPSC-derived cortical neurons (see "Methods"). We observed an accurate prediction in these independent cell lines (mean neuronal proportion = 94.8%, s.d. = 1.1%; Additional file 1: Figure S4a). We also ascertained the cellular composition of mRNA extracted from the barrel cortex neurons isolated by TRAP in 24 mice. TRAP is a method that captures cell-type-specific mRNA translation by purifying tagged ribosomal subunit and capturing the mRNA it bound to [45]. We observed an average of neuronal proportion = 96.7% and s.d. = 1.2% (Additional file 1: Figure S4b). Similarly, we assessed the RNA-seq data generated for iPSC-derived microglia (n = 10) deposited in the AMP-AD portal (synapse ID: syn7203233) and inferred their cellular population structure and observed a mean

microglia proportion = 86.6% and s.d. = 7.1% (Additional file 1: Figure S4c).

To evaluate the accuracy of digital deconvolution for measuring cell-type proportion from cell-type admixtures, we simulated RNA-seq libraries by pooling reads from individual cell types into well-defined proportions. We combined randomly sampled reads from neurons, astrocytes, oligodendrocytes, and microglia to create chimeric libraries that mimic bulk RNA-seq from brain, but with a range of pre-defined cell-type distributions (Additional file 1: Figure S3). We then quantified the gene expression for the chimeric libraries and inferred the cell-type distribution (employing for the reference panel samples that did not contribute reads to the chimeric libraries). This process was repeated 23,040 times, choosing distinct human samples to represent each cell type and varying the proportions in 32 alternative distributions (see "Methods" and Additional file 1: Table S4). The overall error (RMSE) compared to known proportions = 0.08.

Finally, we evaluated whether any gene included in the reference panel was dominating the inference of cell proportions. We re-calculated the cell-type distributions of the chimeric libraries but dropping each of the genes from the reference panel one at a time. We observed a negligible difference between the cellular population structure inferred using the full reference and the gene-dropped panels (average RMSE = 0.022, s.d. < 0.01). In this way, we verified that the proportions inferred using the reference panel are not driven by the expression of a single gene. This reassured us the inference should be robust to any bias introduced by the potential association of a single gene included in the reference panel with a particular trait.

Deconvolution of bulk RNA-seq of non-demented and AD brains shows a characteristic signature for neurodegeneration

Pathologically, AD is associated with neuronal death and gliosis specifically in the cerebral cortex. We evaluated whether we could exploit deconvolution methods using our reference panel to detect altered cellular population structure from the bulk RNA-seq and whether this corresponded to known pathological alterations.

We initially analyzed the RNA-seq from the Mayo Clinic Brain Bank that includes bulk RNA-seq from the TC and CB for 191 participants [18] (Table 1). In the TC, we observed a significant higher astrocyte relative proportion ($\beta = 0.23$; $p = 5.01 \times 10^{-09}$; Table 2; Fig. 2; Additional file 1: Table S6) in AD brains compared to control brains. We also found a significant lower relative proportion of neurons ($\beta = -0.17$; $p = 1.58 \times 10^{-07}$; Table 2; Fig. 2; Additional file 1: Table S6) and oligodendrocytes ($\beta = -0.07$; $p = 1.8 \times 10^{-02}$; Table 2; Additional file 1: Figure S5; Additional file 1: Table S6). As expected given the absence of pathology, we did not observe a significant difference in the cell-type composition in the CB (Table 2).

The distribution of microglia was similar in the TC and CB from AD and control brains (Table 2; Additional file 1: Figure S5). The proportion of microglia was lower than any other cell types. The Mayo dataset also includes brains from individuals with PA (Table 1); which is neuropathologically defined by amyloid-beta (Aβ) senile plaque deposits but little or no neurofibrillary tau pathology [18, 63]. We observed a significant lower relative proportion of microglia in PA brains compared to AD in both TC and CB (Additional file 1: Table S7; Additional file 1: Figure S6). Therefore, we speculated that the lack of changes in the AD microglial population was neither due to low statistical power nor the inability of our method to estimate the microglial proportions but reflected unaltered neuropathological observations in AD brains.

We also analyzed data from the MSBB, which contains bulk RNA-seq for four additional cerebral cortex areas (APC, STG, PHG, IFG). Replicating our findings from the Mayo dataset, we observed a significant lower relative proportion in neurons and increase in astrocytes in all four areas (Table 2; Fig. 2; and Additional file 1: Table S6). The strongest effect size was detected in the PHG and STG ($p < 3.49 \times 10^{-07}$) (Table 2; Additional file 1: Table S8). Neuropathological studies have described that the PHG is one of the first brain areas in which AD pathology occurs [64–66]. We also observed a significant and strong correlation between neuronal and astrocyte relative proportions and the last ascertained clinical status (CDR), the number of amyloid plaques and Braak staging (Table 2; Fig. 2; Additional file 1: Figure S7).

The cellular population structure differs between ADAD vs LOAD

While the loss of neurons is a common feature of AD, it is not clear whether the mechanism holds true across different forms of AD or AD cases carrying different genetic risk variants. Therefore, we investigated whether AD with distinct etiologies showed different cellular compositions. We generated RNA-seq data from the parietal lobe of participants enrolled in Knight-ADRC (84 LOAD, 3 ADAD, and 16 neuropath-free controls) and DIAN (19 ADAD) studies (Table 1; Additional file 1: Table S1). We selected the LOAD and ADAD participants to match for CDR at death, brain weight, and sex distributions (see Additional file 1: Table S1).

Using digital deconvolution, we determined the cellular composition for these brains. We observed a significant lower relative proportion of neurons ($\beta = -0.02$, $p = 2.66 \times 10^{-02}$) and significant higher relative proportion of astrocyte in AD ($\beta = 0.03$, $p = 5.48 \times 10^{-03}$) for the combined LOAD and ADAD brains compared to controls (Table 3; Fig. 3; Additional file 1: Table S9), consistent with our findings in the Mayo and MSBB datasets. Similarly, the joint analysis of the brains from Knight-ADRC and DIAN showed significant associations between the neuronal and astrocyte relative proportions and neuropathological measures (Braak staging: $\beta = -0.03$, $p = 8.51 \times 10^{-06}$ for neurons and $\beta = 0.03$, $p = 3.83 \times 10^{-06}$ for astrocytes; Table 3; Fig. 3b) as well as for clinical measures (CDR: $\beta = -0.02$, $p = 2.66 \times 10^{-02}$ for neurons and $\beta = 0.03$ and $p = 5.48 \times 10^{-03}$ for astrocytes; Table 3; Fig. 3c). We did not observe a significant difference in the compositions of microglia or oligodendrocytes (Table 3; Additional file 1: Figure S8).

Next, we compared the cell proportion of LOAD vs ADAD and found that the cell composition differs between them. We first selected the LOAD brains ($n = 25$) to match the Braak staging distribution of ADAD brains ($n = 17$). The ADAD brains showed a significant lower relative neuronal proportion compared to LOAD brains ($\beta = -0.08$; $p = 1.03 \times 10^{-02}$; Table 3) and an increased relative astrocyte proportion ($\beta = 0.11$; $p = 9.26 \times 10^{-04}$; Table 3). Then, we analyzed the entire Knight-ADRC LOAD brains, by extending the model to correct for Braak stages. We also observed significant lower relative neuronal proportion ($\beta = -0.09$; $p = 4.71 \times 10^{-03}$; Table 3; Fig. 3a; Additional file 1: Table S9) and increased relative astrocyte proportion ($\beta = 0.11$; $p = 5.24 \times 10^{-04}$; Table 3; Fig. 3a; Additional file 1: Table S9) in ADAD brains compared to LOAD. We observed the same cellular differences when we corrected for CDR at death ($\beta = -0.12$; $p = 2.11 \times 10^{-03}$ for neurons and $\beta = 0.13$; $p = 6.29 \times 10^{-04}$ for astrocytes; Table 3; Fig. 3b, c). In summary, our results indicate that ADAD individuals present a higher neuronal loss even in the same stage of the disease, suggesting that in ADAD neuronal death plays a more important role in pathogenesis compared to sporadic AD, in which other factors such as inflammation or immune response may be involved.

Table 2 Comparison of the cellular population structure (AD vs neuropath-free controls) from the brains in the Mayo Clinic and Mount Sinai Brain Bank

Brain regions		Sample size	Neuron		Astrocyte		Oligodendrocyte		Microglia	
		n	Effect	p value	Effect	p value	Effect	p value	Effect	p value
Mayo	AD vs Control									
	CB	119	-0.03	2.74×10^{-01}	0.05	8.65×10^{-02}	-0.02	1.07×10^{-01}	-3.19×10^{-04}	9.19×10^{-01}
	TC	119	-0.17	1.58×10^{-07}	0.23	5.01×10^{-09}	-0.07	1.8×10^{-02}	-2.03×10^{-03}	5.48×10^{-01}
Mount Sinai Brain Bank	AD vs Control									
	APC	184	-0.04	8.14×10^{-04}	0.06	8.11×10^{-05}	-0.01	3.36×10^{-02}	-3.18×10^{-03}	1.12×10^{-02}
	STG	167	-0.08	3.49×10^{-07}	0.1	1.45×10^{-07}	-0.01	5.8×10^{-02}	-3.17×10^{-03}	5.78×10^{-02}
	PHG	160	-0.11	1.35×10^{-08}	0.13	5.48×10^{-10}	-0.02	1.79×10^{-03}	-3.18×10^{-03}	1.35×10^{-01}
	IFG	159	-0.04	3.12×10^{-03}	0.06	3.58×10^{-04}	-0.01	4.39×10^{-02}	-3.98×10^{-03}	1.64×10^{-02}
	Clinical Dementia Rating									
	APC	184	-0.02	9.38×10^{-04}	0.02	2.07×10^{-04}	-3.43×10^{-03}	1.25×10^{-01}	-1.46×10^{-03}	4.95×10^{-03}
	STG	167	-0.03	1.87×10^{-06}	0.04	3.33×10^{-07}	-0.01	2.1×10^{-02}	-1.02×10^{-03}	1.49×10^{-01}
	PHG	160	-0.04	8.56×10^{-06}	0.04	2.85×10^{-06}	-0.01	8.7×10^{-02}	-1.94×10^{-03}	2.53×10^{-02}
	IFG	159	-0.02	8.29×10^{-05}	0.03	1.4×10^{-05}	-4.64×10^{-03}	6.7×10^{-02}	-1.46×10^{-03}	3.11×10^{-02}
	Braak staging									
	APC	173	-0.01	1.21×10^{-02}	0.01	1.27×10^{-03}	-3.09×10^{-03}	2.77×10^{-02}	-7.04×10^{-04}	3.12×10^{-02}
	STG	158	-0.02	2.22×10^{-07}	0.02	2.77×10^{-07}	-2.91×10^{-03}	1.17×10^{-01}	-5.47×10^{-04}	1.97×10^{-01}
	PHG	147	-0.02	1.83×10^{-06}	0.03	9.6×10^{-08}	-0.01	1.49×10^{-03}	-3.71×10^{-04}	4.97×10^{-01}
	IFG	152	-0.01	1.01×10^{-02}	0.01	8.56×10^{-04}	-3.55×10^{-03}	2.37×10^{-02}	-1.01×10^{-03}	1.74×10^{-02}
	Mean amyloid plaques									
	APC	184	-1.88×10^{-03}	3.6×10^{-03}	2.82×10^{-03}	1.03×10^{-04}	-7.99×10^{-04}	2.13×10^{-03}	-1.46×10^{-04}	1.72×10^{-02}
	STG	167	-4.2×10^{-03}	7.73×10^{-08}	0.01	4.63×10^{-08}	-6.08×10^{-04}	9.01×10^{-02}	-2.04×10^{-04}	1.5×10^{-02}
	PHG	160	-4.96×10^{-03}	5.05×10^{-09}	0.01	1.26×10^{-10}	-9.99×10^{-04}	1.85×10^{-03}	-2.1×10^{-04}	2.58×10^{-02}
	IFG	159	-2.58×10^{-03}	3.82×10^{-04}	3.53×10^{-03}	1.96×10^{-05}	-7.41×10^{-04}	1.51×10^{-02}	-2.04×10^{-04}	1.26×10^{-02}

The cell-type proportions from AD cases and control were inferred from bulk RNA-seq using the ssNMF method. Effects of AD and associations with additional clinical and pathological phenotypes in cell-type distributions were estimated using linear regression model

CB cerebellum, TC temporal cortex, APC anterior prefrontal cortex, SGT superior temporal gyrus, PHG parahippocampal gyrus, IFG inferior frontal gyrus

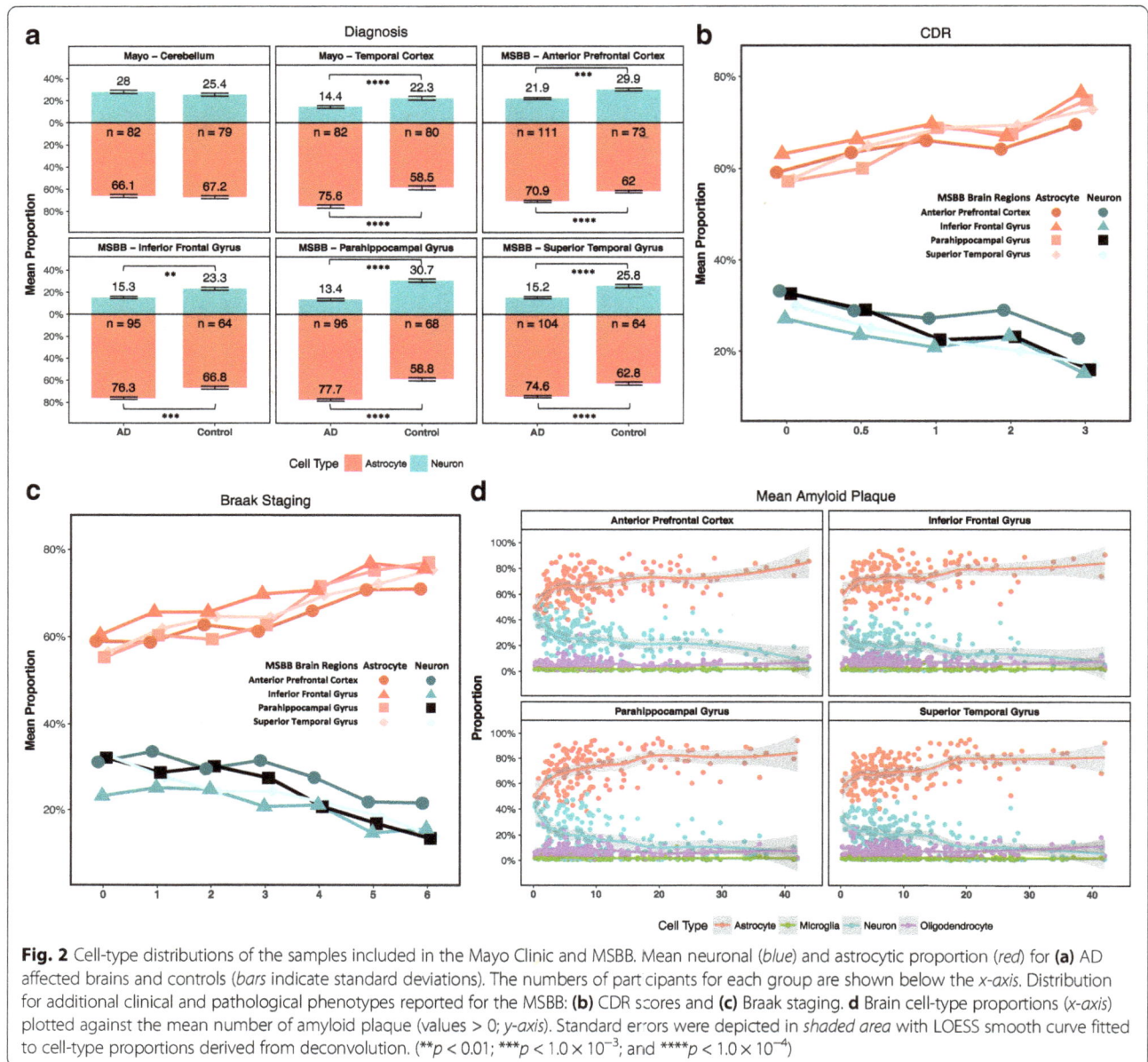

Fig. 2 Cell-type distributions of the samples included in the Mayo Clinic and MSBB. Mean neuronal (*blue*) and astrocytic proportion (*red*) for **(a)** AD affected brains and controls (*bars* indicate standard deviations). The numbers of part cipants for each group are shown below the *x-axis*. Distribution for additional clinical and pathological phenotypes reported for the MSBB: **(b)** CDR scores and **(c)** Braak staging. **d** Brain cell-type proportions (*x-axis*) plotted against the mean number of amyloid plaque (values > 0; *y-axis*). Standard errors were depicted in *shaded area* with LOESS smooth curve fitted to cell-type proportions derived from deconvolution. (*******p* < 0.01; ********p* < 1.0 × 10⁻³; and *********p* < 1.0 × 10⁻⁴)

Specific genetic variants confer a distinctive cell composition profile

A variety of genetic variants increase risk of LOAD; however, it is unclear if the cellular mechanisms are the same across these distinct risk factors. Therefore, we tested the hypothesis that distinct genetic causes of LOAD have characteristic cellular population signatures.

We initially ascertained the effect of *APOE* ε4 on the cell-type composition. We observed a significant lower relative proportion of neurons ($\beta = -0.06$ for each of the ε4 alleles; $p = 9.91 \times 10^{-03}$) and increase of relative proportion of astrocytes ($\beta = 0.10$; $p = 4.15 \times 10^{-02}$) from the TC included in the Mayo Clinic dataset (Additional file 1: Table S10; Fig. 4a; Additional file 1: Figure S9a). This

finding was replicated when we performed a multi-area analysis of the MSBB dataset ($\beta = -0.04$; $p = 2.60 \times 10^{-03}$ and $\beta = 0.05$; $p = 1.31 \times 10^{-03}$ for neurons and astrocytes, respectively; Table 4; Fig. 4a; Additional file 1: Table S10; Additional file 1: Figure S9a). Given the strong risk conferred by the *APOE* ε4 allele [4], we studied its effects on the cell-type composition by restricting our analysis to AD brains. We observed a significant association in the multi-area analysis of the MSBB dataset ($\beta = -0.03$ $p = 4.01 \times 10^{-02}$; Table 4; Fig. 4b; Additional file 1: Table S11; Additional file 1: Figure S9b) and also a significant increase in relative proportion of astrocytes ($\beta = 0.03$; $p = 1.23 \times 10^{-02}$; Table 4; Fig. 4b; Additional file 1: Table S11; Additional file 1: Figure S9b). We also

Table 3 Cellular population structure altered in the parietal lobe from AD brains in the DIAN study and Knight-ADRC brain bank

Disease status	Sample size	Neuron		Astrocyte		Oligodendrocyte		Microglia	
	n	Effect	p value	Effect	p value	Effect	p value	Effect	p value
AD status									
AD[a] vs Control	122	−0.11	5.52×10^{-04}	0.14	2.48×10^{-05}	−0.03	6.5×10^{-02}	-2.64×10^{-03}	2.49×10^{-01}
ADAD vs Control	38	−0.19	3.94×10^{-07}	0.24	1.57×10^{-10}	−0.04	8.5×10^{-03}	−0.01	7.77×10^{-05}
LOAD vs Control	100	−0.09	5.67×10^{-03}	0.12	3.34×10^{-04}	−0.02	1.06×10^{-01}	-1.70×10^{-03}	4.57×10^{-01}
ADAD vs LOAD									
Braak matched	42	−0.08	1.03×10^{-02}	0.11	9.26×10^{-04}	−0.03	7.1×10^{-02}	-1.46×10^{-03}	7.01×10^{-01}
Braak corrected	91	−0.09	4.71×10^{-03}	0.11	5.24×10^{-04}	−0.02	1.77×10^{-01}	-2.41×10^{-03}	4.25×10^{-01}
CDR corrected	94	−0.12	2.11×10^{-03}	0.13	6.29×10^{-04}	−0.02	3.8×10^{-01}	-3.11×10^{-03}	2.41×10^{-01}
Clinical Dementia Rating									
AD[a] and Controls	110	−0.02	2.66×10^{-02}	0.03	5.48×10^{-03}	−0.01	2×10^{-01}	-4.63×10^{-04}	4.77×10^{-01}
ADAD and Controls	26	−0.08	4.12×10^{-04}	0.11	1.78×10^{-07}	0.01	4.03×10^{-03}	-1.55×10^{-03}	1.75×10^{-08}
LOAD and Controls	100	−0.02	3.22×10^{-02}	0.03	7.01×10^{-03}	−0.01	1.81×10^{-01}	-4.64×10^{-04}	5.11×10^{-01}
Braak staging									
AD[a] and Controls	106	−0.03	8.51×10^{-06}	0.03	3.83×10^{-06}	-4.24×10^{-03}	2.04×10^{-01}	-2.52×10^{-04}	6.81×10^{-01}
ADAD and Controls	33	−0.05	2.37×10^{-05}	0.06	2.45×10^{-05}	−0.01	2.29×10^{-01}	-7.2×10^{-04}	4.89×10^{-01}
LOAD and Controls	88	−0.03	7.41×10^{-04}	0.03	4.63×10^{-04}	-3.72×10^{-03}	3.29×10^{-01}	-1.66×10^{-04}	7.86×10^{-01}

[a] AD includes both autosomal dominant AD (ADAD) and late-onset AD (LOAD)

The cellular population structure was inferred using the ssNMF method. Effects and p-values for the association with disease status, clinical dementia rating and Braak staging using generalized mixed models. We identified similar trends with approximately the same significance levels

AD Alzheimer's disease, *ADAD* autosomal dominant AD, *LOAD* late-onset AD

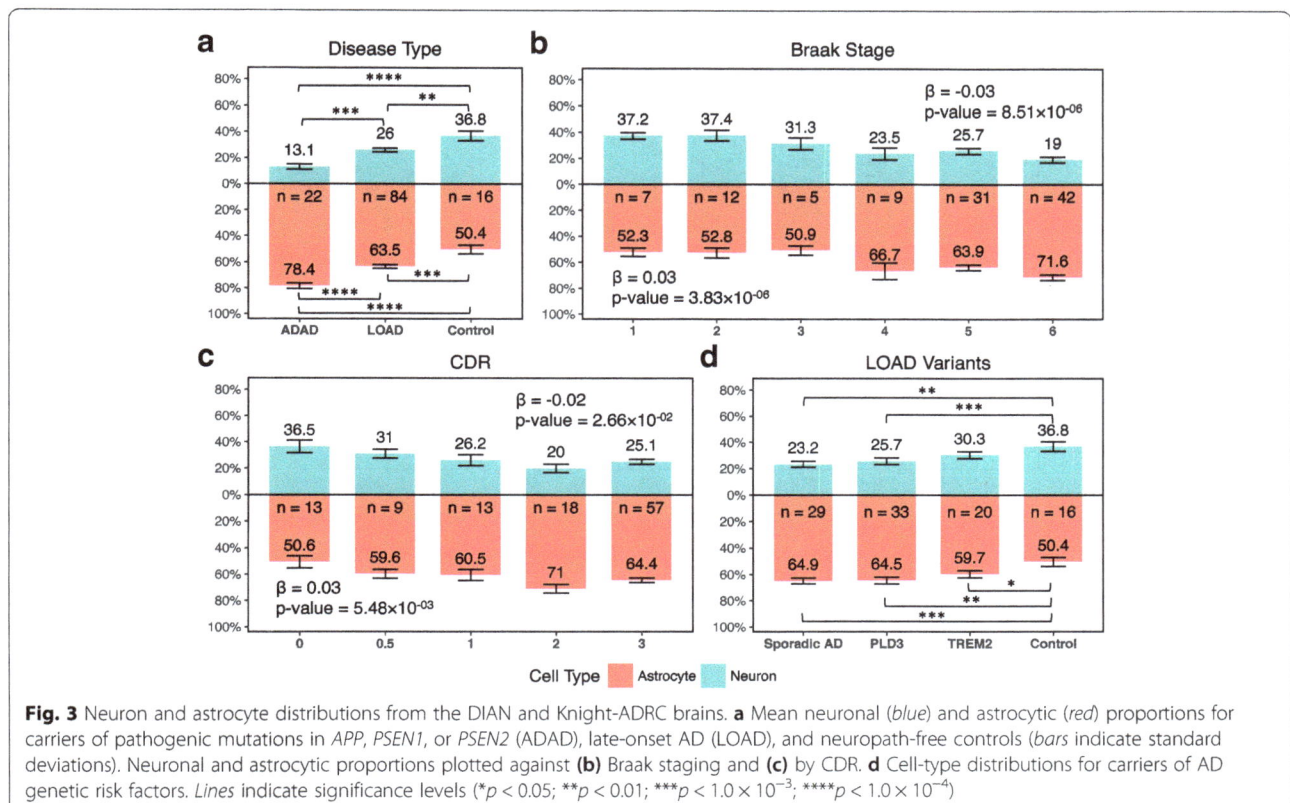

Fig. 3 Neuron and astrocyte distributions from the DIAN and Knight-ADRC brains. **a** Mean neuronal (*blue*) and astrocytic (*red*) proportions for carriers of pathogenic mutations in *APP*, *PSEN1*, or *PSEN2* (ADAD), late-onset AD (LOAD), and neuropath-free controls (*bars* indicate standard deviations). Neuronal and astrocytic proportions plotted against **(b)** Braak staging and **(c)** by CDR. **d** Cell-type distributions for carriers of AD genetic risk factors. *Lines* indicate significance levels (**p* < 0.05; ***p* < 0.01; ****p* < 1.0×10^{-3}; *****p* < 1.0×10^{-4})

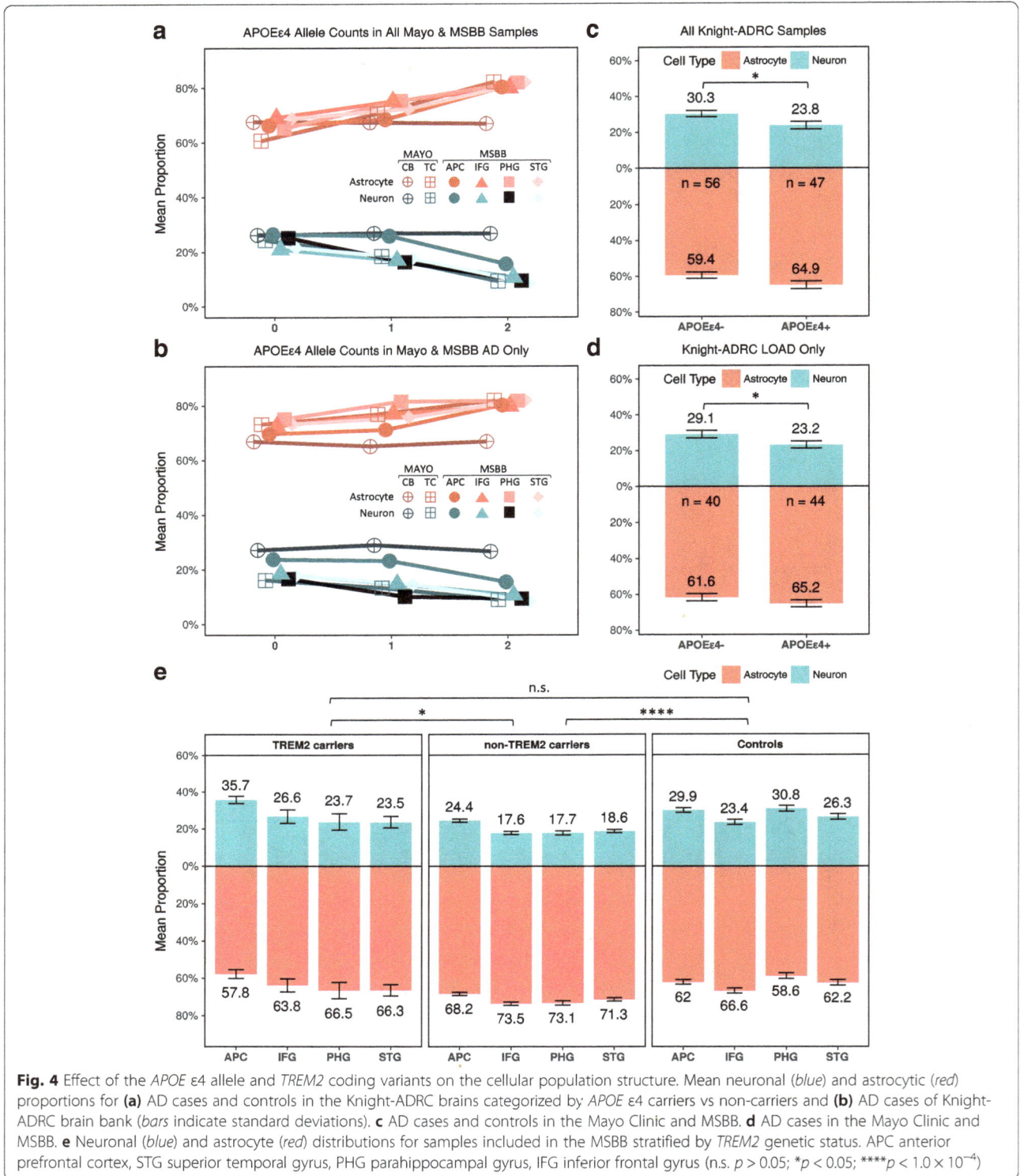

Fig. 4 Effect of the *APOE* ε4 allele and *TREM2* coding variants on the cellular population structure. Mean neuronal (*blue*) and astrocytic (*red*) proportions for **(a)** AD cases and controls in the Knight-ADRC brains categorized by *APOE* ε4 carriers vs non-carriers and **(b)** AD cases of Knight-ADRC brain bank (*bars* indicate standard deviations). **c** AD cases and controls in the Mayo Clinic and MSBB. **d** AD cases in the Mayo Clinic and MSBB. **e** Neuronal (*blue*) and astrocyte (*red*) distributions for samples included in the MSBB stratified by *TREM2* genetic status. APC anterior prefrontal cortex, STG superior temporal gyrus, PHG parahippocampal gyrus, IFG inferior frontal gyrus (n.s. $p > 0.05$; *$p < 0.05$; ****$p < 1.0 \times 10^{-4}$)

observed a significant decrease in relative proportion of neurons ($\beta = -0.06$; $p = 2.11 \times 10^{-02}$; Table 4; Fig. 4c) when we analyzed the LOAD and control brains from the Knight-ADRC. When we restricted the analysis to

AD brains from the Knight-ADRC and compared the *APOE* ε4 carriers ($n = 44$) to non-carriers ($n = 40$) we also observed a decreased relative neuronal proportion ($\beta = -0.06$; $p = 2.69 \times 10^{-02}$; Table 4; Fig. 4d). We

Table 4 Gene-specific cellular proportion analysis for Knight-ADRC and Mount Sinai Brain Bank studies

Variant carriers	Sample size	Neuron		Astrocyte		Oligodendrocyte		Microglia	
	n	Effect	p value	Effect	p value	Effect	p value	Effect	p value
Knight-ADRC									
PLD3 vs Control	49	−0.1	1.6×10^{-04}	0.13	2.84×10^{-03}	−0.03	6.17×10^{-02}	7.05×10^{-04}	7.89×10^{-01}
TREM2 vs Control	36	−0.07	7.93×10^{-02}	0.11	1.05×10^{-02}	−0.03	4.9×10^{-02}	1.65×10^{-03}	5.84×10^{-01}
Sporadic AD vs Control	45	−0.11	5.45×10^{-03}	0.13	2.95×10^{-04}	−0.02	4.55×10^{-01}	-3.48×10^{-03}	1.13×10^{-01}
APOEε4+ vs APOEε4- LOAD cases & controls	100	−0.06	2.11×10^{-02}	0.05	5.35×10^{-02}	0.01	3.72×10^{-01}	-8.09×10^{-04}	6.31×10^{-01}
APOEε4+ vs APOEε4- LOAD cases only	84	−0.06	2.69×10^{-02}	0.03	2×10^{-01}	0.03	1.4×10^{-02}	-8.31×10^{-04}	6.21×10^{-01}
CDR corrected	84	−0.06	2.78×10^{-02}	0.03	2.05×10^{-01}	0.03	1.16×10^{-02}	-1.05×10^{-03}	5.37×10^{-01}
Braak corrected	73	−0.06	3.66×10^{-02}	0.03	3.72×10^{-01}	0.03	4.51×10^{-03}	-1.14×10^{-03}	5.93×10^{-01}
Mount Sinai Brain Bank - Multi-region									
AD TREM2 carriers vs Control	301	−0.03	3.57×10^{-01}	0.03	3.19×10^{-01}	-2.08×10^{-03}	7.87×10^{-01}	-2.68×10^{-03}	8.67×10^{-02}
AD non-carriers TREM2 vs Control	882	−0.07	1.91×10^{-08}	0.08	1.25×10^{-08}	-3.36×10^{-03}	4.79×10^{-01}	-2.89×10^{-04}	7.97×10^{-01}
AD TREM2 vs AD non-TREM2	673	0.05	1.98×10^{-02}	−0.05	1.58×10^{-02}	2.12×10^{-03}	7.76×10^{-01}	-2.13×10^{-03}	1.74×10^{-01}
CDR corrected	673	0.04	5.83×10^{-02}	−0.04	4.46×10^{-02}	1.68×10^{-03}	8.19×10^{-01}	-1.92×10^{-03}	2.22×10^{-01}
Braak corrected	642	0.05	1.3×10^{-02}	−0.05	2.7×10^{-02}	-1.82×10^{-03}	8.13×10^{-01}	-2.66×10^{-03}	1.28×10^{-01}
Mean plaque counts corrected	673	0.05	2×10^{-02}	−0.05	1.59×10^{-02}	1.73×10^{-03}	8.15×10^{-01}	-2.2×10^{-03}	1.5×10^{-01}
APOEε4 counts all samples	556	−0.04	2.6×10^{-03}	0.05	1.31×10^{-03}	−0.01	4.47×10^{-02}	-3.58×10^{-04}	6.53×10^{-01}
APOEε4 counts AD cases	225	−0.03	4.01×10^{-02}	0.03	4.23×10^{-02}	-4.52×10^{-03}	3.73×10^{-01}	-5.13×10^{-04}	6.78×10^{-01}
CDR corrected	225	−0.03	2.02×10^{-02}	0.03	2.03×10^{-02}	-4.86×10^{-03}	3.19×10^{-01}	-4.91×10^{-04}	6.93×10^{-01}
Braak corrected	198	−0.03	7.35×10^{-02}	0.04	4.89×10^{-02}	−0.01	8.54×10^{-02}	-1.08×10^{-03}	4.12×10^{-01}

AD Alzheimer's disease, ADAD autosomal dominant AD, LOAD late-onset AD, CDR Clinical Dementia Rating

extended the models to correct for the Braak stages and observed a significant association for the relative proportion of neurons with the *APOE* ε4 allele in the Knight-ADRC dataset (β = − 0.06; $p = 3.66 \times 10^{-02}$; Table 4) and a significant association for the relative proportion of astrocytes in the MSBB (β = 0.04; $p = 4.89 \times 10^{-02}$; Table 4). Furthermore, we performed a meta-analysis to combine the evidence of both studies and observed a significant association of the relative neuronal proportion with *APOE* ε4 allele ($p = 1.86 \times 10^{-02}$) and marginally significant association for the relative astrocytic relative proportion ($p = 0.09$).

Next, we analyzed the cellular composition in *PLD3* carriers ($n = 33$). *PLD3* carriers exhibited significantly lower relative proportion of neurons compared to controls (β = − 0.10; $p = 1.60 \times 10^{-04}$; Fig. 3d) and a significant higher relative proportion of astrocytes (β = 0.13; $p = 2.84 \times 10^{-03}$; Table 4; Fig. 3d). Sporadic AD non-carrier cases also exhibited significantly lower relative proportion of neurons compared to controls (β = − 0.11; $p = 5.45 \times 10^{-03}$) and significant higher relative proportion of astrocytes (β = 0.13; $p = 2.95 \times 10^{-04}$; Table 4; Fig. 3d). The cell proportion between sporadic AD non-carriers and *PLD3* carriers did not show any significant difference ($p > 0.05$).

Finally, we performed similar analyses with *TREM2* carriers. *TREM2* is involved in the immune response and its role in amyloid-β deposition or clearance remains controversial [67]. Our analysis on the Knight-ADRC data showed significantly higher relative astrocytic proportion in AD affected *TREM2* carriers (n = 20) compared to controls (β = 0.11; $p = 1.05 \times 10^{-02}$; Table 4; Fig. 3d). Despite *TREM2* carriers presenting lower neuron relative proportion compared to controls, this difference was not statistically significant ($p > 0.05$; Table 4; Fig. 3d). We analyzed whether the *TREM2* carriers provided sufficient power to detect a significant association. Our empirical estimates showed that *TREM2* sample size provides 96% of power to detect an association with an effect size comparable to that observed for sporadic AD (β = − 0.11). We also investigated the cellular proportion of the 11 *TREM2* carriers in the MSBB dataset. The multi-region analysis showed *TREM2* carriers do not show a significant difference in relative neuronal proportion compared to controls ($p > 0.05$; Table 4; Fig. 4e), whereas in the AD *TREM2* non-carriers the relative neuronal and astrocytic proportions are significantly different from controls (β = − 0.07; $p = 1.91 \times 10^{-08}$; and β = 0.08; $p = 1.25 \times 10^{-08}$ respectively; Table 4; Fig. 4e).

In fact, our analyses indicate that *TREM2* carriers have a unique cellular brain composition distinct than the other AD cases. *TREM2* brains showed significantly higher relative neuronal proportion (β = 0.05; $p = 1.98 \times 10^{-02}$) and significantly lower relative astrocyte proportion than the AD *non*-carries (β = − 0.05; $p = 1.58 \times 10^{-02}$; Table 4). The distribution of CDR, mean number of amyloid plaques, and Braak staging do not differ between strata. Nonetheless, we verified that the cellular proportions were still significantly different after correcting for each of those variables (Table 4). These results suggested that the mechanism that lead to disease in *TREM2* carriers is less neuron-centric than in the general AD population.

Discussion

We have developed, optimized, and validated a digital deconvolution approach to infer cell composition from bulk brain gene expression that integrates publicly available cell-type specific expression data while addressing the heterogeneity of the phenotypic differences of samples and technical characteristics of transcriptome ascertainment. We acknowledge that the accuracy of this platform might be affected by the phenotypic diversity of the reference panel or the disease-induced dysregulation of genes it includes. However, the deconvolution approach proved to be robust to the genes included in the reference panel, as we demonstrated that the proportions it inferred are not driven by the expression of any single gene. This platform produced reliable cell proportion estimates, as was shown by the evaluation of independent datasets of iPSC-derived neurons and microglia, mice cortical neurons (Additional file 1: Figure S4), and simulated chimeric libraries.

We used this approach to deconvolve studies that include large numbers of neuropathologically defined AD and control brains with their transcriptome ascertained in distinct brain regions. We observed consistently significant lower relative neuronal proportion and increased relative astrocyte proportions in the cerebral cortex suggesting neuronal loss and astrocytosis. Compatible with other studies, we also identified that the altered cellular proportion is also significantly associated with decline in cognition and Braak staging [68]. In contrast, we did not identify a significant difference in the cellular population structure in the cerebellum, a region not affected in AD (Table 2; Fig. 2a).

We generated RNA-seq data from brains carrying pathogenic mutations in *APP, PSEN1*, and *PSEN2*, which cause alterations in Aβ processing and lead to ADAD, and also generated RNA-seq from brains of LOAD and neuropath-free controls. We observed altered cell composition in both ADAD and LOAD compared to controls. However, we identified that ADAD brains have a different cell-type composition than disease-stage-matched LOAD, as the ADAD has a significantly lower relative neuronal proportion and more pronounced astrocytosis. Given the specific cellular population structure of the *TREM2* carriers, we compared the neuronal and astrocytic relative proportion of ADAD to that of LOAD non-carriers of variants in *TREM2* and observed significant differences ($\beta = -0.09$ and $p = 6.89 \times 10^{-03}$ for neurons and $\beta = 0.10$; $p = 1.49 \times 10^{-03}$ for astrocytes). This indicates that the difference of the relative proportion between ADAD and LOAD are not driven by *TREM2* carrier brains. Based on our results, we would hypothesize that this change in Aβ processing of ADAD would lead to more direct to neuronal death than the pathological processes of LOAD. Similarly, decreased neuronal and increased astrocyte relative proportions were significantly associated with *APOE ε4* allele. It has been reported *APOE ε4* allele increases the risk for AD by affecting APP metabolism or Aβ clearance [69, 70], suggesting a direct link between APP metabolism and neuronal death.

In contrast, the analysis of the Knight-ADRC brains showed that the neuronal relative proportion decrease is less pronounced in *TREM2* carriers than in other LOAD cases. We replicated this finding in a multi-area analysis from the MSBB dataset. These results may implicate that *TREM2* risk variants lead to a cascade of pathological events that differ from those occurring in sporadic AD cases, which is also consistent with the known biology of *TREM2*. Further longitudinal neuroimaging analysis is required to validate our findings. *TREM2* is involved in AD pathology through microglia mediated pathways, implicated on altered immune response and inflammation [71]. Recent studies in *TREM2* knock-out animals showed that fewer microglia cells were found surrounding Aβ plaques with impaired microgliosis [72]. Furthermore, *TREM2* deficiency was reported to attenuate tauopathy against brain atrophy [73]. We found no significant difference in the proportion of microglia between AD cases and controls. However, we found significantly decreased microglia in brains exhibiting PA (Additional file 1: Table S7; Additional file 1: Figure S6), proving that these studies are sufficiently powered to identify significant differences. In any case, we cannot rule out the possibility of a change in the activation stage of microglia in these individuals. Overall, these results suggest that *TREM2* affects AD risk through a slightly different mechanism to that of ADAD or LOAD in general. Therefore, other pathogenic mechanisms should contribute to disease. We believe that a detailed modeling of immune response cells, reflecting the alternative microglia activation states, will generate more accurate profiles to elucidate the immune cell distribution in AD.

Conclusions

There is a large interest in the scientific community to use brain expression studies to try to identity novel pathogenic mechanisms in AD and to identify novel therapeutic targets. These efforts are generating a large amount of bulk RNA-seq data, as single-cell RNA (scRNA-seq) from human brain tissue in large sample sizes is not feasible. Single-cell sorting needs to be performed with fresh tissue [74], which restrains the analysis of highly characterized fresh-frozen brains collected by AD research centers. Our results indicate that digital deconvolution methods can accurately infer relative cell distributions from brain bulk RNA-seq data, but we recognize the importance of obtaining traditional neuropathological measures to validate the results we observed. Having this approach validated for AD can have an important impact in the community, because digital deconvolution analyses can: (1) reveal distinct cellular composition patterns underlying different disease etiologies; (2) provide additional insights about the overall pathologic mechanisms underlying different mutations carriers for variants as in genes such as *TREM2*, *APOE*, *APP*, *PSEN1*, and *PSEN2*; (3) correct the effect that altered cell composition and genetic statuses have in addition to downstream transcriptomic analyses and lead to novel and informative results; and (4) help the analysis of highly informative frozen brains collected over the years.

In conclusion, our study provides a reliable approach to enhance our understanding of the fundamental cellular mechanisms involved in AD and enable the analysis of large bulk RNA-seq data that may lead to novel discoveries and insights into neurodegeneration.

Abbreviations
AD: Alzheimer's disease; ADAD: Autosomal dominant Alzheimer's disease; AMP-AD: Advanced Medicines Partnership - Alzheimer's disease; APC: Anterior prefrontal cortex; Aβ: Amyloid-beta; CB: Cerebellum; CDR: Clinical Dementia Rating; DIAN: Dominantly Inherited Alzheimer Network; DSA: Digital sorting algorithm; IFG: Inferior frontal gyrus; iPSC: Induced pluripotent stem cell; Knight-ADRC: Charles F. and Joanne Knight Alzheimer's Disease Research Center (Knight ADRC); LOAD: Late-onset Alzheimer's disease; meanProfile: Implementation of method Population-Specific Expression Analysis; MSBB: Mount Sinai Brain Bank; PA: Pathological aging; PCA: Principal component analyses; PHG: Parahippocampal gyrus; PSEA: Population-Specific Expression Analysis; RIN: RNA integrity number; RMSE: Root-mean-square error; ssNMF: Semi-supervised non-negative matrix factorization; STG: Superior temporal gyrus; TC: Temporal cortex; TRAP-seq: Translating ribosome affinity purification sequencing

Acknowledgements
We thank all participants and their families for their commitment and dedication to helping advance research into the early detection and causation of AD; and the Knight-ADRC research and support staff at each of the participating sites for their contributions to this study.
This manuscript has been reviewed by DIAN Study investigators for scientific content and consistency of data interpretation with previous DIAN Study publications. We acknowledge the altruism of the participants and their families and contributions of the DIAN research and support staff at each of the participating sites for their contributions to this study.
We would like to thank the operations staff at the Elizabeth H. and James S. McDonnell III Genome Institute at Washington University with their assistance

in constructing the RNA-seq libraries and generating sequence data for our project. This work was also supported by accessing to equipment made possible by the Hope Center for Neurological Disorders and the Departments of Neurology and Psychiatry at Washington University School of Medicine. We also thank Allison M. Lake for her comments and suggestions.
The results published here are in whole or in part based on data obtained from the AMP-AD Knowledge Portal accessed at doi:https://doi.org/10.7303/syn2580853. Mayo Clinic RNA-seq data were provided by the following sources: The Mayo Clinic Alzheimer's Disease Genetic Studies, led by Dr. Nilufer Taner and Dr. Steven G. Younkin, Mayo Clinic, Jacksonville, FL using samples from the Mayo Clinic Study of Aging, the Mayo Clinic Alzheimer's Disease Research Center, and the Mayo Clinic Brain Bank. MSBB RNA-seq data were generated from postmortem brain tissue collected through the Mount Sinai VA Medical Center Brain Bank and were provided by Dr. Eric Schadt from Mount Sinai School of Medicine. MSSMiPSC data were generated by Kristen Brennand, a New York Stem Cell Foundation - Robertson Investigator.

Funding

This work was supported by grants from the National Institutes of Health (R01-AG044546, P01-AG003991, RF1AG053303, R01-AG035083, and R01-NS085419) and the Alzheimer's Association (NIRG-11-200110). This research was conducted while CC was a recipient of a New Investigator Award in Alzheimer's disease from the American Federation for Aging Research. CC and CMK are recipient of a BrightFocus Foundation Alzheimer's Disease Research Grant (A2013359S). This work was supported in part by NIH K01AG046374 awarded to CMK, and also the Tau Consortium (CMK). JDD is supported by the Brain and Behavior Research Foundation and the NIH (R01NS102272). The recruitment and clinical characterization of research participants at Washington University were supported by NIH P50 AG005681, P01 AG003991, and P01 AG026276.
DIAN data collection and sharing for this project were supported by The Dominantly Inherited Alzheimer's Network (DIAN, U19AG032438) funded by the National Institute on Aging (NIA), the German Center for Neurodegenerative Diseases (DZNE), Raul Carrea Institute for Neurological Research (FLENI), Partial support by the Research and Development Grants for Dementia from Japan Agency for Medical Research and Development, AMED, and the Korea Health Technology R&D Project through the Korea Health Industry Development Institute (KHIDI).
Mayo Clinic RNA-seq data collection was supported through funding by NIA grants P50 AG016574, R01 AG032990, U01 AG046139, R01 AG018023, U01 AG006576, U01 AG006786, R01 AG025711, R01 AG017216, R01 AG003949, NINDS grant R01 NS080820, CurePSP Foundation, and support from the Mayo Foundation. Study data include samples collected through the Sun Health Research Institute Brain and Body Donation Program of Sun City, Arizona. The Brain and Body Donation Program is supported by the National Institute of Neurological Disorders and Stroke (U24 NS072026 National Brain and Tissue Resource for Parkinson's Disease and Related Disorders), the National Institute on Aging (P30 AG19610 Arizona Alzheimer's Disease Core Center), the Arizona Department of Health Services (contract 211002, Arizona Alzheimer's Research Center), the Arizona Biomedical Research Commission (contracts 4001, 0011, 05–901, and 1001 to the Arizona Parkinson's Disease Consortium), and the Michael J. Fox Foundation for Parkinson's Research. MSSMiPSC data collection was supported by the Brain and Behavior Research Foundation, NIH grant R01 MH101454, and the New York Stem Cell Foundation. We analyzed iPSC-derived microglia RNA-seq data funded by NIH U01AG046170.

Authors' contributions

ZL performed the analyses, contributed to the study design and data interpretation. JDA, UD, JB, RM, KB, QB, NC, JDD, JML, JCM, RJB, and CMK contributed by data collection, data processing, QC, and cleaning. CC and OH designed the study, collected data, supervised the analyses, performed data interpretation, and wrote the manuscript. All the authors read and provide input to the manuscript.

Ethics approval and consent to participate

All research participants contributing clinical, genetic, or tissue samples for genet c analysis to this study provided written informed consent, subject to oversight by the Washington University in St. Louis, Mayo clinic or Mount Sinai School of Medicine review boards. All procedures of the Knight-ADRC (2011C5102) and DIAN (201106339) studies were approved by the Washington University Human Research Protection Office and written informed consent was obtained from each participant. The study was conducted according to the principles of the Declaration of Helsinki. All animal procedures were performed in accordance with the guidelines of Washington University's Institutional Animal Care and Use Committee.

Competing interests

The authors declare that they have no competing interests.

Author details

[1]Department of Psychiatry, Washington University School of Medicine, 660 S. Euclid Ave. B8134, St. Louis, MO 63110, USA. [2]Medical Scientist Training Program, Washington University School of Medicine, 660 S. Euclid Ave, St. Louis, MO 63110, USA. [3]Department of Neurology, Washington University School of Medicine, 660 S. Euclid Ave, St. Louis, MO 63110, USA. [4]Department of Pathology & Immunology, Washington University in St. Louis, School of Medicine, 510 S. Kingshighway, MC 8131, Saint Louis, MO 63110, USA. [5]Knight Alzheimer's Disease Research Center, Washington University School of Medicine, 660 S. Euclid Ave, St. Louis, MO 63110, USA. [6]Hope Center for Neurological Disorders, Washington University School of Medicine, 660 S. Euclid Ave. B8111, St. Louis, MO 63110, USA. [7]Department of Genetics, Washington University School of Medicine, 660 S. Euclid Ave, St. Louis, MO 63110, USA.

References

1. LaFerla FM, Oddo S. Alzheimer's disease: Abeta, tau and synaptic dysfunction. Trends Mol Med. 2005;11:170–6.
2. De Strooper B, Annaert W. Novel research horizons for presenilins and gamma-secretases in cell biology and disease. Annu Rev Cell Dev Biol. 2010; 26:235–60.
3. Selkoe DJ. Alzheimer's disease: genes, proteins, and therapy. Physiol Rev. 2001;81:741–66.
4. Corder EH, Saunders AM, Strittmatter WJ, Schmechel DE, Gaskell PC, Small GW, et al. Gene dose of apolipoprotein E type 4 allele and the risk of Alzheimer's disease in late onset families. Science. 1993;261:921–3.
5. Benitez BA, Cruchaga C. TREM2 and neurodegenerative disease. N Engl J Med. 2013;369:1567–8.
6. Guerreiro R, Wojtas A, Bras J, Carrasquillo M, Rogaeva E, Majounie E, et al. TREM2 variants in Alzheimer's disease. N Engl J Med. 2013;368:117–27.
7. Cruchaga C, Karch CM, Jin SC, Benitez BA, Cai Y, Guerreiro R, et al. Rare coding variants in the phospholipase D3 gene confer risk for Alzheimer's disease. Nature. 2014;505:550–4.
8. Steinberg S, Stefansson H, Jonsson T, Johannsdottir H, Ingason A, Helgason H, et al. Loss-of-function variants in ABCA7 confer risk of Alzheimer's disease. Nat Genet. 2015;47:445–7.
9. Del-Aguila JL, Fernandez MV, Jimenez J, Black K, Ma SM, Deming Y, Carrell D, Saef B, Howells B, Budde J, Cruchaga C. Role of ABCA7 loss-of-function variant in Alzheimer's disease: a replication study in European-Americans. Alzheimers Res Ther. 2015;7:73.
10. Rogaeva E, Meng Y, Lee JH, Gu Y, Kawarai T, Zou F, et al. The neuronal sortilin-related receptor SORL1 is genetically associated with Alzheimer disease. Nat Genet. 2007;39:168–77.
11. Fernandez MV, Black K, Carrell D, Saef B, Budde J, Deming Y, et al. SORL1 variants across Alzheimer's disease European American cohorts. Eur J Hum Genet. 2016;24:1828–30.
12. Tang M, Ryman DC, McDade E, Jasielec MS, Buckles VD, Cairns NJ, et al. Neurological manifestations of autosomal dominant familial Alzheimer's disease: a comparison of the published literature with the Dominantly Inherited Alzheimer Network observational study (DIAN-OBS). Lancet Neurol. 2016;15:1317–25.

13. Ryan NS, Nicholas JM, Weston PS, Liang Y, Lashley T, Guerreiro R, et al. Clinical phenotype and genetic associations in autosomal dominant familial Alzheimer's disease: a case series. Lancet Neurol. 2016;15:1326–35.

14. Padurariu M, Ciobica A, Mavroudis I, Fotiou D, Baloyannis S. Hippocampal neuronal loss in the CA1 and CA3 areas of Alzheimer's disease patients. Psychiatr Danub. 2012;24:152–8.

15. Wright AL, Zinn R, Hohensinn B, Konen LM, Beynon SB, Tan RP. Neuroinflammation and neuronal loss precede Abeta plaque deposition in the hAPP-J20 mouse model of Alzheimer's disease. PLoS One. 2013;8:e59586.

16. Holtzman DM, Morris JC, Goate AM. Alzheimer's disease: the challenge of the second century. Sci Transl Med. 2011;3:77sr71.

17. Golub VM, Brewer J, Wu X, Kuruba R, Short J, Manchi M. Neurostereology protocol for unbiased quantification of neuronal injury and neurodegeneration. Front Aging Neurosci. 2015;7:196.

18. Allen M, Carrasquillo MM, Funk C, Heavner BD, Zou F, Younkin CS, et al. Human whole genome genotype and transcriptome data for Alzheimer's and other neurodegenerative diseases. Sci Data. 2016;3:160089.

19. Narayanan M, Huynh JL, Wang K, Yang X, Yoo S, McElwee J, et al. Common dysregulation network in the human prefrontal cortex underlies two neurodegenerative diseases. Mol Syst Biol. 2014;10:743.

20. Srinivasan K, Friedman BA, Larson JL, Lauffer BE, Goldstein LD, Appling LL, et al. Untangling the brain's neuroinflammatory and neurodegenerative transcriptional responses. Nat Commun. 2016;7:11295.

21. Zhang B, Gaiteri C, Bodea LG, Wang Z, McElwee J, Podtelezhnikov AA, et al. Integrated systems approach identifies genetic nodes and networks in late-onset Alzheimer's disease. Cell. 2013;153:707–20.

22. Chan G, White CC, Winn PA, Cimpean M, Replogle JM, Glick LR, et al. CD33 modulates TREM2: convergence of Alzheimer loci. Nat Neurosci. 2015;18:1556–8.

23. Miller JA, Woltjer RL, Goodenbour JM, Horvath S, Geschwind DH. Genes and pathways underlying regional and cell type changes in Alzheimer's disease. Genome Med. 2013;5:48.

24. Parikshak NN, Gandal MJ, Geschwind DH. Systems biology and gene networks in neurodevelopmental and neurodegenerative disorders. Nat Rev Genet. 2015;16:441–58.

25. Gaiteri C, Mostafavi S, Honey CJ, De Jager PL, Bennett DA. Genetic variants in Alzheimer disease - molecular and brain network approaches. Nat Rev Neurol. 2016;12:413–27.

26. Newman AM, Liu CL, Green MR, Gentles AJ, Feng W, Xu Y. Robust enumeration of cell subsets from tissue expression profiles. Nat Methods. 2015;12:453–7.

27. Zhong Y, Wan YW, Pang K, Chow LM, Liu Z. Digital sorting of complex tissues for cell type-specific gene expression profiles. BMC Bioinformatics. 2013;14:89.

28. Shen-Orr SS, Gaujoux R. Computational deconvolution: extracting cell type-specific information from heterogeneous samples. Curr Opin Immunol. 2013;25:571–8.

29. Kuhn A, Thu D, Waldvogel HJ, Faull RL, Luthi-Carter R. Population-specific expression analysis (PSEA) reveals molecular changes in diseased brain. Nat Methods. 2011;8:945–7.

30. Zhang Y, Chen K, Sloan SA, Bennett ML, Scholze AR, O'Keeffe S, et al. An RNA-sequencing transcriptome and splicing database of glia, neurons, and vascular cells of the cerebral cortex. J Neurosci. 2014;34:11929–47.

31. Zhang Y, Sloan SA, Clarke LE, Caneda C, Plaza CA, Blumenthal PD, et al. Purification and characterization of progenitor and mature human astrocytes reveals transcriptional and functional differences with mouse. Neuron. 2016;89:37–53.

32. Brennand KJ, Simone A, Jou J, Gelboin-Burkhart C, Tran N, Sangar S, et al. Modelling schizophrenia using human induced pluripotent stem cells. Nature 2011, 473:221–225.

33. Knight-Alzheimer's Disease Research Center [http://alzheimer.wustl.edu/].

34. Dominantly Inherited Alzheimer Network [https://dian.wustl.edu//].

35. Mirra SS, Heyman A, McKeel D, Sumi SM, Crain BJ, Brownlee LM, et al. The Consortium to Establish a Registry for Alzheimer's Disease (CERAD). Part II. Standardization of the neuropathologic assessment of Alzheimer's disease. Neurology. 1991;41:479–86.

36. Morris JC. Clinical dementia rating: a reliable and valid diagnostic and staging measure for dementia of the Alzheimer type. Int Psychogeriatr. 1997;9(Suppl 1):173–6. discussion 177-178

37. Braak H, Braak E. Staging of Alzheimer's disease-related neurofibrillary changes. Neurobiol Aging. 1995;16:271 8. discussion 278-284

38. AMPAD Knowledge Portal Mayo Clinic RNAseq [https://www.synapse.org/#!Synapse:syn5550404].

39. AMPAD Knowledge Portal Mount Sinai Brain Bank RNAseq [https://www.synapse.org/#!Synapse:syn3157743].

40. Takahashi K, Yamanaka S. Induction of pluripotent stem cells from mouse embryonic and adult fibroblast cultures by defined factors. Cell. 2006;126:663–76.

41. van de Leemput J, Boles NC, Kiehl TR, Corneo B, Lederman P, Menon V, et al. CORTECON: a temporal transcriptome analysis of in vitro human cerebral cortex development from human embryonic stem cells. Neuron. 2014;83:51–68.

42. UConn StemCell Core Broad iPSC deposited in the AMP-AD [https://www.synapse.org/#!Synapse:syn3607401].

43. Zhou P, Zhang Y, Ma Q, Gu F, Day DS, He A, et al. Interrogating translational efficiency and lineage-specific transcriptomes using ribosome affinity purification. Proc Natl Acad Sci U S A. 2013;110:15395–400.

44. Hippenmeyer S, Vrieseling E, Sigrist M, Portmann T, Laengle C, Ladle DR, et al. A developmental switch in the response of DRG neurons to ETS transcription factor signaling. PLoS Biol. 2005;3:e159.

45. Heiman M, Kulicke R, Fenster RJ, Greengard P, Heintz N. Cell type-specific mRNA purification by translating ribosome affinity purification (TRAP). Nat Protoc. 2014;9:1282–91.

46. Douvaras P, Sun B, Wang M, Kruglikov I, Lallos G, Zimmer M, et al. Directed differentiation of human pluripotent stem cells to microglia. Stem Cell Reports. 2017;8:1516–24.

47. Andrews S. FastQC: a quality control tool for high throughput sequence data. 2010. Available online at http://www.bioinformatics.babraham.ac.uk/projects/fastqc.

48. Dobin A, Davis CA, Schlesinger F, Drenkow J, Zaleski C, Jha S, et al. STAR: ultrafast universal RNA-seq aligner. Bioinformatics. 2013;29:15–21.

49. Broad Institute The Picard Pipeline [http://broadinstitute.github.io/picard/].

50. Robinson JT, Thorvaldsdottir H, Winckler W, Guttman M, Lander ES, Getz G, et al. Integrative genomics viewer. Nat Biotechnol. 2011;29:24–6.

51. Li H, Durbin R. Fast and accurate short read alignment with Burrows-Wheeler transform. Bioinformatics. 2009;25:1754–60.

52. McKenna A, Hanna M, Banks E, Sivachenko A, Cibulskis K, Kernytsky A, et al. The Genome Analysis Toolkit: a MapReduce framework for analyzing next-generation DNA sequencing data. Genome Res. 2010;20:1297–303.

53. Patro R, Duggal G, Love MI, Irizarry RA, Kingsford C. Salmon provides fast and bias-aware quantification of transcript expression. Nat Methods. 2017;14:417–9.

54. Brennand KJ. The hiPSC Neurons and NPCs study (MSSMiPSC) deposited in the AMP-AD. https://www.synapse.org/#!Synapse:syn5986884.

55. Cahoy JD, Emery B, Kaushal A, Foo LC, Zamanian JL, Christopherson KS, et al. A transcriptome database for astrocytes, neurons, and oligodendrocytes: a new resource for understanding brain development and function. J Neurosci. 2008;28:264–78.

56. Holtman IR, Raj DD, Miller JA, Schaafsma W, Yin Z, Brouwer N, et al. Induction of a common microglia gene expression signature by aging and neurodegenerative conditions: a co-expression meta-analysis. Acta Neuropathol Commun. 2015;3:31.

57. Gaujoux R, Seoighe C. Semi-supervised Nonnegative Matrix Factorization for gene expression deconvolution: a case study. Infect Genet Evol. 2012;12:913–21.

58. Abbas AR, Wolslegel K, Seshasayee D, Modrusan Z, Clark HF. Deconvolution of blood microarray data identifies cellular activation patterns in systemic lupus erythematosus. PLoS One. 2009;4:e6098.

59. Gong T, Hartmann N, Kohane IS, Brinkmann V, Staedtler F, Letzkus M, et al. Optimal deconvolution of transcriptional profiling data using quadratic programming with application to complex clinical blood samples. PLoS One. 2011;6:e27156.

60. Chikina M, Zaslavsky E, Sealfon SC. CellCODE: a robust latent variable approach to differential expression analysis for heterogeneous cell populations. Bioinformatics. 2015;31:1584–91.

61. Sul JH, Han B, Ye C, Choi T, Eskin E. Effectively identifying eQTLs from multiple tissues by combining mixed model and meta-analytic approaches. PLoS Genet. 2013;9:e1003491.

62. Gaujoux R, Seoighe C. CellMix: a comprehensive toolbox for gene expression deconvolution. Bioinformatics. 2013;29:2211–2.

63. Murray ME, Dickson DW. Is pathological aging a successful resistance against amyloid-beta or preclinical Alzheimer's disease? Alzheimers Res Ther. 2014;6:24.

64. Echavarri C, Aalten P, Uylings HB, Jacobs HI, Visser PJ, Gronenschild EH, et al. Atrophy in the parahippocampal gyrus as an early biomarker of Alzheimer's disease. Brain Struct Funct. 2011;215:265–71.

65. Braak H, Braak E. Neurofibrillary changes confined to the entorhinal region and an abundance of cortical amyloid in cases of presenile and senile dementia. Acta Neuropathol. 1990;80:479–86.

66. Van Hoesen GW, Augustinack JC, Dierking J, Redman SJ, Thangavel R. The parahippocampal gyrus in Alzheimer's disease. Clinical and preclinical neuroanatomical correlates. Ann N Y Acad Sci. 2000;911:254–74.

67. Ulrich JD, Ulland TK, Colonna M, Holtzman DM. Elucidating the role of TREM2 in Alzheimer's disease. Neuron. 2017;94:237–48.

68. Serrano-Pozo A, Frosch MP, Masliah E, Hyman BT. Neuropathological alterations in Alzheimer disease. Cold Spring Harb Perspect Med. 2011;1:a006189.

69. Castellano JM, Kim J, Stewart FR, Jiang H, DeMattos RB, Patterson BW, et al. Human apoE isoforms differentially regulate brain amyloid-beta peptide clearance. Sci Transl Med. 2011;3:89ra57.

70. Kim J, Basak JM, Holtzman DM. The role of apolipoprotein E in Alzheimer's disease. Neuron. 2009;63:287–303.

71. Colonna M. TREMs in the immune system and beyond. Nat Rev Immunol. 2003;3:445–53.

72. Wang Y, Ulland TK, Ulrich JD, Song W, Tzaferis JA, Hole JT, et al. TREM2-mediated early microglial response limits diffusion and toxicity of amyloid plaques. J Exp Med. 2016;213:667–75.

73. Leyns CEG, Ulrich JD, Finn MB, Stewart FR, Koscal LJ, Remolina Serrano J, Robinson GO, Anderson E, Colonna M, Holtzman DM. TREM2 deficiency attenuates neuroinflammation and protects against neurodegeneration in a mouse model of tauopathy. Proc Natl Acad Sci. 2017; 114:11524-29.

74. Habib N, Avraham-Davidi I, Basu A, Burks T, Shekhar K, Hofree M, et al. Massively parallel single-nucleus RNA-seq with DroNc-seq. Nat Methods. 2017;14:955–8.

5

Rare variants in *SOX17* are associated with pulmonary arterial hypertension with congenital heart disease

Na Zhu[1,2†], Carrie L. Welch[1†], Jiayao Wang[1,2], Philip M. Allen[1], Claudia Gonzaga-Jauregui[3], Lijiang Ma[1], Alejandra K. King[3], Usha Krishnan[1], Erika B. Rosenzweig[1,4], D. Dunbar Ivy[5], Eric D. Austin[6], Rizwan Hamid[6], Michael W. Pauciulo[7,8], Katie A. Lutz[7], William C. Nichols[7,8], Jeffrey G. Reid[3], John D. Overton[3], Aris Baras[3], Frederick E. Dewey[3], Yufeng Shen[2,9] and Wendy K. Chung[1,4,10,11*]

Abstract

Background: Pulmonary arterial hypertension (PAH) is a rare disease characterized by distinctive changes in pulmonary arterioles that lead to progressive pulmonary arterial pressures, right-sided heart failure, and a high mortality rate. Up to 30% of adult and 75% of pediatric PAH cases are associated with congenital heart disease (PAH-CHD), and the underlying etiology is largely unknown. There are no known major risk genes for PAH-CHD.

Methods: To identify novel genetic causes of PAH-CHD, we performed whole exome sequencing in 256 PAH-CHD patients. We performed a case-control gene-based association test of rare deleterious variants using 7509 gnomAD whole genome sequencing population controls. We then screened a separate cohort of 413 idiopathic and familial PAH patients without CHD for rare deleterious variants in the top association gene.

Results: We identified *SOX17* as a novel candidate risk gene ($p = 5.5e{-}7$). *SOX17* is highly constrained and encodes a transcription factor involved in Wnt/β-catenin and Notch signaling during development. We estimate that rare deleterious variants contribute to approximately 3.2% of PAH-CHD cases. The coding variants identified include likely gene-disrupting (LGD) and deleterious missense, with most of the missense variants occurring in a highly conserved HMG-box protein domain. We further observed an enrichment of rare deleterious variants in putative targets of SOX17, many of which are highly expressed in developing heart and pulmonary vasculature. In the cohort of PAH without CHD, rare deleterious variants of *SOX17* were observed in 0.7% of cases.

Conclusions: These data strongly implicate *SOX17* as a new risk gene contributing to PAH-CHD as well as idiopathic/familial PAH. Replication in other PAH cohorts and further characterization of the clinical phenotype will be important to confirm the precise role of *SOX17* and better estimate the contribution of genes regulated by SOX17.

Keywords: Pulmonary hypertension, Congenital heart disease, Exome sequencing, Genetic association study

Background

Pulmonary arterial hypertension (PAH[MIM:178600]) is a rare disease characterized by distinctive changes in pulmonary arterioles that lead to progressive pulmonary arterial pressures, right-sided heart failure and a high mortality rate.

Up to 30% of adult- [1, 2] and 75% of pediatric-onset PAH cases [3] are associated with congenital heart disease (PAH-CHD), and due to improved treatments, the number of adults with PAH-CHD is rising [1, 4]. Congenital heart defects can result in left-to-right (systemic-to-pulmonary) shunts leading to increased pulmonary blood flow and risk of PAH. However, not all patients are exposed to prolonged periods of increased pulmonary flow. PAH may persist following surgical repair of cardiac defects or recur many years after repair. Thus, the underlying etiology is heterogeneous and may include increased pulmonary blood flow,

* Correspondence: wkc15@cumc.columbia.edu; wkc15@columbia.edu
†Na Zhu and Carrie L. Welch contributed equally to this work.
¹Department of Pediatrics, Columbia University Medical Center, New York, NY, USA
⁴Department of Medicine, Columbia University Medical Center, New York, NY, USA
Full list of author information is available at the end of the article

pulmonary vasculature abnormalities, or a combination. In addition to environmental factors, genetic factors likely play an important role in PAH-CHD although no major risk gene has been identified to date [1].

Genetic studies of PAH alone have identified 11 known risk genes for PAH [5–8]. Several of the risk genes encode members of the transforming growth factor beta/bone morphogenetic protein (TGF-β/BMP) signaling pathway, important in both vasculogenesis and embryonic heart development. For example, mutations in bone morphogenetic protein receptor type 2 (BMPR2) are found in approximately 70% of familial and 10–40% of idiopathic PAH cases. Estimates of the frequency of BMPR2 mutations in PAH-CHD are considerably lower than for PAH alone [9–11]. Mutations in other TGFβ family member genes—activin A, receptor type II-like 1 (ACVRL1), endoglin (ENG), BMP receptor type 1A (BMPR1A) and type 1B (BMPR1B)—as well as caveolin-1 (CAV1), eukaryotic initiation translation factor 2 alpha kinase 4 (EIF2AK4), potassium two-pore-domain channel subfamily K member 3 (KCNK3), SMAD family members 4 and 9 (SMAD4 and SMAD9), and T-box4 (TBX4) have all been identified as less frequent or rare causes of PAH [5–8]. The genetics of CHD are complex and no single major risk gene accounts for more than 1% of cases [12, 13]. Aneuploidies and copy number variations underlie up to 23% of CHD cases [14, 15]. Rare, inherited, and de novo variants in hundreds of genes encoding transcription factors, chromatin regulators, signal transduction proteins, and cardiac structural proteins have been implicated in ~ 10% of CHD cases [12, 16–19].

To identify novel genetic causes of PAH-CHD, we performed exome sequencing in a patient cohort of PAH-CHD. Association analysis using population controls identified SOX17, a member of the SRY-related HMG-box family of transcription factors, as a new candidate risk gene.

Methods

An overview of the experimental design and workflow is provided in Additional file 1: Figure S1.

Patients

PAH-CHD patients were recruited from the pulmonary hypertension centers at Columbia University and Children's Hospital of Colorado (via enrollment in the PAH Biobank at Cincinnati Children's Hospital Medical Center). Patients were diagnosed according to the World Health Organization (WHO) pulmonary hypertension group I classification [20]. The diagnosis of PAH-CHD was confirmed by medical record review including right heart catheterization and echocardiogram to define the cardiac anatomy. The cohort included 15 familial cases, 160 singletons with no family history of PAH, 61 trios

(proband and two unaffected biological parents), and 20 duos (proband and one unaffected parent). Written informed consent (and assent when appropriate) was obtained under a protocol approved by the institutional review board at Columbia University Medical Center or Children's Hospital of Colorado.

Whole exome sequencing (WES)

Familial cases were screened for BMPR2 and ACVRL1 mutations by Sanger sequencing and multiplex ligation-dependent probe amplification (MLPA). Familial cases without mutations in the two risk genes and all other samples were exome sequenced. DNA was extracted from peripheral blood leukocytes using Puregene reagents (Gentra Systems Inc., Minnesota, USA). Exome sequencing was performed in collaboration with the Regeneron Genetics Center (RGC) or at the Children's Hospital of Cincinnati. In brief, genomic DNA processed at the RGC was prepared with a customized reagent kit from Kapa Biosystems and captured using the SeqCap VCRome 2 exome capture reagent or xGen lockdown probes. Patient DNA samples sequenced at the PAH Biobank/Cincinnati Children's Hospital Medical Center were prepared with the Clontech Advantage II kit and enriched using the SeqCap EZ exome V2 capture reagent. All samples were sequenced on the Illumina HiSeq 2500 platform, generating 76-bp paired-end reads. Read-depth coverage was ≥ 15× in ≥ 95% of targeted regions for all exome sequencing samples.

WES data analysis

The workflow is outlined in Additional file 1: Figure S1A. We used a previously established bioinformatics procedure [18] to process and analyze exome sequence data. Specifically, we used BWA-MEM (Burrows-Wheeler Aligner) [21] to map and align paired-end reads to the human reference genome (version GRCh37/hg19), Picard MarkDuplicates to identify and flag PCR duplicate reads, GATK HaplotypeCaller (version 3) [22, 23] to call genetic variants, and GATK variant quality score recalibration (VQSR) to estimate accuracy of variant calls. We used heuristic filters to minimize potential technical artifacts, excluding variants that met any of the following conditions: missingness > 10%, minimum read depth ≤ 8 reads, allele balance ≤ 20% [24], genotype quality < 30, mappability < 1 (based on 150 bp fragments), or GATK VQSR < 99.6. Only variants with FILTER "PASS" in gnomAD WGS and restricted to the captured protein coding region were kept.

We used ANNOVAR [25] to annotate the variants and aggregate information about allele frequencies (AF) and in silico predictions of deleteriousness. We used population AF from public databases: Exome Aggregation Consortium (ExAC) [26] and Genome Aggregation Database (gnomAD). Rare variants were defined by AF < 0.01% in both ExAC and gnomAD WES datasets. We employed multiple in silico prediction algorithms including PolyPhen 2, metaSVM [27], Combined Annotation Dependent Depletion (CADD) [28], and REVEL (rare exome variant ensemble learner) [29]. We noted that REVEL outperformed other ensemble methods in pathogenicity prediction in a recent comparison using clinical genetic data [30]. We performed further evaluation of the prediction toolkits using de novo missense variants published in a recent CHD study [19] and published de novo variants of unaffected siblings of Simons Simplex Collection [31] as controls. We observed that REVEL-predicted damaging missense de novo variants reached the highest enrichment rate in cases compared to controls (Additional file 1: Figure S1B). Thus, we ultimately used REVEL to define damaging missense variants (D-mis, REVEL > 0.5) in this study.

We identified de novo variants in a set of 60 PAH-CHD trios using methods described previously [18, 32], and manually inspected all candidate de novo variants using the Integrative Genomics Viewer (IGV) [33] to exclude potential false positives.

Identification of rare, deleterious variants in established risk genes

We screened for variants in 11 known risk genes for PAH [5–8]: *ACVRL1*, *BMPR1A*, *BMPR1B*, *BMPR2*, *CAV1*, *EIF2AK4*, *ENG*, *KCNK3*, *SMAD4*, *SMAD9*, and *TBX4*. We also screened for variants in the recently curated list of 253 candidate risk genes for CHD [19]. Variants identified in the PAH-CHD cohort were compared to mutations reported in the literature and in genetic databases (Online Mendelian Inheritance in Man database, Human Genome Mutation Database [34] and ClinVar [35]). We defined deleterious variants as likely gene-disrupting (LGD) (including premature stopgain, frameshift indels, canonical splicing variants, and deletion of exons) or damaging missense with REVEL score > 0.5 (D-mis). Insertion/deletion variants in known risk genes were confirmed with Sanger sequencing and tested for disease segregation when family DNA samples were available.

Statistical analysis

To identify novel candidate risk genes, we performed a case-control association test comparing frequency of rare deleterious variants in each gene in PAH-CHD cases with gnomAD whole genome sequencing (WGS) subjects as population controls. To control for ethnicity, we selected cases of European ancestry ($n = 144$) using principal components analysis (PCA) (*Peddy* software package) [36] (Additional file 1: Figure S1C) and gnomAD subjects of non-Finnish European (NFE) ancestry ($n = 7509$). Since cases and controls were sequenced using different platforms, we assessed the batch effect based on the burden of rare synonymous variants, a variant class that is mostly neutral with respect to disease status. We observed that the frequency of rare

synonymous variants in cases and controls was virtually identical (enrichment rate = 1.01, p value = 0.4) (Additional file 1: Table S3a). The analysis of disease-associated genes was confined to gene-specific enrichment of rare, deleterious variants (AF < 0.01%, LGD or D-mis). We assumed that under the null model, the number of rare deleterious variants observed in cases should follow a binomial distribution, given the total number of such variants in cases and controls, and a rate determined by fraction of cases in total number of subjects (cases and controls). The enrichment rate was then determined by the average number of variants in cases over the sum of average number of variants in cases and controls. The statistical significance of enrichment was tested using binom.test in R. We defined the threshold for genome-wide significance by Bonferroni correction for multiple testing ($n = 17,701$, threshold p value = 2.8e −6). We used the Benjamini-Hochberg procedure to estimate false discovery rate (FDR) by p.adjust in R. All *SOX17* variants reported herein were confirmed with Sanger sequencing and inheritance determined when parental DNA samples were available.

To guard against spurious association results due to population differences or batch effects inherent to the use of publicly available gnomAD data, we repeated the association analysis using a set of 1319 European control subjects with individual level data obtained from the same analytical pipeline and called jointly with the PAH-CHD cases. These controls were comprised of unrelated, unaffected European parents from the Pediatric Cardiac Genomics Consortium [18]. The data were captured using NimbleGen V2.0. We performed principle components analysis of ethnicity with cases and controls together.

To estimate the burden of de novo variants in cases, we calculated the background mutation rate using a previously published tri-nucleotide change table [32, 37] and calculated the rate in protein-coding regions that are uniquely mappable. We assumed that the number of de novo variants of various types (e.g., synonymous, missense, LGD) expected by chance in gene sets or all genes followed a Poisson distribution [32]. For a given type of de novo variant in a gene set, we set the observed number of cases to m1, the expected number to m0, estimated the enrichment rate by (m1/m0), and tested for significance using an exact Poisson test (poisson.test in R) with m0 as the expectation.

Results

Characteristics of the PAH-CHD cohort are shown in Table 1. The cohort included 15 familial and 241 sporadic cases, including 61 parent-child trios and 20 duos. The majority of cases (56%) had an age of PAH onset < 18 years (pediatric-onset). There were more females among both pediatric-onset ($n = 91/53$, 1.7:1 female-to-male ratio)

Table 1 PAH-CHD patient population

	Pediatric	Adult
Male, n (%)	53 (36.8)	24 (21.4)
Female, n (%)	91 (63.2)	88 (78.6)
Total, n (%)	144 (56.3)	112 (43.7)
Female-to-male ratio	1.7:1	3.7:1[a]
Ancestry, n (%)		
East Asian	7 (4.9)	7 (6.3)
Hispanic	30 (20.8)	27 (24.1)
African	13 (9)	6 (5.4)
South Asian	10 (6.9)	7 (6.3)
European	81 (56.3)	63 (56.3)
Unknown	3 (2.1)	2 (1.8)
Primary cardiac defect, %		
Atrial septal defect (ASD)	33.8	55.7
Ventricular septal defect (VSD)	22.5	17.7
ASD + VSD	13.8	7.6
Atrioventricular canal defect	7.5	6.3
Tetralogy of Fallot	5.6	1.3
Transposition of the great vessels	3.8	3.8
Hypoplastic left heart syndrome	1.3	0
Coarctation of the artery	0.6	0
Other/complex	11.3	7.6

[a]Fisher's exact test, $p = 0.009$, indicating a higher female-to-male ratio in adult-onset cases compared to pediatric-onset cases

and adult-onset ($n = 88/24$, 3.7:1) patients, with a significant ~ 2-fold enrichment of females for adult- compared to pediatric-onset PAH ($p = 0.009$) (Table 1). Fifty-six percent of the patients were of European ancestry, 26% Hispanic, and 5–7% each of African, East Asian, or South Asian. The most common cardiac defects were atrial and ventricular septum defects; however, more severe defects were more frequent in pediatric-onset cases.

Rare deleterious variants in known PAH and CHD risk genes

We screened for rare, predicted deleterious variants in 11 known risk genes for PAH and 253 candidate risk genes for CHD (Additional file 1: Table S1). PAH risk gene variants were identified in only 6.4% (16/250) of sporadic PAH-CHD cases and four of 15 familial cases (Additional file 1: Table S2). Of these cases, the majority had pediatric-onset disease (17/144 pediatric vs 3/112 adult, $p = 0.0085$ Fisher's exact test). Most of the rare deleterious variants were identified in BMPR2 ($n = 7$, 6 pediatric) and TBX4 ($n = 7$, all pediatric) with a few variants in BMPR1A (n=1), BMPR1B (1), CAV1 (1), ENG (1), and SMAD9 (2). Parental DNA samples were available for a subset of the cases and three TBX4 variants were

confirmed to be de novo: c.C293G:p.P98R, c.537_546del:p.I801 fs*45, and c.669_671del:p.223_224delF. We performed enrichment analysis for the PAH gene set in all PAH-CHD individuals of European ancestry ($n = 143$), using NFE gnomAD WGS subjects ($n = 7509$) as population controls. Similar frequencies of synonymous variants in cases and controls indicated that potential batch effects were minimal between the two independent datasets (Additional file 1: Table S3a). For the known PAH gene set, we observed a 5.7-fold enrichment of rare deleterious (LGD or D-mis) variants in PAH-CHD ($P = 0.001$) (Additional file 1: Table S3b). In contrast, there was no enrichment of rare deleterious variants in CHD risk genes in cases compared to controls (Additional file 1: Table S3b; Additional file 2: Table S4), indicating that overall these variants contribute little to PAH-CHD risk.

Association analysis identifies transcription factor SOX17 as a new candidate PAH-CHD risk gene

To identify novel risk genes for PAH-CHD, we performed an association analysis comparing per-gene rate of rare deleterious variants in European cases and NFE gnomAD WGS controls. We used a binomial test to assess the significance in 17,701 genes and found SOX17 to be associated with PAH-CHD with genome-wide significance (5/143, 3.3% of cases vs 5/7509, 0.07% of controls; enrichment rate = 52, p value = 5.5e–07) (Fig. 1). Analysis of the depth of coverage in the targeted SOX17 region indicated nearly 100% of gnomAD samples and a slightly lower percentage of PAH-CHD samples attained read depths of at least 10 (Additional file 1: Figure S2), excluding the possibility that the association is driven by coverage difference between cases and population data. No other genes reached the threshold for genome-wide significance. The top associations with a Benjamini-Hochberg FDR < 1.0 are listed in Fig. 1b. Notably, three of these genes (BZW2, FTSJ3, BAZ1B) encode putative SOX17 downstream targets [38] and two have been implicated in CHD (BAZ1B [39]) or cardiac defects associated with syndromic intellectual ability (THOC3 [40]). Similar results were obtained using a smaller cohort of European controls with individual-level data, called and annotated together with the PAH-CHD cases (Additional file 1: Figure S3). Based on the different frequencies between cases and population controls, we estimate that rare deleterious variants in SOX17 contribute to about 3.2% of European PAH-CHD patients.

We then searched for SOX17 variants in the non-European cases in the PAH-CHD cohort, and an additional cohort of 413 idiopathic and familial PAH patients without CHD (IPAH/HPAH) [41]. We identified two additional rare LGD and three additional rare D-mis variants in the PAH-CHD cohort, and one additional rare LGD (Table 2) and two rare D-mis variants in the IPAH/HPAH cohort. Variant c.C398T:p.133L, from a European

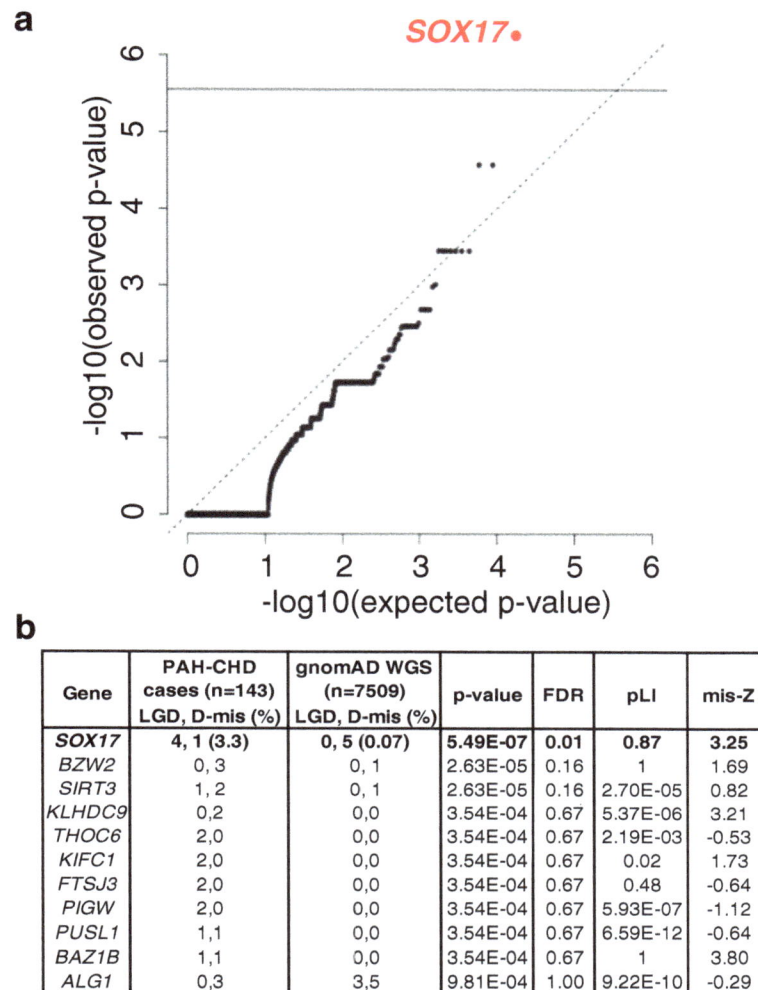

Fig. 1 Significant association of *SOX17* with PAH-CHD. **a** Quantile-quantile plot showing results of test of rare variant association in 17,701 genes, using 143 cases of European ancestry and 7509 gnomAD whole genome sequencing subjects of non-Finnish European ancestry. The association of *SOX17* is genome-wide significant following Bonferroni correction for multiple testing. **b** Table of all genes with *p* value < 0.001 in the association tests. False discovery rate (FDR) was estimated using Benjamini-Hochberg procedure. LGD, likely gene-disrupting; D-mis, damaging missense defined as REVEL score > 0.5

patient, was not included in the initial association analysis due to in silico quality control failure but was later confirmed by Sanger sequencing. Frameshift variant c.489_510del/ p.Q163fs was observed in three unrelated patients of European or Hispanic ancestry. Closer examination of the sequence revealed a 10-bp repeat, once at the start of the deletion and once just downstream (data not shown), suggesting that a replication error may explain the recurrence. Among these three c.489_510del/p.Q163fs mutations, one was a de novo variant and another inherited from an asymptomatic parent (Table 2). Five of the six missense mutations occur within a highly conserved DNA-binding HMG-box domain (Fig. 2a). Three-dimensional modeling indicates that three of these mutations (M76V, N95S, W106L) localize within the DNA binding pocket (Fig. 2b). Comparative sequence

analysis shows that all six of the missense variants are in sites highly conserved between species, including vertebrates and invertebrates (Fig. 2c).

We hypothesized that deleterious variants in *SOX17* confer PAH-CHD risk through dysregulation of SOX17 target genes and some of these genes may contribute to PAH-CHD risk directly, independent of *SOX17*. Therefore, we tested for enrichment of rare variants in 1947 putative *SOX17* target genes identified by genome-wide ChIP-X experiments [38] in European cases compared to NFE gnomAD WGS subjects. We observed a moderate but significant enrichment of rare missense variants (enrichment rate = 1.16, *p* value = 3.4e–4) (Additional file 1: Table S5). Since there are 618 rare missense variants in these genes in 143 cases, even a moderate enrichment suggests a large number

Table 2 Rare deleterious *SOX17* variants identified in 258 PAH-CHD and ⩽13 IPAH/HPAH samples

Proband ID	Gender	Age at dx (years)	Disease class	Heart defect[a]	Ancestry	*SOX17* exon[b]	Nucleotide change	AA change	Inheritance	Allele frequency (gnomAD)	CADD	REVEL score[c]
JM0016	M	5	PAH-CHD	ASD	European	2	c.C398T	p.P133L	Paternal	–	32.0	0.91
JM0025	M	7 months	PAH-CHD	VSD	European	2	c.489_510del	p.Q163fs	De novo	–	33	N/A
JM1277	F	30	PAH-CHD	ASD	Asian	2	c.1203delC	p.D401fs	Unknown	–	24.1	N/A
JM1417	F	3	PAH-CHD	ASD	European	2	c.489_510del	p.Q163fs	Paternal or de novo	–	33	N/A
JM174	F	14	PAH-CHD	ASD	European	2	c.344delG	p.R115fs	Maternal	–	35	N/A
JM654	M	1	PAH-CHD	PDA	Hispanic	1	c.A284G	p.N95S	Unknown	–	24.7	0.93
JM673	M	34	PAH-CHD	ASD	European	2	c.C388T	p.Q130X	Unknown	–	39.0	N/A
JM887	F	3	PAH-CHD	PDA	European	1	c.A226G	p.M76V	Unknown	–	28.7	0.97
JM951	M	9	PAH-CHD	ASD, VSD, AV canal defect, sinus inversus, mitral cleft	Hispanic	2	c.C664G	p.P222A	Unknown	–	26.1	0.57
SPH1070EW5480	F	38	PAH-CHD	Unknown	Hispanic	2	c.A392G	p.D131G	Unknown	–	22.4	0.89
SPH831KB5173	F	32	IPAH	N/A	European	2	c.G317T	p.W106L	Unknown	–	28.4	0.9
JM1363	F	5	IPAH	N/A	Hispanic	2	c.489_510del	p.Q163fs	Maternal	–	33	N/A
FPPH126-01	M	3	HPAH	N/A	European	1	c.72_76del	p.M24fs	Unknown	–	33	N/A

[a]ASD, atrial septal defect; PDA, patent ductus arteriosus; VSD, ventricular septal defect; AV, atrioventricular
[b]*SOX17* variants identified from transcript NM_022454
[c]Rare, deleterious variants defined as gnomAD AF < 0.01% and REVEL > 0.5

of rare variants in *SOX17*-regulated genes may contribute to PAH-CHD risk. Using publicly available gene expression data for developing heart [17] and adult pulmonary artery endothelial cells (ENCODE RNA-seq data, ENCBS024RNA), we found that the majority of the SOX17 target genes with rare deleterious variants are expressed in one or both of these tissue/cell types, with 28% (42/149) having top quartile expression in *both* tissue/cell types (Additional file 1: Table S6 and Fig. S4a). We assessed the statistical significance of this expression pattern by building a background distribution with randomly selected sets of 149 genes that carry at least one rare LGD or D-mis variant in cases and counted the number of genes with top quartile ranked expression in both tissues. Based on 100,000 simulations, the number of observed genes in the top quartile of developing heart and PAEC expression in the SOX17 targets (42 out of 149) is significantly larger than expectation by chance ($p \leq 10{-}5$) (Additional file 1: Figure S4b), supporting functional relevance of these SOX17 target genes. Pathway enrichment analysis using Reactome 2016 [42, 43] through Enrichr (amp.pharm.mssm.edu/Enrichr/enrich) showed that the SOX17 target genes with deleterious variants are over-represented (FDR-adjusted p value < 0.05) in (1) developmental processes, (2) transmembrane transport of small molecules and ion homeostasis, and (3) extracellular matrix interactions (Additional file 1: Table S7).

Contribution of de novo mutations to PAH-CHD

We have previously reported an enrichment of de novo predicted deleterious variants in a CHD cohort ascertained without considering PAH [17, 18]. We tested for a role of de novo mutations in PAH-CHD in 60 cases with WES data of biological parents ("trios"). The complete list of 60 rare de novo variants is provided in Additional file 1: Table S8. As mentioned previously, three de novo variants were identified in PAH risk gene *TBX4* and one variant each in CHD risk genes *NOTCH1* and *PTPN11*. However, testing for enrichment of all rare de novo variants in PAH-CHD trio probands compared to an estimated background mutation rate indicated no overall enrichment, likely due to the small sample size.

Discussion

Exome sequencing in our cohort of 256 PAH-CHD patients indicated that the genetic contribution of known/ candidate risk genes for PAH or CHD alone is minimal. An unbiased, gene-based association analysis of rare deleterious variants identified *SOX17* as a novel PAH-CHD candidate risk gene, explaining up to 3.2% of cases. A recent study of 1038 PAH cases (not including PAH-CHD) also found an association of *SOX17* with IPAH but with a smaller effect size (relative risk ∼ 2.9) [44]. The observed frequency of rare variants was ∼ 0.9% of PAH cases [44], similar to our observation of *SOX17* variants in ∼ 0.7% of IPAH/HPAH patients without CHD. Of note, no rare deleterious *SOX17* variants were identified in a recently published cohort of 1200 patients with CHD [18]. Additionally, we observed an enrichment of rare variants in putative target genes of SOX17. There was no

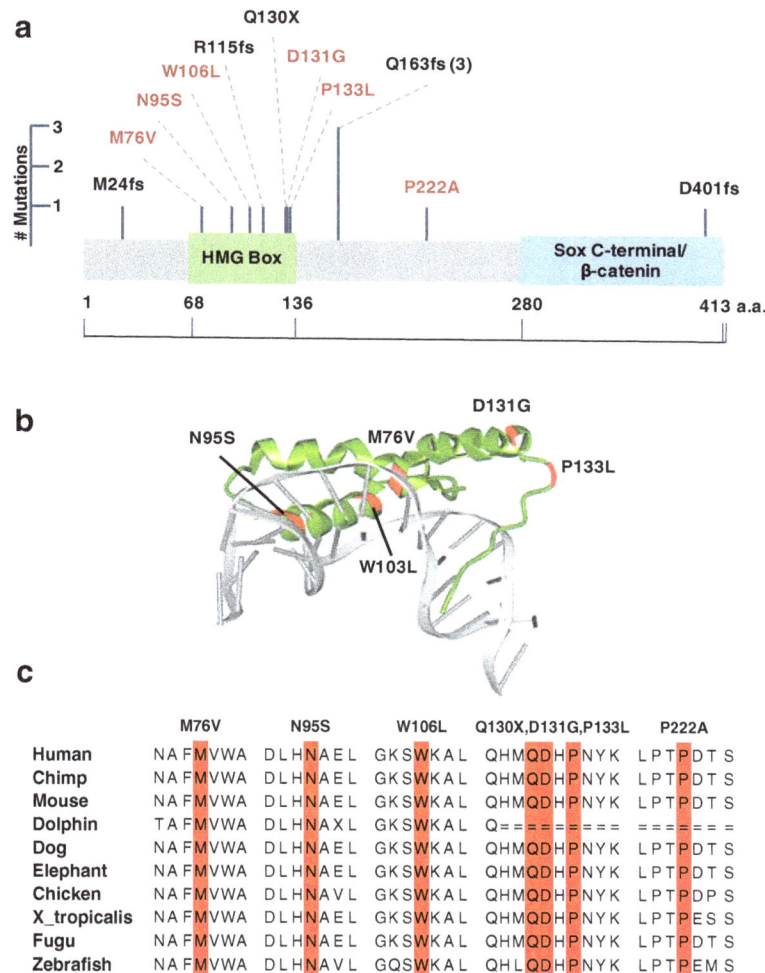

Fig. 2 Rare deleterious variants in *SOX17*. **a** Linear schematic of the *SOX17* encoded protein and location of genetic variants identified by WES. LGD variants are in black, D-mis variants in red. **b** Three-dimensional structure of the *SOX17* HMG box domain, comprised of three alpha-helices, bound to the minor groove of DNA (Protein Data Bank 3F27). Localization of the five patient D-mis variants (red) indicates that three reside within the DNA binding pocket. **c** Multiple sequence alignment indicating a high degree of sequence conservation across species at the locations of *SOX17* missense variants

enrichment of de novo mutations in this cohort, possibly due to the relatively small number of available trios.

SOX17 is a member of the conserved *SOX* family of transcription factors widely expressed in development, and the subgroup of *SOXF* genes (including *SOX7*, *SOX17*, and *SOX18*) participate in vasculogenesis and re-modeling [45]. In the embryonic vasculature, *SOX17* is selectively expressed in arterial endothelial cells [46–48]. Early studies of *Sox17* knock-out mice did not find obvious abnormalities in embryonic vasculature [49, 50], at least partially explained by functional redundancy and compensatory roles of *Sox17* and *Sox18* [50, 51]. Subsequent genetic studies revealed that gene compensation and phenotypic effects were dependent on strain background [52]. Recent endothelial-specific inactivation of *Sox17* in murine embryo or postnatal retina led to impaired arterial specification and embryonic death or arterial-venous malformations, respectively [46]. *SOX17* has also been associated with intracranial aneurysms in genome-wide association studies [53–55], and endothelial-specific *Sox17* deficiency was subsequently shown to induce intracranial aneurysm pathology in an angiotensin II infusion mouse model [56]. Finally, conditional deletion of *Sox17* in mesenchymal progenitor cells demonstrated that SOX17 is required for normal pulmonary vasculature morphogenesis in utero and deficiency results in postnatal cardiac defects [57].

Cardiogenesis occurs in a highly conserved and regulated manner in the developing embryo [58]. Precise temporal and spatial control of gene expression is controlled by master transcription factors such as GATA4, MEF2C, TBX5, and NKX2–5 [59], In addition, signaling pathways, including canonical and non-canonical WNT/

β-catenin [60, 61] and NOTCH [62] signaling cascades, drive cardiac morphogenesis and differentiation. *SOX17* is a direct transcriptional target of GATA4, giving rise to SOX17-positive endoderm from embryonic stem cells [63] and the two proteins co-localize in the primitive endoderm [64, 65]. *SOX17* induction inhibits WNT/ β-catenin signaling by direct protein interaction with β-catenin through a carboxyl terminal domain of SOX17 required for transactivation of target genes [66, 67]. *NOTCH1* has recently been shown to be a direct transcriptional target of SOX17 in early arterial development [68]. Thus, it is possible that impaired functional interactions between these molecules during embryogenesis could provide an underlying mechanism for the development of CHD in some PAH-CHD patients.

SOX17 is a highly constrained gene depleted of LGD and missense variants in a large population data set (ExAC pLI = 0.87, missense Z-score = 3.25) [26]. About half of the observed rare, deleterious variants in cases are LGD variants, and most of the missense variants are located in a conserved HMG box domain. The HMG box is a 79-amino acid domain that binds in a sequence-specific manner within the minor groove of DNA causing bending and facilitating assembly of nucleoprotein complexes [45]. Localization of the five HMG box missense variants within a three-dimensional model of the protein domain interacting with DNA indicated that three of the patient missense mutations (M76V, N95S, W106L) localize to the DNA binding pocket (Fig. 2b). Previously reported site-directed mutagenesis studies indicate that similar point mutations within this region (M76A, G103R) can impair both direct DNA binding [69] and complex nucleoprotein interactions, including SOX17/β-catenin protein complexes, at target gene promoters [70, 71]. This suggests that haploinsufficiency with loss of function alleles is the likely mechanism of *SOX17* risk in PAH-CHD.

Some variants in SOX17 downstream target genes may be predicted to mimic some of the consequences of *SOX17* loss of function mutations or haploinsufficiency. We identified 163 rare deleterious variants (131 D-mis and 32 LGD) in 149 putative target genes. Using published gene expression data, we found that most of these genes are expressed in developing heart and/or pulmonary artery endothelial cells, with significant enrichment of top quartile expression in both tissue/cell types compared to randomly selected sets of genes carrying deleterious variants in European PAH-CHD cases. Additionally, we showed that these target genes are overrepresented in pathways related to developmental biology, ion transport/homeostasis, and extracellular matrix interactions. A wide range of transmembrane small molecule transporters/channels/pumps are expressed in developing heart and pulmonary vasculature, and some have been shown to be differentially expressed in lung tissue from PAH patients compared to non-disease controls or PH with interstitial fibrosis [72]. As key regulators of vascular tone, some of these molecules function as targets of vasodilatory pharmacotherapy [73]. We recently identified the potassium channel gene, *KCNK3*, as a risk gene for PAH using exome sequencing [74]. Extracellular matrix proteins, including laminins, play key roles in embryonic development of both pulmonary vasculature and heart [75]. Thus, it is likely that mutations in *SOX17*, and possibly downstream target genes, may increase risk for PAH-CHD via multiple pathways.

The striking clinical finding was that nine out of 13 patients had pediatric-onset disease. The mean age of PAH onset for all patients with rare *SOX17* variants was 14.2 years. Most of the congenital heart defects were simple (i.e., atrial septal defect, ventricular septal defect, or patent ductus arteriosus). However, most of the patients had severe PAH with systemic or supersystemic resting pulmonary arterial pressures, right ventricular hypertrophy with diminished right ventricular function, and requiring chronic intravenous vasodilator treatment. Severe PAH was observed in all patients carrying variants in the HMG-box domain or the recurrent c.489_510del/ p.Q163fs variant.

Conclusions

Together, these data strongly implicate *SOX17* as a new risk gene contributing to ~ 3% of PAH-CHD cases and suggest that rare variants in genes regulated by SOX17 also contribute to PAH-CHD. Expansion of the number of PAH-CHD patients assessed and characterization of the clinical phenotypes will be important to confirm the role of *SOX17* in PAH-CHD and IPAH, and more precisely estimate the contribution of genes regulated by SOX17 and de novo mutations.

Abbreviations

ACVRL1: Activin A receptor-like 1; AF: Allele frequency; *BMPR1A*: Bone morphogenetic protein receptor type 1A; *BMPR1B*: Bone morphogenetic protein receptor type 1B; *BMPR2*: Bone morphogenetic protein receptor type 2; bp: Base pair; BWA-MEM: Burrows-Wheeler Aligner; CADD: Combined Annotation Dependent Depletion; *CAV1*: Caveolin-1; CHD: Congenital heart disease; D-mis: Damaging missense variants; *EIF2AK4*: Eukaryotic initiation translation factor 2 alpha kinase 4; *ENG*: Endoglin; ExAC: Exome Aggregation Consortium; FDR: False discovery rate; gnomAD: Genome Aggregation Database; IGV: Integrative Genomics Viewer; IPAH: Idiopathic pulmonary arterial hypertension; *KCNK3*: Potassium two-pore-domain channel subfamily K member 3; LGD: Likely gene-disrupting; MLPA: Multiplex ligation-dependent probe amplification; NFE: Non-Finnish Europeans; *NOTCH1*: Notch (Drosophila) homolog 1; PAH: Pulmonary arterial hypertension; PAH-CHD: Pulmonary arterial hypertension associated with congenital heart disease; PCA: Principal components analysis; *PTPN11*: Protein tyrosine phosphatase non-receptor type 11; REVEL: Rare exome variant ensemble learner; RGC: Regeneron Genetics Center; SMAD4: SMAD family member 4; SMAD9: SMAD family member 9; *SOX17*: SRY-related HMG-box family member 17; *TBX4*: T-box 4; TGF-β/BMP: Transforming growth factor beta/bone morphogenetic protein; VQSR: Variant quality score recalibration; WES: Whole exome sequencing; WGS: Whole genome sequencing; WHO: World Health Organization

Acknowledgements
We thank the patients and their families for their generous contribution. Robyn Barst and Jane Morse were critical members of the team to enroll and clinically characterize patients. Patricia Lanzano provided oversight of the Columbia biorepository. Hongjian Qi provided helpful discussions on bioinformatics analysis of WES data.

Funding
Funding support was provided by NHLBI HL060056 (to WKC), NIH/NCATS Colorado Clinical and Translational Science Award UL1 TR001082 (DDI), and The Jayden de Luca Foundation (DDI). Funding for the PAH Biobank was provided by NHLBI R24HL105333 (WCN). Y.S. was partly supported by NIH grant R01GM120609.

Authors' contributions
WKC conceived and designed the study. NZ, YS, WKC, CW, JW, and PMA analyzed and interpreted the data. CW, YS, WKC, NZ, CG-J, and FED wrote the manuscript. LM, UK, and EBR collected the samples and clinical information. DDI, EDA, RH, WCN, MWP, and KAL collected the samples and provided the WES data and clinical information. JDO, AKK, JGR, and AB provided the WES data. All authors contributed to and discussed the results and critically reviewed the manuscript. All authors read and approved the final manuscript.

Competing interests
CG-J, AKK, JGR, JDO, AB, and FD are full time employees of Regeneron Pharmaceuticals Inc. and receive stock options as part of compensation. The remaining authors declare that they have no competing interests.

Author details
[1]Department of Pediatrics, Columbia University Medical Center, New York, NY, USA. [2]Department of Systems Biology, Columbia University Medical Center, New York, NY, USA. [3]Regeneron Genetics Center, Regeneron Pharmaceuticals, Tarrytown, New York, USA. [4]Department of Medicine, Columbia University Medical Center, New York, NY, USA. [5]Department of Pediatric Cardiology, Children's Hospital Colorado, Denver, CO, USA. [6]Department of Pediatrics, Vanderbilt University School of Medicine, Nashville, TN, USA. [7]Division of Human Genetics, Cincinnati Children's Hospital Medical Center, Cincinnati, OH, USA. [8]Department of Pediatrics, University of CincinnatiCollege of Medicine, Cincinnati, OH, USA. [9]Department of Biomedical Informatics, Columbia University, New York, NY, USA. [10]Herbert Irving Comprehensive Cancer Center, Columbia University Medical Center, New York, NY, USA. [11]New York, USA.

References
1. van Dissel AC, Mulder BJ, Bouma BJ. The changing landscape of pulmonary arterial hypertension in the adult with congenital heart disease. J Clin Med. 2017;6(4)
2. Dimopoulos K, Wort SJ, Gatzoulis MA. Pulmonary hypertension related to congenital heart disease: a call for action. Eur Heart J. 2014;35(11):691–700.
3. Li L, Jick S, Breitenstein S, Hernandez G, Michel A, Vizcaya D. Pulmonary arterial hypertension in the USA: an epidemiological study in a large insured pediatric population. Pulm Circ. 2017;7(1):126–36.
4. Marelli AJ, Ionescu-Ittu R, Mackie AS, Guo L, Dendukuri N, Kaouache M. Lifetime prevalence of congenital heart disease in the general population from 2000 to 2010. Circulation. 2014;130(9):749–56.
5. Best DH, Austin ED, Chung WK, Elliott CG. Genetics of pulmonary hypertension. Curr Opin Cardiol. 2014;29(6):520–7.
6. Chida A, Shintani M, Nakayama T, Furutani Y, Hayama E, Inai K, et al. Missense mutations of the BMPR1B (ALK6) gene in childhood idiopathic pulmonary arterial hypertension. Circ J. 2012;76(6):1501–8.
7. Nasim MT, Ogo T, Ahmed M, Randall R, Chowdhury HM, Snape KM, et al. Molecular genetic characterization of SMAD signaling molecules in pulmonary arterial hypertension. Hum Mutat. 2011;32(12):1385–9.
8. Kerstjens-Frederikse WS, Bongers EMHF, Roofthooft MTR, Leter EM, Douwes JM, Van Dijk A, et al. TBX4 mutations (small patella syndrome) are associated with childhood-onset pulmonary arterial hypertension. J Med Genet. 2013;50(8):500–6.
9. Roberts KE, McElroy JJ, Wong WP, Yen E, Widlitz A, Barst RJ, et al. BMPR2 mutations in pulmonary arterial hypertension with congenital heart disease. Eur Respir J. 2004;24(3):371–4.
10. Pfarr N, Fischer C, Ehlken N, Becker-Grunig T, Lopez-Gonzalez V, Gorenflo M, et al. Hemodynamic and genetic analysis in children with idiopathic, heritable, and congenital heart disease associated pulmonary arterial hypertension. Respir Res. 2013;14:3.
11. Levy M, Eyries M, Szezepanski I, Ladouceur M, Nadaud S, Bonnet D, et al. Genetic analyses in a cohort of children with pulmonary hypertension. Eur Respir J. 2016;48(4):1118–26.
12. Vecoli C, Pulignani S, Foffa I, Andreassi MG. Congenital heart disease: the crossroads of genetics, epigenetics and environment. Curr Genomics. 2014;15(5):390–9.
13. Zaidi S, Brueckner M. Genetics and genomics of congenital heart disease. Circ Res. 2017;120(6):923–40.
14. Soemedi R, Wilson IJ, Bentham J, Darlay R, Topf A, Zelenika D, et al. Contribution of global rare copy-number variants to the risk of sporadic congenital heart disease. Am J Hum Genet. 2012;91(3):489–501.
15. Glessner JT, Bick AG, Ito K, Homsy J, Rodriguez-Murillo L, Fromer M, et al. Increased frequency of de novo copy number variants in congenital heart disease by integrative analysis of single nucleotide polymorphism array and exome sequence data. Circ Res. 2014;115(10):884–96.
16. Fahed AC, Gelb BD, Seidman JG, Seidman CE. Genetics of congenital heart disease: the glass half empty. Circ Res. 2013;112(4):707–20.
17. Zaidi S, Choi M, Wakimoto H, Ma L, Jiang J, Overton JD, et al. De novo mutations in histone-modifying genes in congenital heart disease. Nature. 2013;498(7453):220–3.
18. Homsy J, Zaidi S, Shen Y, Ware JS, Samocha KE, Karczewski KJ, et al. De novo mutations in congenital heart disease with neurodevelopmental and other congenital anomalies. Science. 2015;350(6265):1262–6.
19. Jin SC, Homsy J, Zaidi S, Lu Q, Morton S, DePalma SR, et al. Contribution of rare inherited and de novo variants in 2,871 congenital heart disease probands. Nat Genet. 2017;49(11):1593–601.
20. Simonneau G, Robbins IM, Beghetti M, Channick RN, Delcroix M, Denton CP, et al. Updated clinical classification of pulmonary hypertension. J Am Coll Cardiol. 2009;54(1 Suppl):S43–54.
21. Li H, Ruan J, Durbin R. Mapping short DNA sequencing reads and calling variants using mapping quality scores. Genome Res. 2008;18(11):1851–8.

22. DePristo MA, Banks E, Poplin R, Garimella KV, Maguire JR, Hartl C, et al. A framework for variation discovery and genotyping using next-generation DNA sequencing data. Nat Genet. 2011;43(5):491–8.

23. Van der Auwera GA, Carneiro MO, Hartl C, Poplin R, Del Angel G, Levy-Moonshine A, et al. From FastQ data to high confidence variant calls: the Genome Analysis Toolkit best practices pipeline. Curr Protoc Bioinformatics. 2013;43:11 0 1–33.

24. Krumm N, Turner TN, Baker C, Vives L, Mohajeri K, Witherspoon K, et al. Excess of rare, inherited truncating mutations in autism. Nat Genet. 2015; 47(6):582–8.

25. Wang K, Li M, Hakonarson H. ANNOVAR: functional annotation of genetic variants from high-throughput sequencing data. Nucleic Acids Res. 2010; 38(16):e164.

26. Lek M, Karczewski KJ, Minikel EV, Samocha KE, Banks E, Fennell T, et al. Analysis of protein-coding genetic variation in 60,706 humans. Nature. 2016; 536(7616):285–91.

27. Dong C, Wei P, Jian X, Gibbs R, Boerwinkle E, Wang K, et al. Comparison and integration of deleteriousness prediction methods for nonsynonymous SNVs in whole exome sequencing studies. Hum Mol Genet. 2015;24(8): 2125–37.

28. Kircher M, Witten DM, Jain P, O'Roak BJ, Cooper GM, Shendure J. A general framework for estimating the relative pathogenicity of human genetic variants. Nat Genet. 2014;46(3):310–5.

29. Ioannidis NM, Rothstein JH, Pejaver V, Middha S, McDonnell SK, Baheti S, et al. REVEL: an ensemble method for predicting the pathogenicity of rare missense variants. Am J Hum Genet. 2016;99(4):877–85.

30. Ghosh RO, N. Oak, and Plon, S.E. Evaluation of in silico algorithms for use with ACMG/AMP clinical variant interpretation guidelines. bioRxiv. 2017.

31. Iossifov I, O'Roak BJ, Sanders SJ, Ronemus M, Krumm N, Levy D, et al. The contribution of de novo coding mutations to autism spectrum disorder. Nature. 2014;515(7526):216–21.

32. Samocha KE, Robinson EB, Sanders SJ, Stevens C, Sabo A, McGrath LM, et al. A framework for the interpretation of de novo mutation in human disease. Nat Genet. 2014;46(9):944–50.

33. Thorvaldsdottir H, Robinson JT, Mesirov JP. Integrative genomics viewer (IGV): high-performance genomics data visualization and exploration. Brief Bioinform. 2013;14(2):178–92.

34. Stenson PD, Ball EV, Mort M, Phillips AD, Shiel JA, Thomas NS, et al. Human Gene Mutation Database (HGMD): 2003 update. Hum Mutat. 2003;21(6):577–81.

35. Landrum MJ, Lee JM, Riley GR, Jang W, Rubinstein WS, Church DM, et al. ClinVar: public archive of relationships among sequence variation and human phenotype. Nucleic Acids Res. 2014;42(Database issue):D980–5.

36. Pedersen BS, Quinlan AR. Who's who? Detecting and resolving sample anomalies in human DNA sequencing studies with Peddy. Am J Hum Genet. 2017;100(3):406–13.

37. Ware JS, Samocha KE, Homsy J, Daly MJ. Interpreting de novo variation in human disease using denovolyzeR. Curr Protoc Hum Genet. 2015;87:7 25 1–7 15. editorial board, Jonathan L Haines [et al]

38. Lachmann A, Xu H, Krishnan J, Berger SI, Mazloom AR, Ma'ayan A. ChEA: transcription factor regulation inferred from integrating genome-wide ChIP-X experiments. Bioinformatics. 2010;26(19):2438–44.

39. Andersen TA, Troelsen Kde L, Larsen LA. Of mice and men: molecular genetics of congenital heart disease. Cell Mol Life Sci. 2014;71(8):1327–52.

40. Amos JS, Huang L, Thevenon J, Kariminedjad A, Beaulieu CL, Masurel-Paulet A, et al. Autosomal recessive mutations in THOC6 cause intellectual disability: syndrome delineation requiring forward and reverse phenotyping. Clin Genet. 2017;91(1):92–9.

41. Zhu N, Gonzaga-Jauregui C, Welch CL, Ma L, Qi H, King AK, et al. Exome sequencing in children with pulmonary arterial hypertension demonstrates differences compared with adults. Circ Genom Precis Med. 2018;11(4):e001887.

42. Croft D, Mundo AF, Haw R, Milacic M, Weiser J, Wu G, et al. The Reactome pathway knowledgebase. Nucleic Acids Res. 2014;42(Database issue):D472–7.

43. Fabregat A, Sidiropoulos K, Viteri G, Forner O, Marin-Garcia P, Arnau V, et al. Reactome pathway analysis: a high-performance in-memory approach. BMC Bioinformatics. 2017;18(1):142.

44. Graf S, Haimel M, Bleda M, Hadinnapola C, Southgate L, Li W, et al. Identification of rare sequence variation underlying heritable pulmonary arterial hypertension. Nat Commun. 9(1):2018, 1416.

45. Francois M, Koopman P, Beltrame M. SoxF genes: key players in the development of the cardio-vascular system. Int J Biochem Cell Biol. 2010; 42(3):445–8.

46. Corada M, Orsenigo F, Morini MF, Pitulescu ME, Bhat G, Nyqvist D, et al. Sox17 is indispensable for acquisition and maintenance of arterial identity. Nat Commun. 2013;4:2609.

47. Liao WP, Uetzmann L, Burtscher I, Lickert H. Generation of a mouse line expressing Sox17-driven Cre recombinase with specific activity in arteries. Genesis. 2009;47(7):476–83.

48. Sacilotto N, Monteiro R, Fritzsche M, Becker PW, Sanchez-Del-Campo L, Liu K, et al. Analysis of Dll4 regulation reveals a combinatorial role for sox and notch in arterial development. Proc Natl Acad Sci U S A. 2013;110(29): 11893–8.

49. Kanai-Azuma M, Kanai Y, Gad JM, Tajima Y, Taya C, Kurohmaru M, et al. Depletion of definitive gut endoderm in Sox17-null mutant mice. Development. 2002;129(10):2367–79.

50. Sakamoto Y, Hara K, Kanai-Azuma M, Matsui T, Miura Y, Tsunekawa N, et al. Redundant roles of Sox17 and Sox18 in early cardiovascular development of mouse embryos. Biochem Biophys Res Commun. 2007;360(3):539–44.

51. Matsui T, Kanai-Azuma M, Hara K, Matoba S, Hiramatsu R, Kawakami H, et al. Redundant roles of Sox17 and Sox18 in postnatal angiogenesis in mice. J Cell Sci. 2006;119(Pt 17):3513–26.

52. Hosking B, Francois M, Wilhelm D, Orsenigo F, Caprini A, Svingen T, et al. Sox7 and Sox17 are strain-specific modifiers of the lymphangiogenic defects caused by Sox18 dysfunction in mice. Development. 2009;136(14):2385–91.

53. Bilguvar K, Yasuno K, Niemela M, Ruigrok YM, von Und Zu Fraunberg M, van Duijn CM, et al. Susceptibility loci for intracranial aneurysm in European and Japanese populations. Nat Genet. 2008;40(12):1472–7.

54. Yasuno K, Bilguvar K, Bijlenga P, Low SK, Krischek B, Auburger G, et al. Genome-wide association study of intracranial aneurysm identifies three new risk loci. Nat Genet. 2010;42(5):420–5.

55. Foroud T, Koller DL, Lai D, Sauerbeck L, Anderson C, Ko N, et al. Genome-wide association study of intracranial aneurysms confirms role of Anril and SOX17 in disease risk. Stroke. 2012;43(11):2846–52.

56. Lee S, Kim IK, Ahn JS, Woo DC, Kim ST, Song S, et al. Deficiency of endothelium-specific transcription factor Sox17 induces intracranial aneurysm. Circulation. 2015;131(11):995–1005.

57. Lange AW, Haitchi HM, LeCras TD, Sridharan A, Xu Y, Wert SE, et al. Sox17 is required for normal pulmonary vascular morphogenesis. Dev Biol. 2014; 387(1):109–20.

58. Li X, Martinez-Fernandez A, Hartjes KA, Kocher JP, Olson TM, Terzic A, et al. Transcriptional atlas of cardiogenesis maps congenital heart disease interactome. Physiol Genomics. 2014;46(13):482–95.

59. McCulley DJ, Black BL. Transcription factor pathways and congenital heart disease. Curr Top Dev Biol. 2012;100:253–77.

60. Gillers BS, Chiplunkar A, Aly H, Valenta T, Basler K, Christoffels VM, et al. Canonical wnt signaling regulates atrioventricular junction programming and electrophysiological properties. Circ Res. 2015;116(3):398–406.

61. Klaus A, Muller M, Schulz H, Saga Y, Martin JF, Birchmeier W. Wnt/beta-catenin and Bmp signals control distinct sets of transcription factors in cardiac progenitor cells. Proc Natl Acad Sci U S A. 2012;109(27):10921–6.

62. Luxan G, D'Amato G, MacGrogan D, de la Pompa JL. Endocardial notch signaling in cardiac development and disease. Circ Res. 2016;118(1):e1–e18.

63. Holtzinger A, Rosenfeld GE, Evans T. Gata4 directs development of cardiac-inducing endoderm from ES cells. Dev Biol. 2010;337(1):63–73.

64. Artus J, Piliszek A, Hadjantonakis AK. The primitive endoderm lineage of the mouse blastocyst: sequential transcription factor activation and regulation of differentiation by Sox17. Dev Biol. 2011;350(2):393–404.

65. Viotti M, Nowotschin S, Hadjantonakis AK. SOX17 links gut endoderm morphogenesis and germ layer segregation. Nat Cell Biol. 2014;16(12):1146–56.

66. Morrison G, Scognamiglio R, Trumpp A, Smith A. Convergence of cMyc and beta-catenin on Tcf7l1 enables endoderm specification. EMBO J. 2016;35(3):356–68.

67. Zorn AM, Barish GD, Williams BO, Lavender P, Klymkowsky MW, Varmus HE. Regulation of Wnt signaling by Sox proteins: XSox17 alpha/beta and XSox3 physically interact with beta-catenin. Mol Cell. 1999;4(4):487–98.

68. Chiang IK, Fritzsche M, Pichol-Thievend C, Neal A, Holmes K, Lagendijk A, et al. SoxF factors induce Notch1 expression via direct transcriptional regulation during early arterial development. Development. 2017;144(14):2629–39.

69. Sinner D, Kordich JJ, Spence JR, Opoka R, Rankin S, Lin SC, et al. Sox17 and Sox4 differentially regulate beta-catenin/T-cell factor activity and proliferation of colon carcinoma cells. Mol Cell Biol. 2007;27(22):7802–15.

70. Liu X, Luo M, Xie W, Wells JM, Goodheart MJ, Engelhardt JF. Sox17 modulates Wnt3A/beta-catenin-mediated transcriptional activation of the Lef-1 promoter. Am J Physiol Lung Cell Mol Physiol. 2010;299(5):L694–710.

71. Banerjee A, Ray S. Structural insight, mutation and interactions in human beta-catenin and SOX17 protein: a molecular-level outlook for organogenesis. Gene. 2017;610:118–26.
72. Rajkumar R, Konishi K, Richards TJ, Ishizawar DC, Wiechert AC, Kaminski N, et al. Genomewide RNA expression profiling in lung identifies distinct signatures in idiopathic pulmonary arterial hypertension and secondary pulmonary hypertension. Am J Physiol Heart Circ Physiol. 2010;298(4): H1235–48.
73. Olschewski A, Papp R, Nagaraj C, Olschewski H. Ion channels and transporters as therapeutic targets in the pulmonary circulation. Pharmacol Ther. 2014;144(3):349–68.
74. Piovan E, Yu J, Tosello V, Herranz D, Ambesi-Impiombato A, Da Silva AC, et al. Direct reversal of glucocorticoid resistance by AKT inhibition in acute lymphoblastic leukemia. Cancer Cell. 2013;24(6):766–76.
75. Durbeej M. Laminins. Cell Tissue Res. 2010;339(1):259–68.

6

Integrated biology approach reveals molecular and pathological interactions among Alzheimer's A β42, Tau, TREM2, and TYROBP in *Drosophila* models

Michiko Sekiya[1†], Minghui Wang[2,3†], Naoki Fujisaki[1,4], Yasufumi Sakakibara[1], Xiuming Quan[1], Michelle E. Ehrlich[2,5,6], Philip L. De Jager[7,8], David A. Bennett[9], Eric E. Schadt[2,3], Sam Gandy[5,10,11,12], Kanae Ando[13], Bin Zhang[2,3,14*] and Koichi M. Iijima[1,4*]

Abstract

Background: Cerebral amyloidosis, neuroinflammation, and tauopathy are key features of Alzheimer's disease (AD), but interactions among these features remain poorly understood. Our previous multiscale molecular network models of AD revealed *TYROBP* as a key driver of an immune- and microglia-specific network that was robustly associated with AD pathophysiology. Recent genetic studies of AD further identified pathogenic mutations in both *TREM2* and *TYROBP*.

Methods: In this study, we systematically examined molecular and pathological interactions among Aβ, tau, TREM2, and TYROBP by integrating signatures from transgenic *Drosophila* models of AD and transcriptome-wide gene co-expression networks from two human AD cohorts.

Results: Glial expression of TREM2/TYROBP exacerbated tau-mediated neurodegeneration and synergistically affected pathways underlying late-onset AD pathology, while neuronal Aβ42 and glial TREM2/TYROBP synergistically altered expression of the genes in synaptic function and immune modules in AD.

Conclusions: The comprehensive pathological and molecular data generated through this study strongly validate the causal role of *TREM2/TYROBP* in driving molecular networks in AD and AD-related phenotypes in flies.

Keywords: Alzheimer's disease, Amyloid-β (Aβ) peptides, Microtubule-associated protein tau, *TYROBP* (tyrosine kinase binding protein), *TREM2* (triggering receptor expressed on myeloid cells 2), Differential expression, Gene co-expression network, Gene module, Synaptophagy, Immune function, Neurodegeneration

Background

Alzheimer's disease (AD) is the leading cause of neurodegeneration and dementia. At the level of neuropathology, AD is characterized by aggregation and accumulation of two proteins, β-amyloid peptides (Aβ) and the microtubule-associated protein tau [1]. It is accompanied by the activation of multiple neuroinflammatory pathways [2]. Lines of evidence from laboratories and clinics worldwide support the concept that accumulation of Aβ peptides can be an initiating factor and can lie upstream of tau to drive synaptic dysfunction, neuron death and cognitive impairment [3–7].

A new model was developed to account for the fact that up to one-third of patients with clinically diagnosed AD have no evidence of amyloidosis on brain amyloid imaging [8]. Alternatively, some older individuals with neuropathological AD were asymptomatic during their lifetime [9]. These clinicopathological studies indicate that disease progression is a complex process resulting from the interplay of a number of genetic and

* Correspondence: bin.zhang@mssm.edu; iijimakm@ncgg.go.jp
†Equal contributors
²Department of Genetics & Genomic Sciences, Icahn School of Medicine at Mount Sinai, 1470 Madison Avenue, Room 8-111, Box 1498, New York, NY 10029, USA
¹Department of Alzheimer's Disease Research, National Center for Geriatrics and Gerontology, 7-430 Morioka-cho, Obu, Aichi 474-8511, Japan
Full list of author information is available at the end of the article

environmental factors, some of which modulate accumulation of neuropathology while others modulate synaptic and neuronal resilience [10]. System-level analyses of large datasets from patients have emerged as powerful tools for understanding complex diseases such as AD. Gene expression datasets, along with genomic and clinical information from multiple studies, continue to accumulate and data interpretation is becoming a difficult challenge in these "omics" approaches.

Gene regulatory network analysis is a powerful tool in identifying gene modules pathologically related to human complex diseases including AD [11, 12]. We employed an integrative multiscale network analysis approach to identify key molecular interactions of cellular pathways and causal regulators underlying pathological changes in AD. This approach identified *TYROBP* (tyrosine kinase binding protein, also known as *DAP12*), the intracellular adaptor of *TREM2* (triggering receptor expressed on myeloid cells 2), as a key driver of immune- and microglia-specific networks that are associated with LOAD pathology [11, 13]. Genome-wide association studies (GWAS) revealed that *TREM2*, a *TYROBP*-binding protein, is a risk gene for late-onset sporadic AD [14–16]. More recently, *TYROBP*-coding sequence genetic variants were found to contribute to an increased risk of early-onset AD [17]. Moreover, TREM2/TYROBP signaling is upregulated by plaque-associated myeloid cells in AD brains and in APP transgenic mice [18–20]. An ectodomain of TREM2 is cleaved and released into the extracellular space as a soluble form (sTREM2) and sTREM2 levels in CSF are elevated in the early symptomatic phase of AD [21–23]. Interestingly, this cleavage of TREM2 is reduced by pathogenic mutations for AD [24, 25]. These reports underscore the role of *TREM2/TYROBP* in AD pathogenesis.

TREM2 encodes a receptor expressed exclusively in the immune cells in the brain [26, 27]. Studies with *TREM2*-deficient AD model mice suggest that TREM2 may influence phagocytosis of Aβ-lipid complexes as well as microglial survival [28] and metabolic fitness [29]. Microglia forms a barrier to restrict Aβ plaque growth and diffusion of soluble Aβ oligomers [30], thereby ameliorating tau pathology in AD mouse models [31–33]. *TREM2* deficiency or the AD-associated R47H mutation in *TREM2* significantly reduced accumulation of microglia around Aβ plaques [28, 34]. A recent study also shows that some effects of *TREM2* on Aβ pathology may be disease-stage-dependent [33].

By contrast, activation of microglia can play not only beneficial but also detrimental roles in plaque-related neuropathology. Microglia in adult brains engulf spines and other synaptic processes; exposure to Aβ may inappropriately activate this process to mediate synapse loss [35]. This "synaptophagy" involves complement and CR3, which, like TREM2, can provide an ectodomain

protein that interacts with TYROBP [36]. Intriguingly, *TYROBP* deficiency in APPswe/PS1dE9 mice reduces plaque-associated microglia with improved electrophysiological and learning behavior effects [37]. In addition, TREM2 overexpression failed to improve neuropathology and cognitive impairment in aged APPswe/PS1dE9 mice [38]. More recent studies demonstrate that TREM2 pathway promotes the transition from homeostatic to disease-associated microglia in brains of AD model mice [39, 40].

These reports are consistent with a model wherein TREM2/TYROBP signaling is activated as a protective response against Aβ pathology; however, sustained TREM2/TYROBP activation may ultimately aggravate inflammatory and synapse-related pathologies, thereby driving AD progression. Thus, elucidation of the molecular basis for various interrelationships involving Aβ, TREM2/TYROBP, and tau may fill some gaps in our understanding of AD pathogenesis.

In this study, we aimed to decipher molecular interactions among Aβ, TREM2/TYROBP, and tau by integrating gene expression signatures associated with TREM2/TYROBP from AD *Drosophila* models and transcriptome-wide gene co-expression networks from two human AD cohorts including Harvard Brain Tissue Resource Center (HBTRC) [11], and the Religious Orders Study and the Rush Memory and Aging Project (ROSMAP) [41, 42]. The impact of an AD-associated TREM2 R47H variant on these molecular interactions was also analyzed. Our data demonstrate that co-expression of neuronal Aβ42 with glial TREM2^{R47H}/TYROBP led to synergistic downregulation of genes associated with synaptic function modules in fly brains. Moreover, glial expression of both TREM2^{WT}/TYROBP and TREM2^{R47H}/TYROBP exacerbated tau toxicity and synergistically affected the pathways implicated in AD-related neurodegeneration. Thus, gene regulatory networks highlighted by this unbiased, cross species analysis appeared to recapitulate some key features of AD progression and support a key driver role for *TREM2/TYROBP* in AD pathogenesis.

Methods
Drosophila genetics
Flies were maintained in standard cornmeal media at 25 °C. Complementary DNA (cDNA) encoding the full length of *TREM2* (NM_018965, RC221132) and *TYROBP* (NM_198125, RC203771) with Myc-DDK tag were obtained from OriGene Technologies, Inc. These constructs were subcloned into a pJFRC19-13XLexAop2 vector (Addgene #26224). *TREM2R47H* mutation was introduced by using site-directed mutagenesis kit (Takara Bio Inc.). Transgenic flies were generated by PhiC31 integrase-mediated transgenesis systems (Best Gene Inc.). Transgenic fly lines carrying UAS-Aβ42 and UAS-tau were previously described [43–45]. Repo-LexA

(#67096), Elav-GAL4 (#458), GMR-GAL4 (#1104), UAS-para RNAi (#31626), and UAS-mcherry RNAi (#35785) were obtained from the Bloomington Stock Center. For RNA sequencing (RNA-seq), around seven-day-old male flies were used. All experiments were performed using age-matched male flies.

Western blotting

Fly heads for each genotype were homogenized in appropriate buffer and subjected to western blotting or co-immunoprecipitation. Details for western blotting and sequential extractions of Aβ42 were performed as previously described [44]. Anti-FLAG (Sigma-Aldrich), anti-TREM2 (Cell signaling), anti-tau (Millipore), anti-non phospho tau (Merck Millipore), anti-pThr231 tau (Thermo Fisher Scientific), anti-pSer262 tau (Abcam), and anti-tubulin (Sigma-Aldrich) for western blotting were purchased.

Histological analysis

Heads of male or female flies were fixed in 4% paraformaldehyde for 24 h at 4 °C and embedded in paraffin. Serial sections (6-μm thickness) through the entire heads were prepared, stained with hematoxylin and eosin (Sigma-Aldrich), and examined by bright-field microscopy. Images of the sections were captured with Axio-Cam 105 color (Carl Zeiss); the vacuole area was measured using Image J (NIH).

Climbing assay

Approximately 25 flies were placed in an empty plastic vial. The vial was then gently tapped to knock all of the flies to the bottom. The numbers of flies in the top, middle, or bottom thirds of the vial were scored after 10 s. The percentages of flies that stayed at the bottom were subjected to statistical analyses. Experiments were repeated more than three times and a representative result was shown.

Courtship-conditioning assay

Courtship-conditioning assay was performed using the method by Ishimoto et al. [46, 47]. Unreceptive, mated-females were prepared as "trainers" one day before the conditioning. For training, a three- to five-day-old virgin male was placed with a trainer female in the courtship chamber (15 mm in diameter × 5 mm in depth) for 1 h. Trained males and non-trained naïve males were tested with freeze-killed virgin females as a courtship target in the courtship chamber 1 h after training. The courtship index (CI) was defined as the proportion of time spent in courtship behavior during 10 min observation period. We used more than 60 flies for each genotype. CIs for conditioned males and naïve controls were analyzed by Mann–Whitney U test. To compare the memory performances of each genotype, experimental data are presented as the performance index (PI), which was calculated using the following formula. $PI = 100 \times (CI^{\text{average for naïve}} - CI^{\text{conditioned}})/CI^{\text{average for naïve}}$, after CIs were subjected to arcsine square root transformation to approximate normal distributions.

Reverse transcription polymerase chain reaction (RT-PCR) and quantitative reverse transcription polymerase chain reaction (qRT-PCR)

RNA extraction was described below (RNA-seq and analyses). Total RNA was reverse-transcribed using PrimeScript RT-PCR kit (TaKaRa Bio) and the resulting cDNA was used as a template for PCR (Veriti, Applied Biosystems). PCR products were analyzed by 1% agarose gel.

qRT-PCR was performed using PowerSYBR (Thermo Fisher Scientific) on a CFX96 real-time PCR detection system (Bio-Rad Laboratories). The average threshold cycle value (CT) was calculated from at least three replicates per sample. Expression of genes of interest was standardized relative to GAPDH1. Relative expression values were determined by the ΔΔCT method. Primers were designed using Primer-Blast (NIH) or FlyPrimer-Bank [48] as described in Additional file 1: Table S11.

RNA sequencing and analyses

More than 100 flies for each genotype were collected and frozen. Heads were mechanically isolated and total RNA was extracted using TRIzol Reagent (Invitrogen, Thermo Fisher Scientific) according to the manufacturer's protocol with an additional centrifugation step (16,000 × g for 10 min) to remove cuticle membranes before the addition of chloroform. Total RNA was purified using phenol-chloroform reagents after treatment with DNAaseI.

Preparation of samples for RNA-seq analysis was performed using the TruSeq RNA Sample Preparation Kit v2 (Illumina). Briefly, ribosomal RNA was depleted from total RNA using the Ribo-Zero rRNA Removal Kit (Human/Mouse/Rat) (Illumina) to enrich for coding RNA and long non-coding RNA. The cDNA was synthesized using random hexamers, end-repaired, and ligated with appropriate adaptors for sequencing. The library then underwent size selection and purification using AMPure XP beads (Beckman Coulter). The appropriate Illumina recommended 6-bp bar-code bases are introduced at one end of the adaptors during PCR amplification step. The size and concentration of the RNA-seq libraries were measured by Bioanalyzer (Agilent) and Qubit fluorometry (Life Technologies, Thermo Fisher Scientific) before loading onto the sequencer. The Ribo-Zero libraries were sequenced on the Illumina HiSeq 2500 System with 100 nucleotide single-end reads, according to the standard manufacturer's protocol (Illumina).

Single-ended RNA-seq data were generated with the Illumina HiSeq 2500 platform following the Illumina protocol. The raw sequencing reads were aligned to fly genome BDGP6 using star aligner (version 2.5.0b). Following read alignment, featureCounts [49] was used to quantify the gene expression at the gene level based on Ensembl gene model. Genes with at least 5 reads in at least one sample were considered expressed and hence retained for further analysis, otherwise removed. The gene level read counts data were normalized using trimmed mean of M-values normalization (TMM) method [50] to adjust for sequencing library size difference.

Differential gene expression between different genotypes was predicted by linear model analysis using Bioconductor package LIMMA [51]. RNA integrity number (RIN) score was incorporated as a covariate in the linear model to control for sample quality. To adjust for multiple tests, false discovery rate (FDR) of the differential expression test was estimated using the Benjamini–Hochberg (BH) method [52]. Genes with FDR < 0.05 and log2 fold change > 1 or < − 1 were considered significant.

Functional enrichment analysis (FEA)

For FEA of differential expression gene signatures, the gene ontology (GO) annotations were obtained from the flyBase database. Then the enrichment analysis was carried out using Fisher's exact test (FET), assuming the genes in different sets were identically independently sampled from the genome-wide genes profiled. The BH approach was employed to constrain the FDR.

ROSMAP AD cohort network analysis

We utilized large-scale RNA-seq data of the ROSMAP AD cohort to build a gene co-expression network to capture the coordinated regulation of gene expression traits in brain samples. This dataset profiled gene expression of postmortem brain samples from two longitudinal studies of aging and AD [41, 42]. In both studies, participants enroll without dementia and agree to annual clinical evaluation and organ donation at death. As a result, most decedents are old, without dementia and few participants reach end stage dementia before death. They differ from the types of cases obtained in tertiary care clinics [53]. In the ROSMAP dataset, there were 1059 samples including 362 AD cases and 697 controls. We downloaded preprocessed RNA-seq FPKM gene expression abundance data, SNP genotype data, and DNA methylation data from Synapse (https://doi.org/10.7303/syn3219045). We downloaded preprocessed RNA-seq FPKM gene expression abundance data from Synapse (https://doi.org/10.7303/syn3388564). Genes with at least 1 FPKM in at least 10% of the samples were selected and then the data were corrected for confounding factors including batch, PMI, sex, and RIN score. Co-expression network was constructed by using R package WINA [12], which implements a computationally optimized procedure for weighted gene co-expression network analysis (WGCNA) [54]. In WINA analysis, we used power $\beta = 6$ with other parameters set by default. Thirty-five modules (i.e. clusters of gene showing highly correlated expression profiles across samples) were identified, which were annotated by the mostly enriched gene ontology/canonical pathway term. The modules were rank sorted in relation to AD pathology by multiple sorting features computed from the ROSMAP data, including module-trait correlations and enrichment for AD-related disease gene signatures including DEGs and trait-correlated genes (TCGs) regarding neuropathological/clinical traits such as Braak staging, cognitive score, CERAD neuropathological category, and NIA-Reagan score.

Bayesian causal network was constructed by integrating genome-wide gene expression, SNP genotype, DNA methylation, and known transcription factor (TF)-target relationships. Briefly, we first computed expression quantitative trait loci (eQTLs) and then employed a formal statistical causal inference test (CIT) [55] to infer the causal probability between gene pairs associated with the same eQTL. With a similar strategy, we also computed causal probability of gene pairs mediated or regulated by a DNA methylation site. The causal relationships inferred were combined with TF-target relationships, and together they were subsequently used as priors for building a causal network through a Monte Carlo Markov Chain (MCMC) simulation-based procedure [56].

Statistical analysis for biological assay

All results were expressed as mean ± SEM. Unpaired Student's t-test (Prism7, GraphPad Software Inc.) was used to determine statistical significance as indicated in the figure legends. * indicates $p < 0.05$, ** indicates $p < 0.01$ and *** indicates $p < 0.001$ for biological assays throughout the manuscript.

Data availability

RNA-seq raw data have been deposited in the Gene Expression Omnibus (GEO) database under accession number GSE99012.

Results

The hypothesis underlying this work was that TREM2/TYROBP plays a causal role in driving molecular networks in AD [11]. To test this hypothesis, we used *Drosophila* to identify molecular interactions between neuronal expression of Aβ42 or tau and glial expression of TREM2/TYROBP.

Figure 1 shows an overview of the design and data analysis in the present paper. Briefly, we developed

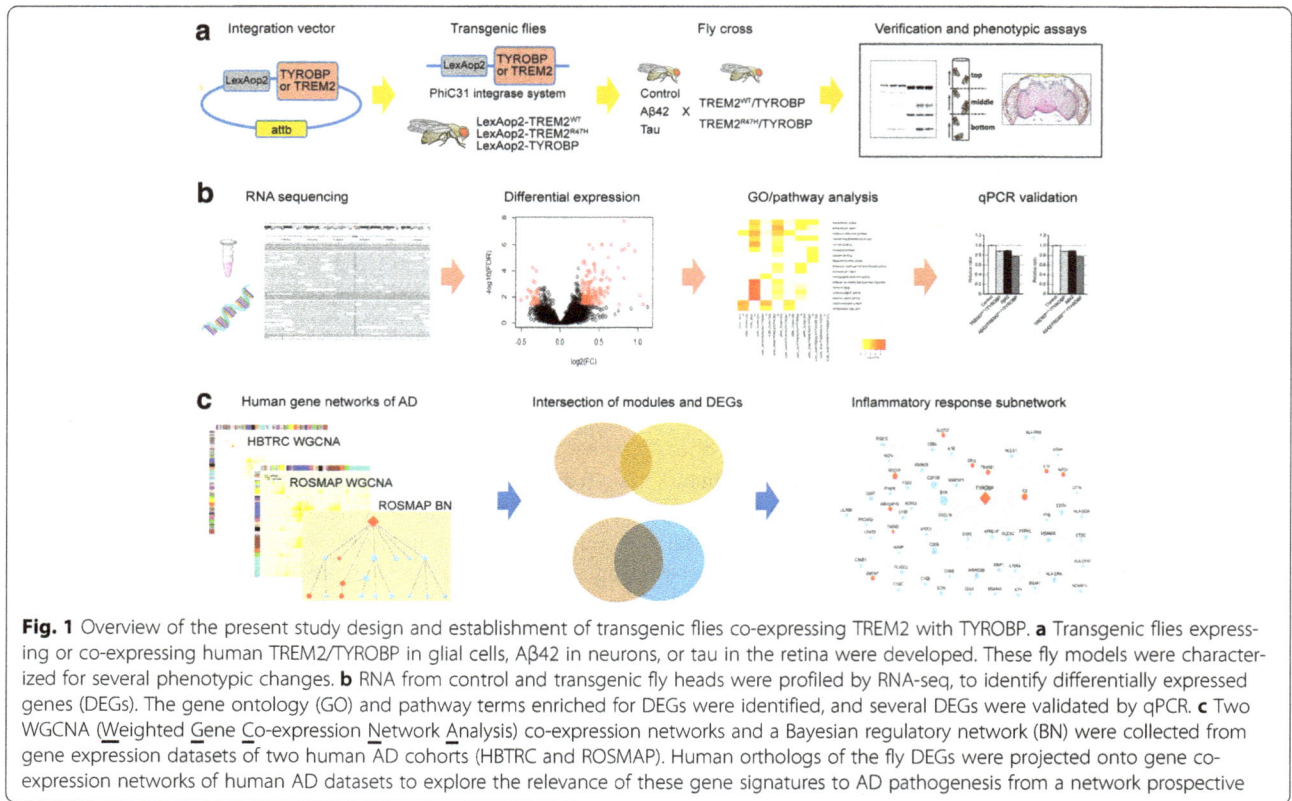

Fig. 1 Overview of the present study design and establishment of transgenic flies co-expressing TREM2 with TYROBP. **a** Transgenic flies express-ing or co-expressing human TREM2/TYROBP in glial cells, Aβ42 in neurons, or tau in the retina were developed. These fly models were character-ized for several phenotypic changes. **b** RNA from control and transgenic fly heads were profiled by RNA-seq, to identify differentially expressed genes (DEGs). The gene ontology (GO) and pathway terms enriched for DEGs were identified, and several DEGs were validated by qPCR. **c** Two WGCNA (Weighted Gene Co-expression Network Analysis) co-expression networks and a Bayesian regulatory network (BN) were collected from gene expression datasets of two human AD cohorts (HBTRC and ROSMAP). Human orthologs of the fly DEGs were projected onto gene co-expression networks of human AD datasets to explore the relevance of these gene signatures to AD pathogenesis from a network prospective

transgenic fly models expressing or co-expressing hu-man TREM2^{WT}/TYROBP or TREM2^{R47H}/TYROBP in glial cells, Aβ42 in neurons, or tau in the retina. These transgenic fly models were characterized for several phenotypic changes including Aβ42 accumulation, the status of tau phosphorylation levels, behavioral deficits, and neurodegeneration. Then transcriptome-wide gene expression in control and transgenic fly heads were pro-filed by RNA-seq to identify differentially expressed gene (DEG) signatures between different genotype groups. The GO and pathway terms enriched in the DEG signa-tures were identified. Several DEGs were validated by qPCR. Lastly, human orthologs of the fly DEG signatures were projected onto gene networks from human AD datasets to explore the relevance of these gene signa-tures to AD pathogenesis from a network prospective. Gene regulatory relationship was characterized for a highlighted inflammatory response subnetwork using Bayesian network analysis.

Establishment of transgenic flies co-expressing TREM2 (TREM2^{WT}) or TREM2 with pathogenic R47H variant (TREM2^{R47H}) with TYROBP in glial cells

In order to co-express human TREM2 and TYROBP in fly glial cells, we generated transgenic flies carrying wild-

type (WT) human TREM2 (TREM2^{WT}), TREM2 with AD-related R47H variant (TREM2^{R47H}), or TYROBP under the control of a tissue-specific LexA operator [57]. Expression of each transgene was driven by a pan-glial driver Repo-LexA, and their messenger RNA (mRNA) ex-pression was confirmed by RT-PCR analysis (Fig. 2a).

We found that, while the expression of TYROBP pro-teins was readily detectable by western blotting, TREM2 protein levels were undetectable, raising the possibility that ectopically expressed human TREM2 proteins may be unstable in fly glial cells perhaps because a binding partner that is required to stabilize TREM2 protein was absent (Fig. 2b). Indeed, when TREM2 and TYROBP transgenes were combined and co-expressed in fly glial cells, TREM2 proteins became readily detectable (Fig. 2c). A prior report showed that R47H mutation reduced the stability of TREM2 proteins [58]. We compared protein levels of TREM2^{WT} and TREM2^{R47H} in fly brains and found no significant difference between them (Fig. 2c). When TYROBP was immunoprecipitated from the lysate of bigenic fly brains co-expressing TYROBP and TREM2, TREM2 proteins (both TREM2^{WT} and TREM2^{R47H}) were also precipitated, indicating that TREM2 and TYROBP proteins interact and stabilize each other in fly glial cells (Fig. 2d).

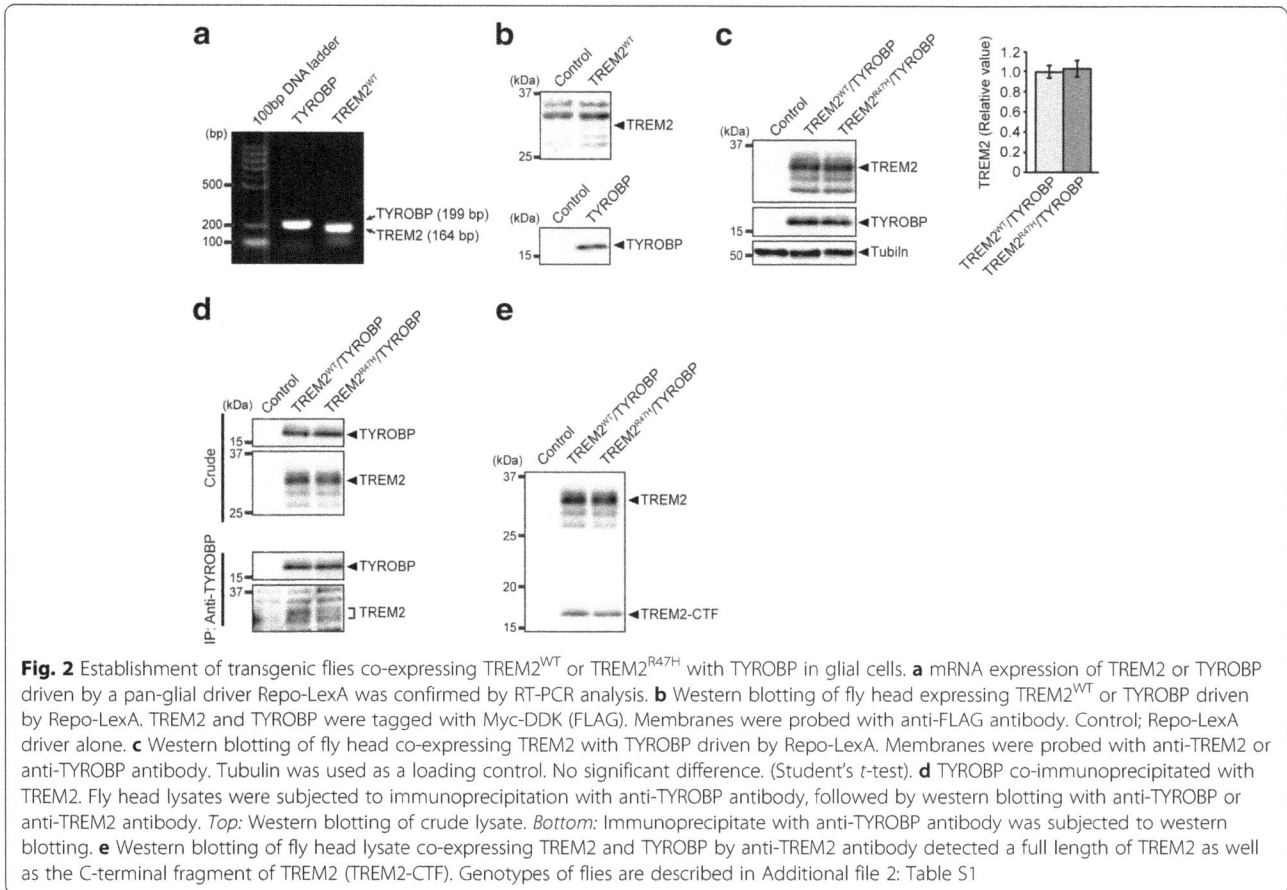

Fig. 2 Establishment of transgenic flies co-expressing TREM2^WT^ or TREM2^R47H^ with TYROBP in glial cells. **a** mRNA expression of TREM2 or TYROBP driven by a pan-glial driver Repo-LexA was confirmed by RT-PCR analysis. **b** Western blotting of fly head expressing TREM2^WT^ or TYROBP driven by Repo-LexA. TREM2 and TYROBP were tagged with Myc-DDK (FLAG). Membranes were probed with anti-FLAG antibody. Control; Repo-LexA driver alone. **c** Western blotting of fly head co-expressing TREM2 with TYROBP driven by Repo-LexA. Membranes were probed with anti-TREM2 or anti-TYROBP antibody. Tubulin was used as a loading control. No significant difference. (Student's t-test). **d** TYROBP co-immunoprecipitated with TREM2. Fly head lysates were subjected to immunoprecipitation with anti-TYROBP antibody, followed by western blotting with anti-TYROBP or anti-TREM2 antibody. *Top:* Western blotting of crude lysate. *Bottom:* Immunoprecipitate with anti-TYROBP antibody was subjected to western blotting. **e** Western blotting of fly head lysate co-expressing TREM2 and TYROBP by anti-TREM2 antibody detected a full length of TREM2 as well as the C-terminal fragment of TREM2 (TREM2-CTF). Genotypes of flies are described in Additional file 2: Table S1

In mammalian cells, TREM2 is cleaved by α-secretase, which results in production of N- and C-terminal fragments of TREM2 [59]. The N-terminal fragments of TREM2 are secreted (sTREM2) and promote inflammatory responses [60], while C-terminal fragments of TREM2 are further processed by γ-secretase [59]. Western blotting using an anti-TREM2 antibody detected the C-terminal fragment of both TREM2^WT^ and TREM2^R47H^ (Fig. 2e), suggesting that TREM2 is processed and that sTREM2 is produced in fly glial cells in a manner similar to that observed in mammalian cells.

FEA revealed that significant overlap between molecular pathways affected by neuronal expression of Aβ42 and those affected by glial expression of TREM2^WT^/TYROBP in fly brains

To gain insights into the effects of glial expression of TREM2/TYROBP in the fly brains at the molecular level, we generated RNA-seq data from the brain samples in control flies (control) and flies with co-expression of TREM2^WT^ and TYROBP (TREM2^WT^/TYROBP). Differentially expressed genes between control and TREM2/TYROBP flies were identified using two criteria including fold change > 1.2 and a FDR < 0.05 in an analysis using

linear models implemented using the R package LIMMA [61]. Expression of TREM2^WT^/TYROBP resulted in upregulation of 239 genes and downregulation of 373 genes (Fig. 3a and Additional file 2: Table S1).

Since TREM2/TYROBP signaling is known to promote survival of microglial cells [28], we evaluated whether ectopic expression of TREM2 and TYROBP induced any structural changes in the fly brain and/or significantly altered the number of glial cells or neurons. No significant alteration in the size or gross morphology of brain structures was observed in TREM2^WT^/TYROBP bigenic flies (Additional file 1: Figure S1). In addition, immunostaining of fly brains against a glial marker protein, Repo, or a neuronal marker, Elav, revealed that the numbers of glial cells or neurons were not significantly different between control and TREM2^WT^/TYROBP bigenic fly brains (Additional file 1: Figure S1). These results suggest that gene expression changes induced by ectopic expression of TREM2^WT^/TYROBP are not due to either structural defects or altered number of neurons or glial cells in the fly brain.

To identify the biological pathways that are affected by glial expression of TREM2^WT^/TYROBP, we performed functional enrichment analysis (FEA) for the DEG

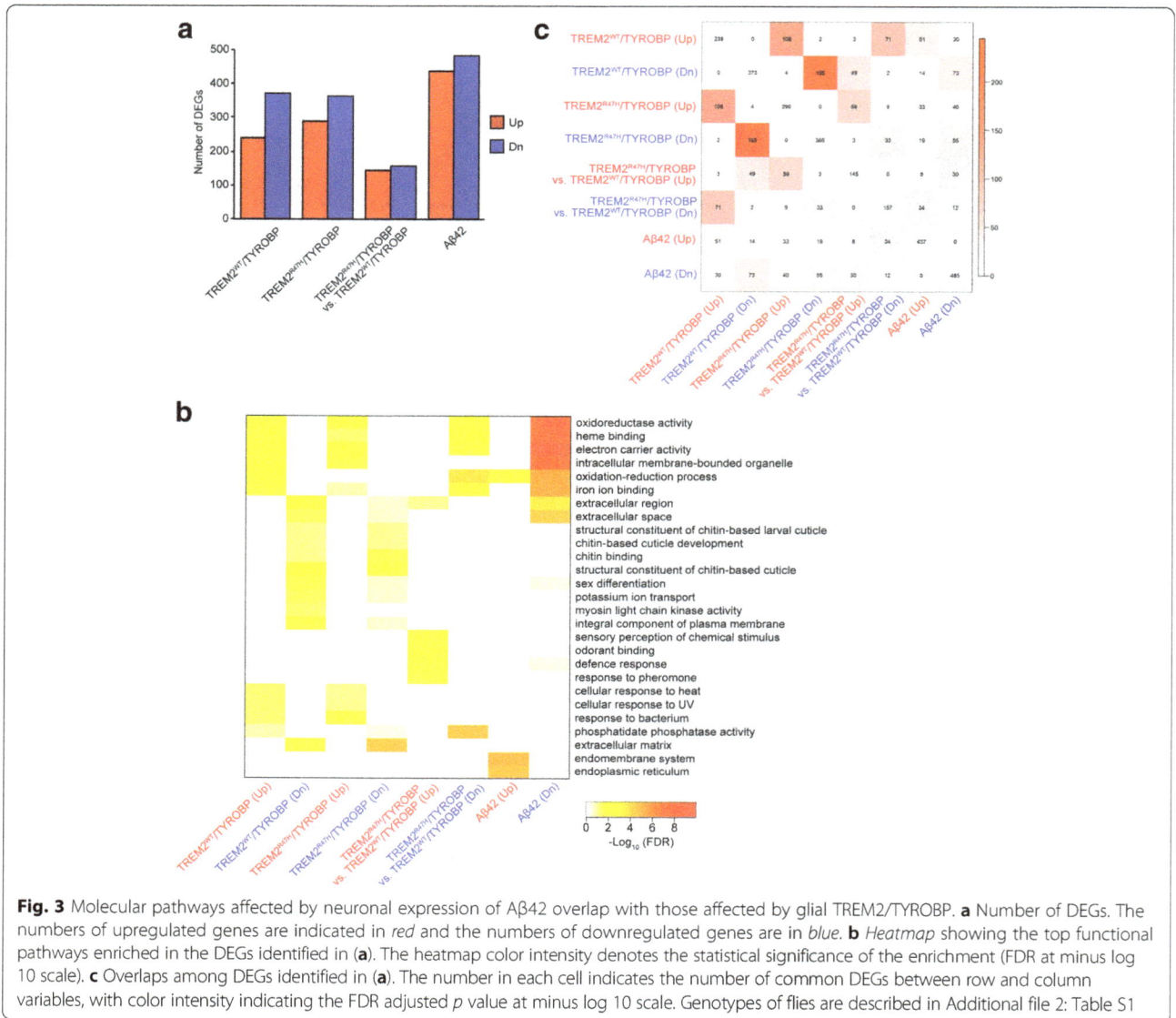

Fig. 3 Molecular pathways affected by neuronal expression of Aβ42 overlap with those affected by glial TREM2/TYROBP. **a** Number of DEGs. The numbers of upregulated genes are indicated in *red* and the numbers of downregulated genes are in *blue*. **b** *Heatmap* showing the top functional pathways enriched in the DEGs identified in (**a**). The heatmap color intensity denotes the statistical significance of the enrichment (FDR at minus log 10 scale). **c** Overlaps among DEGs identified in (**a**). The number in each cell indicates the number of common DEGs between row and column variables, with color intensity indicating the FDR adjusted *p* value at minus log 10 scale. Genotypes of flies are described in Additional file 2: Table S1

signatures using GO annotation. The genes upregulated by the expression of TREM2^{WT}/TYROBP were significantly enriched (multiple testing corrected FET *p* value < 0.05) for pathways designated as "oxidoreductase activity, acting on paired donors, with incorporation or reduction of molecular oxygen," "intracellular membrane-bounded organelle," "electron carrier activity," "heme binding," "iron ion binding," "oxidation-reduction process," and "cellular response to heat" (Fig. 3b and Additional file 3: Table S2). In contrast, the genes downregulated by the expression of TREM2^{WT}/TYROBP were enriched (corrected FET *p* < 0.05) in the pathways including "integral component of plasma membrane," "extracellular region," "extracellular matrix," "structural constituent of chitin-based cuticle," "extracellular space," "potassium ion transport," and "myosin light chain kinase activity" (Fig. 3b and Additional file 3: Table S2).

We next compared molecular pathways affected by glial expression of TREM2^{WT}/TYROBP and those affected by neuronal expression of Aβ42 in fly brains. In mammals, the majority of Aβ peptides are produced from amyloid precursor protein (APP) in the late secretory pathway [62]. In our Aβ42 fly model, a signal sequence was fused to the N-terminus of Aβ42 [43] to target the peptide to the secretory pathway of neurons. Western blot analysis detected monomeric forms of Aβ42 as 4 kDa signals (Fig. 4a and [43]) and immunoprecipitation followed by mass spectrometry analysis confirmed that the fused signal peptide was correctly cleaved and intact Aβ42 peptides were produced [43]. Although this Aβ42 fly model directly expressed Aβ42 peptides in the endoplasmic reticulum, immuno-electron microscopy (Immuno-EM) detected Aβ42 signals in the secretory

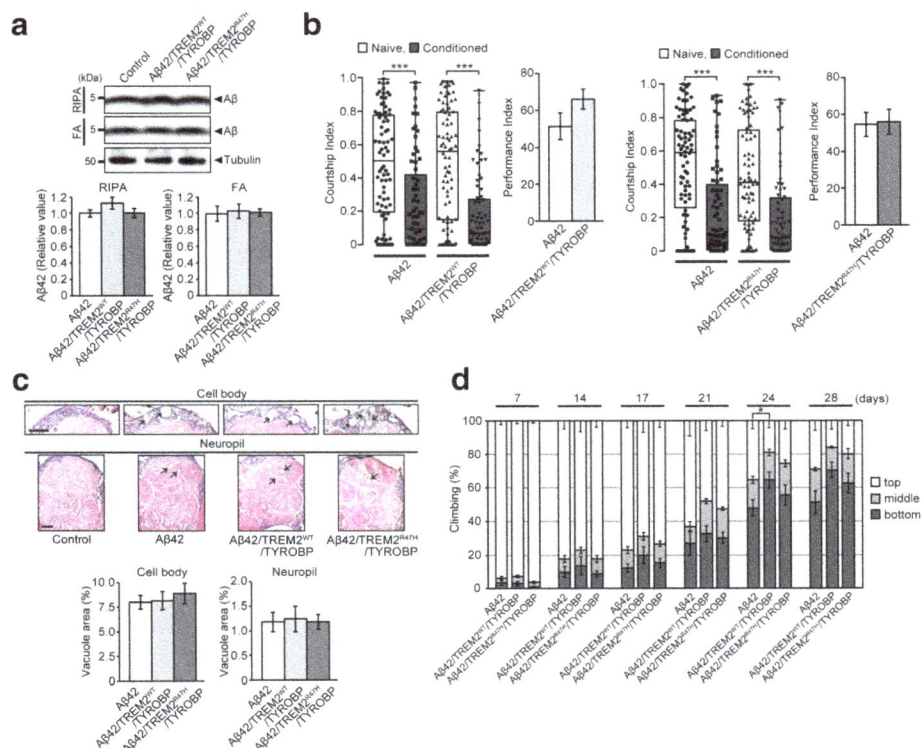

Fig. 4 Effects of glial overexpression of TREM2/TYROBP on Aβ42 levels, Aβ42-mediated neurodegeneration, and Aβ42-induced behavioral deficits. **a** Western blotting of detergent-soluble (RIPA) and -insoluble/formic acid (FA) fractions from fly head lysates with neuronal expression of Aβ42 alone (Aβ42), neuronal expression of Aβ42 and glial expression of TREM2^{WT}/TYROBP (Aβ42/TREM2^{WT}/TYROBP), and neuronal expression of Aβ42 and glial expression of TREM2^{R47H}/TYROBP (Aβ42/TREM2^{R47H}/TYROBP) with anti-Aβ antibody. Tubulin was used as a loading control. **b** Courtship-conditioning assay. Courtship index values are represented by *box plot*. Performance indexes were calculated from courtship indexes. $n = 67–80$, ***$p < 0.001$, naïve vs conditioned by Mann–Whitney U test. Genotypes of flies are described in Additional file 2: Table S1. **c** Brain sections of flies with neuronal expression of Aβ42 alone (Aβ42), neuronal expression of Aβ42 and glial expression of TREM2^{WT}/TYROBP (Aβ42/TREM2^{WT}/TYROBP), and neuronal expression of Aβ42 and glial expression of TREM2^{R47H}/TYROBP (Aβ42/TREM2^{R47H}/TYROBP). Cell body regions (*top*) and neuropil regions (*middle*) of flies are shown. Control; Repo-LexA driver alone. Percentages of vacuole areas (indicated by *arrows*) in fly cortices are shown at the *bottom*. Scale bar: 100 μm. Mean ± SEM, $n = 9–12$ hemispheres. **d** Climbing assay. Average percentages of flies that climbed to the top (*white*) or middle (*light gray*), or stayed at the bottom (*dark gray*), of the vials. Ages (days after eclosion) are indicated on the *top* of the graph. Percentages of flies that stayed at the bottom were subjected to statistical analyses. Mean ± SEM, $n = 5$, *$p < 0.05$ by Student's t-test

pathway, including ER, Golgi, and lysosomes [44], with minimal signals in the mitochondria and cytoplasm of neurons in Aβ42 fly brains. Moreover, secretion of Aβ peptides occurred in *Drosophila* cultured cells [44] and, in *Drosophila* brains, immuno-EM analysis occasionally detected Aβ42 accumulation in glial cells, suggesting that Aβ42 peptides were secreted from neurons and then taken up by glial cells [44]. The expression of Aβ42 in this model caused learning deficits followed by locomotor dysfunction and neurodegeneration with accumulation of detergent-insoluble Aβ42, in the brains. These results suggest that our Aβ42 fly model may recapitulate some aspects of Aβ42-mediated toxicity. Similar approaches have been utilized to generate transgenic Aβ42 fly models by other groups with consistent neurodegenerative phenotypes [63–65].

RNA sequence analysis in our Aβ42 fly model identified that neuronal expression of Aβ42 upregulated 437 genes and downregulated 485 genes in heads as compared to control flies (Fig. 3a, Additional file 2: Table S1). The upregulated DEGs were enriched in pathways including "endomembrane system," "endoplasmic reticulum," and "oxidation-reduction process" (Fig. 3b and Additional file 3: Table S2). By contrast, the downregulated DEGs were enriched in "electron carrier activity," "oxidoreductase activity, acting on paired donors, with incorporation or reduction of molecular oxygen," "intracellular membrane-bounded organelle," "heme binding," "oxidation-reduction process," "iron ion binding," "extracellular space," "transferase activity, transferring phosphorus-containing groups," "extracellular region," "metabolic process," "carboxylic ester hydrolase activity," "cuticle pigmentation," and "melanin biosynthetic process" (Fig. 3b and Additional file 3: Table S2).

Interestingly, this analysis revealed that eight of the 15 pathways (13 pathways for DEGs downregulated by Aβ42, three pathways for DEGs upregulated by Aβ42, one pathway is overlapped) enriched for the Aβ42 DEGs were also enriched for the TREM2^{WT}/TYROBP DEGs in the same or opposite direction (Fig. 3b and Additional file 3: Table S2). For example, the pathways "extracellular space" and "extracellular region" were enriched for the genes downregulated by Aβ42 and by TREM2^{WT}/TYROBP, while "oxidoreductase activity, acting on paired donors, with incorporation or reduction of molecular oxygen," "oxidation-reduction process," "electron carrier activity," "heme binding," "iron ion binding," and "intracellular membrane-bounded organelle" were enriched for the genes downregulated by Aβ42 and for the genes upregulated by TREM2^{WT}/TYROBP.

These unbiased analyses revealed that gene expression changes induced by neuronal expression of Aβ42 and glial expression of TREM2^{WT}/TYROBP merged onto the same molecular pathways. However, in fly genome, there is no clear ortholog of either TREM2 or TYROBP. One possibility could be that glial cells sense Aβ42 and/or associated neuronal damages and then induce gene expression changes through endogenous signaling pathways. Ectopically expressed human TREM2/TYROBP may sense these damage-associated signals and impact the overlapping molecular pathways.

TREM2^{R47H}/TYROBP induces gene expression changes similar to those by TREM2^{WT}/TYROBP in the fly brains

TREM2 variants were originally identified as causative mutations in patients with Nasu-Hakola disease [66]. However, recent genetic analysis revealed that R47H variant of TREM2 is associated with a three- to fourfold increased risk for AD [14, 15]. To examine the impact of glial expression of TREM2^{R47H}/TYROBP in the fly brains at the molecular level, we generated RNA-seq data from the head samples in flies with the co-expression of TREM2^{R47H} and TYROBP (TREM2^{R47H}/TYROBP) as described above [61]. Expression of TREM2^{R47H}/TYROBP resulted in 290 upregulated genes and 365 downregulated ones (Fig. 3a and Additional file 2: Table S1). No significant alteration in either the size, gross morphology of brain structures, the numbers of glial cells, or neurons was observed in TREM2^{R47H}/TYROBP bigenic flies (Additional file 1: Figure S1), suggesting that gene expression changes induced by ectopic expression of TREM2^{R47H}/TYROBP is not due to either structural changes or altered number of neurons or glial cells in the fly brain.

At the pathway level, FEA using GO annotation revealed that genes upregulated or downregulated by TREM2^{R47H}/TYROBP were enriched in the same categories as those with TREM2^{WT}/TYROBP (Fig. 3b and Additional file 3: Table S2), although some of the pathways that were enriched in the DEGs in TREM2^{WT}/TYROBP, such as "iron ion binding," "myosin light chain kinase activity," and "cellular response to heat," were not significantly enriched in the DEGs in TREM2^{R47H}/TYROBP (Fig. 3b and Additional file 3: Table S2). The DEG signatures from TREM2^{WT}/TYROBP and TREM2^{R47H}/TYROBP flies shared about half of their members and that 98% of those overlapped genes changed in the same direction (corrected FET p = 2.0 × 10^{-246}, 25.1-fold for downregulated genes; corrected FET p = 1.9 × 10^{-133}, 27.4-fold for upregulated genes) (Fig. 3c).

To quantify differences in gene expression induced by TREM2^{WT}/TYROBP and TREM2^{R47H}/TYROBP, we directly compared mRNA expression levels between these two groups and identified 145 upregulated genes and 157 downregulated genes in TREM2^{R47H}/TYROBP compared to TREM2^{WT}/TYROBP (Fig. 3a). Interestingly, at an FDR of 5%, the upregulated DEGs are significantly enriched for "odorant binding," "sensory perception of chemical stimulus," "defense response," and "response to pheromone," suggesting that these functional pathways were activated by R47H mutation in TREM2 (Fig. 3b and Additional file 3: Table S2). Among these genes, *Drosophila* Toll-4 gene (the closest ortholog of human TLR7) detected in the "defense response" module is of particular interest, since TREM2 family proteins are known to modulate Toll-like receptor signaling in mammals [67, 68].

We also compared molecular pathways affected by neuronal expression of Aβ42 and those affected by glial expression of TREM2^{R47H}/TYROBP (Fig. 3a, Additional file 2: Table S1). At the pathway levels, four of the above 15 pathways enriched in the Aβ42 DEGs were enriched in the TREM2^{R47H}/TYROBP DEGs. At the gene level, a significant overlap between Aβ42 DEGs and TREM2^{R47H}/TYROBP DEGs was observed (Fig. 3c, corrected p value ≤ 1.0 × 10^{-32}, ≥ 7-fold).

Taken all together, biological pathways affected by glial expression of TREM2^{WT}/TYROBP or TREM2^{R47H}/TYROBP in fly heads are similar but about 300 genes show significant difference in mRNA expression. Moreover, glial expression of TREM2^{R47H}/TYROBP impacts several common molecular pathways affected by neuronal expression of Aβ42, though TREM2^{WT}/TYROBP appears to impact many more other common pathways affected by neuronal expression of Aβ42.

Expression of TREM2/TYROBP in glial cells modifies molecular signatures induced by Aβ42 expression in neurons in fly brains

To investigate the effects of TREM2^{WT}/TYROBP on phenotypes as well as gene expression signatures induced by Aβ42, we achieved neuronal expression of Aβ42 and glial expression of TREM2^{WT}/TYROBP in fly brains by using two tissue-specific transgenes expression systems in *Drosophila* (Additional file 1: Figure S2A). Phenotypic characterization revealed that glial overexpression of TREM2^{WT}/TYROBP did not affect either Aβ42 accumulation levels (Fig. 4a), courtship learning and memory (Fig. 4b), or Aβ42-mediated neurodegeneration (Fig. 4c); however, some exacerbation of Aβ42-mediated behavioral deficits was observed (Fig. 4d and Additional file 1: Figure S2B).

We next analyzed the effects of glial expression of TREM2^{WT}/TYROBP on gene expression signatures induced by neuronal expression of Aβ42 in fly brains. RNA sequence analyses revealed that expression of Aβ42/TREM2^{WT}/TYROBP resulted in upregulation of 533 genes and downregulation of 727 genes compared to control flies (Additional file 1: Figure S2C). Interestingly, comparison of FEA results between Aβ42/TREM2^{WT}/TYROBP and Aβ42 flies revealed that seven of the 15 pathways enriched for the Aβ42 DEGs disappeared when TREM2^{WT}/TYROBP was expressed in glia (Additional file 1: Figure S2D and Additional file 4: Table S3). These pathways include "electron carrier activity," "oxidoreductase activity, acting on paired donors, with incorporation or reduction of molecular oxygen," and "heme binding," which were enriched in the DEGs downregulated by Aβ42 and in the DEGs upregulated by TREM2^{WT}/TYROBP (Fig. 3b and Additional file 3: Table S2).

Using the same strategy, we also analyzed the effects of glial expression of TREM2^{R47H}/TYROBP on phenotypes as well as gene expression signatures induced by neuronal expression of Aβ42 in fly brains (Additional file 1: Figure S2A). Similar to TREM2^{WT}/TYROBP, glial overexpression of TREM2^{R47H}/TYROBP did not affect Aβ42 accumulation levels (Fig. 4a), courtship learning and memory (Fig. 4b), or Aβ42-mediated neurodegeneration (Fig. 4c); although there is a trend toward subtle exacerbation of Aβ42-mediated behavioral deficits (Fig. 4d and Additional file 1: Figure S2B).

RNA sequence analyses revealed that expression of Aβ42/TREM2^{R47H}/TYROBP resulted in upregulation of 661 genes and downregulation of 846 genes (Additional file 1: Figure S2C and Additional file 2: Table S1). Comparison of FEA results between Aβ42/TREM2^{R47H}/TYROBP and Aβ42 flies revealed that nine of the 15 pathways enriched in the Aβ42 DEGs disappeared following glial expression of TREM2^{R47H}/TYROBP (Additional file 1: Figure S2D and Additional file 4: Table S3). Among these nine pathways, six pathways were also disappeared following glial expression of TREM2^{WT}/TYROBP, suggesting that the effects of TREM2^{R47H}/TYROBP on Aβ42 were similar to that of TREM2^{WT}/TYROBP by this analysis.

Taken together, glial expression of TREM2/TYROBP modifies molecular signatures induced by neuronal expression of Aβ42. Since glial expression of TREM2/TYROBP did not reduce Aβ42 levels (Fig. 4a), the observed changes in FEA results are not simply due to reduced response to Aβ42 in fly brains. In addition, since TREM2/TYROBP proteins are expressed in glial cells and Aβ42 peptides are expressed in neurons (Additional file 1: Figure S2A), this modulatory action likely reflects non-cell autonomous effects by TREM2/TYROBP.

Neuronal Aβ42 and glial TREM2^{R47H}/TYROBP synergistically downregulated genes associated with synaptic and immune function modules of the co-expressed gene networks from human AD brains

Gene co-expression network analysis has uncovered a number of co-expressed gene modules pathologically related to human complex diseases including AD [11]. To investigate the relevance of the gene expression signatures in Aβ42, TREM2^{WT}/TYROBP, TREM2^{R47H}/TYROBP, Aβ42/TREM2^{WT}/TYROBP, and Aβ42/TREM2^{R47H}/TYROBP fly brains to AD, we investigated their association with the 111 co-expressed gene modules derived from co-regulation analyses of brain gene expression in the Harvard Brain Tissue Resource Center (HBTRC) AD and controls. The modules were annotated by the GO or pathways that the modules were enriched for. To do this, the fly DEGs were first converted to human orthologs by using DIOPT (DIOPT score > 1) [69]. The enrichment analysis shows that the genes upregulated by Aβ42 were enriched in the modules associated with "extracellular region" and "chaperone" (Fig. 5a and Additional file 5: Table S4a) while no module was enriched for the downregulated DEGs (Additional file 5: Table S4a). Neither the TREM2^{WT}/TYROBP nor the TREM2^{R47H}/TYROBP DEG signature showed significant enrichment in any of the HBTRC modules. By contrast, the DEGs upregulated by Aβ42/TREM2^{WT}/TYROBP were enriched in the "chaperone" module (FET p = 0.022, 3.2-fold; Fig. 5a, Additional file 5: Table S4a) while Aβ42/TREM2^{R47H}/TYROBP expression was associated with downregulation of genes enriched in synaptic transmission, neuronal activities, and transmission of nerve impulses, with FET p = 0.001 (2.1-fold), 0.024 (1.9-fold), and 0.024 (1.6-fold), respectively (Fig. 5a, Additional file 5: Table S4a). These results indicate that neuronal expression of Aβ42 and glial expression of TREM2^{R47H}/TYROBP synergistically downregulated genes known to be associated with AD pathology [11], thus supporting the prediction that TREM2/TYROBP play roles in AD pathogenesis.

To validate these findings, we performed qPCR analyses in five DEGs from the "synaptic transmission" module with known functions related to neuronal activity; Sh, SK, Shab, para, and Nmdar2 (fly orthologs for potassium voltage-gated channel subfamily A, potassium

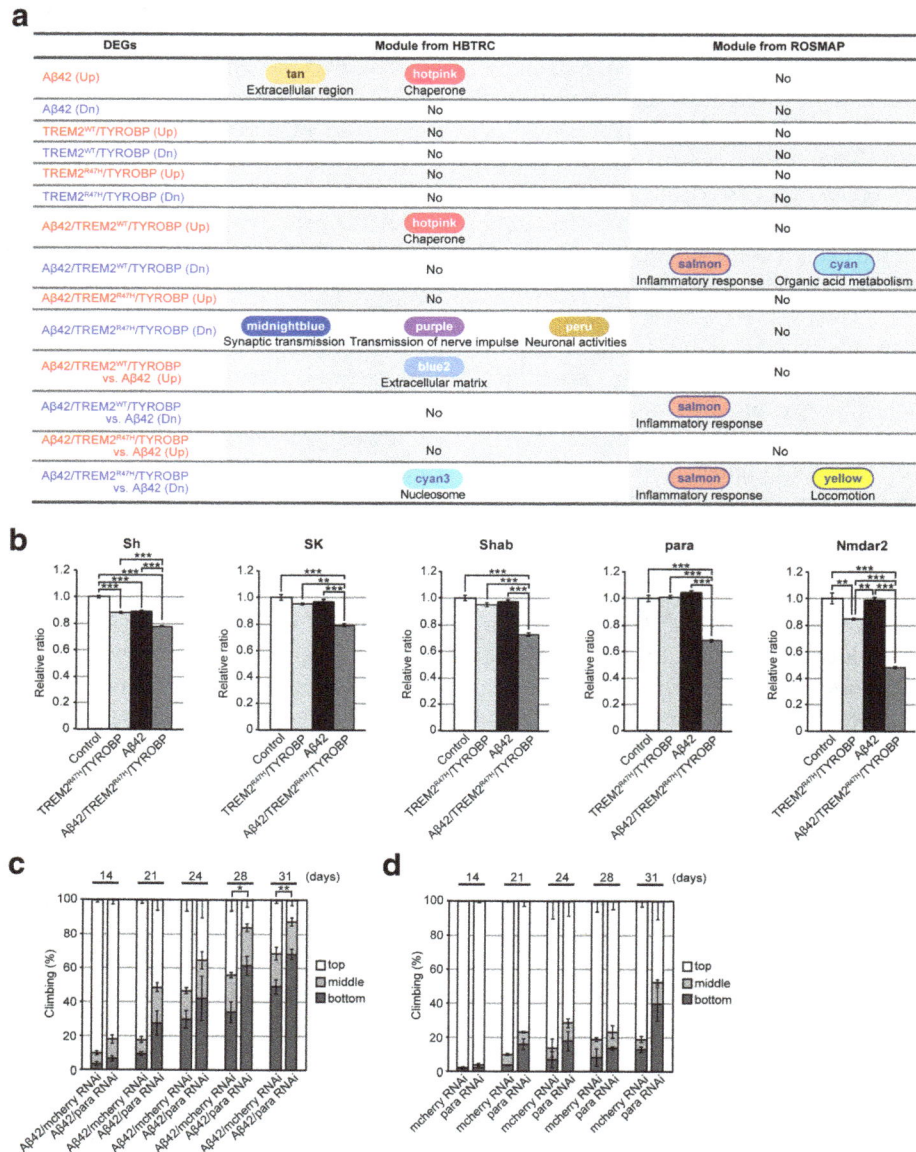

Fig. 5 Gene regulatory network analysis of gene expression signatures in Aβ42/TREM2/TYROBP flies with human AD WGCNA. **a** Overlap between HBTRC or ROSMAP human AD WGCNA co-expression network modules and DEGs identified in (Fig. 3a and Additional file 1: Figure S2C). **b** mRNA expression levels of genes from "synaptic transmission" module validated by qPCR. mRNA levels in the heads of flies with neuronal expression of Aβ42 alone (Aβ42), glial expression of TREM2^R47H/TYROBP (TREM2^R47H/TYROBP) alone and neuronal expression of Aβ42 and glial expression of TREM2^R47H/TYROBP (Aβ42/TREM2^R47H/TYROBP) were analyzed by qRT-PCR. Control; drivers alone. Mean ± SEM, $n = 4$, $*p < 0.05$, $**p < 0.01$, and $***p < 0.001$ by one-way ANOVA with post-hoc Tukey's test. **c** Neuronal knockdown of para worsened Aβ42-induced locomotor deficits as revealed by climbing assay. **d** Neuronal knockdown of para by itself caused modest decline in locomotor functions upon aging. Mean ± SEM, $n = 3–5$, $*p < 0.05$ and $**p < 0.01$ by Student's t-test. Genotypes of flies are described in Additional file 2: Table S1

calcium-activated channel subfamily N, potassium voltage-gated channel subfamily B, sodium voltage-gated channel alpha subunits, and glutamate ionotropic receptor NMDA type subunits, respectively). We found that expression levels of Sh were slightly downregulated by Aβ42 expression alone, while those of Sh and Nmdar2 were slightly downregulated by

expression of TREM2^R47H/TYROBP alone (Fig. 5b). By contrast, expression levels of all five genes were significantly downregulated in Aβ42/TREM2^R47H/TYROBP flies.

We further examined whether downregulation of para, a fly ortholog for sodium voltage-gated channel alpha subunits, modifies neuronal dysfunction in Aβ42 flies.

Neuronal knockdown of para by RNAi significantly worsened Aβ42-induced locomotor deficits (Fig. 5c). Moreover, neuronal knockdown of para by itself caused modest decline in locomotor functions in flies (Fig. 5d).

Taken altogether, these network analysis results suggest that genes associated with synaptic transmission were synergistically downregulated by co-expression of Aβ42 and TREM2^{R47H}/TYROBP, which may lead to neuronal dysfunction.

To further explore the association of the DEG signatures with early phases of AD, we intersect them with the co-expression network modules from an independent cohort in the ROSMAP study. Again, the modules were annotated by the GO/pathways that the modules were most enriched for. The result is summarized in Fig. 5a and Additional file 5: Table S4b. The genes downregulated by Aβ42/TREM2^{WT}/TYROBP were enriched for an "inflammatory response" module (salmon; corrected FET $p = 0.005$, 2.6-fold) and an "organic acid metabolism" module (cyan; corrected FET $p = 0.014$, 2.5-fold). Note that the "inflammatory response" module salmon was ranked number 7 in relation to AD pathology after ranking ROSMAP modules using multiple sorting features, including module-trait correlations and enrichment for genes correlated with or differentially expressed regarding neuropathological and clinical traits Braak staging, global cognition, CERAD neuropathological category (and, by extension, NIA-Reagan score). Importantly, this inflammatory module is not enriched for the DEGs by either Aβ42 alone or TREM2^{WT}/TYROBP alone, suggesting interactions between Aβ42 and TREM2^{WT}/TYROBP at the level of gene expression.

When gene expression levels were compared between Aβ42/TREM2^{WT}/TYROBP and Aβ42 alone, the downregulated genes in Aβ42/TREM2^{WT}/TYROBP were enriched in the "inflammatory response" module (salmon; corrected FET $p = 0.015$, 3.5-fold), while downregulated genes in Aβ42/TREM2^{R47H}/TYROBP were enriched in the same "inflammatory response" module (salmon; corrected FET $p = 5 \times 10^{-4}$, 3.4-fold) and a "locomotion" module (yellow; ranked number 9; corrected FET $p = 0.034$, 1.9-fold).

In summary, for both TREM2^{WT}/TYROBP and TREM2^{R47H}/TYROBP, interaction with Aβ42 affected the "inflammatory response" pathway in flies. This is an interesting observation since neuroinflammation is implicated as a significant contributor to AD pathogenesis and is also consistent with the proposed anti-inflammatory consequences of TREM2 signaling in human microglia.

To test if the enrichment of synaptic transmission and inflammatory response modules was biased by the conserveness of these two pathways between fly and human, we analyzed the enrichment of known GO categories (based on the MSigDB gene sets) in the human

orthologs of fly genes. As shown in Additional file 6: Table S5, the mostly enriched gene sets are big pathways including cytoplasm, metabolic process, nucleus, organelle part, and macromolecular complex, which account for 14. 6%, 12.2%, 10%, 8.8%, and 7.2% of the 10,938 high confidence human orthologous genes (DIOPT score > 1; http:// www.flyrnai.org/cgi-bin/DRSC_orthologs.pl) accordingly, with FDR adjusted FET p value < 1.2E-58. In contrast, the immune system genes only account for < 1.1% of the orthologs and were not enriched (FET p value ≥ 0.54), while synaptic transmission accounted for 1.0% of the orthologs and was marginally enriched (FET p value = 0.004). Thus, it is unlikely that the significant correlation with the inflammatory and synaptic modules in fly signatures were caused by an artifact of overrepresentation of these pathways in the fly-human orthologous genes.

In summary, since Aβ42 accumulation, TREM2/TYROBP activation, altered inflammatory response, and synaptic dysfunctions are all implicated in early phases of AD pathogenesis, Aβ42/TREM2/TYROBP flies may recapitulate some molecular signatures relevant to early stages of AD.

Molecular pathways affected by neuronal expression of tau do not overlap with those affected by glial expression of TREM2/TYROBP in fly brains

In the pathogenesis of AD, abnormal accumulation and toxicity of tau is believed to play a critical role in neurodegeneration. Thus, identification of molecular signatures induced by simultaneous activation of TREM2/TYROBP axis and accumulation of tau may provide important information underlying neurodegenerative process in AD.

We first compared molecular pathways affected by neuronal expression of tau and those affected by glial expression of TREM2/TYROBP in fly heads. We performed RNA sequence analyses and characterized gene expression signatures using an established fly model of human tau toxicity [70] in which expression of human tau causes progressive degeneration of photoreceptor neurons in the retina [71]. Expression of tau in photoreceptor neurons using GMR-GAL4 driver upregulated 384 genes and downregulated 418 genes in the heads compared to control flies (Additional file 1: Figure S3A and Additional file 2: Table S1). The upregulated DEGs in tau fly heads were associated with "endosome transport via multivesicular body sorting pathway," "ESCRT III complex," and "vacuolar transport" (Additional file 1: Figure S3B and Additional file 7: Table S6). In contrast, downregulated DEGs in tau fly heads were significantly enriched in "rhabdomere" and "striated muscle thin filament" (Additional file 1: Figure S3B and Additional file 7: Table S6).

We also analyzed gene expression changes caused by pan-glial expression of TREM2^{WT}/TYROBP or TREM2^{R47H}/

TYROBP in the same genetic background carrying the GMR-GAL4 driver. Glial expression of TREM2^{WT}/TYROBP upregulated 448 genes and downregulated 306 genes while TREM2^{R47H}/TYROBP upregulated 475 genes and downregulated 426 genes (Additional file 1: Figure S3A and Additional file 2: Table S1). There were 29–52 genes common between tau DEGs and TREM2/TYROBP DEGs (Additional file 1: Figure S3C, corrected p value $\leq 10^{-10}$, ≥ 3. 9-fold). However, we observed no pathway that was enriched in both DEG signatures (Additional file 1: Figure S3B and Additional file 7: Table S6).

Taken together, these results suggest that molecular signatures induced by expression of tau are dissimilar to those induced by TREM2/TYROBP in fly heads at the functional pathway level.

Glial expression of TREM2/TYROBP exacerbated tau-mediated neurodegeneration

Next, we examined the effects of glial expression of TREM2/TYROBP on gene expression signatures as well as neurodegenerative phenotypes induced by tau expression. In order to achieve expression of tau in photoreceptor neurons and expression of the TREM2/TYROBP complex in glial cells simultaneously, we utilized two tissue-specific transgenes expression systems in *Drosophila* (Additional file 1: Figure S4A).

Expression of human tau in photoreceptor neurons causes progressive neurodegeneration in the lamina [71], the first synaptic neuropil of the optic lobe containing photoreceptor axons and abundant glial cells [72]. We observed that pan-glial expression of both TREM2^{WT}/TYROBP and TREM2^{R47H}/TYROBP significantly exacerbated this neurodegeneration, while pan-glial expression of TREM2/TYROBP alone (i.e. in the absence of neuronal tau expression) did not show neurodegeneration (Fig. 6a). We also examined whether glial expression of TREM2/TYROBP increased the levels of tau and/or tau phosphorylated at AD-related sites. Western blot analyses with pan-tau or phospho-tau specific antibodies did not detect significant increase in either tau levels or phosphorylation status of tau by glial expression of TREM2/TYROBP (Fig. 6b). These results suggest that glial expression of TREM2/TYROBP exacerbates tau-mediated neurodegeneration without affecting tau accumulation or phosphorylation status, consistent with recent report using TREM2 deficiency mice [73].

Analysis of the gene regulatory network in AD brains revealed that tau and TREM2/TYROBP synergistically downregulated genes overrepresented in the modules related to immune systems associated with AD pathogenesis

We generated RNA-seq data from tau/TREM2^{WT}/TYROBP and tau/TREM2^{R47H}/TYROBP flies and identified gene expression signatures in comparison with control flies. Expression of tau/TREM2^{WT}/TYROBP upregulated 377 genes and downregulated 476 genes, while expression of tau/TREM2^{R47H}/TYROBP upregulated 596 genes and downregulated 601 genes (Additional file 1: Figure S4B and Additional file 2: Table S1).

Most of the pathways enriched in these DEGs (Additional file 1: Figure S4C and Additional file 8: Table S7) were the same as those detected in either TREM2/TYROBP alone or tau alone (Additional file 1: Figure S3B and Additional file 7: Table S6). However, we observed that "proteolysis" and "UDP-glycosyltransferase activity" were uniquely enriched in the DEGs downregulated by tau/TREM2^{WT}/TYROBP and tau/TREM2^{R47H}/TYROBP, respectively (Additional file 1: Figure S3B and Additional file 8: Table S7). The "proteolysis" pathway contains proteases including angiotensin-converting enzyme (ACE), which have been associated with AD [74], and UDP-glycosyltransferases, enzymes associated with oligodendrocyte myelination, disruption of which has been implicated in neurodegeneration in AD [12].

To further explore the relevance of the gene expression signatures in tau, TREM2^{WT}/TYROBP, TREM2^{R47H}/TYROBP, tau/TREM2^{WT}/TYROBP, and tau/TREM2^{R47H}/TYROBP flies to AD, we investigated their association with the 111 co-expressed gene modules derived from co-regulation analyses of brain gene expression in the HBTRC AD and controls [11]. The enrichment analysis shows that no module was enriched for tau DEG signature. Moreover, neither the TREM2^{WT}/TYROBP nor the TREM2^{R47H}/TYROBP DEG signature showed significant enrichment in any of the HBTRC modules.

By contrast, the downregulated DEG signatures in tau/TREM2^{WT}/TYROBP and tau/TREM2^{R47H}/TYROBP were enriched in the "cadherin" module (corrected FET $p = 0$. 035, 1.6-fold; Fig. 7a, Additional file 9: Table S8a) and the "extracellular region" module (corrected FET $p = 0.023$, 2. 0-fold; Fig. 7a, Additional file 9: Table S8a), respectively. Since these two modules are predicted to be highly associated with AD pathology [11], our data suggest pathological interactions between tau and TREM2/TYROBP at the level of gene expression in flies.

In the co-expression network from ROSMAP, the DEGs downregulated by tau/TREM2^{WT}/TYROBP and tau/TREM2^{R47H}/TYROBP significantly overlapped with three modules (Fig. 7a, Additional file 9: Table S8b): the "inflammatory response" module (salmon; ranked number 7) (corrected FET $p = 9.0 \times 10^{-4}$, 3.3-fold and corrected FET $p = 3.7 \times 10^{-4}$, 3.0-fold, respectively); "locomotion" (yellow; ranked number 9) (corrected FET $p = 4.4 \times 10^{-3}$, 2.1-fold and corrected FET $p = 0.04$, 1.7-fold, respectively); and "organic acid metabolism" (cyan; ranked number 24) (corrected FET $p = 5.7 \times 10^{-3}$, 3.1-fold and corrected FET $p = 0.02$, 2.5-fold, respectively).

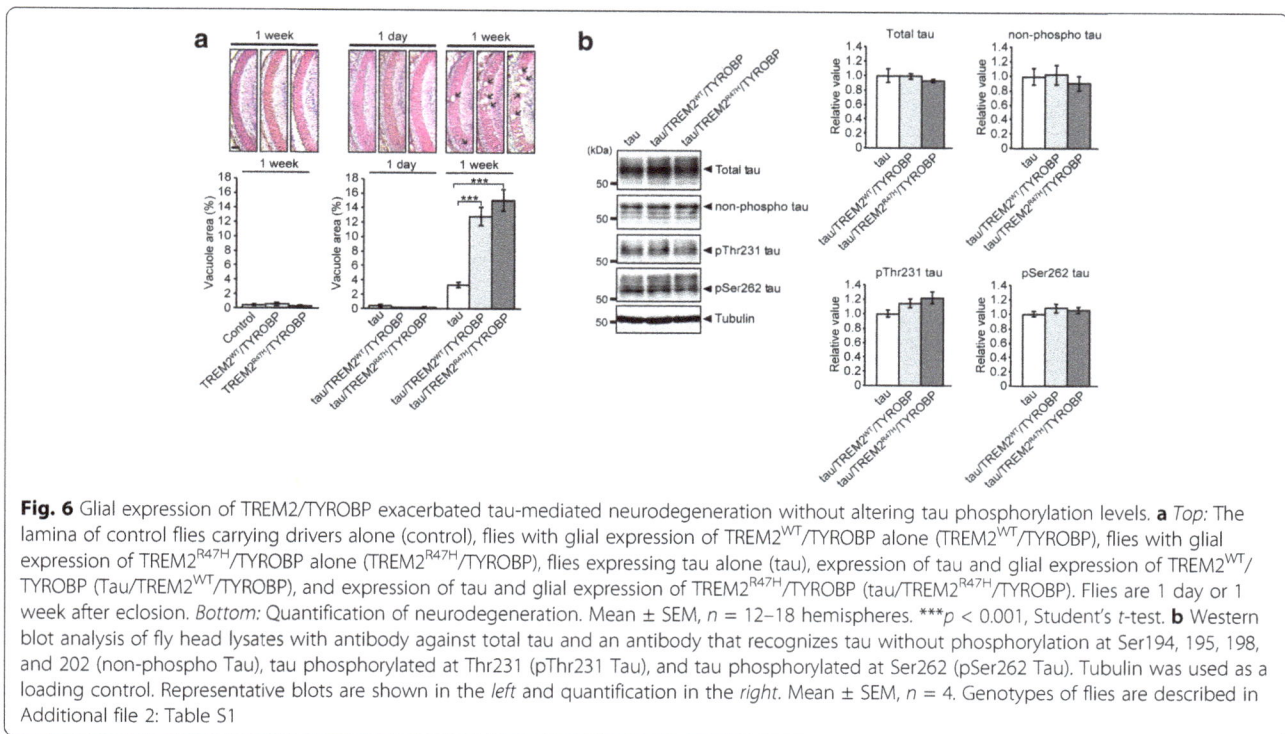

Fig. 6 Glial expression of TREM2/TYROBP exacerbated tau-mediated neurodegeneration without altering tau phosphorylation levels. **a** *Top:* The lamina of control flies carrying drivers alone (control), flies with glial expression of TREM2^{WT}/TYROBP alone (TREM2^{WT}/TYROBP), flies with glial expression of TREM2^{R47H}/TYROBP alone (TREM2^{R47H}/TYROBP), flies expressing tau alone and glial expression of TREM2^{WT}/TYROBP (Tau/TREM2^{WT}/TYROBP), and expression of tau and glial expression of TREM2^{R47H}/TYROBP (tau/TREM2^{R47H}/TYROBP). Flies are 1 day or 1 week after eclosion. *Bottom:* Quantification of neurodegeneration. Mean ± SEM, n = 12–18 hemispheres. ***p < 0.001, Student's *t*-test. **b** Western blot analysis of fly head lysates with antibody against total tau and an antibody that recognizes tau without phosphorylation at Ser194, 195, 198, and 202 (non-phospho Tau), tau phosphorylated at Thr231 (pThr231 Tau), and tau phosphorylated at Ser262 (pSer262 Tau). Tubulin was used as a loading control. Representative blots are shown in the *left* and quantification in the *right*. Mean ± SEM, n = 4. Genotypes of flies are described in Additional file 2: Table S1

These three modules also significantly overlapped with the Aβ42-related DEG signatures, as described above (Fig. 5a). The "locomotion" and "organic acid metabolism" modules were also enriched for DEGs downregulated by expression of tau alone (corrected FET p = 0.01, 2.0-fold and corrected FET p = 0.02, 2.8-fold, respectively), while the "inflammatory response" module salmon was enriched in the DEGs downregulated by expression of TREM2^{WT}/TYROBP alone (corrected FET p = 4.1 × 10^{-5}, 4.9-fold). The "inflammatory response" module (or the salmon module, ranked number 7) was also enriched in the DEGs from downregulated by tau/TREM2^{WT}/TYROBP in comparison with tau (corrected FET p = 0.01, 3.6-fold), or by tau/TREM2^{R47H}/TYROBP in comparison with tau (corrected FET p = 0.006, 3.4-fold). In the ROSMAP data (Additional file 10: Table S9), this salmon module had three members downregulated in AD brains, including *GADD45A*, *FABP5*, and *BAALC-AS1*, the first two of which were also downregulated in the present tau/TREM2^{WT}/TYROBP and tau/TREM2^{R47H}/TYROBP flies (FET p = 9.2 × 10^{-5}, 14.7-fold), consistent with the existence of substantial network consistency when human data and fly data are compared.

Of particular interest, the DEGs upregulated by tau/TREM2^{WT}/TYROBP were enriched for another "inflammatory response" module (lightcyan; ranked number 8; corrected FET p = 0.04, 2.9-fold) in the ROSMAP network. This lightcyan module contained five AD GWAS loci, including *CD33*, *INPP5D*, *MS4A4A/MS4A6A*, *RIN3*,

and *TREM2* (Additional file 10: Table S9). Moreover, *TYROBP* was a member of this ROSMAP lightcyan module. This module was not enriched with DEGs upregulated by either tau alone or TREM2^{WT}/TYROBP alone, suggesting that genetic interactions between tau and TREM2^{WT}/TYROBP may induce this gene expression signature. Moreover, significant enrichment was not observed with the DEG signatures in tau/TREM2^{R47H}/TYROBP flies, suggesting that the TREM2^{R47H} variant may have weaker impact on this module than does TREM2^{WT}.

Taken together, these results revealed that different components of the immune response system were either activated or inhibited by the tau/TREM2/TYROBP pathway. Since both the salmon and lightcyan modules were highly ranked for their predicted relationship to AD pathology, the present results highlighted the importance of inflammatory response subnetworks as potential targets for disease intervention.

As shown in Additional file 1: Figure S5, the salmon and lightcyan modules in the ROSMAP network were adjacent to each other in the cluster dendrogram, indicating that the two inflammatory response modules were highly related in the human data, even though they were regulated differently in tau/TREM2/TYROBP flies. Therefore, our fly models provide valuable biological insights into the human data that were not otherwise evident. To investigate the causal regulatory relationships among the inflammatory response module genes, we combined the genes from the two inflammatory response

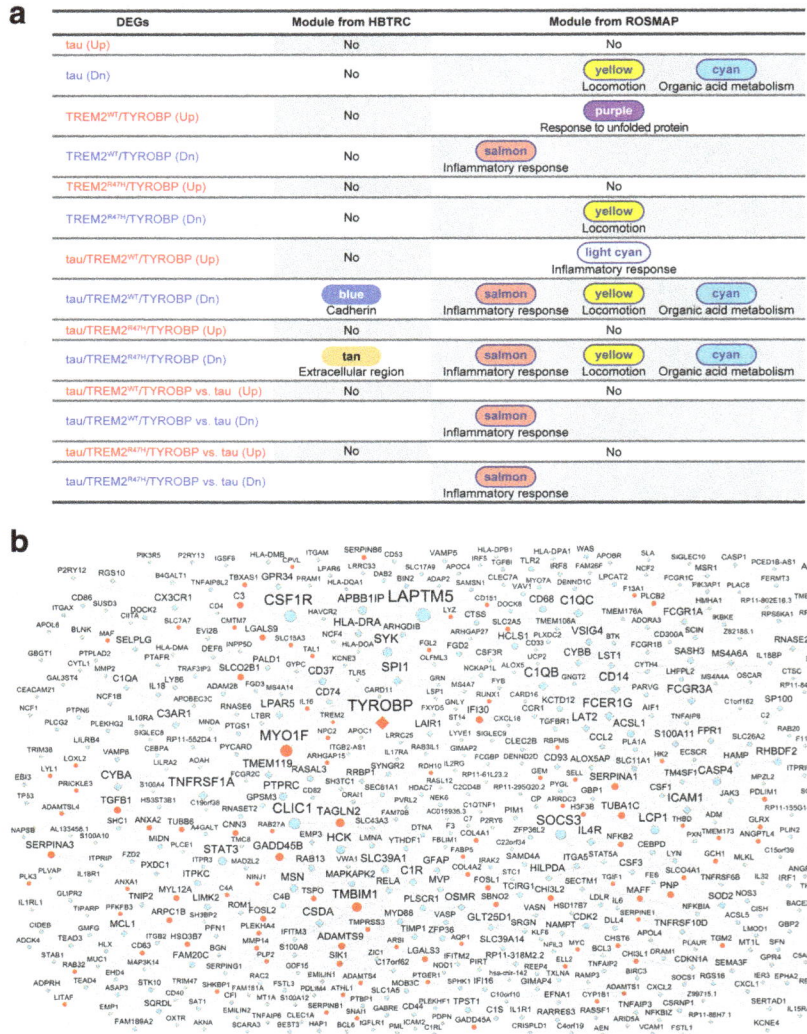

Fig. 7 Gene regulatory network analysis of gene expression signatures in tau/TREM2/TYROBP flies with human AD WGCNA. **a** Overlap between HBTRC or ROSMAP human AD WGCNA co-expression network modules and DEGs identified in (Additional file 1: Figures S3A and S4B). **b** Causal regulatory network of the genes from two inflammatory response modules "salmon" and "lightcyan" identified from the ROSMAP human AD WGCNA co-expression network. DEGs in at least one of the present fly transgenic models are denoted by *red color*, otherwise by *cyan color*. Genes having fly orthologs are in *eclipse shape*, otherwise in *diamond shape*. Node size is proportional to the number of downstream genes. Genotypes of flies are described in Additional file 2: Table S1

modules and overlaid the combined gene set onto a Bayesian causal network constructed from the ROSMAP data by using an approach described in our previous study [11]. Figure 7b shows the network structure of the 604 inflammatory response genes of which 270 genes have fly orthologs. Over one-third (96) of the 270 fly orthologs were differentially expressed in at least one of the fly transgenic models analyzed here, resulting in a 1.3-fold enrichment (p value = 2.5×10^{-4}). *TYROBP* was highlighted as a key regulator for controlling a large number of downstream genes in this inflammatory response network: 17, 36, and 79 genes were in the immediate first, second, and third layer downstream of

TYROBP, respectively. Therefore, the causal network analysis further validated the causal role of TYROBP and informed other novel key regulators, which modulate the inflammatory response pathways, such as, *LAPTM5*, *MYO1F*, *CLIC1*, and *CSF1R*, which were highlighted by a large node size in Fig. 7b.

Discussion

There is an increasing appreciation that immunological mechanisms play important roles in AD pathogenesis, as evidenced by the identification of a number of genes expressed in immune cells of the central nervous system (CNS) carrying genetic variants associated with increased risk for late-onset AD, including *CD33* [75], *TREM2* [14, 15], and *CR1* [76]. Thus, dysregulation of immune response genes and/or pathways are believed to be key factors in the cause and/or progression of AD. The present transcriptomic analysis indicated an overlap between glial expression of TREM2/TYROBP and neuronal expression of Aβ42. FEA of the DEGs suggested a strong overlap of the common pathways regulated by TREM2^{WT}/TYROBP and by Aβ42. More than half of the pathways detected in Aβ42 DEGs were also detected in TREM2^{WT}/TYROBP DEGs with the same or opposite regulation direction (Fig. 3b). In addition, more than half of the pathways regulated by Aβ42 disappeared by glial expression of TREM2^{WT}/TYROBP (Additional file 1: Figure S2D), suggesting that the changes in the TREM2^{WT}/TYROBP signaling pathway might represent a defense reaction to Aβ42 toxicity. This is consistent with the proposed role of TREM2 as a component of the microglial reaction to Aβ-related pathology [18–20].

In order to identify potential modules associated with AD pathogenesis, we overlaid DEGs onto two independent human AD co-expression networks, one from the HBTRC AD cohort and the other from the ROSMAP AD cohort. Synaptic transmission modules from the HBTRC network and inflammatory response modules from the ROSMAP network were among the most interesting subnetworks enriched with different sets of DEGs (Fig. 5a). Different modules emerged from the two networks, possibly due to differences in the distribution of AD severity within each cohort. The ROSMAP cohort contains normal individuals, and patients with mild cognitive impairment (MCI) to mild to moderate stages of dementia with very few individuals with advanced dementia [41, 42], while the HBTRC AD cohort samples were concentrated in more advanced stages of the disease (CDR 3.0 and higher [11]).

When TREM2/TYROBP is expressed in glial cells, three out of the five ROSMAP modules enriched with the DEGs identified from fly models of tau toxicity were also enriched with the DEGs detected from fly models of Aβ42 toxicity (Figs. 5a and 7a). This suggests that changes in these pathways maybe part of the pathological interaction between Aβ and tau toxicity and therefore may have implications for elucidation of the pathogenesis of early phases of AD. In turn, identification of molecules that play roles in early phases of AD may point to novel sites of intervention where progression of AD may be slowed or arrested.

We also found that, while the "inflammatory response" module salmon was enriched in downregulated DEGs from both Aβ42/TREM2^{WT}/TYROBP and tau/TREM2^{WT}/TYROBP genotypes, the "inflammatory response" lightcyan module was enriched in upregulated DEGs from the tau/TREM2^{WT}/TYROBP genotype (Fig. 7a). Activation of this

subnetwork of the inflammatory response pathway may represent an event linked to late stages of AD characterized by tau toxicity and upregulation of TREM2/TYROBP signaling. Interestingly, the lightcyan module was not detected in the tau/TREM2^{R47H}/TYROBP genotype, suggesting that the pathogenic R47H variant may have a negative impact on activating this inflammatory response. The finding has significant implication for selectively and differentially targeting subnetworks of inflammatory response for potential therapeutic intervention. The lightcyan module contained *TYROBP*, as well as several AD GWAS gene loci, including *CD33, INPP5D, MS4A4A/ MS4A6A, RIN3, and TREM2*. In addition, this module was highly enriched for various AD signatures and hence was the top ranked module in relation to AD pathology among all ROSMAP modules. Taken together, these results highlighted the lightcyan module as an interesting target for potential disease intervention from both genetic and the molecular pathway perspectives.

Innate immune response is a conserved biological process that multicellular organisms use for their defense against pathogens and toxic stimuli. In AD brains, there is a sustained increase in innate immune activity. In fruit fly, immune response relies on combined action of both cellular processes, such as the phagocytosis of invading microbials, and humoral immune responses, such as the secretion of antimicrobial peptides (AMPs) into the hemolymph [77]. NF-κB signaling pathways play paramount roles in modulating humoral immune response. We noted that DEGs in the present Aβ or Tau flies with or without TREM2/TYROBP showed a significant overlap with the fly Rel/NF-κB perturbation signatures induced by *Rel* mutation or *Rel* overexpression in Pal *et al.* [78] (Additional file 11: Table S10a). In addition, we found that *Rel* signatures were enriched for the immune response modules in both HBTRC and ROSMAP data (Additional file 11: Table S10b). For example, the *Rel* overexpression genes were enriched for the "yellow" (response to biotic stimulus) module in the HBTRC dataset (2.5-fold, BH adjusted FET *p* value 0.035) and the "salmon" (inflammatory response) module in the ROSMAP dataset (6.4-fold, BH adjusted FET *p* value 0.001). This suggests that fly is a promising model for studying the NF-κB-controlled immune signaling pathways that are implicated in the Aβ or tau pathologies of AD.

Besides the impact on the immune response modules, we systematically examined the impact of the *TREM2^{R47H}* variant on neuronal expression of Aβ42 or tau. Overall, the gene expression changes induced by *TREM2^{R47H}* were similar to those induced by *TREM2^{WT}* in terms of GO function and co-expression network enrichment under conditions with or without Aβ42 or tau. However, we noted a significant enrichment for the synaptic transmission modules with downregulated DEGs in Aβ42/TREM2^{R47H}/TYROBP flies, but not with Aβ42/TREM2^{WT}/TYROBP flies (Fig. 5a and Additional file 5: Table S4a), suggesting a potential role of R47H variant involved in dysregulation of neuronal activities. Direct comparison of mRNA levels between $TREM2^{R47H}$ and $TREM2^{WT}$ under various genotype configurations revealed several consistent GO categories, including upregulation of "odorant binding," "extracellular region," "defense response," and "response to pheromone," downregulation of "phosphatidate phosphatase activity." Among these categories, "extracellular region" was consistently identified to differ except under the tau expression background. "Extracellular region" is of particular interest because the R47H variant is located in the extracellular region of TREM2 protein. It is postulated that the amino acid change by this mutation interferes the normal biological function of TREM2, such as the binding to its ligands, its receptor function and its processing by proteases, leading to impaired biological pathways implicated in the pathogenesis of AD [79]. In addition, "defense response" contains Toll-4, a fly ortholog of mammalian TLR7, suggesting that TREM2 R47H variant may have distinct impact on Toll-like receptor singling. We anticipate that the gene signatures and pathways identified in this study will be a starting point for a complete identification of the exact molecular mechanisms underlying how risk for AD is specified by $TREM2^{R47H}$.

Conclusions

In summary, we constructed novel transgenic fly models of AD in order to study the genetic interactions between glial expression of TREM2/TYROBP and the neuronal expression of Aβ42 or tau, the two hallmark proteins for the characterization of AD neuropathology. Using these novel transgenic fly models of AD, we also investigated the impact of a TREM2 pathogenic R47H variant (rs75932628), for which the observed effect size has been estimated to be comparable to that of the *APOE ε4* allele [15]. To the best of our knowledge, we are the first to systematically analyze phenotypic and genome-wide gene expression changes associated with overexpression of the WT and R47H mutant type TREM2/TYROBP and their interaction with Aβ42- or tau-related pathobiology *in vivo*. A recent work reports that R47H mutation impairs TREM2-mediated microglial response to Aβ pathology [34], while our results demonstrate that $TREM2^{R47H}$ is capable of promoting tau-mediated neurodegeneration. The comprehensive pathological and molecular data generated through this study strongly validate the causal role of *TREM2/TYROBP* in driving molecular networks in AD and AD-related phenotypes

in flies and also provides insight into the role of R47H variant TREM2 in AD pathogenesis.

Additional files

Additional file 1: Figure S1. No significant alteration in either the gross morphology of brain structures or the number of neuronal and glial cells was observed in TREM2/TYROBP flies. **Figure S2.** Molecular pathways affected by neuronal expression of Aβ42 and glial expression of TREM2/TYROBP. **Figure S3.** Molecular pathways affected by tau do not overlap with those affected by glial TREM2/TYROBP. **Figure S4.** Gene expression signatures in tau/TREM2/TYROBP flies. **Figure S5.** Heatmap showing the topological overlapping matrix (TOM) from weighted gene co-expression network analysis. **Table S11.** Primer sequences for RT-PCR and qRT-PCR.

Additional file 2: Table S1. Differentially expressed genes identified from different comparisons under FDR ≤ 0.05 and absolute log2 fold change ≥ 1.2.

Additional file 3: Table S2. Functional enrichment of DEGs identified in TREM2^{WT}/TYROBP, TREM2^{R47H}/TYROBP, and Aβ42 files.

Additional file 4: Table S3. Functional enrichment of DEGs identified in Aβ42, Aβ42/TREM2^{WT}/TYROBP, and Aβ42/TREM2^{R47H}/TYROBP files.

Additional file 5: Table S4a. Overlap between HBTRC human AD co-expression network modules and DEGs identified in Aβ42, Aβ42/TREM2^{WT}/TYROBP. **Table S4b.** Overlap between ROSMAP human AD co-expression network modules and DEGs identified in Aβ42, Aβ42/TREM2^{WT}/TYROBP.

Additional file 6: Table S5. Overlap between MSigDB gene ontology/pathway gene sets and fly-human conserved genes.

Additional file 7: Table S6. Functional enrichment of DEGs identified in TREM2^{WT}/TYROBP, TREM2^{R47H}/TYROBP, and Tau files.

Additional file 8: Table S7. Functional enrichment of DEGs identified in Tau/TREM2^{WT}/TYROBP, Tau/TREM2^{R47H}/TYROBP files.

Additional file 9: Table S8a. Overlap between HBTRC human AD co-expression network modules and DEGs identified in Tau/TREM2^{WT}/TYROBP and Tau/TREM2^{R47H}/TYROBP files. **Table S8b.** Overlap between ROSMAP human AD co-expression network modules and DEGs identified in Tau, Tau/TREM2^{WT}/TYROBP, and Tau/TREM2^{R47H}/TYROBP files.

Additional file 10: Table S9 Module membership from weighted gene co-expression network analysis for ROSMAP gene expression data.

Additional file 11: Table S10a. Overlap between fly Rel mutation or overexpression signatures and DEGs in Aβ and Tau flies. **Table S10b.** Overlap between fly Rel mutation or Rel overexpression signatures and human AD network modules.

Acknowledgements
We thank Dr. T. Awasaki and Dr. H. Ishimoto for their technical advice and the Bloomington Stock Center for fly stocks.

Funding
This work was supported by the NIA/NIH grant U01AG046170 (to KMI, BZ, ES, SG, and ME), the Research Funding for Longevity Science from National Center for Geriatrics and Gerontology, Japan, grant number 28-26 (to KMI), Takeda Science Foundation (JP) (to KMI), the NIA/NIH grants RF1AG054014 (to BZ), RF1AG057440 (to BZ), R01AG057907 (to BZ), U01AG052411 (to BZ), U01AG46152 (to DB and PDJ), P30AG10161 (to DB and PDJ), RF1AG15819 (to DB and PDJ), and R01AG36836 (to DB and PDJ). U01AG046170 and U01AG46152 are components of the AMP-AD Target Discovery and Preclinical Validation Project.

Authors' contributions

Conceptualization: MS, MW, ES, SG, KA, BZ, and KMI; investigation: MS, MW, NF, YS, XQ, BZ, and KMI; writing (original draft): MS, MW, SG, KA, BZ, and KMI; writing (review and editing): ME, PDJ, DB, and ES; supervision: BZ and KMI; funding acquisition: ME, PDJ, DB, ES, SG, BZ, and KMI. All authors read and approved the final manuscript.

Competing interests

The authors declare that they have no competing interests.

Author details

[1]Department of Alzheimer's Disease Research, National Center for Geriatrics and Gerontology, 7-430 Morioka-cho, Obu, Aichi 474-8511, Japan. [2]Department of Genetics & Genomic Sciences, Icahn School of Medicine at Mount Sinai, 1470 Madison Avenue, Room 8-111, Box 1498, New York, NY 10029, USA. [3]Icahn Institute of Genomics and Multiscale Biology, Icahn School of Medicine at Mount Sinai, One Gustave L. Levy Place, New York, NY, USA. [4]Department of Experimental Gerontology, Graduate School of Pharmaceutical Sciences, Nagoya City University, 3-1 Tanabe-dori, Mizuho-ku, Nagoya, Japan. [5]Department of Neurology, Alzheimer's Disease Research Center, Icahn School of Medicine at Mount Sinai, New York, NY, USA. [6]Department of Pediatrics, Icahn School of Medicine at Mount Sinai, New York, NY, USA. [7]Center for translational & Computational Neuroimmunology, Department of Neurology, The Neurological Institute of New York, Columbia University Medical Center, New York, NY, USA. [8]Broad Institute, Cambridge, MA, USA. [9]Rush Alzheimer's Disease Research Center and Department of Neurology, Rush University Medical Center, 1750 W. Congress Parkway, Chicago, IL 60612, USA. [10]Department of Psychiatry and Alzheimer's Disease Research Center, Icahn School of Medicine at Mount Sinai, New York, NY, USA. [11]Center for NFL Neurological Care, Department of Neurology, New York, NY, USA. [12]James J. Peters VA Medical Center, 130 West Kingsbridge Road, New York, NY, USA. [13]Department of Biological Sciences, Graduate School of Science and Engineering, Tokyo Metropolitan University, Tokyo, Japan. [14]Ronald M. Loeb Center for Alzheimer's Disease, Icahn School of Medicine at Mount Sinai, One Gustave L Levy Place, New York, NY, USA.

References

1. Hardy J, Selkoe DJ. The amyloid hypothesis of Alzheimer's disease: progress and problems on the road to therapeutics. Science. 2002;297(5580):353–6.
2. Heneka MT, Carson MJ, El Khoury J, Landreth GE, Brosseron F, Feinstein DL, et al. Neuroinflammation in Alzheimer's disease. Lancet Neurol. 2015;14(4): 388–405.
3. Lewis J, Dickson DW, Lin WL, Chisholm L, Corral A, Jones G, et al. Enhanced neurofibrillary degeneration in transgenic mice expressing mutant tau and APP. Science. 2001;293(5534):1487–91.
4. Oddo S, Billings L, Kesslak JP, Cribbs DH, LaFerla FM. Abeta immunotherapy leads to clearance of early, but not late, hyperphosphorylated tau aggregates via the proteasome. Neuron. 2004;43(3):321–32.
5. Caccamo A, Oddo S, Sugarman MC, Akbari Y, LaFerla FM. Age- and region-dependent alterations in Abeta-degrading enzymes: implications for Abeta-induced disorders. Neurobiol Aging. 2005;26(5):645–54.
6. Chabrier MA, Blurton-Jones M, Agazaryan AA, Nerhus JL, Martinez-Coria H, LaFerla FM. Soluble abeta promotes wild-type tau pathology in vivo. J Neurosci. 2012;32(48):17345–50.
7. Bennett DA, Schneider JA, Wilson RS, Bienias JL, Arnold SE. Neurofibrillary tangles mediate the association of amyloid load with clinical Alzheimer disease and level of cognitive function. Arch Neurol. 2004;61(3):378–84.
8. Jack CR Jr, Wiste HJ, Weigand SD, Knopman DS, Lowe V, Vemuri P, et al. Amyloid-first and neurodegeneration-first profiles characterize incident amyloid PET positivity. Neurology. 2013;81(20):1732–40.
9. Iacono D, Resnick SM, O'Brien R, Zonderman AB, An Y, Pletnikova O, et al. Mild cognitive impairment and asymptomatic Alzheimer disease subjects: equivalent beta-amyloid and tau loads with divergent cognitive outcomes. J Neuropathol Exp Neurol. 2014;73(4):295–304.
10. Arnold SE, Louneva N, Cao K, Wang LS, Han LY, Wolk DA, et al. Cellular, synaptic, and biochemical features of resilient cognition in Alzheimer's disease. Neurobiol Aging. 2013;34(1):157–68.
11. Zhang B, Gaiteri C, Bodea LG, Wang Z, McElwee J, Podtelezhnikov AA, et al. Integrated systems approach identifies genetic nodes and networks in late-onset Alzheimer's disease. Cell. 2013;153(3):707–20.
12. Wang M, Roussos P, McKenzie A, Zhou X, Kajiwara Y, Brennand KJ, et al. Integrative network analysis of nineteen brain regions identifies molecular signatures and networks underlying selective regional vulnerability to Alzheimer's disease. Genome Med. 2016;8(1):104.
13. Forabosco P, Ramasamy A, Trabzuni D, Walker R, Smith C, Bras J, et al. Insights into TREM2 biology by network analysis of human brain gene expression data. Neurobiol Aging. 2013;34(12):2699–714.
14. Guerreiro R, Wojtas A, Bras J, Carrasquillo M, Rogaeva E, Majounie E, et al. TREM2 variants in Alzheimer's disease. N Engl J Med. 2013;368(2):117–27.
15. Jonsson T, Stefansson H, Steinberg S, Jonsdottir I, Jonsson PV, Snaedal J, et al. Variant of TREM2 associated with the risk of Alzheimer's disease. N Engl J Med. 2013;368(2):107–16.
16. Lill CM, Rengmark A, Pihlstrom L, Fogh I, Shatunov A, Sleiman PM, et al. The role of TREM2 R47H as a risk factor for Alzheimer's disease, frontotemporal lobar degeneration, amyotrophic lateral sclerosis, and Parkinson's disease. Alzheimers Dement. 2015;11(12):1407–16.
17. Pottier C, Ravenscroft TA, Brown PH, Finch NA, Baker M, Parsons M, et al. TYROBP genetic variants in early-onset Alzheimer's disease. Neurobiol Aging. 2016;48:2220. e229–2. e215.
18. Frank S, Burbach GJ, Bonin M, Walter M, Streit W, Bechmann I, et al. TREM2 is upregulated in amyloid plaque-associated microglia in aged APP23 transgenic mice. Glia. 2008;56(13):1438–47.
19. Melchior B, Garcia AE, Hsiung BK, Lo KM, Doose JM, Thrash JC, et al. Dual induction of TREM2 and tolerance-related transcript, Tmem176b, in amyloid transgenic mice: implications for vaccine-based therapies for Alzheimer's disease. ASN Neuro. 2010;2(3):e00037.
20. Jay TR, Miller CM, Cheng PJ, Graham LC, Bemiller S, Broihier ML, et al. TREM2 deficiency eliminates TREM2+ inflammatory macrophages and ameliorates pathology in Alzheimer's disease mouse models. J Exp Med. 2015;212(3):287–95.
21. Suarez-Calvet M, Kleinberger G, Araque Caballero MA, Brendel M, Rominger A, Alcolea D, et al. sTREM2 cerebrospinal fluid levels are a potential biomarker for microglia activity in early-stage Alzheimer's disease and associate with neuronal injury markers. EMBO Mol Med. 2016;8(5):466–76.
22. Heslegrave A, Heywood W, Paterson R, Magdalinou N, Svensson J, Johansson P, et al. Increased cerebrospinal fluid soluble TREM2 concentration in Alzheimer's disease. Mol Neurodegener. 2016;11:3.
23. Piccio L, Deming Y, Del-Aguila JL, Ghezzi L, Holtzman DM, Fagan AM, et al. Cerebrospinal fluid soluble TREM2 is higher in Alzheimer disease and associated with mutation status. Acta Neuropathol. 2016;131(6):925–33.
24. Schlepckow K, Kleinberger G, Fukumori A, Feederle R, Lichtenthaler SF, Steiner H, et al. An Alzheimer-associated TREM2 variant occurs at the ADAM cleavage site and affects shedding and phagocytic function. EMBO Mol Med. 2017;9(10):1356–65.
25. Thornton P, Sevalle J, Deery MJ, Fraser G, Zhou Y, Stahl S, et al. TREM2 shedding by cleavage at the H157-S158 bond is accelerated for the Alzheimer's disease-associated H157Y variant. EMBO Mol Med. 2017;9(10):1366–78.
26. Klesney-Tait J, Turnbull IR, Colonna M. The TREM receptor family and signal integration. Nat Immunol. 2006;7(12):1266–73.
27. Linnartz B, Neumann H. Microglial activatory (immunoreceptor tyrosine-based activation motif)- and inhibitory (immunoreceptor tyrosine-based inhibition motif)-signaling receptors for recognition of the neuronal glycocalyx. Glia. 2013;61(1):37–46.
28. Wang Y, Cella M, Mallinson K, Ulrich JD, Young KL, Robinette ML, et al. TREM2 lipid sensing sustains the microglial response in an Alzheimer's disease model. Cell. 2015;160:1061–71.
29. Ulland TK, Song WM, Huang SC, Ulrich JD, Sergushichev A, Beatty WL, et al. TREM2 maintains microglial metabolic fitness in Alzheimer's disease. Cell. 2017;170(4):649–63. e613.

30. Ulrich JD, Ulland TK, Colonna M, Holtzman DM. Elucidating the role of TREM2 in Alzheimer's disease. Neuron. 2017;94(2):237–48.

31. Jiang T, Tan L, Zhu XC, Zhang QQ, Cao L, Tan MS, et al. Upregulation of TREM2 ameliorates neuropathology and rescues spatial cognitive impairment in a transgenic mouse model of Alzheimer's disease. Neuropsychopharmacology. 2014;39(13):2949–62.

32. Yeh FL, Wang Y, Tom I, Gonzalez LC, Sheng M. TREM2 binds to apolipoproteins, including APOE and CLU/APOJ, and thereby facilitates uptake of amyloid-beta by microglia. Neuron. 2016;91(2):328–40.

33. Jay TR, Hirsch AM, Broihier ML, Miller CM, Neilson LE, Ransohoff RM, et al. Disease progression-dependent effects of TREM2 deficiency in a mouse model of Alzheimer's disease. J Neurosci. 2017;37(3):637–47.

34. Song WM, Joshita S, Zhou Y, Ulland TK, Gilfillan S, Colonna M. Humanized TREM2 mice reveal microglia-intrinsic and -extrinsic effects of R47H polymorphism. J Exp Med. 2018;215:745–60.

35. Hong S, Beja-Glasser VF, Nfonoyim BM, Frouin A, Li S, Ramakrishnan S, et al. Complement and microglia mediate early synapse loss in Alzheimer mouse models. Science. 2016;352(6286):712–6.

36. Squarzoni P, Oller G, Hoeffel G, Pont-Lezica L, Rostaing P, Low D, et al. Microglia modulate wiring of the embryonic forebrain. Cell Rep. 2014;8(5):1271–9.

37. Haure-Mirande JV, Audrain M, Fanutza T, Kim SH, Klein WL, Glabe C, et al. Deficiency of TYROBP, an adapter protein for TREM2 and CR3 receptors, is neuroprotective in a mouse model of early Alzheimer's pathology. Acta Neuropathol. 2017;134:769–88.

38. Jiang T, Wan Y, Zhang YD, Zhou JS, Gao Q, Zhu XC, et al. TREM2 Overexpression has no improvement on neuropathology and cognitive impairment in aging APPswe/PS1dE9 mice. Mol Neurobiol. 2017;54(2):855–65.

39. Keren-Shaul H, Spinrad A, Weiner A, Matcovitch-Natan O, Dvir-Szternfeld R, Ulland TK, et al. A unique microglia type associated with restricting development of Alzheimer's disease. Cell. 2017;169(7):1276–90.

40. Krasemann S, Madore C, Cialic R, Baufeld C, Calcagno N, El Fatimy R, et al. The TREM2-APOE pathway drives the transcriptional phenotype of dysfunctional microglia in neurodegenerative diseases. Immunity. 2017; 47(3):566–81. e569.

41. Bennett DA, Schneider JA, Arvanitakis Z, Wilson RS. Overview and findings from the religious orders study. Curr Alzheimer Res. 2012;9(6):628–45.

42. Bennett DA, Schneider JA, Buchman AS, Barnes LL, Boyle PA, Wilson RS. Overview and findings from the rush Memory and Aging Project. Curr Alzheimer Res. 2012;9(6):646–63.

43. Iijima K, Liu HP, Chiang AS, Hearn SA, Konsolaki M, Zhong Y. Dissecting the pathological effects of human Abeta40 and Abeta42 in Drosophila: a potential model for Alzheimer's disease. Proc Natl Acad Sci U S A. 2004; 101(17):6623–8.

44. Iijima K, Chiang HC, Hearn SA, Hakker I, Gatt A, Shenton C, et al. Abeta42 mutants with different aggregation profiles induce distinct pathologies in Drosophila. PLoS One. 2008;3(2):e1703.

45. Sekiya M, Maruko-Otake A, Hearn S, Sakakibara Y, Fujisaki N, Suzuki E, et al. EDEM function in ERAD protects against chronic ER proteinopathy and age-related physiological decline in drosophila. Dev Cell. 2017;41(6):652–64. e655.

46. Ishimoto H, Sakai T, Kitamoto T. Ecdysone signaling regulates the formation of long-term courtship memory in adult Drosophila melanogaster. Proc Natl Acad Sci U S A. 2009;106(15):6381–6.

47. Ishimoto H, Wang Z, Rao Y, Wu CF, Kitamoto T. A novel role for ecdysone in Drosophila conditioned behavior: linking GPCR-mediated non-canonical steroid action to cAMP signaling in the adult brain. PLoS Genet. 2013;9(10): e1003843.

48. Hu Y, Sopko R, Foos M, Kelley C, Flockhart I, Ammeux N, et al. FlyPrimerBank: an online database for Drosophila melanogaster gene expression analysis and knockdown evaluation of RNAi reagents. G3 (Bethesda). 2013;3(9):1607–16.

49. Liao Y, Smyth GK, Shi W. featureCounts: an efficient general purpose program for assigning sequence reads to genomic features. Bioinformatics. 2014;30(7):923–30.

50. Robinson MD, McCarthy DJ, Smyth GK. edgeR: a Bioconductor package for differential expression analysis of digital gene expression data. Bioinformatics. 2010;26(1):139–40.

51. Ritchie ME, Phipson B, Wu D, Hu Y, Law CW, Shi W, et al. limma powers differential expression analyses for RNA-sequencing and microarray studies. Nucleic Acids Res. 2015;43(7):e47.

52. Benjamini Y, Hochberg Y. Controlling the false discovery rate: a practical and powerful approach to multiple testing. J R Stat Soc. 1995;B 57:289–300.

53. Schneider JA, Aggarwal NT, Barnes L, Boyle P, Bennett DA. The neuropathology of older persons with and without dementia from community versus clinic cohorts. J Alzheimers Dis. 2009;18(3):691–701.

54. Zhang B, Horvath S. A general framework for weighted gene co-expression network analysis. Stat Appl Genet Mol Biol. 2005;4(1):Article 17.

55. Millstein J, Zhang B, Zhu J, Schadt EE. Disentangling molecular relationships with a causal inference test. BMC Genet. 2009;10(1):23.

56. Zhu J, Wiener MC, Zhang C, Fridman A, Minch E, Lum PY, et al. Increasing the power to detect causal associations by combining genotypic and expression data in segregating populations. PLoS Comput Biol. 2007; 3(4):e69.

57. Lai SL, Lee T. Genetic mosaic with dual binary transcriptional systems in Drosophila. Nat Neurosci. 2006;9(5):703–9.

58. Kleinberger G, Yamanishi Y, Suarez-Calvet M, Czirr E, Lohmann E, Cuyvers E, et al. TREM2 mutations implicated in neurodegeneration impair cell surface transport and phagocytosis. Sci Transl Med. 2014;6(243):243ra286.

59. Wunderlich P, Glebov K, Kemmerling N, Tien NT, Neumann H, Walter J. Sequential proteolytic processing of the triggering receptor expressed on myeloid cells-2 (TREM2) protein by ectodomain shedding and gamma-secretase-dependent intramembranous cleavage. J Biol Chem. 2013;288(46):33027–36.

60. Zhong L, Chen XF, Wang T, Wang Z, Liao C, Wang Z, et al. Soluble TREM2 induces inflammatory responses and enhances microglial survival. J Exp Med. 2017;214(3):597–607.

61. Smyth GK. Linear models and empirical bayes methods for assessing differential expression in microarray experiments. Stat Appl Genet Mol Biol. 2004;3:Article3.

62. Gandy S. The role of cerebral amyloid beta accumulation in common forms of Alzheimer disease. J Clin Invest. 2005;115(5):1121–9.

63. Crowther DC, Kinghorn KJ, Miranda E, Page R, Curry JA, Duthie FA, et al. Intraneuronal Abeta, non-amyloid aggregates and neurodegeneration in a Drosophila model of Alzheimer's disease. Neuroscience. 2005;132(1):123–35.

64. Schilling S, Zeitschel U, Hoffmann T, Heiser U, Francke M, Kehlen A, et al. Glutaminyl cyclase inhibition attenuates pyroglutamate Abeta and Alzheimer's disease-like pathology. Nat Med. 2008;14(10):1106–11.

65. Casas-Tinto S, Zhang Y, Sanchez-Garcia J, Gomez-Velazquez M, Rincon-Limas DE, Fernandez-Funez P. The ER stress factor XBP1s prevents amyloid-beta neurotoxicity. Hum Mol Genet. 2011;20(11):2144–60.

66. Paloneva J, Manninen T, Christman G, Hovanes K, Mandelin J, Adolfsson R, et al. Mutations in two genes encoding different subunits of a receptor signaling complex result in an identical disease phenotype. Am J Hum Genet. 2002;71(3):656–62.

67. Hamerman JA, Jarjoura JR, Humphrey MB, Nakamura MC, Seaman WE, Lanier LL. Cutting edge: inhibition of TLR and FcR responses in macrophages by triggering receptor expressed on myeloid cells (TREM)-2 and DAP12. J Immunol. 2006;177(4):2051–5.

68. Turnbull IR, Gilfillan S, Cella M, Aoshi T, Miller M, Piccio L, et al. Cutting edge: TREM-2 attenuates macrophage activation. J Immunol. 2006;177(6):3520–4.

69. Hu Y, Flockhart I, Vinayagam A, Bergwitz C, Berger B, Perrimon N, et al. An integrative approach to ortholog prediction for disease-focused and other functional studies. BMC Bioinformatics. 2011;12:357.

70. Wittmann CW, Wszolek MF, Shulman JM, Salvaterra PM, Lewis J, Hutton M, et al. Tauopathy in Drosophila: neurodegeneration without neurofibrillary tangles. Science. 2001;293(5530):711–4.

71. Iijima-Ando K, Sekiya M, Maruko-Otake A, Ohtake Y, Suzuki E, Lu B, et al. Loss of axonal mitochondria promotes tau-mediated neurodegeneration and Alzheimer's disease-related tau phosphorylation via PAR-1. PLoS Genet. 2012;8(8):e1002918.

72. Chotard C, Salecker I. Glial cell development and function in the Drosophila visual system. Neuron Glia Biol. 2007;3(1):17–25.

73. Leyns CEG, Ulrich JD, Finn MB, Stewart FR, Koscal LJ, Remolina Serrano J, et al. TREM2 deficiency attenuates neuroinflammation and protects against neurodegeneration in a mouse model of tauopathy. Proc Natl Acad Sci U S A. 2017;114(43):11524–9.

74. Chou PS, Wu MN, Chou MC, Chien I, Yang YH. Angiotensin-converting enzyme insertion/deletion polymorphism and the longitudinal progression of Alzheimer's disease. Geriatr Gerontol Int. 2017;17:1544–50.

75. Griciuc A, Serrano-Pozo A, Parrado AR, Lesinski AN, Asselin CN, Mullin K, et al. Alzheimer's disease risk gene CD33 inhibits microglial uptake of amyloid beta. Neuron. 2013;78(4):631–43.

76. Crehan H, Holton P, Wray S, Pocock J, Guerreiro R, Hardy J. Complement receptor 1 (CR1) and Alzheimer's disease. Immunobiology. 2012;217(2):244–50.
77. Lemaitre B, Hoffmann J. The host defense of Drosophila melanogaster. Annu Rev Immunol. 2007;25(1):697–743.
78. Pal S, Wu J, Wu LP. Microarray analyses reveal distinct roles for Rel proteins in the Drosophila immune response. Dev Comp Immunol. 2008;32(1):50–60.
79. Park J-S, Ji IJ, Kim D-H, An HJ, Yoon S-Y. The Alzheimer's disease-associated R47H variant of TREM2 has an altered glycosylation pattern and protein stability. Front Neurosci. 2016;10:618.

7

Exome-wide analysis of bi-allelic alterations identifies a Lynch phenotype in The Cancer Genome Atlas

Alexandra R. Buckley[1,2], Trey Ideker[3,4,5], Hannah Carter[3,4,5], Olivier Harismendy[4,6*] and Nicholas J. Schork[2,7,8*]

Abstract

Background: Cancer susceptibility germline variants generally require somatic alteration of the remaining allele to drive oncogenesis and, in some cases, tumor mutational profiles. Whether combined germline and somatic bi-allelic alterations are universally required for germline variation to influence tumor mutational profile is unclear. Here, we performed an exome-wide analysis of the frequency and functional effect of bi-allelic alterations in The Cancer Genome Atlas (TCGA).

Methods: We integrated germline variant, somatic mutation, somatic methylation, and somatic copy number loss data from 7790 individuals from TCGA to identify germline and somatic bi-allelic alterations in all coding genes. We used linear models to test for association between mono- and bi-allelic alterations and somatic microsatellite instability (MSI) and somatic mutational signatures.

Results: We discovered significant enrichment of bi-allelic alterations in mismatch repair (MMR) genes and identified six bi-allelic carriers with elevated MSI, consistent with Lynch syndrome. In contrast, we find little evidence of an effect of mono-allelic germline variation on MSI. Using MSI burden and bi-allelic alteration status, we reclassify two variants of unknown significance in *MSH6* as potentially pathogenic for Lynch syndrome. Extending our analysis of MSI to a set of 127 DNA damage repair (DDR) genes, we identified a novel association between methylation of *SHPRH* and MSI burden.

Conclusions: We find that bi-allelic alterations are infrequent in TCGA but most frequently occur in *BRCA1/2* and MMR genes. Our results support the idea that bi-allelic alteration is required for germline variation to influence tumor mutational profile. Overall, we demonstrate that integrating germline, somatic, and epigenetic alterations provides new understanding of somatic mutational profiles.

Keywords: Cancer genomics, Cancer germline, Cancer predisposition, TCGA, Microsatellite instability, Lynch syndrome, Mutational signatures

Background

In rare familial cancer, inherited variation can both increase cancer risk and influence the molecular landscape of a tumor. For example, Lynch syndrome is characterized by an increased cancer risk and increased burden of somatic microsatellite instability (MSI) [1, 2]. The study of this phenomenon has been recently extended to sporadic cancers. For example, carriers of pathogenic mutations in

BRCA1/2 have both increased cancer risk and molecular evidence of homologous recombination deficiency in their tumors [3, 4]. Novel sequencing and analytical methods can be used to reveal a myriad of molecular phenotypes in the tumor, such as mutational signatures, rearrangement signatures, MSI, and infiltrating immune cell content [5–9]. A number of novel associations between these molecular somatic phenotypes and germline variants have recently been discovered. Rare variants in *BRCA1/2* have been associated with mutational signature 3, a novel rearrangement signature, and an overall increased mutational burden [6, 10–12]. Common variants in the

* Correspondence: oharismendy@ucsd.edu; nschork@jcvi.org
[4]Moores Cancer Center, University of California San Diego, La Jolla, CA, USA
[2]Human Biology Program, J. Craig Venter Institute, La Jolla, CA, USA
Full list of author information is available at the end of the article

APOBEC3 region have been associated with the corresponding *APOBEC* deficient mutational signature, and a haplotype at the 19p13.3 locus has been associated with somatic mutation of *PTEN* [13, 14]. In addition, interestingly, distinct squamous cell carcinomas (SCCs) arising in the same individual have a more similar somatic copy number profile than SCCs that occur between individuals [15]. Taken together, these results demonstrate that both common and rare germline variation can influence the somatic phenotype of sporadic cancers.

Similar to the two-hit mechanism of inactivation of tumor suppressor genes in familial cancer syndromes described by Nordling and then Knudson decades ago, germline and somatic bi-allelic alteration of *BRCA1/2* is required to induce somatic mutational signature 3, a single germline "hit" is not sufficient [10, 11, 16, 17]. Whether a secondary hit is universally required for germline variation to influence somatic phenotype is currently unclear. Here, we address this question using The Cancer Genome Atlas (TCGA) dataset. TCGA is the most comprehensive resource of germline and somatic variation to enable this analysis, as it contains paired tumor and normal sequence data and a number of other molecular somatic phenotypes for 33 cancer types [18]. In contrast with previous studies of TCGA germline variation that focused on specific cancer types or candidate genes, we performed an exome-wide analysis to identify genes affected by both germline and somatic alterations (referred to as bi-allelic alteration) and study their association with somatic phenotypes [10–13, 19]. Specifically, we conducted an integrated study of all genetic factors that contribute to somatic MSI burden and identified six individuals with characteristics consistent with Lynch syndrome: bi-allelic alteration of a MMR gene, elevated somatic MSI, and an earlier age of cancer diagnosis.

Methods
Data acquisition
Approval for access to TCGA case sequence and clinical data were obtained from the database of Genotypes and Phenotypes (project no. 8072, Integrated analysis of germline and somatic perturbation as it relates to tumor phenotypes). Whole exome (WXS) germline variant calls from 8542 individuals were obtained using GATK v3.5 as described previously [20]. The samples prepared using whole genome amplification (WGA) were excluded from the analysis due to previous identification of technical artifacts in both somatic and germline variant calls in WGA samples [20, 21]. Somatic mutation calls obtained using MuTect2 were downloaded from GDC as Mutation Annotation Format (MAF) files [22]. Raw somatic sequence data was downloaded from the Genomic Data Commons (GDC) in Binary Alignment Map (BAM) file

format aligned to the hg19 reference genome. Normalized somatic methylation beta values from the Illumina 450 methylation array for the probes most anti-correlated with gene expression were downloaded from Broad Firehose (release stddata__2016_01_28, file extension: min_exp_corr). A total of 7790 samples and 28 cancer types had germline, somatic, and methylation data available.

Segmented SNP6 array data were downloaded from Broad Firehose (release stddata__2016_01_28, file extension: segmented_scna_hg19). Segments with an estimated fold change value ≤ 0.9, which corresponds to a single chromosome loss in 20% of tumor cells, were considered deletions. RNAseq RSEM abundance estimates normalized by gene were downloaded from Broad Firehose (release 2016_07_15, file extension: RSEM_genes_normalized). For 5931 TCGA WXS samples quantitative MSI burden and binary MSI classification calls were obtained from previous work done by Hause et al. [8]. When used as a quantitative phenotype, MSI is expressed as the percentage of microsatellite regions that display somatic instability; when used as a binary classification, MSI is expressed as MSI high (MSI-H) vs. non-MSI. Aggregate allele frequencies and allele frequencies in seven ancestry groups (African, Admixed American, East Asian, Finnish, non-Finnish European, South Asian, and other) were obtained from ExAC v3.01 [23]. Gene-level expression data from normal tissues was downloaded from the GTEx portal (V7, file extension: RNASeQCv1.1.8_gene_tpm) [24].

Variant annotation and filtering
Raw variant calls were filtered using GATK VQSR TS 99.5 for SNVs and TS 95.0 for indels. Additionally, indels in homopolymer regions, here defined as four or more sequential repeats of the same nucleotide, with a quality by depth (QD) score < 1 were removed.

Putative germline and somatic loss-of-function (LOF) variants were identified using the LOFTEE plugin for VEP and Ensembl release 85 [25]. LOFTEE defines LOF variants as stop-gained, nonsense, frameshift, and splice site disrupting. Default LOFTEE settings were used, and only variants receiving a high confidence LOF prediction were retained. It was further required that LOF variants have an allele frequency < 0.05 in all ancestry groups represented in ExAC. For somatic mutations, LOFTEE output with no additional filters was used. Gene level, CADD score, and ClinVar annotations were obtained using ANNOVAR and ClinVar database v.20170905 [26]. A germline variant was determined to be pathogenic using ClinVar annotations if at least half of the contributing sources rated the variant "Pathogenic" or "Likely Pathogenic." Li-Fraumeni variant annotations were obtained from the IARC-TP53 database [27–29]. Pfam protein domain annotations used in lollipop plots were obtained from Ensembl BioMart [30, 31].

Somatic methylation

For each gene, the methylation probe that was most anti-correlated with gene expression was obtained from Broad Firehose and used for all subsequent analyses. Methylation calls were performed for each gene and each cancer type independently. For each gene, the beta value of the chosen methylation probe was converted to a Z-score within each cancer type. Individuals with a Z-score ≥ 3 were considered hyper methylated ($M = 1$), and all others were considered non-methylated ($M = 0$). To determine if methylation calls were associated with reduced somatic gene expression, a linear model of the form $\log_{10} (E_{ij}) \sim C_i + M_{ij}$ was used, where E_{ij} denotes expression of gene j in tumor i, C_i denotes cancer type of sample i, and M_{ij} denotes binary methylation status of gene j in sample i. Only genes where methylation calls were nominally associated ($p \leq 0.05$) with decreased gene expression were retained. Using this process, we identified 863,798 methylation events affecting 11,744 genes.

Loss of heterozygosity

To assess loss of heterozygosity (LOH) for a given heterozygous germline variant, the somatic allele frequency of the germline variant was obtained from the somatic BAM files using samtools mpileup v1.3.1 (SNPs) or varscan v2.3.9 (indels) [32, 33]. Any germline variant that was not observed in the tumor was excluded from further analysis. A one-way Fisher's exact test comparing reference and alternate read counts was performed to test for allelic imbalance between the normal and tumor sample. Only sites with a nominally significant ($p \leq 0.05$) increase in the germline allelic fraction were retained. To confirm that the observed allelic imbalance was due to somatic loss of the WT allele and not due to somatic amplification of the damaging allele, we required that the region be deleted in the tumor based on TCGA CNV data (fold change value ≤ 0.9). Loci that had a significant Fisher's exact test but were not located in a somatic deletion were considered "allelic imbalance" (AI). Using this method, we observed 3418 LOH events in 1672 genes.

Gene set enrichment analysis

Gene set enrichment analysis was performed using the fgsea R package and the following parameters: minSize = 3, maxSize = 500, nperm = 20,000, and the canonical pathway gene set from MsigDB (c2.cp.v5.0.symbols.gmt) [34, 35]. Genes were ranked according to the fraction of germline LOF variants that acquired a second somatic alteration (number bi-allelic alterations/number germline LOF variants). Genes with fewer than three germline

LOF variants in the entire cohort were excluded from this analysis to reduce noise.

Mutational signature analysis

To identify somatic mutational signatures, counts for each of 96 possible somatic substitutions ± 1 bp context were obtained for all tumor samples. For each sample, mutational signatures were identified using the DeconstructSigs R package, which uses a non-negative least squares regression to estimate the relative contributions of previously identified signatures to the observed somatic mutation matrix [36]. DeconstructSigs was run with default normalization parameters, and relative contributions were estimated for the 30 mutational signatures in COSMIC [37].

To estimate significance of association between germline variants and somatic mutational signature burden, we employed both a pan-cancer Wilcoxon rank sum test and a permutation-based approach to ensure that significance was due to germline variant status and not cancer type. For the permutation approach, the pairing between germline variant status and mutational signature profile was shuffled 10,000×. A Wilcoxon rank sum test was run for each permutation to obtain a null distribution for the test statistic. P values were determined for each signature as the fraction of permutations with a Wilcoxon test statistic greater than or equal to the observed data.

Statistical analyses

Principal component analysis (PCA) was performed on common (allele frequency > 0.01) germline variants using PLINK v1.90b3.29, and the first two principal components obtained from this analysis were used to control for ancestry in all of the regression models we fit to the data [38]. G*Power 3.1 was used to perform a power calculation for the contribution of damaging germline variants to somatic MSI [39]. The following parameters were used: α error probability = 0.05, power = 0.80, effect size = $6.83e^{-4}$, and number of predictors = 20. To assess potential co-occurrence of SHPRH methylation with alterations in other genes, individuals were grouped according to presence (+) or absence (−) of SHPRH methylation. A one-way Fisher's exact test was used to test for an abundance of another alteration of interest in SHPRH methylation positive individuals vs. SHPRH methylation negative individuals. Individuals with > 5000 somatic mutations were excluded from these analyses to exclude potential confounding due to somatic hypermutation.

To test for association between genetic alteration and somatic MSI burden, a linear model of the form $\log_{10} (M_i) \sim G_{ij} + S_{ij} + Me_{ij} + X_i$ was used, where M_i denotes somatic MSI burden of sample i, G_{ij}, S_{ij}, and Me_{ij} are binary indicators for germline, somatic, and methylation alteration status of gene j in sample i, and X_i represents a vector of covariates for sample i (cancer type, PC1, PC2). All analyses using somatic MSI data were performed on a maximum of $n = 4997$ individuals. To test for association between germline alteration and age of diagnosis, a linear model of the form $A_i \sim G_{ij} + X_i$ was used where A_i denotes age of diagnosis for sample i, G_{ij} is a binary indicator for germline alteration status of gene j in sample i, and X_i represents a vector of covariates for sample i (cancer type, PC1, PC2). All analyses using age of diagnosis were performed on a maximum of $n = 8913$ individuals.

Results

The MMR pathway is frequently affected by bi-allelic alteration

To find events most likely to influence a somatic phenotype, we limited our analysis to alterations predicted to be highly disruptive. We therefore only considered loss-of-function (LOF) germline variants, LOF somatic mutations, epigenetic silencing of genes via DNA hyper-methylation, and somatic loss of heterozygosity (LOH) events that select for a germline LOF allele (see "Methods" and Additional file 1: Figure S1 and S2). In total, we analyzed 7790 individuals with germline variant, somatic mutation, and methylation data available, corresponding to 95,601 germline LOF variants, 225,257 somatic LOF mutations, and 863,798 somatic methylation events (Fig. 1). Using this data, we were able to determine the frequency of three types of germline bi-allelic alterations: (1) germline LOF and somatic LOF (germline:somatic), (2) germline LOF and somatic epigenetic silencing (germline:methylation), and (3) germline LOF with somatic LOH.

Surprisingly, we found a low incidence of bi-allelic alterations, with only 4.0% of all germline LOF variants acquiring a secondary somatic alteration via any mechanism. We observed 198 germline:somatic events (0.02% of all germline LOF), 433 germline:methylation events (0.04%), and 3279 LOH events (3.4%). To determine whether bi-allelic alterations affect specific biological processes, we ranked genes by the frequency of bi-allelic alteration and performed a gene set enrichment analysis (GSEA) using 1330 canonical pathway gene sets [34, 35]. The only association significant beyond a

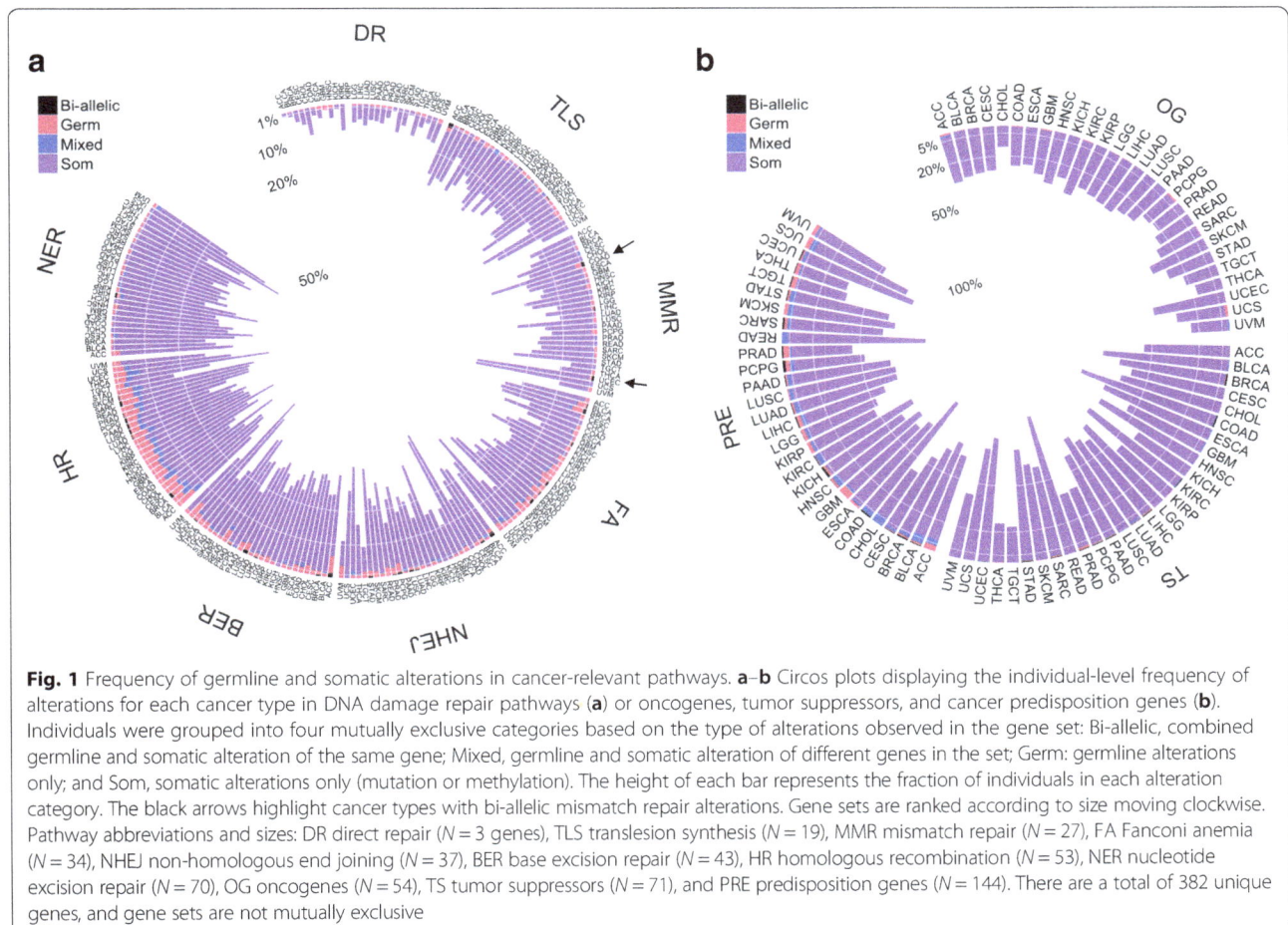

Fig. 1 Frequency of germline and somatic alterations in cancer-relevant pathways. **a–b** Circos plots displaying the individual-level frequency of alterations for each cancer type in DNA damage repair pathways (**a**) or oncogenes, tumor suppressors, and cancer predisposition genes (**b**). Individuals were grouped into four mutually exclusive categories based on the type of alterations observed in the gene set: Bi-allelic, combined germline and somatic alteration of the same gene; Mixed, germline and somatic alteration of different genes in the set; Germ: germline alterations only; and Som, somatic alterations only (mutation or methylation). The height of each bar represents the fraction of individuals in each alteration category. The black arrows highlight cancer types with bi-allelic mismatch repair alterations. Gene sets are ranked according to size moving clockwise. Pathway abbreviations and sizes: DR direct repair ($N = 3$ genes), TLS translesion synthesis ($N = 19$), MMR mismatch repair ($N = 27$), FA Fanconi anemia ($N = 34$), NHEJ non-homologous end joining ($N = 37$), BER base excision repair ($N = 43$), HR homologous recombination ($N = 53$), NER nucleotide excision repair ($N = 70$), OG oncogenes ($N = 54$), TS tumor suppressors ($N = 71$), and PRE predisposition genes ($N = 144$). There are a total of 382 unique genes, and gene sets are not mutually exclusive

multiple hypothesis correction was an enrichment of germline:somatic alterations in the KEGG mismatch repair (MMR) pathway ($q = 0.0056$) (Additional file 1: Figure S3 and Additional file 2: Table S1). To ensure that the lack of enriched pathways was not due to our strict definition of somatic damaging events, we repeated the analysis including all somatic mutations with a CADD score ≥ 20. Though this increased, the number of germline:somatic alterations (376, 0.039%), no additional significantly enriched pathways were found. Similarly, we repeated the analysis using a less restrictive definition of LOH, referred to as "allelic imbalance" (AI), that accommodates other mechanisms such as copy neutral LOH, subclonal LOH, or intra-tumoral SCNA heterogeneity (see "Methods"). We again observed more AI events (7920, 8.2%), but no additional pathways were significantly enriched.

Landscape of germline and somatic alteration of DNA damage repair pathways

Having shown that MMR genes frequently harbor bi-allelic alterations, we next investigated the frequency of germline, somatic, and epigenetic alterations in a panel of 210 DNA damage repair (DDR) genes. While germline variation in DDR genes has previously been studied, only a few studies have considered specific DDR pathway information. DDR genes were assigned to eight gene sets using pathway information: direct repair, translesion synthesis, mismatch repair, Fanconi anemia, non-homologous end joining, base excision repair, homologous recombination, and nucleotide excision repair [40]. We also examined three additional cancer-relevant gene sets: oncogenes, tumor suppressors, and cancer predisposition genes (Additional file 3: Table S2) [41, 42]. For each gene set and cancer type, we calculated the fraction of individuals with bi-allelic, germline, somatic, or epigenetic alteration of any gene in the gene set (Fig. 1).

Consistent with previous studies, the fraction of individuals carrying germline LOF was low for both DDR genes and cancer-relevant gene sets (Fig. 1, Additional file 4: Table S3) [12]. Overall, 16% of individuals carried a germline LOF in any of the genes interrogated, with 5% carrying a germline LOF in a known predisposition gene. For each gene set, we tested for overabundance of germline LOF carriers in each cancer type vs. all other cancer types. We discovered associations between breast cancer and germline alteration of the Fanconi anemia and tumor suppressor gene set, which are likely driven by *BRCA1/2* germline variants (Additional file 1: Figure S4a). We expanded our analysis to include known pathogenic missense variants from the ClinVar database and discovered additional significant associations between pheochromocytoma and paraganglioma (PCPG) and both the predisposition and oncogene sets (Additional file 1: Figure S4b

and Additional file 5: Table S4) [26]. This association is driven by missense variants in *SDHB* and *RET* that predispose to PCPG and have been previously reported in TCGA [43]. Loss of heterozygosity in these PCPG individuals was frequently observed (77% of *SDHB* germline carriers), consistent with *SDHB* acting via a tumor suppressor mechanism [44]. We conclude that there is no cancer type in TCGA that harbors an excess of damaging germline variants in DDR or cancer-relevant genes, with the exception of the well-described predisposition syndrome genes *BRCA1/2*, *SDHB*, and *RET*.

A subset of individuals in TCGA exhibits characteristics of Lynch syndrome

We found that the MMR pathway was significantly enriched for germline:somatic alterations. This association was driven by six individuals who carry a germline:somatic alteration of a MMR gene. In five individuals, the gene affected was a known Lynch syndrome gene (*MLH1*, *MSH2*, *MSH6*, and *PMS2*), which we will refer to as L-MMR genes [2]. The remaining individual carried a germline:somatic alteration of *MSH5* (Fig. 2a, red arrow). While *MSH5* is not known to be a Lynch syndrome gene, we included this individual in further analyses of MMR germline:somatic alteration carriers. Four of the germline:somatic alteration carriers have uterine cancer (UCEC) and two have colon cancer (COAD), cancer type characteristic of Lynch syndrome (Fig. 1b, arrows) [45]. This prompted us to investigate the molecular and clinical phenotype of germline:somatic alteration carriers to determine if they are consistent with Lynch syndrome characteristics. While germline:somatic alteration of MMR genes in TCGA has been previously described, detailed somatic phenotyping of these individuals has not been performed [9]. Using previously published MSI data, we investigated the fraction of microsatellite loci that exhibit instability in the tumor (somatic MSI burden) of individuals carrying alterations in MMR genes [8]. Figure 2a shows germline, somatic, and epigenetic alteration status of L-MMR genes for all individuals classified as MSI high (MSI-H) by Hause et al., with bi-allelic mutation carriers grouped to the left. Interestingly, only 76% of MSI-H individuals have an alteration (germline LOF, somatic LOF, or hyper-methylation) of an MMR gene, indicating that some of the variation in somatic MSI is not explained by the genetic alterations investigated.

Using a linear model controlling for cancer type, we found that the 6 individuals with germline:somatic MMR alterations were diagnosed on average 14 years earlier ($p = 0.0041$) and have 2.8 fold higher somatic MSI ($p = 3.95e^{-15}$) than individuals with any other type of MMR pathway alteration (Fig. 2b, Additional file 1: Tables S5, S6). Of the five individuals with germline:somatic alteration of a L-MMR

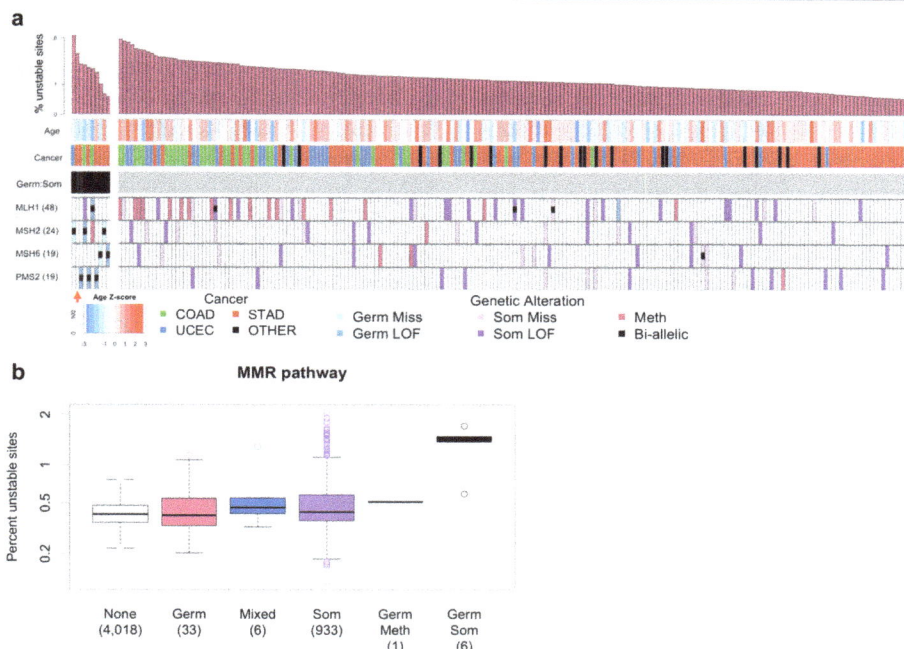

Fig. 2 Genetic and clinical characteristics of MSI-H individuals. **a** CoMut plot displaying germline, somatic, and epigenetic events in L-MMR genes (bottom 4 rows—number of affected individuals in parentheses) for 217 MSI-H individuals (columns). The top histogram represents MSI burden expressed as the fraction of possible microsatellite sites that are unstable. Age of diagnosis was converted to a Z-score using the mean and standard deviation age for each cancer type. Cancer types with fewer than 5 MSI-H individuals are labeled "Other" and include bladder, head and neck, kidney, glioma, lung, liver, prostate, stomach, and rectal cancer. The type of genetic alteration is indicated by color, and bi-allelic events are indicated by a black box. Individuals with bi-allelic (germline:somatic) MMR mutations are grouped to the left. The red arrow highlights an individual with bi-allelic alteration in *MSH5* (not an L-MMR gene). **b** Somatic MSI burden in 4997 TCGA individuals grouped by type of MMR pathway alteration. Categories are the same as those described in Fig. 1: Bi-allelic, combined germline and somatic alteration of the same gene; Mixed, germline and somatic alteration of different genes in the set; Germ, germline alterations only; and Som, somatic alterations only (mutation or methylation). Individuals with bi-allelic alteration occurring via germline:somatic and germline:methylation mechanisms are displayed separately. The number of individuals in each category is indicated in parentheses

gene, four carried a germline LOF variant that is known to be pathogenic for Lynch syndrome, and one carried a LOF variant *MSH6* (p.I855fs) not present in ClinVar (Additional file 1: Table S7). This frameshift *MSH6* VUS is five base pairs upstream of a known pathogenic frameshift variant. This suggests that disruption of the reading frame in this gene region is pathogenic and the novel MSH6 variant likely also predisposes to Lynch syndrome (Additional file 1: Table S8). While a diagnosis of Lynch syndrome requires clinical family history data not available in TCGA, the carriers were diagnosed at an earlier age and exhibit increased somatic MSI characteristic of Lynch syndrome. We note that this result would have gone unnoticed in an analysis of somatic MSI using interaction terms to model bi-allelic alteration at the single gene level, highlighting the value of grouping genes by biological pathway (Additional file 1: Table S9). Interestingly, we observed the identical nonsense mutation in *PMS2* (p.R628X) in two individuals, once

as an inherited variant and once as an acquired somatic mutation (Additional file 1: Figure S5). This overlap between clinically relevant germline variants and somatic mutations suggests that, in some instances, the origin of a mutation is less important than its functional effect.

Using the MSI-H phenotype to identify potentially pathogenic variants

Given the large effect of germline:somatic LOF mutations on somatic MSI, we next asked whether germline:somatic missense mutations produced a similar phenotype. We expanded our analysis to include missense variants known to be pathogenic for Lynch syndrome from ClinVar. We identified one individual with bi-allelic alteration of *MSH2* involving a pathogenic missense germline variant (p.S554 N) and a somatic LOF mutation (Additional file 1: Table S7). Including missense somatic mutations with a CADD score ≥ 20 led to the identification of one individual with bi-allelic alteration of *PMS2* involving a germline LOF variant (p.R563X) and a secondary somatic missense mutation (Additional file 1: Table S8).

We observed a number of missense germline variants in L-MMR genes not present in ClinVar, which we consider variants of unknown significance (VUS). We reasoned that the phenotype of elevated somatic MSI and germline:somatic L-MMR mutation could be used to identify germline VUS likely to be pathogenic for Lynch syndrome. Using 212 individuals classified as MSI-H, we identified 74 individuals with a damaging somatic mutation in a L-MMR gene (Fig. 3a) [8]. Of the individuals with L-MMR somatic mutations, 37 have a germline missense variant in the somatically mutated gene. To identify variants most likely to be damaging, we retained only those with a minor allele frequency < 0.005 in all ancestry groups represented in ExAC. Three individuals met the criteria of having an MSI-H phenotype and a bi-allelic L-MMR mutation involving a likely damaging missense germline variant. One was the previously identified *MSH2* p.S554N variant carrier, the others carried two VUS: *MSH2* (p.P616R) and *MSH6* (p.F432C) (Additional file 1: Table S8).

Closer investigation of the *MSH6* p.F432C variant showed that other amino acid substitutions at the same residue were classified as pathogenic in ClinVar (Additional file 1: Table S8). Should these VUS be pathogenic, we would expect the carriers to have an earlier age of cancer diagnosis. The individual carrying the *MSH6* p.F432C variant was diagnosed earlier than average ($Z = -1.03$) while the individual carrying the *MSH2* p.P616R variant was diagnosed later ($Z = 1.20$). Age of diagnosis cannot be used alone to classify a variant; however, this evidence suggests that *MSH2* p.P616R may not be pathogenic. While validation is required to confirm pathogenicity of this variant as well as the previously mentioned *MSH6* p.I855fs, we offer evidence that these variants may predispose to Lynch syndrome, as well as show evidence suggesting that *MSH2* p.P616R may be benign.

Missense bi-allelic alterations exhibit an attenuated phenotype

Taken together, we have identified ten individuals with germline:somatic MMR alterations, six of which carry a germline variant that is known to be pathogenic for Lynch syndrome (Table 1). With this in mind, we asked whether individuals with germline:somatic LOF mutations have a more severe phenotype than those with combined LOF and missense mutations. Bi-allelic alteration carriers were divided into two groups: those with germline and somatic LOF mutations (Bi-LOF, $n = 6$) and those with missense germline variants or missense somatic mutations (Bi-Miss, $n = 4$). We found that both Bi-LOF ($p = 2.78e^{-15}$) and Bi-Miss ($p = 1.01e^{-10}$)

groups have significantly elevated MSI (Fig. 3b and Additional file 1: Table S10). Bi-Miss and Bi-LOF have a median 1.50 and 2.35 fold higher somatic MSI compared to individuals with somatic MMR alteration alone, demonstrating a synergistic effect between germline variants and somatic mutations. Similarly, both Bi-LOF and Bi-Miss groups had significantly higher contribution of mutational signature 6, a signature associated with mismatch repair defects (Additional file 1: Figure S6) [7]. In contrast, only Bi-LOF individuals were diagnosed at an earlier age (Fig. 3c and Additional file 1: Table S11). These results show that any damaging bi-allelic MMR alterations are sufficient to induce high levels of somatic MSI, but only bi-allelic alterations via dual LOF mutation are associated with an earlier age of diagnosis.

Mono-allelic damaging germline alteration has minimal effect on somatic MSI burden

Having shown that combined germline LOF and missense somatic mutations are sufficient to cause elevated MSI, we hypothesized that damaging germline variation in the absence of somatic mutation could also increase somatic MSI. To maximize power, we expanded our analysis to include all MMR genes as well as two different categories of damaging germline variation: known (ClinVar) and predicted (CADD ≥ 30) pathogenic (Additional file 5: Table S4). Individuals with any somatic alterations in MMR genes were excluded from this analysis to get an accurate estimate of the effect of damaging germline variation alone. There were no significant association between damaging germline variation in the MMR pathway and somatic MSI burden (Additional file 1: Figure S7 and Table S12). Known variants showed the strongest effect (0.02 fold increase in MSI burden), and this was largely driven by *MLH3* p.V741F, a variant with conflicting reports of pathogenicity that is carried by 195 individuals. From this, we conclude that the effect of damaging germline variation without concomitant somatic mutation on somatic MSI is small.

Methylation of *SHPRH* associated with somatic MSI burden

We observe that 24% of MSI-H individuals have no alteration (germline LOF, somatic LOF, or hyper-methylation) of an MMR gene, suggesting that there is variation in somatic MSI burden due to factors outside of known MMR genes (Fig. 3b) [46]. To investigate this further, we extended the search to all DDR genes. We separately assessed the contribution of germline LOF, somatic LOF, and somatic methylation to somatic MSI burden using a gene level linear model. Somatic LOF frameshift mutations that overlap with microsatellite loci were removed from this analysis, as we were unable to

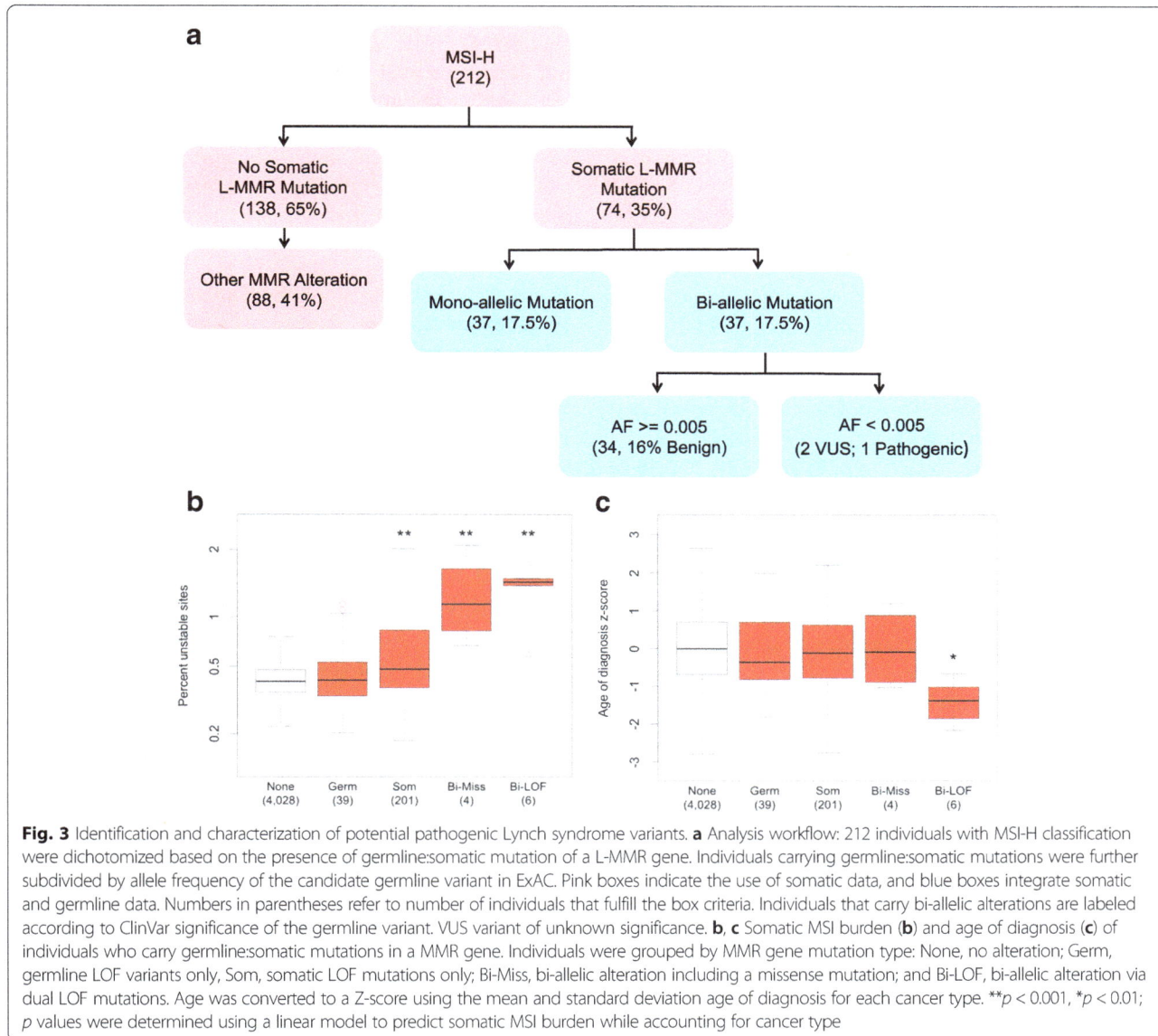

Fig. 3 Identification and characterization of potential pathogenic Lynch syndrome variants. **a** Analysis workflow: 212 individuals with MSI-H classification were dichotomized based on the presence of germline:somatic mutation of a L-MMR gene. Individuals carrying germline:somatic mutations were further subdivided by allele frequency of the candidate germline variant in ExAC. Pink boxes indicate the use of somatic data, and blue boxes integrate somatic and germline data. Numbers in parentheses refer to number of individuals that fulfill the box criteria. Individuals that carry bi-allelic alterations are labeled according to ClinVar significance of the germline variant. VUS variant of unknown significance. **b**, **c** Somatic MSI burden (**b**) and age of diagnosis (**c**) of individuals who carry germline:somatic mutations in a MMR gene. Individuals were grouped by MMR gene mutation type: None, no alteration; Germ, germline LOF variants only, Som, somatic LOF mutations only; Bi-Miss, bi-allelic alteration including a missense mutation; and Bi-LOF, bi-allelic alteration via dual LOF mutations. Age was converted to a Z-score using the mean and standard deviation age of diagnosis for each cancer type. **$**p < 0.001$, *$p < 0.01$; p values were determined using a linear model to predict somatic MSI burden while accounting for cancer type

Table 1 Number of individuals affected by three types of germline:somatic alterations in MMR genes

Gene	Germline LOF somatic LOF	Germline LOF somatic MISS	Germline MISS somatic LOF
MLH1	1*		
MSH2	1*		1,1*
MSH6	1		1
PMS2	2*	1*	
MSH5	1		

*Individual carries a ClinVar pathogenic germline variant

determine the direction of causality between these mutations and overall MSI burden (Additional file 1: Figure S8 and Table S13). Additionally, the MMR bi-allelic alteration carriers were excluded from this analysis to obtain an accurate assessment of mono-allelic germline variation. The results of this analysis are summarized in Fig. 4. Consistent with the lack of association between damaging MMR germline variants and somatic MSI, we found no significant association at the single gene level between germline LOF and somatic MSI (Fig. 4a).

We found that somatic mutation of *MLH1* and *MSH2* and somatic methylation of *MLH1* were associated with increased MSI burden, confirming what has been previously reported (Fig. 4b, c) [46]. In addition, we discovered a novel association between methylation of *SHPRH* and elevated somatic MSI ($p = 1.19e^{-16}$) (Fig. 4c).

SHPRH is a E3 ubiquitin-protein ligase and a member of the translesion synthesis pathway, a pathway that enables DNA replication to traverse regions of DNA damage via specialized polymerases [47]. Methylation of *SHPRH* was associated with a 16% decrease in gene expression in a pan-cancer analysis (Fig. 4d). We observed that methylation of *SHPRH* has the strongest effect both on *SHPRH* expression and somatic MSI burden in uterine cancer (Fig. 4e, f and Additional file 1: Figure S9). Interestingly, *SHPRH* expression is highest in normal ovarian and uterine tissues among 23 tissues examined, suggesting a specific function for *SHPRH* in these organs (Additional file 1: Figure S10) [24]. Methylation of *MLH1* and *SHPRH* are both associated with mutational signature 6, with a stronger association in uterine cancer (Additional file 1: Figure S11).

To confirm that *SHPRH* methylation is the likely causal factor influencing somatic MSI, we performed a co-occurrence analysis to find other somatic events correlated with *SHPRH* methylation (Additional file 1: Figure S12). There were a large number of somatic events significantly correlated with *SHPRH* methylation,

including somatic MMR mutations; however, we found that *SHPRH* methylation remains a significant determinant of somatic MSI even after accounting for other somatic MMR alterations (Additional file 1: Table S14). Furthermore, we found a significant, albeit weaker, association between somatic expression of *SHPRH* and MSI burden, indicating that *SHPRH* methylation likely affects MSI burden via silencing of *SHPRH* (Additional file 1: Table S15).

Mono-allelic germline alterations are not associated with somatic mutational signatures

We demonstrate that bi-allelic alteration is necessary for germline variants to influence somatic MSI. Next, we investigated whether this requirement for bi-allelic alteration applied to other somatic phenotypes, such as mutational signatures. We hypothesized that mono- or bi-allelic alterations in other DDR pathways may also be associated with known mutational signatures, as has been demonstrated between bi-allelic alteration of *BRCA1/2* and mutational signature 3 [10]. We first attempted to replicate the *BRCA1/2* association, but

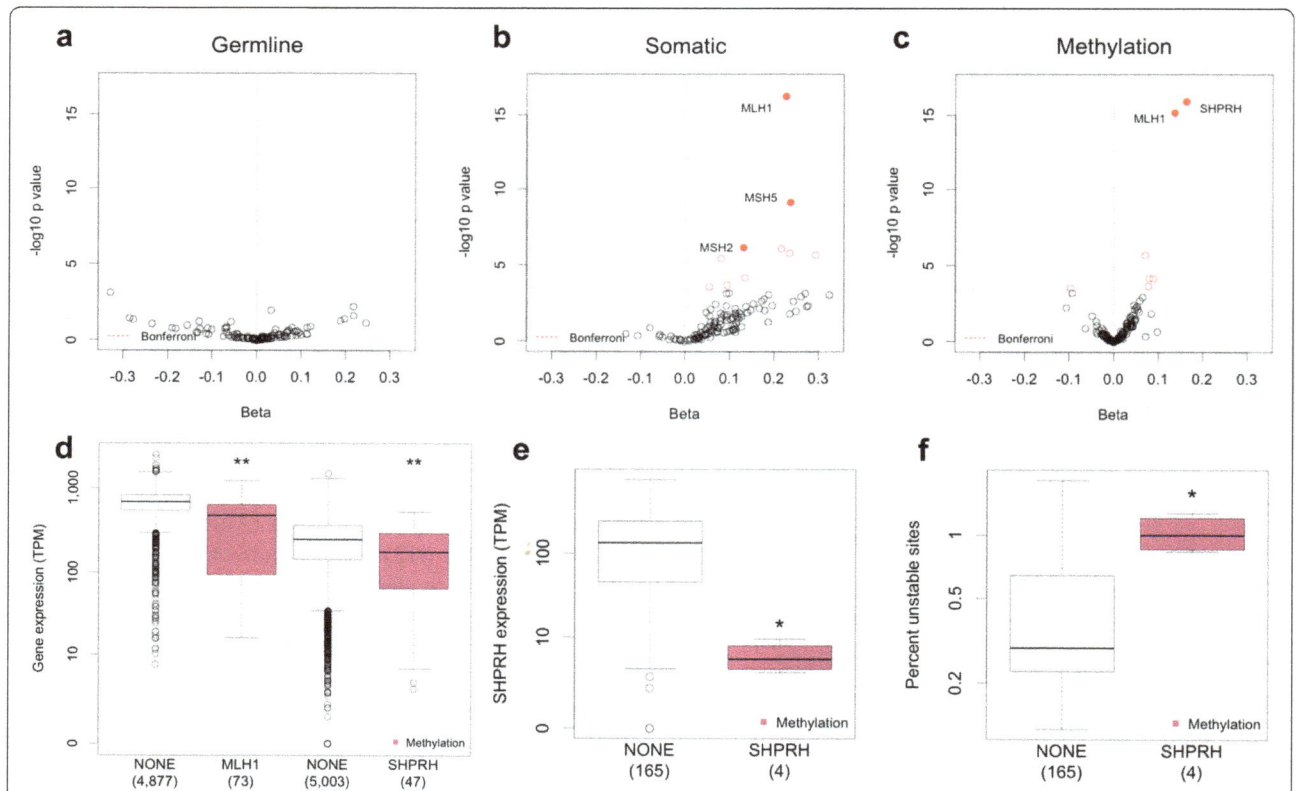

Fig. 4 Germline, somatic, and epigenetic alterations that influence somatic MSI burden. **a–c** Volcano plots of gene-level association testing between germline LOF (**a**) somatic LOF (**b**) and somatic methylation (**c**) and somatic MSI burden. A total of 127 DDR genes were tested in 4987 individuals. Red dotted line represents Bonferroni significance cutoff. **d** Somatic expression of *MLH1* and *SHPRH* in individuals with somatic methylation. **p < 0.001 as determined using a linear model to predict gene expression while accounting for cancer type. **e, f** Somatic *SHPRH* expression is significantly reduced (**e** Wilcox p = 0.0018), and somatic MSI is significantly increased (**f**, Wilcox p = 0.0067) in uterine tumors with *SHPRH* methylation. TPM transcripts per million. The number of individuals in each category is indicated in parentheses

surprisingly found high levels of mutational signature 3 in individuals carrying mono-allelic damaging germline *BRCA1/2* variation. However, when we considered AI events to be bi-allelic alterations, we no longer found a significant association between mono-allelic *BRCA1/2* alterations and somatic mutational signature 3 (Additional file 1: Figure S13 and Additional file 6: Table S16). In contrast to individuals with *BRCA1/2* LOH, we suspect that individuals with AI have subclonal *BRCA1/2* loss, which would explain the lower levels of signature 3 observed. Thus, we demonstrate that variability in LOH calling method can lead to conflicting results.

We next tested for association between 30 somatic mutational signatures from COSMIC and germline bi-allelic alteration in six DDR pathways with more than five individuals carrying bi-allelic alteration (FA, MMR, HR, BER, NHEJ, and TLS) (Additional file 1: Figure S14a) [37]. The only significant association uncovered (FDR < 15%) was between Fanconi anemia and signature 3, which was driven by the known association between *BRCA1/2* alterations and signature 3. We found that when we include all bi-allelic alterations in MMR genes, there was no significant association with signature 6. This was due to the inclusion of germline:methylation events. Limiting our analyses to germline:somatic events led to an association that was statistically significant after multiple hypothesis correction (Additional file 1: Figure S6). This suggests that the mechanism of secondary somatic alteration modulates the effect of germline variation on somatic phenotype. We repeated this analysis expanding to include individuals with mono-allelic germline alteration in DDR pathways and found no significant associations (Additional file 1: Figure S14b). While this analysis is limited due to the small number of individuals carrying pathogenic germline variants, our results are consistent with the previously established idea that bi-allelic alteration is required for the germline to alter somatic mutational phenotypes.

Cancer predisposition syndromes in TCGA

While TCGA is generally thought to represent sporadic adult-onset cancers, our work as well as that of others has shown evidence suggesting that some individuals in TCGA have hereditary cancer predisposition syndromes. Known pathogenic variation in *SDHB/RET*, *BRCA1/2*, and MMR genes is thought to be responsible for a subset of pheochromocytoma and paraganglioma, breast, ovarian, colon, and uterine cancers in TCGA [9, 10, 43, 48]. Another relatively common cancer syndrome that predisposes to cancer types found in TCGA is Li-Fraumeni syndrome (LFS), which arises due to inherited variation in TP53 [1]. Using the IARC-TP53 variant database, we identified 38 individuals carrying a

potential LFS variant (Additional file 5: Table S4). Interestingly, aside from bi-allelic MMR alteration, we observed that pathogenic germline variation in cancer predisposition genes was not associated with an earlier age of diagnosis in 8913 individuals with both germline and age of diagnosis data available. To explore this further, we divided individuals into two groups: those who developed the cancer type expected given the predisposition gene altered and those with another cancer type. Using this approach, we found significant associations between germline alteration status and age of diagnosis for the expected cancer type (Fig. 5a and Additional file 1: Table S17). This suggests that predisposition syndromes can lead to an earlier age of onset in a specific spectrum of cancers, but have no significant effect on other cancer types.

To determine if damaging germline variation in other predisposition genes was associated with earlier age of diagnosis, we examined 75 cancer predisposition genes not included in the previous analysis. We found no significant association between germline alteration status and age of diagnosis in any of these additional genes (Additional file 1: Figure S15 and Table S18). To increase power, we examined these additional genes in aggregate as a gene set ("possible") and compared this gene set to the genes we examined previously ("known," *BRCA1*, *BRCA2*, *MLH1*, *MSH2*, *MSH5*, *MSH6*, *PMS2*, *SDHB*, *RET*, and *TP53*). The known gene set was associated with an earlier age of diagnosis, but the possible gene set was not (Fig. 5b). It is possible that using biological knowledge to group genes or cancer types in a meaningful way could increase power and find new associations. However, we believe much of the variation in age of diagnosis due to germline variation lies in genes associated with prevalent cancer predisposition syndromes.

Discussion

We present an analysis of cancer exomes that integrates germline variation, somatic mutation, somatic LOH, and somatic methylation. To our knowledge, our study is the first exome-wide analysis of the prevalence of bi-allelic alterations across the full spectrum of cancer types represented in TCGA and one of the first to integrate somatic methylation data for a large number of genes. Of all gene sets and bi-allelic alteration mechanism examined, we only discovered a significant enrichment of combined germline and somatic LOF mutations in the MMR pathway. Bi-allelic alteration of the MMR pathway has been previously reported; however, the individuals harboring these alterations were not studied in detail [9]. While a diagnosis of Lynch syndrome cannot be made without a family history, we identified ten individuals with bi-allelic alteration in an MMR gene, elevated somatic MSI burden, and, in individuals with bi-allelic LOF mutations, earlier age of cancer diagnosis.

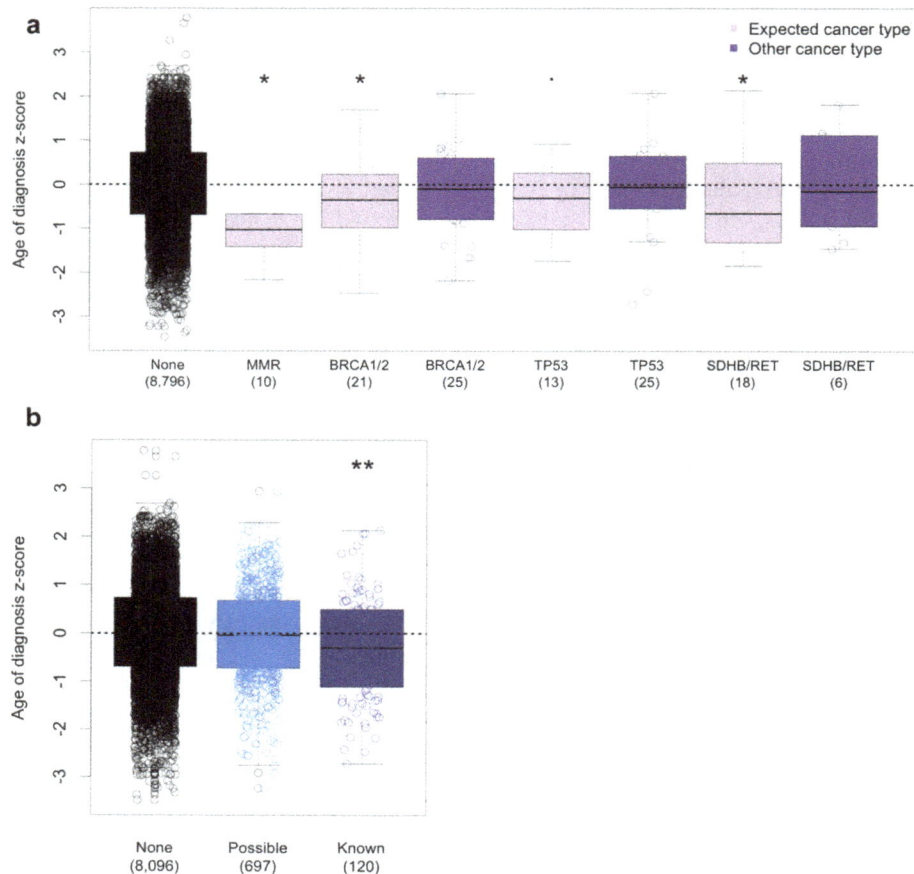

Fig. 5 Cancer predisposition syndromes in TCGA. **a** Age of diagnosis for MMR germline:somatic alteration carriers and individuals carrying ClinVar pathogenic or LOF germline variation in *BRCA1*, *BRCA2*, *TP53*, *SDHB*, and *RET*. Age was converted to a Z-score using the mean and standard deviation age of diagnosis for each cancer type. The expected cancer types for each gene set are MMR, colon, uterine, and stomach; *BRCA1/2*, breast cancer; *TP53*, adrenal cortical carcinoma, glioma, glioblastoma, breast cancer, and sarcoma; and *SDHB/RET*, pheochromocytoma, and paraganglioma. All MMR germline:somatic alteration carriers have the expected cancer type. The number of individuals in each category is displayed in parentheses. **b** Age of diagnosis for individuals carrying ClinVar pathogenic or LOF germline variation in genes described in **a** ("known") compared to a set of 75 other cancer predisposing genes ("possible"). **$p < 0.001$, *$p < 0.05$, $p < 0.1$. p values were determined using a linear model to predict age of onset while accounting for cancer type

The genes harboring bi-allelic alterations by our analyses are predominantly those that are less frequently mutated in Lynch syndrome: *MSH6* and *PMS2*. Similarly, only 20% of the proposed Lynch individuals have colon cancer, the classic Lynch presentation. Thus, it is possible that what we observe is not bona fide Lynch syndrome, but an attenuated form of the disease [45, 49]. The median age of cancer onset in TCGA is 60; thus, the individuals in TCGA carrying cancer predisposing variants may have genetic modifier mechanisms that delay cancer onset and severity. Interestingly, proposed mechanisms of genetic compensation delaying cancer onset have been described previously both for Lynch syndrome and Li-Fraumeni syndrome [50, 51]. We observed six individuals carrying a potentially pathogenic germline variant in a L-MMR gene (two ClinVar pathogenic, four LOF) who did not acquire a second somatic mutation and do not have elevated somatic MSI burden. This is not unexpected as the penetrance of Lynch syndrome variants is often incomplete [2]. We observed that any damaging germline:somatic alteration is sufficient to induce elevated somatic MSI, but only individuals with Bi-LOF mutation have an earlier age of diagnosis. This observation is consistent with the previously proposed idea that bi-allelic MMR mutation is likely not the tumor-initiating event but instead acts to accelerate tumor growth (Fig. 3b, c) [2]. Given our observations, we propose that the less damaging Bi-Miss mutations could lead to slower tumor growth than Bi-LOF mutations.

Recently, Polak et al. demonstrated that somatic mutational signature 3 and *BRCA1/2* LOH bi-allelic inactivation could be used to reclassify *BRCA1/2* germline variants that were previously considered VUS [10]. Here, we provide another example of how somatic phenotype data can be used to reclassify germline VUS. We identify two novel potentially damaging Lynch syndrome variants in *MSH6*. Of note, the ClinVar pathogenic Lynch predisposing *MSH2* variant was not present in the ANNOVAR ClinVar database despite being reported in ClinVar, highlighting the importance of manual curation of potentially pathogenic variants. Further experimental validation of these variants is required. Germline MMR variants can be used to guide therapy and monitoring for patients at risk. For example, the risk of colorectal cancer can be reduced in individuals carrying pathogenic germline MMR variants using a daily aspirin regimen [42, 52]. Distinguishing between sporadic cancer and cancer driven by inherited variation is important both for treatment of the individual as well as for informing relatives who may carry the same inherited predisposition. The novel variants we discovered could increase the knowledge base of variants that predispose to cancer.

A large portion of population-level variation in MSI is not easily explained by germline, somatic, or epigenetic alteration in DDR genes. This could be due to our modeling approach, our strict criteria for defining damaging events, copy number events we did not analyze, measurement error in the evaluation of the MSI phenotype, or the limited focus on DDR genes. Despite these constraints, we successfully identified a novel association between methylation of *SHPRH* and somatic MSI burden, with a particularly strong effect in uterine cancer where *SHPRH* methylated individuals exhibit a 2.4 fold increase in somatic MSI burden. This finding is particularly interesting as outside of *MLH1*, and there is little evidence of other epigenetic alterations associated with somatic MSI burden [53, 54]. Knockdown of *SHPRH* in yeast has previously been shown to increase DNA breaks and genomic instability [55]. To our knowledge, *SHPRH* has not been directly associated with MSI and therefore should motivate further biological validation of this result.

The lack of significant GSEA hits from the exome-wide bi-allelic alteration analysis suggests that there are few novel genes to be found using TCGA that fit the two-hit inactivation model proposed by Nording and Knudson [16, 17]. However, we recognize that our methodology for calling LOH is simplistic and that more sophisticated methods can better identify complex LOH events, for instance copy neutral LOH. We illustrate how differences in LOH calling methodology for germline *BRCA1/2* variants can lead to conflicting conclusions about the frequency of bi-allelic alteration

(Additional file 1: Figure S13). Therefore, it is possible that more sophisticated methods may discover novel genes frequently affected by bi-allelic alteration. Outside of bi-allelic alteration, we find that mono-allelic damaging germline variation has little effect on somatic MSI burden. This is not entirely surprising, as there is conflicting evidence on the effect of MMR haploinsufficiency on mutation rates [45, 56]. Using the effect size of known pathogenic MMR variants, we performed a power calculation and estimated that 11,482 individuals (6485 more than our analysis) would be required to detect the association between mono-allelic damaging germline MMR variants and somatic MSI (see "Methods"). We further found no significant association between mono-allelic damaging germline variants and somatic mutational signatures. Our analysis suggests that the contribution of mono-allelic germline variation to somatic mutational phenotypes is likely to be small.

In addition to individuals with potential Lynch syndrome, we identified individuals who carry germline variants that reportedly predispose to Li-Fraumeni spectrum cancers as well as pheochromocytoma and paraganglioma. While the number of individuals who carry these variants is small, in some cases, their phenotype is extreme enough to confound analyses, as we saw with somatic MSI (Additional file 1: Figure S8b and Table S13). It is important that studies using TCGA as a sporadic cancer control remove potential confounding cases [57]. These individuals may have escaped previous notice due to the fact that many did not develop the cancer type expected based on their germline predisposition. This confirms the variable penetrance of some variants associated with predisposition syndromes: a variant can predispose to one cancer type but have no significant effect on the course of disease of another cancer type [42]. Some individuals with an inherited predisposition variant will not acquire the cancer type they are predisposed toward, but "bad luck" or environmental exposures will lead them to develop a sporadic cancer [58, 59].

Conclusions

The goal of this study was to assess the ability of germline mono-allelic and germline and somatic combined bi-allelic alterations to alter somatic molecular phenotypes. We observed that combined germline and somatic alteration of MMR genes had a synergistic effect on somatic MSI burden, but germline alteration alone showed no effect. We later showed that germline variation in known cancer predisposition genes only led to an earlier age of diagnosis only in a subset of cancer types. From these observations, we conclude that germline variation has the ability to influence both somatic phenotypes and cancer development, but often, this ability is dependent on other somatic alterations or tissue type-specific processes. Our work highlights the importance of integrating germline and somatic data to identify bi-allelic alterations when testing for associations between germline variants and somatic phenotypes.

In this study, we intended to characterize sporadic adult-onset cancers, but in the course of our analyses, we identified individuals that likely have rare cancer predisposition syndromes. Our results and observations shed important light on the issue of incidental findings, not only in the TCGA, but also in any dataset with paired germline variant and phenotype data. We have taken care to be sensitive in our reporting of the data for patient privacy and followed precedents set by others using the TCGA germline data. We believe it will be important moving forward to have a set standard for reporting germline variation, especially given the recent surge of interest in germline variation in cancer.

Additional files

Additional file 1: Figure S1. Calling somatic methylation status. **Figure S2.** Example LOH events. **Figure S3.** Genes frequently affected by germline:somatic alteration. **Figure S4.** Association between germline LOF burden and cancer type. **Figure S5.** Both germline and somatic LOF mutations can alter the same position. **Figure S6.** Mutational signature analysis of germline:somatic MMR alteration carriers. **Figure S7.** Mon-allelic germline variation in MMR pathway not associated with somatic MSI. **Figure S8.** Association testing between germline, somatic, and epigenetic alteration and somatic MSI burden. **Figure S9.** *SHPRH* methylation in uterine cancer. **Figure S10.** *SHPRH* expression in normal tissues. **Figure S11.** Mutational signature analysis of *MLH1* and *SHPRH* methylated samples. **Figure S12.** Co-occurrence testing for *SHPRH* methylation. **Figure S13.** Mutational signature analysis of *BRCA1/2* germline variant carriers. **Figure S14.** Mutational signature analysis of mono- and bi-allelic alteration of DDR pathways. **Figure S15.** Association between damaging germline variants and age of diagnosis. **Table S6.** Association between age of diagnosis and MMR pathway alteration. **Table S7.** ClinVar annotations for germline variants pathogenic for Lynch syndrome. **Table S8.** ClinVar annotations for germline variants of unknown significance. **Table S9.** Modeling a gene-level germline:somatic interaction for L-MMR genes. **Table S10.** Association between type of germline:somatic mutation and somatic MSI burden. **Table S11.** Association between germline:somatic mutation types and age of diagnosis. **Table S12.** Association between mono-allelic germline MMR variants and somatic MSI burden. **Table S13.** MSI linear model results using unfiltered somatic mutations and with germline:somatic MMR alteration carriers included. **Table S14.** Modeling somatic MSI burden using MMR perturbations highly correlated with *SHPRH* methylation. **Table S15.** Modeling somatic MSI burden using *SHPRH* expression. **Table S17.** Association between MMR, *BRCA1/2*, *SDHB/RET*, and *TP53* germline variant carrier status and age of diagnosis. **Table S18.** Association between predisposition gene germline variant carrier status and age of diagnosis. (PDF 2401 kb)

Additional file 2: Table S1. Gene set enrichment analysis on gene-level frequency of bi-allelic alteration. (XLS 90 kb)

Additional file 3: Table S2. List of genes and pathways used. (XLS 27 kb)

Additional file 4: Table S3. Gene-level frequency of mono- and bi-allelic germline alterations. (XLS 44 kb)

Additional file 5: Table S4. List of ClinVar, IARC-TP53, and CADD damaging germline variants used. (XLS 836 kb)

Additional file 6: Table S16. *BRCA1/2* LOH calls using different LOH calling approaches. (XLS 51 kb)

Abbreviations

AI: Allelic imbalance; BER: Base excision repair; COAD: Colon cancer; DDR: DNA damage repair; DR: Direct repair; FA: Fanconi anemia; GDC: Genomic Data Commons; GSEA: Gene set enrichment analysis; HR: Homologous recombination; LFS: Li-Fraumeni syndrome; LOF: Loss-of-function; LOH: Loss of heterozygosity; MAF: Mutation Annotation Format; MMR: Mismatch repair; MSI: Microsatellite instability; MSI-H: MSI high; NER: Nucleotide excision repair; NHEJ: Non-homologous end joining; OG: Oncogenes; PCA: Principal component analysis; PCPG: Pheochromocytoma and paraganglioma; PRE: Predisposition genes; QD: Quality by depth; SCC: Squamous cell carcinoma; TCGA: The Cancer Genome Atlas; TLS: Translesion synthesis; TS: Tumor suppressors; UCEC: Uterine cancer; VUS: Variant of unknown significance

Acknowledgements

All computing was done using the National Resource for Network Biology (NRNB) P41 GM103504. All primary data were accessed from The Cancer Genome Atlas Research Network (cancergenome.nih.gov). We would like to thank Bethany Buckley for her assistance in obtaining ClinVar annotations and interpreting germline variants, and Barry Demchak for his assistance with managing data and setting up analysis pipelines on NRNB.

Funding

AB is supported in part by the National Institute of General Medical Sciences of the National Institutes of Health under the award number T32GM008666 and as a TGen scholar at the University of California San Diego. NJS and his lab are also supported in part by the National Institutes of Health Grants UL1TR001442 (CTSA), U24AG051129, and U19G023122. (Note that the content of this manuscript is solely the responsibility of the authors and does not necessarily represent the official views of the NIH). OH is supported by grant numbers U01CA196406, R21CA192072, UL1TR001442, and P30CA023100.

Authors' contributions

NJS designed and supervised the research. AB performed the statistical analysis, prepared the figures and tables, and drafted the manuscript. AB, OH, and HC designed the experiments. NJS, OH, and HC assisted in writing the manuscript. TI set up high performance computing infrastructure. All authors read and approved the final manuscript.

Competing interests

The authors declare that they have no competing interests.

Author details

[1]Biomedical Sciences Graduate Program, University of California San Diego, La Jolla, CA, USA. [2]Human Biology Program, J. Craig Venter Institute, La Jolla, CA, USA. [3]Division of Medical Genetics, Department of Medicine, University of California San Diego, La Jolla, CA, USA. [4]Moores Cancer Center, University of California San Diego, La Jolla, CA, USA. [5]Cancer Cell Map Initiative (CCMI), University of California San Diego, La Jolla, CA, USA. [6]Division of Biomedical Informatics, Department of Medicine, University of California San Diego, La Jolla, CA, USA. [7]Department of Quantitative Medicine and Systems Biology, The Translational Genomics Research Institute, Phoenix, AZ, USA. [8]Departments of Family Medicine and Public Health and Psychiatry, University of California San Diego, La Jolla, CA, USA.

References

1. Garber JE, Offit K. Hereditary cancer predisposition syndromes. J Clin Oncol. 2005;23:276–92. Available from: http://ascopubs.org/doi/pdfdirect/10.1200/JCO.2005.10.042. [cited 2017 Oct 31].
2. Lynch HT, Smyrk T. Hereditary nonpolyposis colorectal cancer (Lynch syndrome): an updated review. Cancer. 1996;78:1149–67. Available from: http://doi.wiley.com/10.1002/%28SICI%291097-0142%2819960915%2978%3A6%3C1149%3A%3AAID-CNCR1%3E3.0.CO%3B2-5. [cited 2017 Dec 27].
3. Hall J, Lee M, Newman B, Morrow J, Anderson L, Huey B, et al. Linkage of early-onset familial breast cancer to chromosome 17q21. Science. 1990;250:1684–9. Available from: http://www.ncbi.nlm.nih.gov/pubmed/2270482. [cited 2018 Jan 2].
4. Nik-Zainal S, Alexandrov LB, Wedge DC, Van Loo P, Greenman CD, Raine K, et al. Mutational processes molding the genomes of 21 breast cancers. Cell. 2012;149:979–93. Available from: http://www.ncbi.nlm.nih.gov/pubmed/22608084. [cited 2018 Jan 2].
5. Newman AM, Liu CL, Green MR, Gentles AJ, Feng W, Xu Y, et al. Robust enumeration of cell subsets from tissue expression profiles. Nat Methods. 2015;12:453–7. Available from: http://www.nature.com/articles/nmeth.3337. [cited 2018 Jan 2].
6. Nik-Zainal S, Davies H, Staaf J, Ramakrishna M, Glodzik D, Zou X, et al. Landscape of somatic mutations in 560 breast cancer whole-genome sequences. Nature. 2016;534:47–54. Available from: https://www.nature.com/nature/journal/v534/n7605/pdf/nature17676.pdf. [cited 2017 Oct 31].
7. Alexandrov LB, Nik-Zainal S, Wedge DC, Aparicio SAJR, Behjati S, Biankin AV, et al. Signatures of mutational processes in human cancer. Nature. 2013;500:415–21. Available from: https://www.nature.com/nature/journal/v500/n7463/pdf/nature12477.pdf. [cited 2017 Oct 31].
8. Hause RJ, Pritchard CC, Shendure J, Salipante SJ. Classification and characterization of microsatellite instability across 18 cancer types. Nat Med. 2016;22:1342–50. Available from: http://www.nature.com/doifinder/10.1038/nm.4191. [cited 2017 Oct 30].
9. Cortes-Ciriano I, Lee S, Park WY, Kim TM, Park PJ. A molecular portrait of microsatellite instability across multiple cancers. Nat Commun. 2017;8:15180. Available from: https://www.nature.com/articles/ncomms15180.pdf. [cited 2017 Dec 29].
10. Polak P, Kim J, Braunstein LZ, Karlic R, Haradhavala NJ, Tiao G, et al. A mutational signature reveals alterations underlying deficient homologous recombination repair in breast cancer. Nat Genet. 2017;49:1476–86. Available from: http://www.nature.com/doifinder/10.1038/ng.3934. [cited 2018 May 3].
11. Riaz N, Blecua P, Lim RS, Shen R, Higginson DS, Weinhold N, et al. Pan-cancer analysis of bi-allelic alterations in homologous recombination DNA repair genes. Nat Commun. 2017;8:857. Available from: http://www.nature.com/articles/s41467-017-00921-w. [cited 2017 Oct 30].
12. Lu C, Xie M, Wendl MC, Wang J, McLellan MD, Leiserson MDM, et al. Patterns and functional implications of rare germline variants across 12 cancer types. Nat Commun. 2015;6:10086. Available from: http://www.nature.com/doifinder/10.1038/ncomms10086. [cited 2017 Nov 29].
13. Carter H, Marty R, Hofree M, Gross AM, Jensen J, Fisch KM, et al. Interaction landscape of inherited polymorphisms with somatic events in cancer. Cancer Discov. 2017;7:410–23. Available from: http://www.ncbi.nlm.nih.gov/pubmed/28188128. [cited 2017 Oct 31].
14. Middlebrooks CD, Banday AR, Matsuda K, Udquim KI, Onabajo OO, Paquin A, et al. Association of germline variants in the APOBEC3 region with cancer risk and enrichment with APOBEC-signature mutations in tumors. Nat Genet. 2016;48:1330–8. Available from: http://www.nature.com/doifinder/10.1038/ng.3670. [cited 2017 Nov 23].
15. Dworkin AM, Ridd K, Bautista D, Allain DC, Iwenofu OH, Roy R, et al. Germline variation controls the architecture of somatic alterations in tumors. PLoS Genet. 2010;6:e1001136. Available from: http://dx.plos.org/10.1371/journal.pgen.1001136. [cited 2017 Oct 31].
16. Knudson AG. Mutation and cancer: statistical study of retinoblastoma. Proc Natl Acad Sci. 1971;68:820–3. Available from: http://www.ncbi.nlm.nih.gov/pubmed/5279523. [cited 2017 Dec 28].
17. Nordling CO. A new theory on the cancer-inducing mechanism. Br J Cancer. 1953;7:68–72. Available from: http://www.ncbi.nlm.nih.gov/pubmed/13051507. [cited 2018 Jan 31].
18. Cancer Genome Atlas Research Network JN, Weinstein JN, Collisson EA, Mills GB, Shaw KRM, Ozenberger BA, et al. The Cancer Genome Atlas Pan-Cancer analysis project. Nat Genet. 2013;45:1113–20. Available from: http://www.ncbi.nlm.nih.gov/pubmed/24071849. [cited 2017 Oct 30].
19. Verhaak RGW, Hoadley KA, Purdom E, Wang V, Qi Y, Wilkerson MD, et al. Integrated genomic analysis identifies clinically relevant subtypes of glioblastoma characterized by abnormalities in PDGFRA, IDH1, EGFR, and NF1. Cancer Cell. 2010;17:98–110. Available from: http://linkinghub.elsevier.com/retrieve/pii/S1535610809004322. [cited 2017 Dec 27].
20. Buckley AR, Standish KA, Bhutani K, Ideker T, Lasken RS, Carter H, et al. Pan-cancer analysis reveals technical artifacts in TCGA germline variant calls. BMC Genomics. 2017;18:458. Available from: http://bmcgenomics.biomedcentral.com/articles/10.1186/s12864-017-3770-y. [cited 2017 Dec 27].
21. MuTect2 Insertion Artifacts | NCI Genomic Data Commons. Available from: https://gdc.cancer.gov/content/mutect2-insertion-artifacts. [cited 2017 Dec 27].
22. Grossman RL, Heath AP, Ferretti V, Varmus HE, Lowy DR, Kibbe WA, et al. Toward a shared vision for cancer genomic data. N Engl J Med. 2016;375:1109–12. Available from: http://www.nejm.org/doi/10.1056/NEJMp1607591. [cited 2017 24].
23. Lek M, Karczewski KJ, Minikel EV, Samocha KE, Banks E, Fennell T, et al. Analysis of protein-coding genetic variation in 60,706 humans. Nature. 2016;536:285–91. Available from: https://www.nature.com/nature/journal/v536/n7616/pdf/nature19057.pdf. [cited 2017 Oct 31].
24. Carithers LJ, Moore HM. The Genotype-Tissue Expression (GTEx) project. Biopreserv Biobank. 2015;13:307–8. Available from: http://www.ncbi.nlm.nih.gov/pubmed/23715323. [cited 2017 Dec 27].
25. McLaren W, Gil L, Hunt SE, Riat HS, Ritchie GRS, Thormann A, et al. The Ensembl Variant Effect Predictor. Genome Biol. 2016;17:122. Available from: http://genomebiology.biomedcentral.com/articles/10.1186/s13059-016-0974-4. [cited 2017 Oct 30].
26. Landrum MJ, Lee JM, Riley GR, Jang W, Rubinstein WS, Church DM, et al. ClinVar: public archive of relationships among sequence variation and human phenotype. Nucleic Acids Res. 2014;42:D980–5. Available from: http://www.ncbi.nlm.nih.gov/pubmed/24234437. [cited 2018 Jan 31].
27. Wang K, Li M, Hakonarson H. ANNOVAR: functional annotation of genetic variants from high-throughput sequencing data. Nucleic Acids Res. 2010;38:e164. Available from: https://academic.oup.com/nar/article-lookup/doi/10.1093/nar/gkq603. [cited 2017 Oct 30].
28. Bouaoun L, Sonkin D, Ardin M, Hollstein M, Byrnes G, Zavadil J, et al. TP53 variations in human cancers: new lessons from the IARC TP53 database and genomics data. Hum Mutat. 2016;37:865–76. Available from: http://www.ncbi.nlm.nih.gov/pubmed/27328919. [cited 2017 Nov 24].
29. Kircher M, Witten DM, Jain P, O'roak BJ, Cooper GM, Shendure J. A general framework for estimating the relative pathogenicity of human genetic variants. Nat Genet. 2014;46:310–5. Available from: https://www.nature.com/ng/journal/v46/n3/pdf/ng.2892.pdf. [cited 2017 Oct 31].
30. Zerbino DR, Achuthan P, Akanni W, Amode MR, Barrell D, Bhai J, et al. Ensembl 2018. Nucleic Acids Res. 2018;46:D754–61. Available from: http://academic.oup.com/nar/article/doi/10.1093/nar/gkx1098/4634002. [cited 2017 Dec 27].
31. Finn RD, Coggill P, Eberhardt RY, Eddy SR, Mistry J, Mitchell AL, et al. The Pfam protein families database: towards a more sustainable future. Nucleic Acids Res. 2016;44:D279–85. Available from: https://academic.oup.com/nar/article-lookup/doi/10.1093/nar/gkv1344. [cited 2017 Dec 27].
32. Li H, Handsaker B, Wysoker A, Fennell T, Ruan J, Homer N, et al. The sequence alignment/map format and SAMtools. Bioinformatics. 2009;25:2078–9. Available from: http://www.ncbi.nlm.nih.gov/pubmed/19505943. [cited 2017 Oct 30].
33. Koboldt DC, Zhang Q, Larson DE, Shen D, McLellan MD, Lin L, et al. VarScan 2: somatic mutation and copy number alteration discovery in cancer by exome sequencing. Genome Res. 2012;22:568–76. Available from: http://www.ncbi.nlm.nih.gov/pubmed/22300766. [cited 2017 Oct 30].
34. Subramanian A, Tamayo P, Mootha VK, Mukherjee S, Ebert BL, Gillette MA, et al. Gene set enrichment analysis: a knowledge-based approach for interpreting genome-wide expression profiles. Proc Natl Acad Sci. 2005;102:15545–50. Available from: http://www.ncbi.nlm.nih.gov/pubmed/16199517. [cited 2017 Dec 27].
35. Sergushichev A. An algorithm for fast preranked gene set enrichment analysis using cumulative statistic calculation. bioRxiv. 2016:60012. Available from: https://www.biorxiv.org/content/early/2016/06/20/060012. [cited 2017 Dec 27].
36. Rosenthal R, McGranahan N, Herrero J, Taylor BS, Swanton C. deconstructSigs: delineating mutational processes in single tumors distinguishes DNA repair deficiencies and patterns of carcinoma evolution. Genome Biol. 2016;17:31. Available from: http://genomebiology.com/2016/17/1/31. [cited 2017 Oct 30].

37. Forbes SA, Beare D, Boutselakis H, Bamford S, Bindal N, Tate J, et al. COSMIC: somatic cancer genetics at high-resolution. Nucleic Acids Res. 2017;45: D777–83. Available from: https://academic.oup.com/nar/article-lookup/doi/10.1093/nar/gkw1121. [cited 2017 Nov 24].

38. Chang CC, Chow CC, Tellier LC, Vattikuti S, Purcell SM, Lee JJ. Second-generation PLINK: rising to the challenge of larger and richer datasets. Gigascience. 2015;4:7. Available from: https://academic.oup.com/gigascience/article-lookup/doi/10.1186/s13742-015-0047-8. [cited 2017 Oct 30].

39. Faul F, Erdfelder E, Lang A-G, Buchner A. G*Power 3: A flexible statistical power analysis program for the social, behavioral, and biomedical sciences. Behav Res Methods. 2007;39:175–91. Available from: http://www.springerlink.com/index/10.3758/BF03193146.

40. Pearl LH, Schierz AC, Ward SE, Al-Lazikani B, FMG P. Therapeutic opportunities within the DNA damage response. Nat Rev Cancer. 2015;15: 166–80. Available from: https://www.ncbi.nlm.nih.gov/pubmed/25709118. [cited 2017 Oct 31].

41. Vogelstein B, Papadopoulos N, Velculescu VE, Zhou S, Diaz LA, Kinzler KW. Cancer genome landscapes. Science. 2013:1546–58. Available from: http://science.sciencemag.org/content/sci/339/6127/1546.full.pdf. [cited 2017 Oct 31].

42. Rahman N. Realizing the promise of cancer predisposition genes. Nature. 2014;505(7483):302–8..

43. Fishbein L, Leshchiner I, Walter V, Danilova L, Robertson AG, Johnson AR, et al. Comprehensive molecular characterization of pheochromocytoma and paraganglioma. Cancer Cell. 2017;31:181–93. Available from: http://www.sciencedirect.com/science/article/pii/S1535610817300016. [cited 2017 Dec 29].

44. Burnichon N, Brière J-J, Libé R, Vescovo L, Rivière J, Tissier F, et al. SDHA is a tumor suppressor gene causing paraganglioma. Hum Mol Genet. 2010;19: 3011–20. Available from: https://academic.oup.com/hmg/article-lookup/doi/10.1093/hmg/ddq206. [cited 2017 Dec 29].

45. Lynch HT, Snyder CL, Shaw TG, Heinen CD, Hitchins MP. Milestones of Lynch syndrome: 1895–2015. Nat Rev Cancer. 2015;15:181–94..

46. Liu B, Nicolaides NC, Markowitz S, Willson JKV, Parsons RE, Jen J, et al. Mismatch repair gene defects in sporadic colorectal cancers with microsatellite instability. Nat Genet. 1995;9:48–55. Available from: http://www.nature.com/doifinder/10.1038/ng0195-48. [cited 2018 Feb 1].

47. Kunkel TA, Beckman RA, Loeb LA. On the fidelity of DNA synthesis. Pyrophosphate-induced misincorporation allows detection of two proofreading mechanisms. J Biol Chem. 1986;261:13610–6. Available from: http://www.nature.com/articles/cr20084. [cited 2017 Dec 29].

48. Kandoth C, McLellan MD, Vandin F, Ye K, Niu B, Lu C, et al. Mutational landscape and significance across 12 major cancer types. Nature. 2013;502: 333–9. Available from: http://www.nature.com/doifinder/10.1038/nature12634. [cited 2017 Nov 23].

49. Bozzao C, Lastella P, Stella A. Anticipation in Lynch syndrome: where we are where we go. Curr Genomics. 2011;12:451–65. Available from: http://www.ncbi.nlm.nih.gov/pubmed/22547953. [cited 2018 Jan 22].

50. Talseth-Palmer BA, Wijnen JT, Grice DM, Scott RJ. Genetic modifiers of cancer risk in lynch syndrome: a review. Fam Cancer. 2013;12:207–16. Available from: http://www.ncbi.nlm.nih.gov/pubmed/23471748. [cited 2018 Jan 28].

51. Ariffin H, Hainaut P, Puzio-Kuter A, Choong SS, Chan ASL, Tolkunov D, et al. Whole-genome sequencing analysis of phenotypic heterogeneity and anticipation in Li-Fraumeni cancer predisposition syndrome. Proc Natl Acad Sci U S A. 2014;111:15497–501. Available from: http://www.pnas.org/content/111/43/15497.full.pdf. [cited 2018 Jan 22].

52. Burn J, Mathers JC, Bishop DT. Chemoprevention in Lynch syndrome. Fam Cancer. 2013;12:707–18. Available from: http://cgaicc.com/downloads/Capp2_Lynch.pdf. [cited 2018 Apr 11].

53. Cunningham JM, Christensen ER, Tester DJ, Kim CY, Roche PC, Burgart LJ, et al. Hypermethylation of the hMLH1 promoter in colon cancer with microsatellite instability. Cancer Res. 1998;58:3455–60. Available from: http://www.ncbi.nlm.nih.gov/pubmed/9699680. [cited 2018 Feb 6].

54. Esteller M, Toyota M, Sanchez-Cespedes M, Capella G, Peinado MA, Watkins DN, et al. Inactivation of the DNA repair gene O6-Methylguanine-DNA methyltransferase by promoter hypermethylation is associated with G to A mutations in K-ras in colorectal tumorigenesis. Cancer Res. 2000;60:2368–71. Available from: http://www.ncbi.nlm.nih.gov/pubmed/10811111. [cited 2018 Feb 6].

55. Motegi A, Sood R, Moinova H, Markowitz SD, Liu PP, Myung K. Human SHPRH suppresses genomic instability through proliferating cell nuclear antigen polyubiquitination. J Cell Biol. 2006;175:703–8. Available from: http://www.ncbi.nlm.nih.gov/pubmed/17130289. [cited 2017 Dec 29].

56. Coolbaugh-Murphy MI, Xu JP, Ramagli LS, Ramagli BC, Brown BW, Lynch PM, et al. Microsatellite instability in the peripheral blood leukocytes of HNPCC patients. Hum Mutat. 2010;31:317–24. Available from: http://www.ncbi.nlm.nih.gov/pubmed/20052760. [cited 2018 Jan 23].

57. Dominguez-Valentin M, Therkildsen C, Veerla S, Jönsson M, Bernstein I, Borg Å, et al. Distinct gene expression signatures in Lynch syndrome and familial colorectal cancer type X. PLoS One. 2013;8:e71755. Available from: http://www.ncbi.nlm.nih.gov/pubmed/23951239. [cited 2018 Jan 1].

58. Tomasetti C, Li L, Vogelstein B. Stem cell divisions, somatic mutations, cancer etiology, and cancer prevention. Science. 2017;355:1330–4. Available from: http://science.sciencemag.org/content/sci/355/6331/1330.full.pdf. [cited 2018 Apr 18].

59. Tomasetti C, Vogelstein B. Variation in cancer risk among tissues can be explained by the number of stem cell divisions. Science. 2015;347:78–81..

8

KLRD1-expressing natural killer cells predict influenza susceptibility

Erika Bongen[1,2] (iD), Francesco Vallania[1,3], Paul J. Utz[1,2,4] and Purvesh Khatri[1,2,3]*

Abstract

Background: Influenza infects tens of millions of people every year in the USA. Other than notable risk groups, such as children and the elderly, it is difficult to predict what subpopulations are at higher risk of infection. Viral challenge studies, where healthy human volunteers are inoculated with live influenza virus, provide a unique opportunity to study infection susceptibility. Biomarkers predicting influenza susceptibility would be useful for identifying risk groups and designing vaccines.

Methods: We applied cell mixture deconvolution to estimate immune cell proportions from whole blood transcriptome data in four independent influenza challenge studies. We compared immune cell proportions in the blood between symptomatic shedders and asymptomatic nonshedders across three discovery cohorts prior to influenza inoculation and tested results in a held-out validation challenge cohort.

Results: Natural killer (NK) cells were significantly lower in symptomatic shedders at baseline in both discovery and validation cohorts. Hematopoietic stem and progenitor cells (HSPCs) were higher in symptomatic shedders at baseline in discovery cohorts. Although the HSPCs were higher in symptomatic shedders in the validation cohort, the increase was statistically nonsignificant. We observed that a gene associated with NK cells, KLRD1, which encodes CD94, was expressed at lower levels in symptomatic shedders at baseline in discovery and validation cohorts. KLRD1 expression in the blood at baseline negatively correlated with influenza infection symptom severity. KLRD1 expression 8 h post-infection in the nasal epithelium from a rhinovirus challenge study also negatively correlated with symptom severity.

Conclusions: We identified KLRD1-expressing NK cells as a potential biomarker for influenza susceptibility. Expression of KLRD1 was inversely correlated with symptom severity. Our results support a model where an early response by KLRD1-expressing NK cells may control influenza infection.

Keywords: Influenza, Natural killer cells, Hematopoietic stem and progenitor cells, KLRD1, CD94

Background

Influenza is a major public health problem that causes 9 to 35 million illnesses annually in the USA [1]. Children, older adults, pregnant women, and immunocompromised patients are at an increased risk of influenza infection. Within healthy young adults, influenza susceptibility is difficult to predict as responses to influenza exposure vary from no detectable infection to severe disease. A better understanding of the immune determinants of influenza susceptibility is necessary to identify novel high-risk populations and design better vaccines.

Human influenza challenge studies provide a unique opportunity to study influenza susceptibility. In these studies, healthy individuals are inoculated with live influenza virus, and viral shedding titers and self-reported symptom scores are measured over the course of infection. Infected individuals fall into four groups: symptomatic shedders, asymptomatic nonshedders, symptomatic nonshedders, and asymptomatic shedders. Previous challenge studies have used transcriptional data to distinguish symptomatic shedders from asymptomatic nonshedders post-infection [2], detect infection prior to symptom onset [3], develop transcriptional signatures of symptom status [4, 5], and prototype individualized

* Correspondence: pkhatri@stanford.edu
[1]Institute for Immunity, Transplantation and Infection, Stanford University School of Medicine, Stanford, CA 94305, USA
[2]Program in Immunology, Stanford University School of Medicine, Stanford 94305, CA, USA
Full list of author information is available at the end of the article

predictors for infection [6]. However, to our knowledge, no cellular or transcriptional signatures that can predict infection susceptibility prior to inoculation have been reported.

Relatively little work has been done examining how preexisting immune cell populations affect influenza susceptibility. Wilkinson et al. demonstrated in an H3N2 influenza challenge study that higher baseline levels of influenza-specific CD4+ T cells in the blood were associated with reduced viral shedding and less severe symptoms [7]. Sridhar et al. followed healthy adults during two consecutive flu seasons and found that adults with higher baseline levels of influenza-specific CD8+ T cells experienced lower symptom severity [8]. To our knowledge, the role of immune cell frequencies in influenza susceptibility beyond the T cell compartment has not been described.

Cell mixture deconvolution is an established computational approach to estimate immune cell proportions from bulk tissue gene expression data, either from blood or solid tissue [9]. The key assumption of cell mixture deconvolution is that the gene expression of a bulk tissue sample can be explained by the underlying ratio of cell types and the expression profiles of those cell types. Deconvolution methods define specific cell types using a reference matrix, known as a basis matrix, of expected cell type expression. The basis matrix is used by an algorithm, such as linear regression, to predict the proportion of each cell type in bulk tissue samples. Cell mixture deconvolution has been used to profile the immune response to leprosy and across cancers [10, 11]. We have described a deconvolution basis matrix, immunoStates, that accurately estimates cellular proportions for 20 immune cell subsets by reducing biological, methodological, and technical biases [12]. In this study, we used the immunoStates basis matrix with a linear regression model.

We hypothesized that immune cell populations at baseline (i.e., prior to exposure to influenza) may affect influenza susceptibility. To test this hypothesis, we used 4 influenza challenge studies (3 discovery, 1 validation) composed of 52 samples (40 discovery, 12 validation). We estimated proportions of 20 immune cell subsets in each sample using the immunoStates matrix and a linear

regression model. We performed a multi-cohort analysis of estimated immune cell proportions between symptomatic shedders and asymptomatic nonshedders at baseline across the three discovery influenza challenge studies. Symptomatic shedders had lower proportions of natural killer (NK) cells at baseline in discovery cohorts and the held-out validation cohort. Symptomatic shedders had significantly higher proportions of hematopoietic stem and progenitor cells (HSPCs) at baseline. Although the validation cohort demonstrated the same trend, it was not statistically significant. NK cell-associated gene KLRD1 expression was also significantly lower in the blood of symptomatic shedders at baseline in discovery and validation cohorts and correlated negatively with symptom severity. Increased KLRD1 expression may be associated with increased proportions of cytotoxic cells, as KLRD1 expression at baseline correlated with cytotoxic granule-associated genes CCL5, perforin (PRF1), and several granzymes (GZMA, GZMB, and GZMH). We also observed that KLRD1 expression decreased in the blood during the first 48 h of influenza infection. We examined KLRD1 expression in the nasal epithelium in human rhinovirus (HRV) and respiratory syncytial virus (RSV) infection as robust common immune response across these viruses has been described [13]. KLRD1 expression significantly increased in nasal epithelium during infection with HRV or RSV. In an HRV challenge cohort, symptom severity correlated negatively with expression of KLRD1 in the nasal epithelium 8 h post-infection. This data supports a model where a rapid antiviral response by KLRD1-expressing NK cells may control viral infection.

Methods
Identification and preprocessing of cohorts
We identified 4 influenza challenge studies consisting of 52 whole blood samples from the NCBI database Gene Expression Omnibus (GEO) (Table 1). We supplemented the influenza challenge cohorts with 7 acute viral infection studies consisting of 16 cohorts of 771 whole blood, PBMC, and nasal epithelium samples from GEO (Table 2) [14]. We excluded challenge studies with less than five asymptomatic nonshedders or five symptomatic shedders. We used phenotypic labels as reported by

Table 1 Influenza challenge cohorts

Cohort	Group	Virus	Tissue	Asymptomatic nonshedders	Symptomatic shedders	Platform	Citations
GSE73072 challenge A	Discovery challenge	H1N1	Whole blood	6	8	Affymetrix	[2, 3, 6]
GSE73072 challenge B	Discovery challenge	H3N2	Whole blood	6	7	Affymetrix	[2, 3, 6]
GSE73072 challenge C	Discovery challenge	H3N2	Whole blood	6	7	Affymetrix	[6]
GSE61754	Validation challenge	H3N2	Whole blood	5	7	Illumina	[5]
Total		2	1	23	29	2	

Table 2 Additional viral infection cohorts

Cohort	Virus	Tissue	Controls	Acute infection	Platform	Citations
GSE11348	HRV	Nasal scrapings	15	15	Affymetrix	[22]
GSE97742 HRV	HRV	Nasopharyngeal swabs	30	30	Illumina	[23]
GSE97742 RSV	RSV	Nasopharyngeal swabs	38	38	Illumina	[23]
GSE97742 RSVco	RSV co-infected with other viruses	Nasopharyngeal swabs	15	15	Illumina	[23]
GSE61821 mild H1N1	Seasonal H1N1	Whole blood	36	32	Illumina	[40]
GSE61821 mild H3N2	Seasonal H3N2	Whole blood	13	15	Illumina	[40]
GSE61821 severe H1N1	Seasonal H1N1	Whole blood	19	16	Illumina	[40]
GSE61821 severe H3N2	Seasonal H3N2	Whole blood	6	7	Illumina	[40]
GSE61821 pandemic H1N1	Pandemic H1N1	Whole blood	8	10	Illumina	[40]
GSE68310 flu	Influenza A	Whole blood	40	34	Illumina	[24]
GSE43777	Dengue	PBMC	45	45	Affymetrix	[41]
GSE51808	Dengue	Whole blood	9	13	Affymetrix	[42]
GSE68310 HRV	HRV	Whole blood	20	20	Illumina	[24]
GSE97741 HRV	HRV	Whole blood	25	24	Illumina	[23]
GSE67059 RSV	RSV	Whole blood	20	65	Illumina	[43]
GSE97741 RSV	RSV	Whole blood	25	28	Illumina	[23]
Total	8	4	364	407		

the original authors. All datasets used were publicly available (Additional file 1: Supplemental Methods).

Cell mixture deconvolution using immunoStates

We performed cell mixture deconvolution using the immunoStates basis matrix and a linear regression model, as described previously, to estimate the immune cell frequencies for 20 immune cell subsets in blood or nasal epithelium gene expression data [12]. We removed all cell types that were not detected in any samples (Additional file 1: Table S1). If a cell type was detected in a subset of samples, values of zero were set to an arbitrarily low number and each sample was rescaled so that the cell type proportions summed to 100% in each sample.

Integrated multi-cohort analysis of cellular proportions

We performed an integrated multi-cohort analysis using the MetaIntegrator R package [15]. To analyze differences in cell proportions, we utilized random effects inverse variance model-based meta-analysis by combining effect sizes, as described previously [13, 15, 16]. We estimated the change in proportion for each cell type in each cohort between symptomatic shedders and asymptomatic nonshedders as Hedge's adjusted g. We combined the changes in cellular proportion for each cell type into a summary effect size using a linear combination of study-specific effect sizes, where each cohort-specific effect size was weighted by the inverse of that cohort's pooled variance [15, 17]. We performed multiple hypotheses testing

correction using the Benjamini-Hochberg false discovery rate (FDR) [18].

Results

Dataset description

We identified four human influenza challenge studies from the NCBI database Gene Expression Omnibus (GEO) (Table 1 and Fig. 1) [14]. Each of these studies profiled the whole blood transcriptome of healthy individuals inoculated with live H1N1 or H3N2 influenza at baseline and the subsequent 2–7 days. These studies defined viral shedding status based on influenza laboratory tests and symptom status based on self-reported modified Jackson scores [5, 6].

We chose three of the challenge cohorts as discovery cohorts as they were part of a single study and all profiled samples using Affymetrix microarrays [6]. The remaining dataset, GSE61754, profiled samples using Illumina microarrays and was used as a validation cohort [5]. This choice allowed us to ensure that our deconvolution analysis was robust to the microarray platform used. We only included baseline samples from subjects with concordant symptom and shedding status (symptomatic shedders and asymptomatic nonshedders).

Integrated multi-cohort analysis of estimated cell proportions

We hypothesized that the immune cell profiles of symptomatic shedders and asymptomatic nonshedders would be different prior to inoculation. To test this hypothesis,

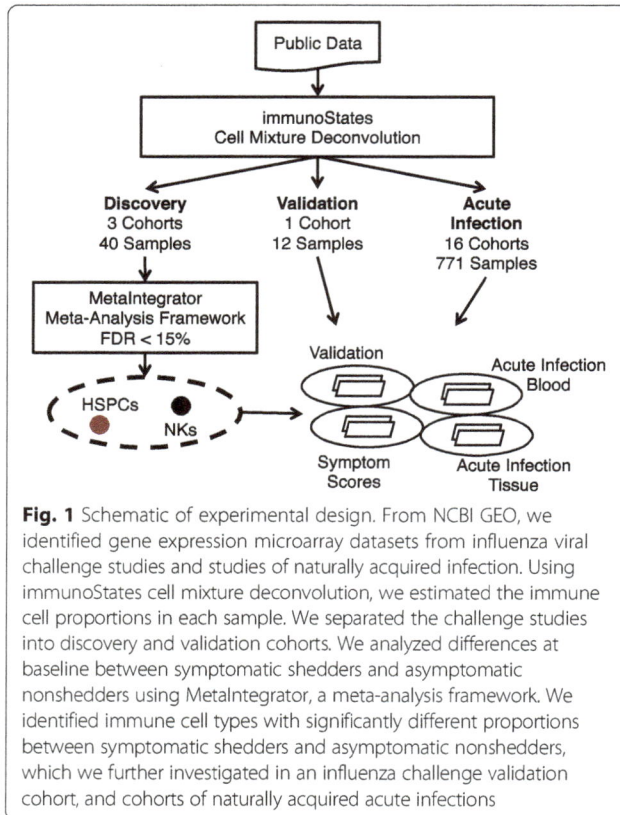

Fig. 1 Schematic of experimental design. From NCBI GEO, we identified gene expression microarray datasets from influenza viral challenge studies and studies of naturally acquired infection. Using immunoStates cell mixture deconvolution, we estimated the immune cell proportions in each sample. We separated the challenge studies into discovery and validation cohorts. We analyzed differences at baseline between symptomatic shedders and asymptomatic nonshedders using MetaIntegrator, a meta-analysis framework. We identified immune cell types with significantly different proportions between symptomatic shedders and asymptomatic nonshedders, which we further investigated in an influenza challenge validation cohort, and cohorts of naturally acquired acute infections

we estimated proportions of 20 immune cell types in each sample in each cohort using immunoStates and a linear regression model [12]. We removed 8 out of 20 cell types from further analysis as they were not detected in at least one dataset (Additional file 1: Table S1). A multi-cohort analysis of estimated cellular proportions for the remaining cell types in discovery cohorts using MetaIntegrator found that proportions of NK cells were significantly lower ($P = 0.012$, FDR < 15%; Fig. 2a), and hematopoietic stem and progenitor cells (HSPCs) were significantly higher ($P = 0.017$, FDR < 15%; Fig. 2b) in symptomatic shedders at baseline. We also observed significantly lower NK cell proportions at baseline in symptomatic shedders in the validation cohort ($P = 0.045$; Fig. 2c). Although the validation cohort exhibited a trend of higher proportions of HSPCs in symptomatic shedders at baseline, this increase was not statistically significant ($P = 0.13$; Fig. 2d).

Identification of *KLRD1* as an NK cell-associated gene relevant to influenza challenge
A basis matrix in deconvolution defines a set of genes as a proxy for the presence of a cell type in a sample. Therefore, a significant reduction in NK cell proportions suggests that a subset of genes in immunoStates representing NK cells should be downregulated at baseline in

symptomatic shedders compared to asymptomatic nonshedders. One of the 19 NK cell-related genes in immunoStates, *KLRD1*, was significantly downregulated in symptomatic shedders in discovery cohorts (summary ES = − 0.54, $P = 0.026$; Fig. 3a) and the validation cohort ($P = 3.3e{-}3$; Fig. 3b). In a validation cohort, *KLRD1* expression in the blood prior to infection differentiated between symptomatic shedders and asymptomatic non-shedders with high accuracy (AUROC = 0.91, 95% CI 0.75–1.0; Fig. 3c). Interestingly, the baseline expression of *KLRD1* was significantly inversely correlated with total symptom scores ($r = − 0.79$, $P = 5.2e{-}4$; Fig. 3d) in the validation cohort and was marginally significant ($r = − 0.48$, $P = 0.07$) in one of the two discovery cohorts where total symptom scores were available (Additional file 1: Figure S1). This suggests that *KLRD1*-expressing NK cells may be important for controlling influenza symptom severity.

KLRD1 baseline expression correlates with KLRC3 and cytotoxic granule associated genes
KLRD1 encodes NK cell receptor CD94 that forms a heterodimer with several *NKG2* family members [19]. To determine whether *KLRD1* expression was associated with a particular *NKG2* family member, we correlated *KLRD1* expression at baseline with three *NKG2* family member encoding genes: *KLRC1*, *KLRC2*, and *KLRC3*. Only *KLRC3*, which encodes protein isoforms NKG2E and NKG2H, significantly correlated with *KLRD1* in the validation cohort ($r = 0.75$, $P = 1.3e{-}3$; Fig. 4a) and discovery cohorts ($r = 0.4$, $P = 7.1e{-}3$; Additional file 1: Figure S2a).

To determine whether expression of *KLRD1* was associated with a cytotoxic transcriptional signature, we correlated expression of *KLRD1* at baseline with genes associated with cytotoxic granules. While releasing cytotoxic granules, NK cells also release CCL5 [20]. *CCL5* expression positively correlated with *KLRD1* in validation ($r = 0.78$, $P = 6e{-}4$; Fig. 4b) and discovery cohorts ($r = 0.74$, $P = 7.3e{-}9$; Additional file 1: Figure S2b). Perforin (*PRF1*) and granzymes (*GZMA, GZMB, GZMH*) are critical components of cytotoxic granules secreted by NK cells to kill target cells [21]. Expression of each cytotoxic granule gene was positively correlated with *KLRD1* expression at baseline in the validation cohort ($0.57 \le r \le 0.62$, $P < 0.03$; Fig. 4c–f) and in the discovery cohorts ($0.76 \le r \le 0.83$, $P < 3e{-}9$; Additional file 1: Figure S2c–f).

KLRD1 expression decreases in the blood and increases in the nasal epithelium after respiratory viral infection
KLRD1 expression further decreased in the blood within the first 48 h of infection in both the discovery (Fig. 5a) and validation (Fig. 5b) cohorts. One possibility for the reduction in *KLRD1* expression in the blood following

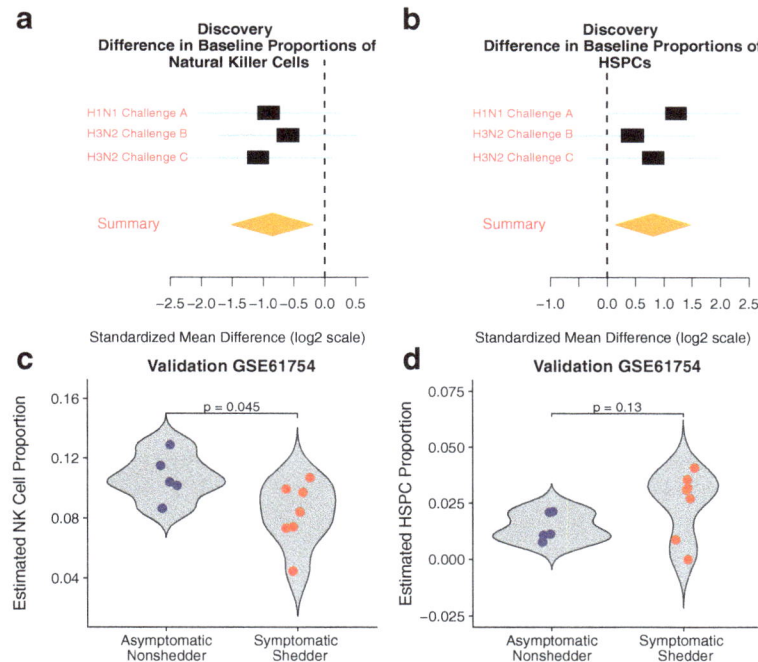

Fig. 2 Differences in estimated cell type proportions between asymptomatic nonshedders and symptomatic shedders before infection. Immune cell proportions were estimated at baseline using cell mixture deconvolution. Forest plots of effect sizes of **a** NK cells (effect size = − 0.85, $P = 0.012$) and **b** HSPCs (effect size = 0.81, $P = 0.017$) in discovery cohorts. Positive effect sizes indicate higher levels while negative effect sizes indicate lower levels for that cell type in symptomatic shedders. The x axes represent standardized mean difference between symptomatic shedders and asymptomatic nonshedders, computed as Hedges' g, in log2 scale. The size of the blue rectangles is proportional to the SEM difference in the study. Whiskers represent the 95% confidence interval. The yellow diamonds represent overall, combined mean difference for a given cell type. Width of the yellow diamonds represents the 95% confidence interval of overall mean difference. Violin plots of estimated cell proportions of **c** NK cells (effect size = − 1.18, $P = 0.045$) and **d** HSPCs (effect size = 0.79, $P = 0.13$) at baseline in validation cohort GSE61754. NK, natural killer. HSPC, hematopoietic stem and progenitor cells

infection is that *KLRD1*-expressing NK cells are trafficking to the site of infection. Therefore, we sought to examine expression of *KLRD1* in nasal epithelium during acute influenza infection. However, no publicly available studies to our knowledge have profiled human nasal epithelium expression during influenza infection. We have previously described a robust common host immune response to acute respiratory viral infection including influenza, human rhinovirus (HRV), and respiratory syncytial virus (RSV) [13]. Therefore, we utilized a HRV challenge study (GSE11348), and a cohort of children naturally infected with HRV, RSV, or RSV co-infected with other pathogens (RSVco) (GSE97742) [22, 23]. *KLRD1* was expressed at significantly higher levels in virally infected nasal epithelium samples (effect size = 0.77, $P = 0.0011$; Fig. 5c).

In the HRV challenge study (GSE11348), *KLRD1* expression at 8 h post-infection was significantly inversely correlated with symptom severity ($r = − 0.6$, $P = 0.031$; Fig. 5d) similar to influenza challenge studies. We also observed significant positive correlations between *KLRD1* expression and expression of *KLRC3* ($r = 0.82$, $P = 6.5e–4$, Fig. 5e) and *HLA-E* ($r = 0.76$, $p = 0.0028$,

Fig. 5f). This data suggests a model where a rapid response by *KLRD1*- and *KLRC3*-expressing NK cells with concurrent upregulation of *HLA-E* by the surrounding tissue may reduce viral infection severity.

HSPCs decrease in the blood during naturally acquired viral infections

Although the difference in HSPC proportions was not statistically significant in validation cohort GSE61754, we observed a trend for higher proportions of HSPCs in symptomatic shedders at baseline (effect size = 0.79, $P = 0.13$; Fig. 2d). It was surprising that HSPCs demonstrated any association with influenza susceptibility, as very little is known about the role of circulating HSPCs in acute infection, particularly in humans. Thus, we investigated changes in HSPC proportions in the blood during acute viral infection. We extended our analysis by performing a meta-analysis of estimated HSPC proportions from naturally acquired influenza cohorts with 236 samples. Individuals with acute influenza infection had consistently lower proportions of HSPCs in the blood than the control time point (summary effect size = − 2.0, $P < 1e–13$; Fig. 6a). To determine whether this

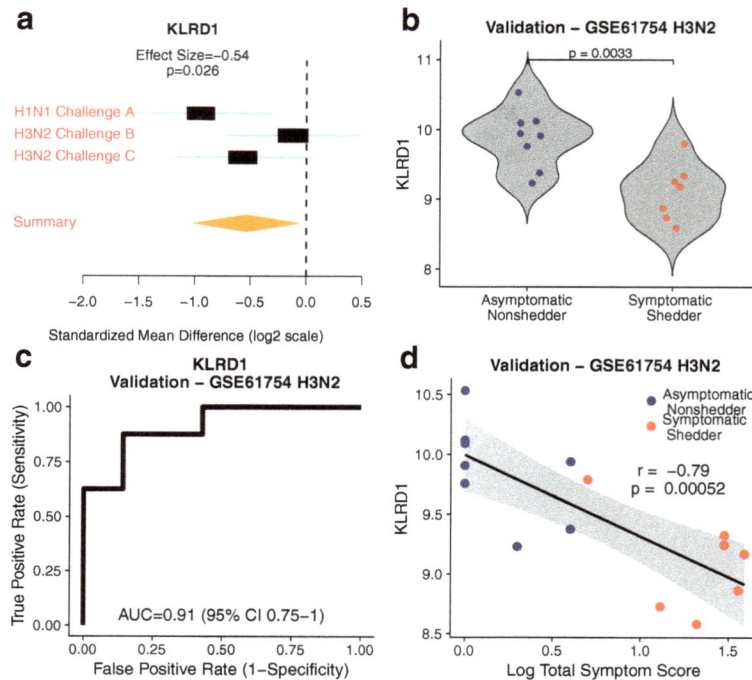

Fig. 3 CD94 encoding gene *KLRD1* is differentially expressed between asymptomatic nonshedders and symptomatic shedders and correlates with symptom severity at baseline. **a** Forest plot of effect sizes of baseline *KLRD1* expression in discovery cohorts (summary effect size = − 0.54, *P* = 0.026). The *x* axes represent standardized mean difference between symptomatic shedders and asymptomatic nonshedders, computed as Hedges' *g*, in log2 scale. The size of the blue rectangles is proportional to the SEM difference in the study. Whiskers represent the 95% confidence interval. The yellow diamonds represent overall, combined mean difference for a given gene. Width of the yellow diamonds represents the 95% confidence interval of overall mean difference. **b** Violin plot of *KLRD1* expression at baseline in validation cohort GSE61754 (*P* = 0.0033). **c** ROC plot of performance of *KLRD1* expression to differentiate asymptomatic nonshedders and symptomatic shedders at baseline (AUC = 0.91, 95% CI 0.75–1.0). **d** Correlation between baseline *KLRD1* expression and logged total symptom score in validation cohort GSE61754 (*r* = − 0.79, *p* = 0.00052)

was influenza-specific, we performed a meta-analysis of estimated HSPC proportions from naturally occurring non-influenza acute viral cohorts. We included six cohorts of acute dengue, HRV, and RSV infection (339 samples total). We observed a significant decrease in HSPC proportions in acute non-influenza viral infection (effect size = 0.5, $P < 0.001$; Fig. 6b).

We further investigated the dynamics of changes in HSPC proportions in the blood during influenza infection using GSE68310, where individuals provided a baseline healthy sample at the beginning of the flu season, and returned to the clinic within 48 h of symptom onset (day 0) [24]. We observed a significant decrease in HSPC proportions ($p < 0.0001$; Fig. 6c). This decrease in HSPC proportions continued through day 6, and HSPC proportions returned to baseline levels by day 21 (Fig. 6c).

HSPC proportions decrease in nasal epithelium over the course of rhinovirus challenge and correlate with increases in mDC and M1 macrophage proportions

To study the presence of HSPCs at the site of infection, we examined HSPC proportions from nasal scrapings of

human volunteers inoculated with HRV (GSE11348) [22]. HSPC proportions sharply decreased 48 h post-infection in nasal scrapings ($P = 1.3e−5$; Fig. 6d). This decrease could result from trafficking, cell death, or differentiation of HSPCs into mature myeloid cells. To test the hypothesis that HSPCs differentiate into mature cells during viral infection, we correlated the changes in HSPC proportions with the changes of myeloid dendritic cell (mDC) and M1 macrophage proportions between pre-infection and 48 h post-infection. Reductions of HSPC proportions strongly correlated with increased proportions of M1 macrophages ($r = − 0.84$, $p = 9.3e−5$; Fig. 6e) and mDCs ($r = − 0.84$, $P = 8.5e−5$; Fig. 6f), both of which derive from the hematopoietic lineage. This finding is supported by data derived from a cohort of children acutely infected with HRV, RSV, or a co-infection of RSV and other pathogens [23]. We observed in this additional cohort that proportions of HSPCs during acute infection from nasopharyngeal swabs negatively correlated with proportions of M1 macrophages and mDCs ($− 0.82 < r < − 0.22$; $2e−4 < p < 0.24$; Additional file 1: Figure S3). As the samples with the lowest proportions of HSPCs were the samples with

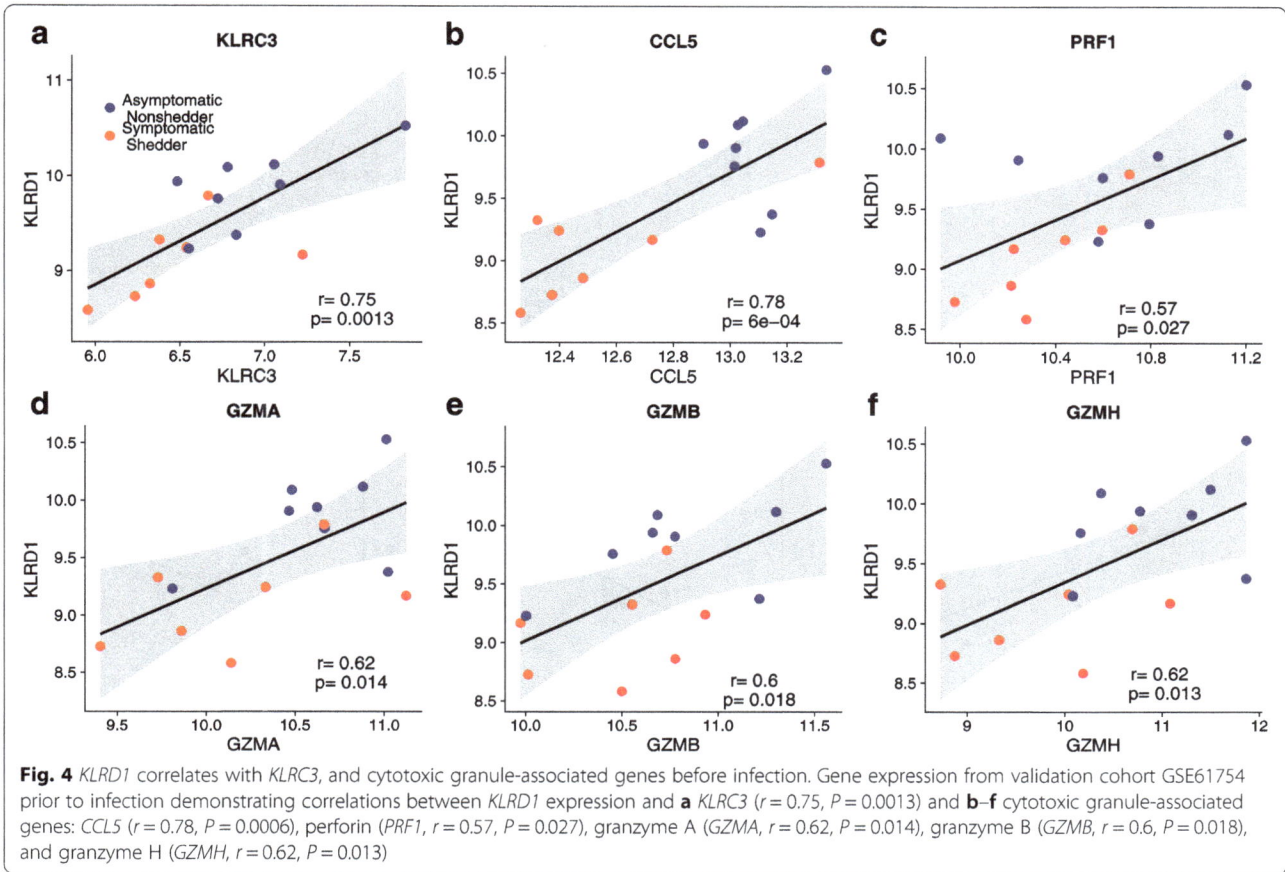

Fig. 4 *KLRD1* correlates with *KLRC3*, and cytotoxic granule-associated genes before infection. Gene expression from validation cohort GSE61754 prior to infection demonstrating correlations between *KLRD1* expression and **a** *KLRC3* ($r = 0.75$, $P = 0.0013$) and **b–f** cytotoxic granule-associated genes: *CCL5* ($r = 0.78$, $P = 0.0006$), perforin (*PRF1*, $r = 0.57$, $P = 0.027$), granzyme A (*GZMA*, $r = 0.62$, $P = 0.014$), granzyme B (*GZMB*, $r = 0.6$, $P = 0.018$), and granzyme H (*GZMH*, $r = 0.62$, $P = 0.013$)

the highest proportions of M1 macrophages and mDCs, this supports a model where HSPCs differentiate into M1 macrophages and mDCs at the site of infection in humans.

Discussion

Here, we tested a hypothesis that the baseline immune profile prior to influenza inoculation can predict which subject will become infected. We applied cell mixture deconvolution of whole blood transcriptome profiles from four independent influenza challenge studies. Symptomatic shedders had lower NK cell proportions prior to influenza inoculation both in discovery and validation cohorts. Symptomatic shedders had significantly higher HSPC proportions in discovery cohorts with a statistically non-significant trend in the validation cohort. NK cell-associated gene *KLRD1* (CD94) was expressed in the blood at lower levels in symptomatic shedders at baseline in both discovery and validation cohorts, which likely reflects differences in NK cell proportions as *KLRD1* was one of the genes used in immunoStates for estimating proportions of NK cells. Baseline *KLRD1* levels negatively correlated with symptom severity and positively correlated with expression of cytotoxic

granule-associated genes. Our results support a model where a rapid response by *KLRD1*-expressing NK cells can lessen severity of or may prevent influenza infection.

NK cells are innate immune cells that can recognize and lyse malignant or virally infected cells [28]. NK cells express a variety of activating and inhibitory receptors that lead to a diverse pool of NK cell phenotypes [26]. *KLRD1* encodes NK cell receptor CD94, which forms a heterodimer with an NKG2 family member, and recognizes HLA-E on target cells [26]. Whether the CD94/NKG2 complex is activating or inhibitory depends on the NKG2 family member involved. The NKG2 family includes inhibitory receptors NKG2A and NKG2B, activating receptor NKG2C, and poorly understood members NKG2E and NKG2H [19, 25]. NKG2E is not expressed on NK cell surface [26], whereas NKG2H is expressed on the surface of a small fraction of human NK cells [27]. By surveying HLA-E levels on target cells, the CD94/NKG2 complex is thought to detect general down-regulation of HLA complexes by viruses or cancer [19].

The CD94/NKG2E receptor complex has been shown to be essential for mouse survival when exposed to mousepox [28]. On the other hand, CD94-deficient mice are not susceptible to mouse cytomegalovirus,

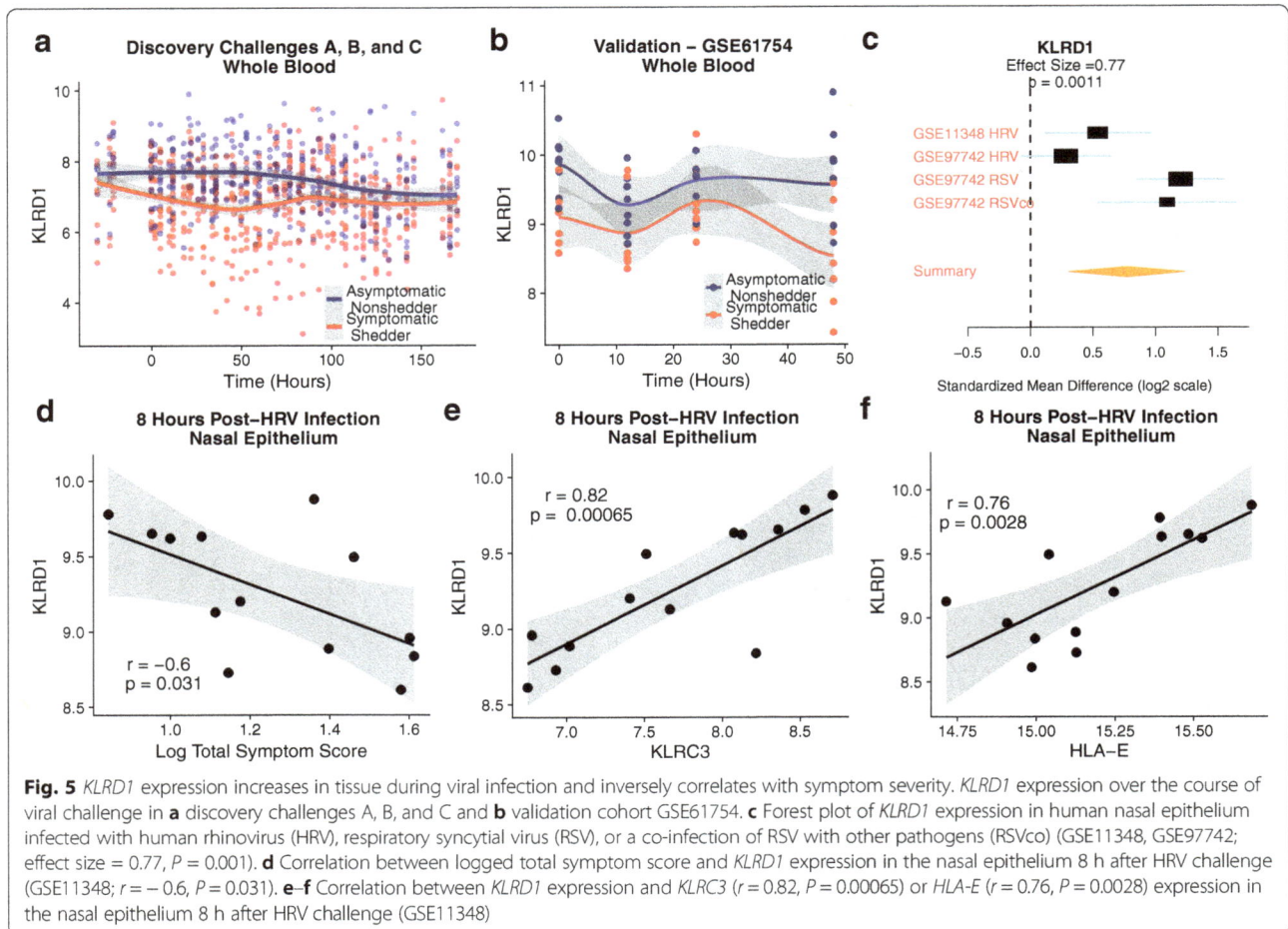

Fig. 5 *KLRD1* expression increases in tissue during viral infection and inversely correlates with symptom severity. *KLRD1* expression over the course of viral challenge in **a** discovery challenges A, B, and C and **b** validation cohort GSE61754. **c** Forest plot of *KLRD1* expression in human nasal epithelium infected with human rhinovirus (HRV), respiratory syncytial virus (RSV), or a co-infection of RSV with other pathogens (RSVco) (GSE11348, GSE97742; effect size = 0.77, P = 0.001). **d** Correlation between logged total symptom score and *KLRD1* expression in the nasal epithelium 8 h after HRV challenge (GSE11348; r = − 0.6, P = 0.031). **e–f** Correlation between *KLRD1* expression and *KLRC3* (r = 0.82, P = 0.00065) or *HLA-E* (r = 0.76, P = 0.0028) expression in the nasal epithelium 8 h after HRV challenge (GSE11348)

lymphocytic choriomeningitis virus, vaccinia virus, *Listeria monocytogenes*, or lethal influenza challenge [29, 30]. Importantly, mouse studies have shown that NK cells are harmful upon lethal challenge by promoting excessive lung inflammation, but beneficial during sublethal influenza challenge by promoting the antiviral immune response [21, 31, 32]. These observations in mouse studies further support our results as human challenge studies are most similar to sublethal mouse influenza models.

We observed that *KLRD1* expression in the blood is downregulated in symptomatic shedders at baseline and inversely correlated with symptom severity in a validation cohort. As *KLRD1* expression in the blood reflects NK cell numbers, this suggests that *KLRD1*-expressing NK cells are protective against influenza infection in humans. Furthermore, *KLRD1* expression in the blood correlated with expression of cytotoxic granule-associated genes: *CCL5*, perforin (*PRF1*), and several granzymes (*GZMA*, *GZMB*, *GZMH*). Thus, having a higher proportion of NK cells in the blood may be protective by increasing the proportions of

cells with cytotoxic capabilities. Importantly, our analysis focused on transcriptome data. These findings should be further confirmed at the protein level.

The role of *KLRD1* (CD94) in influenza susceptibility cannot be fully understood without considering which NKG2 family members are involved. Although bulk transcriptomic data cannot definitively answer this question, we correlated expression of *KLRD1* with genes encoding NKG2 family members known to form dimers with CD94: *KLRC1*, *KLRC2*, and *KLRC3*. Only *KLRC3*, which encodes two poorly understood isoforms, NKG2E and NKG2H, correlated with *KLRD1* expression at baseline. In mice, the CD94/NKG2E receptor complex is critical for recognizing and clearing mousepox infection [32]. Orbelyan and colleagues have shown that while human NKG2E has functional signaling domains and can form a complex with CD94 and DAP12, CD94/NKG2E is located in the endoplasmic reticulum, not the plasma membrane [30]. Although studies have not yet been published to address the biological relevance of this observation, this raises the possibility that human NKG2E

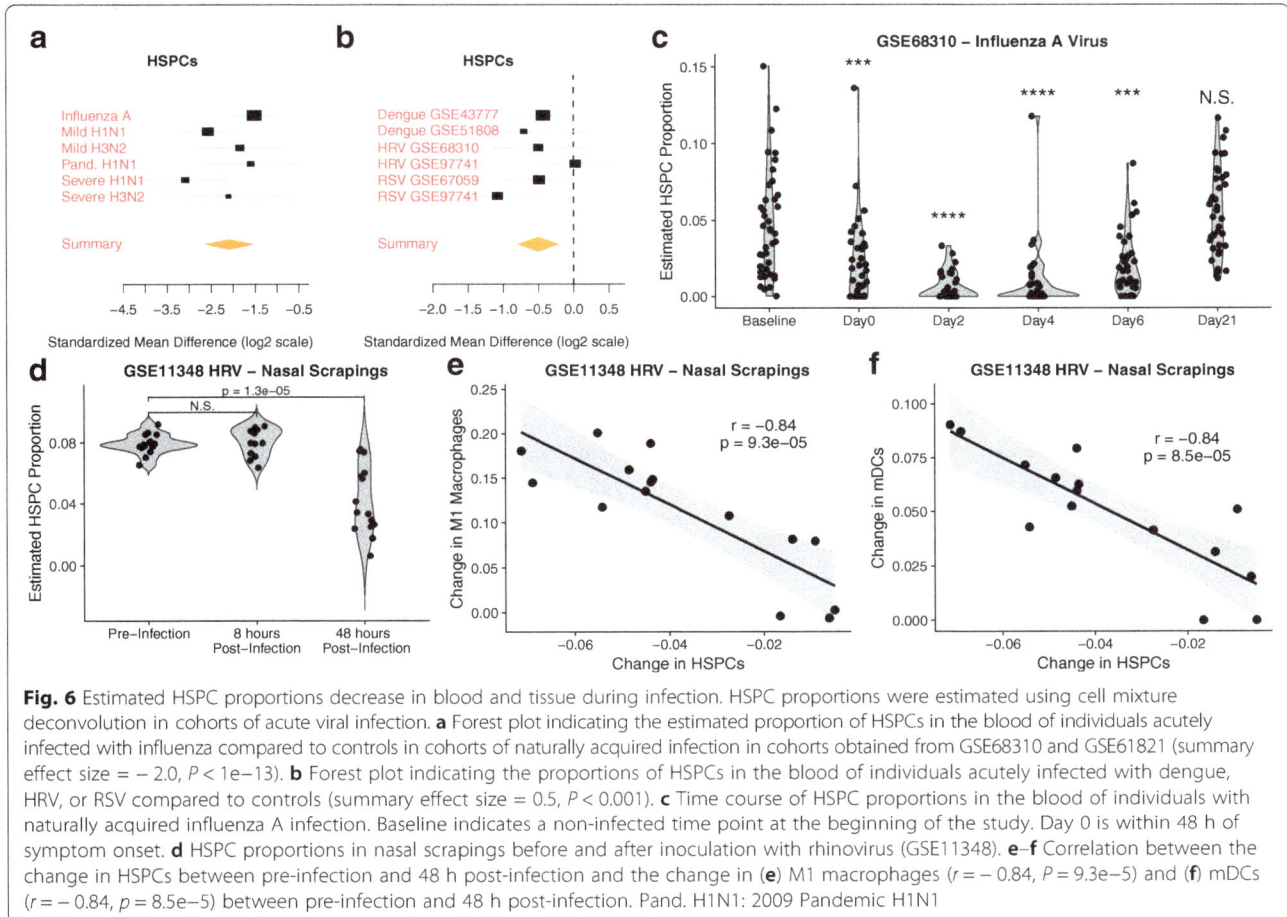

Fig. 6 Estimated HSPC proportions decrease in blood and tissue during infection. HSPC proportions were estimated using cell mixture deconvolution in cohorts of acute viral infection. **a** Forest plot indicating the estimated proportion of HSPCs in the blood of individuals acutely infected with influenza compared to controls in cohorts of naturally acquired infection in cohorts obtained from GSE68310 and GSE61821 (summary effect size = − 2.0, P < 1e−13). **b** Forest plot indicating the proportions of HSPCs in the blood of individuals acutely infected with dengue, HRV, or RSV compared to controls (summary effect size = 0.5, P < 0.001). **c** Time course of HSPC proportions in the blood of individuals with naturally acquired influenza A infection. Baseline indicates a non-infected time point at the beginning of the study. Day 0 is within 48 h of symptom onset. **d** HSPC proportions in nasal scrapings before and after inoculation with rhinovirus (GSE11348). **e−f** Correlation between the change in HSPCs between pre-infection and 48 h post-infection and the change in (**e**) M1 macrophages (r = − 0.84, P = 9.3e−5) and (**f**) mDCs (r = − 0.84, p = 8.5e−5) between pre-infection and 48 h post-infection. Pand. H1N1: 2009 Pandemic H1N1

activates NK cells through an unknown intracellular pathway or inhibits NK cells by restricting the amount of DAP12 available at the cell surface. Less is known about isoform NKG2H, which to the best of our knowledge, has not been studied functionally in NK cells. A larger proportion of human T cells express NKG2H on the cell surface than NK cells, and co-crosslinking NKG2H with a NKG2H-specific monoclonal antibody prevents in vitro activation of T cells through an unknown mechanism [27].

These studies have interesting implications for interpreting our finding that *KLRD1* is associated with influenza resistance and *KLRD1* expression positively correlates with *KLRC3* expression in the blood. Individuals with high levels of *KLRD1* (CD94) also have high levels of *KLRC3* (NKG2E or NKG2H) expression. One interpretation of this observation is that there is a higher probability of forming CD94/NKG2E or CD94/NKG2H receptor complexes, based on stoichiometry. These receptor complexes could lead to influenza resistance through unidentified signaling pathways that activate NK cells. However, it is also possible that *KLRC3*

expression in the blood simply reflects the number of NK cells present and that *KLRD1*-expressing NK cells are protective against influenza using a mechanism independent of NKG2E or NKG2H signaling.

We also investigated the temporal expression of *KLRD1* during influenza infection. We observed that expression of *KLRD1* decreased in symptomatic shedders 48 h post-influenza inoculation. Therefore, we hypothesized that *KLRD1*-expressing cells rapidly traffic to the site of infection. However, no publicly available dataset has profiled expression from the respiratory tract of human influenza patients. Based on our previous report describing a robust common host immune response to acute respiratory viral infection including influenza, HRV, and RSV, we hypothesized that *KLRD1* expression will change in the nasal epithelium of individuals infected with HRV or RSV [13]. In a HRV challenge study, *KLRD1* expression in nasal scrapings 8 h after infection negatively correlated with symptom severity. *KLRD1* expression also correlated with *KLRC3* (NKG2E or NKG2H) and *HLA-E* expression. As *KLRD1* and *KLRC3* encode CD94/NKG2 receptor complexes, these results support a model where a rapid response by CD94/NKG2+ NK cells coupled with high expression of HLA-E by infected target cells leads to rapid viral clearance. Increased expression of KLRD1 and KLRC3 in nasal epithelium samples and reduced frequency of NK cells in peripheral blood samples are consistent with our hypothesis that the NK cells are actively recruited to the site of infection. Alternatively, it is possible that KLRD1 and/or KLRC3 are upregulated on NK cells in lungs of patients with respiratory viral infection or that KLRD1/KLRC3-expressing lung NK cells proliferate vigorously at that site.

Our results suggest that KLRD1 expressing NK cells may be protective against influenza. However, this is undoubtedly only one aspect of influenza susceptibility. Influenza challenge studies routinely exclude individuals with existing antibody titers to the challenge strain, meaning the results may not be directly applicable to individuals with existing B cell memory responses [3, 5]. CD4+ T cell and CD8+ T cell cross-reactive memory responses have also been shown to affect influenza infection susceptibility and severity [7, 8]. Hence, the role of KLRD1-expressing NK cells within broader immune system memory must be further studied.

Hematopoietic stem cells (HSCs) have the unique capacity of self-renewal [33]. HSCs differentiate into hematopoietic progenitor cells (HPCs), with varying differentiation capabilities. HSCs and HPCs are difficult to distinguish experimentally and share expression of the surface marker CD34. Thus, we use the term hematopoietic stem and progenitor cells (HSPCs) to encompass both groups. While HSPCs reside primarily in the bone marrow, it has been shown in mice that HSPCs constantly circulate from the bone marrow, through the blood, into the periphery, and finally through the lymphatic system return to the bone marrow [34]. HSPCs express Toll-like receptors (TLR), such as TLR4 and TLR2, enabling them to recognize and respond to infection [35]. In mice, TLR-stimulated HSPCs have been observed to differentiate into myeloid cell types in the periphery, including dendritic cells and macrophages [34].

Our results demonstrate that during acute viral infection, HSPC proportions decrease in the blood, which may reflect emergency myelopoiesis, a process by which hematopoiesis favors the production of myeloid cells at the expense of the lymphoid compartment to replenish myeloid cells during infection [36]. HSPC proportions may decrease in the blood during infection because HSPCs differentiate into myeloid cells in the bone marrow rather than enter circulation. Furthermore, our results demonstrate that HSPC proportions decrease in nasal scrapings upon rhinovirus challenge, and the decrease in HSPCs correlates with an increase in both M1 macrophages and mDCs. This result supports a model

where human HSPCs take an active role in the immune response at the site of infection by differentiating into myeloid cells.

We identified a nonsignificant trend of reduced proportions of HSPCs in asymptomatic nonshedders prior to influenza exposure. It is possible that the asymptomatic nonshedders were protected due to a recent inflammatory event that promoted HSPC differentiation into protective M1 macrophages and mDCs. However, the likelihood of a recent inflammatory event in challenge study participants is low as subjects are often excluded from a challenge study for having had a recent flu-like illness [37]. It is also possible that the difference in HSPC proportions is due to normal variation observed in the healthy population. Further studies are needed to identify factors driving HSPC proportion variation.

Our study was limited due to our dependence on publicly available challenge study data. Arguably, the number of samples in the challenge studies used here were low. A post hoc statistical power analysis indicated we had sufficient power to detect NK cell and HSPC immune cell proportion differences [38]. We only included symptomatic shedders and asymptomatic nonshedders in our analysis. It is unclear whether our results are applicable to symptomatic nonshedders and asymptomatic shedders. Participants across all challenge studies were healthy young adults. Our results may not be applicable to children or the elderly and need to be investigated in these groups. Furthermore, we only had access to transcriptomic data. Additional studies should confirm whether symptomatic shedders have lower proportions of NK cells at baseline and whether high expression of KLRD1 in the blood directly correlates with greater numbers of CD94+ NK cells via flow cytometry.

Conclusions

In conclusion, we identified KLRD1-expressing NK cells as a novel biomarker for influenza susceptibility. We found that KLRD1 expression correlated with expression of cytotoxic granule-associated genes, suggesting that higher KLRD1 expression may correlate with increased proportions of cytotoxic immune cells. We showed that higher KLRD1 expression in the nasal epithelium 8 h after HRV infection was associated with reduced symptom severity. Our results imply that an early response by KLRD1-expressing NK cells may reduce symptom severity and possibly prevent influenza infection entirely. The seasonal influenza vaccine has already been shown to stimulate memory-like NK cell responses in humans [39]. Future vaccination strategies may benefit from not only targeting B cells and T cells but also enhancing *KLRD1*-expressing NK cell responses.

Abbreviations
FDR: False discovery rate; GEO: Gene Expression Omnibus; HPC: Hematopoietic progenitor cell; HRV: Human rhinovirus; HSC: Hematopoietic stem cell; HSPC: Hematopoietic stem and progenitor cell; mDC: Myeloid dendritic cell; NCBI: National Center for Biotechnology Information; NK: Natural Killer; RSV: Respiratory syncytial virus; SEM: Standard error of mean

Acknowledgements
We thank Catherine Blish and Winston Haynes for the helpful discussions, and Jonathan Wosen for helping with the manuscript revision.

Funding
E.B. was supported by the Stanford Gabilan Graduate Fellowship in Science and Engineering and the Stanford Women and Sex Differences in Medicine (WSDM) Seed Grant. F.V. was supported by NIH K12 Career Award 5K12HL120001–02. P.J.U. was funded by the Donald E. and Delia B. Baxter Foundation; the Henry Gustav Floren Trust; a gift from Elizabeth F. Adler; R01 AI125197-0; and the Autoimmunity Center of Excellence grant U19-AI110491. The Autoimmunity Centers of Excellence is a research consortium supported by the National Institute of Allergy and Infectious disease (NIAID/NIH). P.K. was supported in part by grants from Bill Melinda Gates Foundation, R01 AI125197-01, 1U19AI109662, U19AI057229, U19AI090019. Funding bodies were not involved in design, interpretation, or writing of the manuscript.

Authors' contributions
EB and PK conceived the study. PK and FV developed the immunoStates. EB, PJU, and PK designed experiments. EB performed the data analysis under the supervision of PJU and PK. FV assisted with the analysis and interpretation of the data. EB, PJU, and PK jointly interpreted the results and wrote the manuscript with contributions from all co-authors. All authors read and approved the final manuscript.

Competing interests
The authors declare that they have no competing interests.

Author details
[1]Institute for Immunity, Transplantation and Infection, Stanford University School of Medicine, Stanford, CA 94305, USA. [2]Program in Immunology, Stanford University School of Medicine, Stanford 94305, CA, USA. [3]Department of Medicine, Division of Biomedical Informatics Research, Stanford University School of Medicine, Stanford, CA 94305, USA. [4]Department of Medicine, Division of Immunology and Rheumatology, Stanford University School of Medicine, Stanford, CA 94305, USA.

References
1. CDC: Disease Burden of Influenza [https://www.cdc.gov/flu/about/disease/burden.htm].
2. Zaas AK, Chen M, Varkey J, Veldman T, Hero AO 3rd, Lucas J, Huang Y, Turner R, Gilbert A, Lambkin-Williams R, et al. Gene expression signatures diagnose influenza and other symptomatic respiratory viral infections in humans. Cell Host Microbe. 2009;6(3):207–17.
3. Woods CW, McClain MT, Chen M, Zaas AK, Nicholson BP, Varkey J, Veldman T, Kingsmore SF, Huang Y, Lambkin-Williams R, et al. A host transcriptional signature for presymptomatic detection of infection in humans exposed to influenza H1N1 or H3N2. PLoS One. 2013;8(1):e52198.
4. Muller J, Parizotto E, Antrobus R, Francis J, Bunce C, Stranks A, Nichols M, McClain M, Hill AVS, Ramasamy A, et al. Development of an objective gene expression panel as an alternative to self-reported symptom scores in human influenza challenge trials. J Transl Med. 2017;15(1):134.
5. Davenport EE, Antrobus RD, Lillie PJ, Gilbert S, Knight JC. Transcriptomic profiling facilitates classification of response to influenza challenge. J Mol (Berlin). 2015;93(1):105–14.
6. Liu TY, Burke T, Park LP, Woods CW, Zaas AK, Ginsburg GS, Hero AO. An individualized predictor of health and disease using paired reference and target samples. BMC bioinformatics. 2016;17:47.
7. Wilkinson TM, Li CK, Chui CS, Huang AK, Perkins M, Liebner JC, Lambkin-Williams R, Gilbert A, Oxford J, Nicholas B, et al. Preexisting influenza-specific CD4+ T cells correlate with disease protection against influenza challenge in humans. Nat Med. 2012;18(2):274–80.
8. Sridhar S, Begom S, Bermingham A, Hoschler K, Adamson W, Carman W, Bean T, Barclay W, Deeks JJ, Lalvani A. Cellular immune correlates of protection against symptomatic pandemic influenza. Nat Med. 2013;19(10):1305–12.
9. Shen-Orr SS, Gaujoux R. Computational deconvolution: extracting cell type-specific information from heterogeneous samples. Curr Opin Immunol. 2013;25(5):571–8.
10. Inkeles MS, Teles RM, Pouldar D, Andrade PR, Madigan CA, Lopez D, Ambrose M, Noursadeghi M, Sarno EN, Rea TH, et al. Cell-type deconvolution with immune pathways identifies gene networks of host defense and immunopathology in leprosy. JCI insight. 2016;1(15):e88843.
11. Gentles AJ, Newman AM, Liu CL, Bratman SV, Feng W, Kim D, Nair VS, Xu Y, Khuong A, Hoang CD, et al. The prognostic landscape of genes and infiltrating immune cells across human cancers. Nat Med. 2015;21(8):938–45.
12. Vallania F, Tam A, Lofgren S, Schaffert S, Azad TD, Bongen E, Alsup M, Alonso M, Davis M, Engleman E, et al. Leveraging heterogeneity across multiple data sets increases accuracy of cell-mixture deconvolution and reduces biological and technical biases. In: bioRxiv; 2017.
13. Andres-Terre M, McGuire Helen M, Pouliot Y, Bongen E, Sweeney Timothy E, Tato Cristina M, Khatri P. Integrated, multi-cohort analysis identifies conserved transcriptional signatures across multiple respiratory viruses. Immunity. 2015;43(6):1199–211.
14. Edgar R, Domrachev M, Lash AE. Gene Expression Omnibus: NCBI gene expression and hybridization array data repository. Nucleic Acids Res. 2002;30(1):207–10.
15. Haynes WA, Vallania F, Liu C, Bongen E, Tomczak A, Andres-Terre M, Lofgren S, Tam A, Deisseroth CA, Li MD, et al. Empowering multi-cohort gene expression analysis to increase reproducibility. Pac Symp Biocomput. 2017;22:144–53.
16. Lofgren S, Hinchcliff M, Carns M, Wood T, Aren K, Arroyo E, Cheung P, Kuo A, Valenzuela A, Haemel A, et al. Integrated, multicohort analysis of systemic sclerosis identifies robust transcriptional signature of disease severity. JCI insight. 2016;1(21):e89073.
17. Sweeney TE, Haynes WA, Vallania F, Ioannidis JP, Khatri P. Methods to increase reproducibility in differential gene expression via meta-analysis. Nucleic Acids Res. 2017;45(1):e1-e1.
18. Benjamini Y, Hochberg Y. Controlling the false discovery rate: a practical and powerful approach to multiple testing. J R Statist Soc. 1995;B57:289–300.
19. Martinet L, Smyth MJ. Balancing natural killer cell activation through paired receptors. Nat Rev Immunol. 2015;15(4):243–54.
20. Kumar D, Hosse J, von Toerne C, Noessner E, Nelson PJ. JNK MAPK pathway regulates constitutive transcription of CCL5 by human NK cells through SP1. J Immunol. 2009;182(2):1011–20.

21. Lam VC, Lanier LL. NK cells in host responses to viral infections. Curr Opin Immunol. 2017;44:43–51.

22. Proud D, Turner RB, Winther B, Wiehler S, Tiesman JP, Reichling TD, Juhlin KD, Fulmer AW, Ho BY, Walanski AA, et al. Gene expression profiles during in vivo human rhinovirus infection: insights into the host response. Am J Respir Crit Care Med. 2008;178(9):962–8.

23. Do LAH, Pellet J, van Doorn HR, Tran AT, Nguyen BH, Tran TTL, Tran QH, Vo QB, Tran Dac NA, Trinh HN, et al. Host transcription profile in nasal epithelium and whole blood of hospitalized children under 2 years of age with respiratory syncytial virus infection. J Infect Dis. 2017;217(1):134–46.

24. Zhai Y, Franco LM, Atmar RL, Quarles JM, Arden N, Bucasas KL, Wells JM, Nino D, Wang X, Zapata GE, et al. Host transcriptional response to influenza and other acute respiratory viral infections—a prospective cohort study. PLoS Pathog. 2015;11(6):e1004869.

25. Lieto LD, Maasho K, West D, Borrego F, Coligan JE. The human CD94 gene encodes multiple, expressible transcripts including a new partner of NKG2A/B. Genes Immun. 2006;7(1):36–43.

26. Orbelyan GA, Tang F, Sally B, Solus J, Meresse B, Ciszewski C, Grenier JC, Barreiro LB, Lanier LL, Jabri B. Human NKG2E is expressed and forms an intracytoplasmic complex with CD94 and DAP12. J Immunol. 2014;193(2):610–6.

27. Dukovska D, Fernandez-Soto D, Vales-Gomez M, Reyburn HT. NKG2H-expressing T cells negatively regulate immune responses. Front Immunol. 2018;9:390.

28. Fang M, Orr MT, Spee P, Egebjerg T, Lanier LL, Sigal LJ. CD94 is essential for NK cell-mediated resistance to a lethal viral disease. Immunity. 2011;34(4):579–89.

29. Shin DL, Pandey AK, Ziebarth JD, Mulligan MK, Williams RW, Geffers R, Hatesuer B, Schughart K, Wilk E. Segregation of a spontaneous Klrd1 (CD94) mutation in DBA/2 mouse substrains. G3 (Bethesda). 2014;5(2):235–9.

30. Orr MT, Wu J, Fang M, Sigal LJ, Spee P, Egebjerg T, Dissen E, Fossum S, Phillips JH, Lanier LL. Development and function of CD94-deficient natural killer cells. PLoS One. 2010;5(12):e15184.

31. Abdul-Careem MF, Mian MF, Yue G, Gillgrass A, Chenoweth MJ, Barra NG, Chew MV, Chan T, Al-Garawi AA, Jordana M, et al. Critical role of natural killer cells in lung immunopathology during influenza infection in mice. J Infect Dis. 2012;206(2):167–77.

32. Ge MQ, Ho AW, Tang Y, Wong KH, Chua BY, Gasser S, Kemeny DM. NK cells regulate CD8+ T cell priming and dendritic cell migration during influenza A infection by IFN-gamma and perforin-dependent mechanisms. J Immunol. 2012;189(5):2099–109.

33. Mazo IB, Massberg S, von Andrian UH. Hematopoietic stem and progenitor cell trafficking. Trends Immunol. 2011;32(10):493–503.

34. Massberg S, Schaerli P, Knezevic-Maramica I, Kollnberger M, Tubo N, Moseman EA, Huff IV, Junt T, Wagers AJ, Mazo IB, et al. Immunosurveillance by hematopoietic progenitor cells trafficking through blood, lymph, and peripheral tissues. Cell. 2007;131(5):994–1008.

35. Nagai Y, Garrett KP, Ohta S, Bahrun U, Kouro T, Akira S, Takatsu K, Kincade PW. Toll-like receptors on hematopoietic progenitor cells stimulate innate immune system replenishment. Immunity. 2006;24(6):801–12.

36. Takizawa H, Boettcher S, Manz MG. Demand-adapted regulation of early hematopoiesis in infection and inflammation. Blood. 2012;119(13):2991–3002.

37. Lillie PJ, Berthoud TK, Powell TJ, Lambe T, Mullarkey C, Spencer AJ, Hamill M, Peng Y, Blais ME, Duncan CJ, et al. Preliminary assessment of the efficacy of a T-cell-based influenza vaccine, MVA-NP+M1, in humans. Clin Infect Dis. 2012;55(1):19–25.

38. Valentine JC, Pigott TD, Rothstein HR. How many studies do you need?:a primer on statistical power for meta-analysis. J Educ Behav Stat. 2010;35(2):215–47.

39. Dou Y, Fu B, Sun R, Li W, Hu W, Tian Z, Wei H. Influenza vaccine induces intracellular immune memory of human NK cells. PLoS One. 2015;10(3):e0121258.

40. Hoang LT, Tolfvenstam T, Ooi EE, Khor CC, Naim AN, Ho EX, Ong SH, Wertheim HF, Fox A, Van Vinh Nguyen C, et al. Patient-based transcriptome-wide analysis identify interferon and ubiquination pathways as potential predictors of influenza A disease severity. PLoS One. 2014;9(11):e111640.

41. Sun P, Garcia J, Comach G, Vahey MT, Wang Z, Forshey BM, Morrison AC, Sierra G, Bazan I, Rocha C, et al. Sequential waves of gene expression in patients with clinically defined dengue illnesses reveal subtle disease phases and predict disease severity. PLoS Negl Trop Dis. 2013;7(7):e2298.

42. Kwissa M, Nakaya HI, Onlamoon N, Wrammert J, Villinger F, Perng GC, Yoksan S, Pattanapanyasat K, Chokephaibulkit K, Ahmed R, et al. Dengue virus infection induces expansion of a CD14(+)CD16(+) monocyte population that stimulates plasmablast differentiation. Cell Host Microbe. 2014;16(1):115–27.

43. Heinonen S, Jartti T, Garcia C, Oliva S, Smitherman C, Anguiano E, de Steenhuijsen Piters WA, Vuorinen T, Ruuskanen O, Dimo B, et al. Rhinovirus detection in symptomatic and asymptomatic children: value of host transcriptome analysis. Am J Respir Crit Care Med. 2016;193(7):772–82.

9

Tracking key virulence loci encoding aerobactin and salmochelin siderophore synthesis in *Klebsiella pneumoniae*

Margaret M. C. Lam[1], Kelly L. Wyres[1], Louise M. Judd[1], Ryan R. Wick[1], Adam Jenney[3], Sylvain Brisse[2] and Kathryn E. Holt[1,4]*

Abstract

Background: *Klebsiella pneumoniae* is a recognised agent of multidrug-resistant (MDR) healthcare-associated infections; however, individual strains vary in their virulence potential due to the presence of mobile accessory genes. In particular, gene clusters encoding the biosynthesis of siderophores aerobactin (*iuc*) and salmochelin (*iro*) are associated with invasive disease and are common amongst hypervirulent *K. pneumoniae* clones that cause severe community-associated infections such as liver abscess and pneumonia. Concerningly, *iuc* has also been reported in MDR strains in the hospital setting, where it was associated with increased mortality, highlighting the need to understand, detect and track the mobility of these virulence loci in the *K. pneumoniae* population.

Methods: Here, we examined the genetic diversity, distribution and mobilisation of *iuc* and *iro* loci amongst 2503 *K. pneumoniae* genomes using comparative genomics approaches and developed tools for tracking them via genomic surveillance.

Results: *Iro* and *iuc* were detected at low prevalence (< 10%). Considerable genetic diversity was observed, resolving into five *iro* and six *iuc* lineages that show distinct patterns of mobilisation and dissemination in the *K. pneumoniae* population. The major burden of *iuc* and *iro* amongst the genomes analysed was due to two linked lineages (*iuc1/iro1* 74% and *iuc2/iro2* 14%), each carried by a distinct non-self-transmissible IncFIB_K virulence plasmid type that we designate KpVP-1 and KpVP-2. These dominant types also carry hypermucoidy (*rmpA*) determinants and include all previously described virulence plasmids of *K. pneumoniae*. The other *iuc* and *iro* lineages were associated with diverse plasmids, including some carrying IncFII conjugative transfer regions and some imported from *Escherichia coli*; the exceptions were *iro3* (mobilised by ICE*Kp1*) and *iuc4* (fixed in the chromosome of *K. pneumoniae* subspecies *rhinoscleromatis*). *Iro/iuc* mobile genetic elements (MGEs) appear to be stably maintained at high frequency within known hypervirulent strains (ST23, ST86, etc.) but were also detected at low prevalence in others such as MDR strain ST258.

Conclusions: *Iuc* and *iro* are mobilised in *K. pneumoniae* via a limited number of MGEs. This study provides a framework for identifying and tracking these important virulence loci, which will be important for genomic surveillance efforts including monitoring for the emergence of hypervirulent MDR *K. pneumoniae* strains.

Keywords: *Klebsiella pneumoniae*, Virulence, Hypervirulence, Salmochelin, Aerobactin, Virulence plasmids, Plasmids, Invasive disease, Genomic surveillance

* Correspondence: kat.holt@lshtm.ac.uk
[1]Department of Biochemistry and Molecular Biology, Bio21 Molecular Science and Biotechnology Institute, University of Melbourne, Parkville, Victoria 3010, Australia
[4]London School of Hygiene & Tropical Medicine, London WC1E 7HT, UK
Full list of author information is available at the end of the article

Background

The enteric opportunistic bacterial pathogen *Klebsiella pneumoniae* imposes an increasing infection burden worldwide [1, 2]. These infections typically fall into one of two distinct categories: healthcare-associated (HA) infections caused by strains that are frequently multidrug-resistant (MDR) and community-associated (CA) infections arising from the so-called hypervirulent strains that can cause highly invasive infections such as liver abscess but are usually drug sensitive [2, 3]. The antimicrobial resistance (AMR) and/or virulence determinants possessed by the associated bacteria are generally found on mobile genetic elements (MGEs) that transmit between *K. pneumoniae* cells via horizontal gene transfer (HGT) [4]. These MGEs, most typically plasmids and integrative and conjugative elements (ICEs), are therefore important constituents of the accessory genome that imbue *K. pneumoniae* organisms with their distinct HA or CA clinical profiles.

It is apparent that a wide diversity of *K. pneumoniae* can cause infections in hospitalised patients [3, 5, 6] and that basic pathogenicity factors such as lipopolysaccharide, capsular polysaccharide, type 3 fimbriae and the siderophore enterobactin (Ent) are common to all *K. pneumoniae* and conserved in the chromosome as core genes [1, 3]. However, enhanced virulence or 'hypervirulence' is associated with specific capsular serotypes (K1, K2, K5) and with MGE-encoded accessory genes that are much rarer in the *K. pneumoniae* population [3]. Of particular importance are those encoding additional siderophore systems, namely yersiniabactin (Ybt) [3, 7, 8], aerobactin (Iuc) [9] and salmochelin (Iro) [10].

Synthesis of acquired siderophores contributes to *K. pneumoniae* virulence via multiple mechanisms. However, iron assimilation via the conserved siderophore Ent is hampered by human neutrophils and epithelial cells through the secretion of lipocalin-2 (Lcn2), which binds, and thus inhibits bacterial uptake of, iron-loaded Ent [11]. Ybt, Iro and Iuc on the other hand are not subject to Lcn2 binding; Iro is a glycosylated derivative of Ent, while Ybt and Iuc possess an entirely distinct structure from Ent. The ability of salmochelin to counter Lcn2 binding is important for bacterial growth and has been shown to correlate with enhanced virulence in a mouse sepsis model [12]. The association between aerobactin and virulence has long been recognised, with multiple studies demonstrating its key role in an increased iron acquisition, bacterial growth and/or virulence in various murine models, human ascites fluid and blood [9, 13–15]. Even in strains that possess all four siderophore-encoding loci, Iuc appears to play the most critical role in virulence both in vitro and in vivo [13] and serves as an important biomarker for identifying hypervirulent isolates [16].

In *K. pneumoniae*, Ybt biosynthesis is encoded by the *ybt* locus, which is typically located on a chromosomal ICE known as ICE*Kp* (of which there are at least 14 distinct variants) and was recently also reported on plasmids [7, 8, 17]. A screen of 2500 *K. pneumoniae* genomes showed *ybt* to be prevalent in one third of the sequenced population and associated with hundreds of putative ICE*Kp* acquisition events across the chromosomes of both hypervirulent and MDR lineages [8]. In contrast, Iuc and Iro synthesis is encoded by loci (*iuc* and *iro*, depicted in Fig. 1), that are typically co-located on the so-called 'virulence plasmids' of *K. pneumoniae*. The best characterised virulence plasmids are the 224 kbp plasmid pK2044 from serotype K1, sequence type (ST) 23 strain NTUH-K2044 [18]; the 219 kbp plasmid pLVPK from K2, ST86 strain CG43 [19]; and the 121 kbp plasmid Kp52.145pII from serotype K2, ST66 strain Kp52.145 (strain also known as 52145 or B5055; plasmid also known as pKP100) [9, 20]. These plasmids also carry additional virulence determinants including *rmpA* genes that upregulate capsule production, conferring a hypermucoid phenotype that is considered a hallmark of hypervirulent strains [21], other gene clusters associated with iron uptake and utilisation and other loci encoding resistance to heavy metals such as copper (*pco-pbr*), silver (*sil*) and tellurite (*ter*) [4]. In addition to the virulence plasmid-encoded *iro* and *rmpA* genes, the ST23 strain NTUH-K2044 also carries a chromosomal copy of *iro* and *rmpA* located within ICE*Kp1* [7]; however, this is not a typical feature of ST23 [22].

The majority of *K. pneumoniae* lineages associated with liver abscess and other invasive community-acquired infections (e.g. clonal group (CG) 23, CG86, CG380) carry virulence plasmids encoding *iro*, *iuc* and *rmpA* [3, 9, 16, 23–25]. However, while virulence and AMR genes are both transmitted within the *K. pneumoniae* population via plasmids, until recently, these plasmids have mainly been segregated in non-overlapping populations such that the virulence plasmids encoding *iuc* and *iro* have rarely been detected in MDR populations that cause HA infections and outbreaks [3, 4, 26]. However, the virulence plasmid Kp52.145pII has been shown experimentally to be mobilisable [21], and there are emerging reports of MDR clones such as ST11, ST147 and ST15 acquiring virulence plasmids [27, 28]. The combination of hypervirulence and MDR can result in invasive infections that are very difficult to treat. This can result in dangerous hospital outbreaks; for example, an aerobactin-producing carbapenemase-producing ST11 strain recently caused a fatal outbreak of ventilator-associated pneumonia in a Chinese intensive care unit, with 100% mortality [27, 29]. AMR plasmids are also occasionally acquired by ST23 and other hypervirulent *K. pneumoniae* clones [25, 30, 31].

The ease with which virulence plasmids spread in the *K. pneumoniae* population poses a significant global health threat, highlighting the importance of understanding and

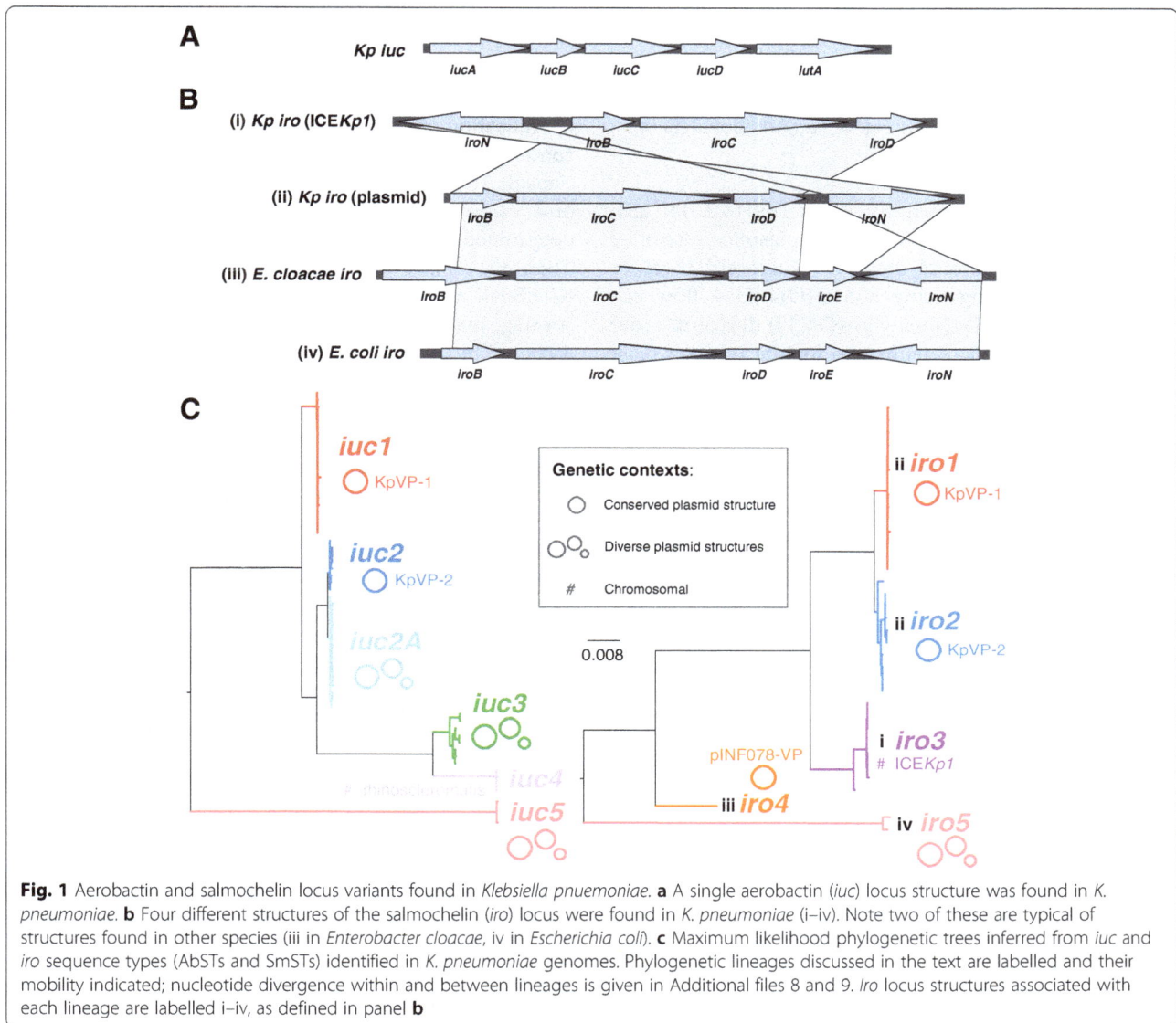

Fig. 1 Aerobactin and salmochelin locus variants found in *Klebsiella pnuemoniae*. **a** A single aerobactin (*iuc*) locus structure was found in *K. pneumoniae*. **b** Four different structures of the salmochelin (*iro*) locus were found in *K. pneumoniae* (i–iv). Note two of these are typical of structures found in other species (iii in *Enterobacter cloacae*, iv in *Escherichia coli*). **c** Maximum likelihood phylogenetic trees inferred from *iuc* and *iro* sequence types (AbSTs and SmSTs) identified in *K. pneumoniae* genomes. Phylogenetic lineages discussed in the text are labelled and their mobility indicated; nucleotide divergence within and between lineages is given in Additional files 8 and 9. *Iro* locus structures associated with each lineage are labelled i–iv, as defined in panel **b**

monitoring the movement of these loci between different strains and clones. Here, we investigate the diversity of aerobactin and salmochelin synthesis loci in 2733 *K. pneumoniae* complex genomes, aiming to understand the diversity and distribution of these virulence loci in the population and to develop a framework for their inclusion in genomic surveillance efforts.

Methods

Bacterial genome sequences

2733 genomes of the *K. pneumoniae* complex, including isolates collected from diverse sources and geographical locations, were analysed in this study (see Additional file 1). The genomes represent a convenience sample of our own isolate collections from clinical and species diversity studies [5, 8, 22, 32], as well as sequences that were publicly

available in GenBank or via the NCTC 3000 project (https://www.sanger.ac.uk/resources/downloads/bacteria/nctc/) at the commencement of the study (June 2017). The majority of these genomes were also included in our previous genome study screening for yersiniabactin and colibactin [8].

For *n* = 1847 genomes (see Additional file 1), Illumina short reads were available, and these were used to generate consistently optimised de novo assembly graphs using Unicycler v0.3.0b with SPAdes v3.8.1 [33, 34]. The remaining *n* = 886 genomes were publicly available only in the form of draft genome assemblies, i.e. with no reads available for direct analysis. All genome assemblies were re-annotated using Prokka [35] to allow for standardised comparison. All genomes were assigned to species by comparison to a curated set of Enterobacteriaceae genomes using mash (implemented in Kleborate, https://github.com/katholt/Kleborate); this confirmed 2503 *K. pneumoniae*, 12 *Klebsiella quasipneumoniae* subsp. *quasipneumoniae*, 59 *K. quasipneumoniae* subsp. *similipneumoniae*, 158 *Klebsiella variicola* and 1 *Klebsiella quasivariicola* (Additional file 1).

Long-read sequencing of isolates

Three isolates in our own collection (INF078, INF151, INF237) carried novel *iuc* and/or *iro* plasmids identified from short-read Illumina data. We subjected these to long-read sequencing using a MinION R9.4 flow cell (Oxford Nanopore Technologies (ONT)) device in order to resolve the complete sequences for the relevant plasmids. Overnight cultures of each isolate were prepared in LB broth at 37 °C, and DNA extracted using Agencourt Genfind v2 (Beckman Coulter) according to a previously described protocol (doi: https://doi.org/10.17504/protocols.io.p5mdq46). Sequencing libraries were prepared using a 1D ligation library (SQK-LSK108) and native barcoding (EXP-NBD103) as previously described [22, 36]. The resulting reads were combined with their respective Illumina reads to generate a hybrid assembly using our Unicycler software v0.4.4-beta [33, 36]. Note this approach uses ONT reads to bridge together contig sequences constructed from Illumina data, followed by consensus base call polishing with both types of reads. Annotations for the hybrid assemblies were generated as described above, and the annotated sequences submitted to GenBank under accession numbers QWFT01000001-QWFT01000009, and CP032831-CP032838 (Additional files 1, 2 and 3).

Multi-locus sequence typing

Chromosomal sequence types were determined for each genome assembly using the BIGSdb-*Kp* seven-locus multilocus sequence typing (MLST) scheme [37] screened using Kleborate (https://github.com/katholt/Kleborate). A novel ST (ST3370) was identified and added to the BIGSdb-*Kp* MLST database.

To facilitate the development of MLST schemes for the aerobactin and salmochelin biosynthesis loci *iuc* and *iro*, alleles for genes belonging to each locus (i.e. *iucABCD*, *iutA*; and *iroBCDN*; respectively) from genomes with 'typeable' loci (defined as those in which all genes in the locus had high-quality consensus base calls when mapping with SRST2) were extracted by comparison to known alleles in the BIGSdb-*Kp* virulence database (http://bigsdb.pasteur.fr/klebsiella/klebsiella.html) [25], using SRST2 v0.2.0 [38] to screen Illumina read sets where available and BLAST+ v2.2.30 to screen assemblies. Incomplete, 'non-typeable' *iro* and *iuc* loci were excluded from the MLST scheme (marked NT in Additional file 1). Each unique combination of alleles was assigned an aerobactin sequence type (AbST) or salmochelin sequence type (SmST), defined in Additional files 4 and 5. The AbST

and SmST schemes, profiles and corresponding alleles are also available in the BIGSdb-*Kp* database and in the Kleborate Github repository (see links above).

Identification of other genes of interest and genetic context of *iuc* and *iro* loci

Capsule (K) loci were identified in each assembled genome using Kaptive [39]. *RmpA* gene copy number was determined by BLASTn search of all genome assemblies using the *rmpA* and *rmpA2* sequences from pK2044 (GenBank accession AP006726.1) as queries with > 90% coverage and > 90% nucleotide identity. Similarly, BLASTn was used to screen the genome assemblies for the IncFIB$_K$ *repA* sequence from virulence plasmids pK2044 and Kp52.145 pII (GenBank accession FO834905.1), with IncFIB$_K$ presence defined as > 90% coverage and > 80% nucleotide identity to these query sequences (to ensure inclusion of known IncFIB$_K$ sequences while excluding detection of non-FIB$_K$ sequences such as the IncFIB sequences frequently detected in other Enterobacteriaceae bacteria). IncFII replicons were identified using BLASTn search of the PlasmidFinder database [40].

Assemblies of all *iuc+* or *iro+* genomes were manually inspected to determine whether the loci of interest were located on the chromosome or on previously described virulence plasmids (pK2044 and Kp52.145pII). This confirmed most to be located in the chromosome (*iro3* in ICE*Kp1* or *iuc4* in the subspecies *rhinoscleromatis* lineage) or one of the known plasmids. For the remaining genomes, annotated contigs containing the *iuc* and/or *iro* loci were checked for known chromosomal or plasmid features, aided by BLASTn searching against the NCBI non-redundant nucleotide database and inspection of the assembly graphs using Bandage v0.8.0 [41].

Phylogenetic analyses

Maximum likelihood phylogenetic trees capturing the relationships between AbSTs or SmSTs were constructed by aligning the allele nucleotide sequences corresponding to each sequence type within each scheme using MUSCLE v3.8.31 [42] then using each of the two alignments (one for AbSTs, one for SmSTs) as input for phylogenetic inference in RAxML v7.7.2 [43]. For each alignment, RAxML was run five times with the generalised time-reversible model and a gamma distribution, and the trees with the highest likelihood were selected. Lineages were defined as monophyletic groups of AbSTs or SmSTs, which were each associated with a unique MGE structure; STs within lineages shared ≥ 2 alleles (for SmSTs) or ≥ 3 alleles (for AbST), whereas no alleles were shared between lineages.

Maximum likelihood phylogenies were similarly constructed for (i) aerobactin and salmochelin locus alignments populated by sequences extracted from BLAST hits amongst representatives of the wider Enterobacterales order (representatives listed in Additional file 6) and (ii) IncFIB$_K$ replicon sequence alignments constructed by mapping *iuc*-positive (*iuc+*) and *iro*-positive (*iro+*) genomes to a reference IncFIB$_K$ sequence (coordinates 128130 to 132007, spanning *repA* to *sopB*, of the pK2044 plasmid sequence; GenBank accession AP006726.1).

Plasmid comparisons

Twelve representative plasmids (10 complete, including *n* = 3 generated from hybrid long- and short-read assemblies detailed above, and 2 partial) were chosen for comparative analysis (these are available as a set in FigShare under doi: https://doi.org/10.6084/m9.figshare.6839981; and see Additional file 2 for list of sources and GenBank accession numbers). Six of these representative plasmids were sourced from the NCTC 3000 project (https://www.sanger.ac.uk/resources/downloads/bacteria/nctc/). As no complete plasmid sequences from *K. pneumoniae* were available with *iuc5*, we used plasmid p3PCN033 from *E. coli* as the reference for *iuc5*. We consider this appropriate in the circumstances since the *K. pneumoniae iuc5* plasmids shared with p3PCN033 the IncFII replicon (native to *E. coli*) and the *iuc* and *iro* sequences and structural variants typical of *E. coli*; the *iuc5* contigs from *K. pneumoniae* showed 99.19–99.95% sequence identity with p3PCN033, and IncFII plasmids while considered native to *E. coli* have been detected in *Klebsiella pneumoniae* alongside other Enterobacteriaceae members [44, 45].

The representative plasmid sequences were compared using Mauve v2.4.0 [46], in order to identify homology blocks conserved amongst subsets of the plasmids. BLASTn comparisons of related plasmids were plotted using GenoPlotR v0.8.7 package [47] for R. All *iuc+* or *iro+* genomes were mapped against all 12 representative plasmids in order to calculate the coverage of each plasmid in each genome. This was done using Bowtie2 v2.2.9 [48] to map Illumina reads where available, and 100 bp reads simulated from draft assemblies where raw sequence reads were not available, using the RedDog pipeline (https://github.com/katholt/RedDog). For every gene annotated within each reference plasmid, the proportion of isolates within each group of genomes sharing the same *iuc/iro* lineage carrying the gene was calculated using the gene presence/absence table reported by RedDog (presence defined as ≥ 95% of the length of the gene being covered by at least five reads) and plotted as circular heatmaps using ggplot2 in R (using geom_tile to achieve a heatmap grid and polar_coord to circularise).

Results

Prevalence of *iuc* and *iro* in *K. pneumoniae*

Iuc and *iro* were detected only in *K. pneumoniae* genomes, and not in other members of the *K. pneumoniae* species complex. Of the 2503 *K. pneumoniae* genomes screened, *iuc* was detected in 8.7% (*n* = 217) and *iro* in 7.2% (*n* = 181; listed in Additional file 1, excluding those with a partial *iro* locus as discussed below). The presence of intact *iro* and *iuc* loci was strongly associated (odds ratio (OR) 711, 95% confidence interval (CI) 386–1458, $p < 1 \times 10^{-16}$), co-occurring in 162 genomes (6.5% of the genomes tested). The *iro* locus appears to be susceptible to deletion; partial *iro* loci were observed in *n* = 50 *K. pneumoniae* isolates (noted as *iro** in Additional file 1), mostly those that were isolated from historical collections prior to 1960. Of 39 isolates collected prior to 1960 and with any *iro* genes present, 36 (92%) carried deletion variants of the locus, compared to 4/163 (2.5%) amongst isolates from 1975 onwards (OR 416, 95% CI 88–3297, $p < 2 \times 10^{-16}$). As expected, the presence of *iuc* and *iro* was each strongly associated with the presence of *rmpA*, with 157 genomes carrying all three loci (excluding partial *iro*). A total of 238 genomes (9.5%) carried *rmpA* genes: *n* = 110 (4.4%) carried one, *n* = 127 (5.1%) carried two, and a single genome, ST23 NTUH-K2044, carried three (as described previously [7, 18], see Additional file 1).

Genetic diversity of *iuc* and *iro* in *K. pneumoniae*

Next, we explored nucleotide diversity of the genes comprising the *iro* and *iuc* loci in *K. pneumoniae*. The five genes comprising the *iuc* locus (Fig. 1a) and four genes of the *K. pneumoniae* forms of the *iro* locus (Fig. 1b) were screened for sequence variation, and each unique gene sequence variant was assigned an allele number. Of the *n* = 209 genomes carrying a typeable *iuc* locus, 62 unique *iuc* allele combinations were observed and assigned a unique aerobactin sequence type or AbST (see Additional file 4 for AbST definitions and Additional file 1 for AbSTs assigned to each genome). The *iutA* alleles present in the *iuc* locus showed > 28% nucleotide divergence from a core chromosomal paralog of *iutA* encoding a TonB-dependent siderophore receptor (positions 2043670–2045871 in NTUH-K2044), which we observed in 96.4% of all genomes; the alleles of this core chromosomal gene are not included in the aerobactin MLST scheme. Typeable *iro* loci were identified in *n* = 164 genomes, comprising 35 unique salmochelin sequence types or SmSTs (defined in Additional file 5, see Additional file 1 for SmSTs assigned to each genome). Maximum likelihood phylogenetic analyses of the AbST and SmST sequences, and their translated amino acid sequences, revealed five highly distinct *iuc* lineages and five *iro* lineages (labelled *iro1*, *iro2* etc.; see Fig. 1c, Additional file 7). Nucleotide divergence between lineages was 1–11% (20–1000 substitutions), and no alleles were shared between lineages (Additional files 8 and 9). Nucleotide divergence within lineages was low, with mean divergence of 0.001–0.40% (*iro*) and 0.013–0.50% (*iuc*) (Additional files 8 and 9) and at least two (*iro*) or three (*iuc*) shared alleles between members of the same lineage. Of note, the *iro4*, *iro5* and *iuc5* loci were quite distant from other lineages (each showing > 5.5% nucleotide divergence from all other lineages vs < 4.6% divergence amongst the other lineages; Fig. 1, Additional files 8 and 9). Comparison to *iuc* and *iro* genes present in other bacteria (all of which were members of the order Enterobacterales, see Additional files 10 and 11), and the presence of the additional *iroE* gene that we observed in other bacteria (all of which were members of family Enterobacteriaceae, see Fig. 1b), suggests that these more distant lineages derive from outside *Klebsiella*, most likely *Enterobacter* (*iro4*) and *E. coli* (*iro5*, *iuc5*). Note that genotyping of *rmpA* was not performed since most *rmpA*-positive genomes carry two copies of the gene, which complicates allele typing from short-read data; however, *rmpA* copy number per genome is reported in Additional file 1.

Mobile genetic elements associated with *iuc* and *iro* loci

Inspection of the genetic context surrounding the *iuc* and *iro* sequences revealed that the various *iuc* and *iro* lineages were associated with distinct MGEs, with the exception of *iuc4* which was restricted to the chromosome of *K. pneumoniae* subspecies *rhinoscleromatis* (ST67) (Fig. 1c, Table 1). Most common were *iuc1* and *iro1*; these were both associated with pK2044-like plasmids (hereafter called KpVP1-1, see below) and the presence of two *rmpA* genes and accounted for 74% of all *iuc+iro+* genomes. These were followed by *iuc2* and *iro2*, which were associated with Kp52.145 pII-like plasmids (hereafter called KpVP-2, see below), the presence of one *rmpA* gene, and accounted for 14% of all *iuc+iro* + genomes. A sister clade of *iuc2*, which we named *iuc2a*, was associated with diverse plasmids that shared some homology with Kp52.145 pII (36–70% coverage,

99% nucleotide identity). Most *iuc2a*+ isolates carried a single *rmpA* gene (*n* = 38, 88.4%), and all lacked an intact *iro* locus (*n* = 26, 60.5% had a partial *iro* locus). Lineage *iuc3* was related to the *iuc4* lineage encoded on the *rhinoscleromatis* chromosome but was present on novel plasmids. *Iro3* was located within the chromosomally integrated ICE*Kp1*, along with *rmpA*. Four genomes carried *iuc5* (two of these also carried *iro5*; all lacked *rmpA*). The *iuc5* sequences were distantly related to *iuc1* and *iuc2* (> 8.9% nucleotide divergence) but were identical to sequences found in *E. coli* and located on contigs that matched closely to *E. coli* AMR plasmids (e.g. strain PCN033 plasmid p3PCN033, accession CP006635.1 [49], which showed > 99% nucleotide identity to the best assembled of *iuc5*+ *K. pneumoniae* contigs). *Iro4* was identified in a single genome (which lacked *rmpA*) and was > 6.1% divergent from *iro1* and *iro2* sequences. Its closest known relatives are *iro* sequences present in the chromosomes of *Enterobacter cloacae* and *Enterobacter hormaechei* (strains AR_0065, accession CP020053.1, and 34977, accession CP010376.2, respectively; 95% identity). Lineages *iro4* and *iro5* follow the gene configuration typical of non-*K. pneumoniae* Enterobacteriaceae *iro* loci, from which the *K. pneumoniae iro1*, *iro2* and *iro3* differ by lack of *iroE* and inversion of *iroN* (see Fig. 1b).

To examine the gene content and replicon differences between the various *K. pneumoniae* plasmids associated with *iuc* and/or *iro*, 12 representative plasmids associated with the various lineages were selected for comparison (Fig. 2, Additional file 2). These include six complete *K. pneumoniae* plasmid sequences identified from finished genomes: *iuc1*/*iro1* (*n* = 1), *iuc2*/*iro2* (*n* = 1), *iuc2a* (*n* = 3), *iuc3* (*n* = 1); three novel complete *K. pneumoniae* plasmid sequences that we generated for this study, carrying *iuc2a* (*n* = 2) and *iro4* (*n* = 1); and two large contigs that we

Table 1 Summary of *iuc* and/or *iro* plasmid lineages

Lineage(s)	N	Mobile genetic element	Reference(s)
iuc1 (+ *iro1*)	121 (119)	*K. pneumoniae* VP-1, type I IncFIB$_K$ + IncHI1B, *rmpA*+*rmpA2*	pK2044 (accession AP006726.1)
iuc2 (+ *iro2*)	23 (23)	*K. pneumoniae* VP-2, type II IncFIB$_K$, *rmpA*	Kp52.145 plasmid II (accession FO384905.1)
iuc2a	43	Novel, diverse plasmids IncFIB$_K$ + other IncF replicons, sometimes IncFII *tra*	Many distinct types Novel examples: pINF151_01-VP (accession QWFT01000004), pINF237_01-VP (accession CP032834)
iuc3	11	Novel, diverse plasmids IncFIB$_K$ + IncFII *tra*	NCTC11676, NCTC11697
iuc4	7	Chromosomal integration	*K. pneumoniae rhinoscleromatis*, e.g. strain SB3432 (accession FO203501.1)
iuc5 (+*iro5*)	4 (2)	*E. coli* IncFII *tra* plasmid *E. coli iroBCDEN* + AMR	*E. coli* strain PCN033 plasmid p3PCN033 (accession CP006635.1)
iro3	16	Chromosomal ICE*Kp1*	*K. pneumoniae* NTUH-K2044 ICE*Kp1* (accession AB298504.1)
iro4	1	Novel plasmid IncFIB$_K$ + IncFII *tra* *E. cloacae*/*E. hormaechei iroBCDEN* (× 13 copies)	pINF078-VP (accession CP032832)

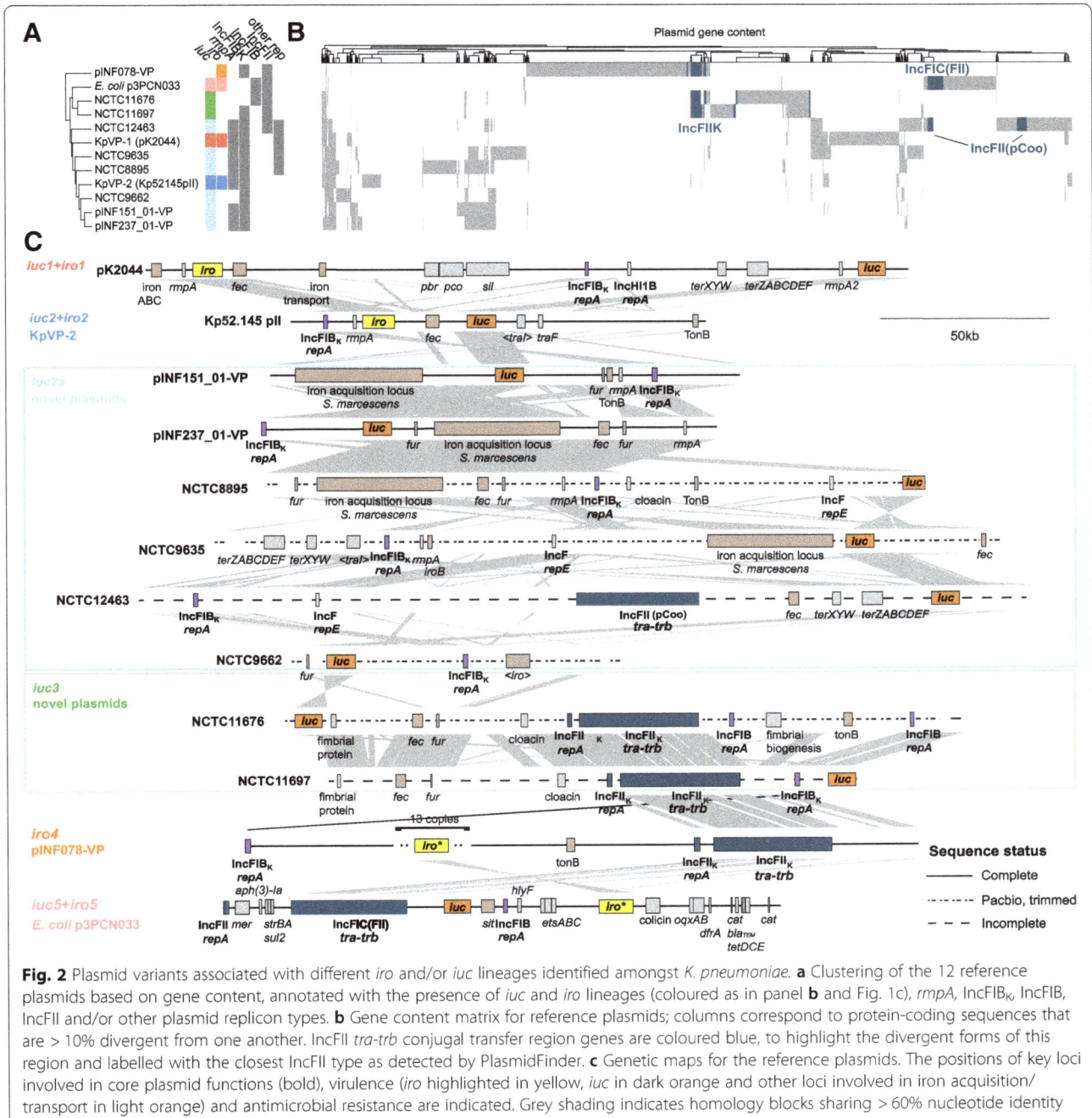

Fig. 2 Plasmid variants associated with different *iro* and/or *iuc* lineages identified amongst *K. pneumoniae*. **a** Clustering of the 12 reference plasmids based on gene content, annotated with the presence of *iuc* and *iro* lineages (coloured as in panel **b** and Fig. 1c), *rmpA*, IncFIB$_K$, IncFIB, IncFII and/or other plasmid replicon types. **b** Gene content matrix for reference plasmids; columns correspond to protein-coding sequences that are > 10% divergent from one another. IncFII *tra-trb* conjugal transfer region genes are coloured blue, to highlight the divergent forms of this region and labelled with the closest IncFII type as detected by PlasmidFinder. **c** Genetic maps for the reference plasmids. The positions of key loci involved in core plasmid functions (bold), virulence (*iro* highlighted in yellow, *iuc* in dark orange and other loci involved in iron acquisition/transport in light orange) and antimicrobial resistance are indicated. Grey shading indicates homology blocks sharing > 60% nucleotide identity

identified from public *K. pneumoniae* genome data representing partial sequences for additional plasmids carrying *iuc2a* (*n* = 1) and *iuc3* (*n* = 1) (Fig. 2). The *K. pneumoniae* genomes in which *iuc5/iro5* were identified were available only as draft assemblies deposited in public databases, and the associated plasmid sequences were fragmented in these assemblies; hence, we used *E. coli* strain PCN033 plasmid p3PCN033 [49] as the representative for *iuc5/iro5*. The representative plasmid sequences differed substantially in their structure and gene content between and within the different lineages (Fig. 2b, c).

All representative *iuc* or *iro* plasmids harboured an IncFIB$_K$ (*n* = 9) or IncFIB (*n* = 3) replicon, including the *repA* replication gene, *oriT* origin of transfer and *sopAB* partitioning genes (presence of these replicons in each plasmid is indicated purple in Fig. 2c and listed in Additional file 2). The IncFIB$_K$ replicon was present in *n* = 202/208 (97%) of isolates with plasmid-encoded *iuc* or *iro*, including 100% of *iuc1/iro1*, *iuc2/iro2*, *iuc2a* and *iro4* isolates, and 82% of *iuc3* isolates. Each of these *iuc/iro* lineages was associated with a unique sequence variant of the IncFIB$_K$ replicon (see tree in Fig. 3 and nucleotide identity with the IncFIB$_K$ *rep* sequences from KpVP-1 and KpVP-2 listed in Additional file 1), supporting the segregation of the *iuc* and *iro* loci with distinct FIB$_K$ plasmid backbones. However, the IncFIB$_K$ replicon was also widely detected amongst isolates that do not carry *iro* and *iuc* (77% of all *K. pneumoniae* genomes and 69% amongst other species in the complex; see Additional file 1), including MDR *K. pneumoniae* lineages such as CG258, and is known to be associated with AMR plasmids [44, 50]. IncFIB replicons, which are common amongst *E. coli* and display > 39% nucleotide divergence from the IncFIB$_K$ replicon, were found in all *K. pneumoniae* isolates carrying the *E. coli* variant *iuc5* (100%) and also detected in two isolates carrying *iuc3* plasmids (18%; marked in Fig. 2a, c), suggesting the transfer of these *iuc* variants into *K. pneumoniae* via such plasmids.

In order to explore structural conservation of plasmids amongst isolates with each *iro* or *iuc* lineage, we mapped the sequence data from all isolates carrying either of these loci against the 12 representative plasmid sequences (Fig. 4). This revealed that plasmid structures were largely conserved amongst isolates sharing the same *iuc* or *iro* lineages, although plasmids associated with *iuc2a* and *iuc3* showed more diversity than others (Fig. 4 and see below). The distribution of *iuc* and *iro* variants with respect to the clonal group of the host strain, identified by chromosomal MLST, shows that each follows quite distinct patterns of dissemination in the *K. pneumoniae* population (Fig. 5).

Iuc/iro lineages 1 and 2 are associated with two dominant *K. pneumoniae* virulence plasmids, KpVP-1 and KpVP-2

Iuc/iro lineages 1 and 2 accounted for 64% of *K. pneumoniae* isolates carrying any aerobactin or salmochelin synthesis loci, and 88% of isolates carrying both. While it was not possible to resolve the complete sequences for all plasmids associated with these lineages, read mapping to pK2044 and Kp52.145 pII reference sequences strongly supported the presence of pK2044-like plasmids in *iro1* +*iuc1*+ genomes (mean plasmid coverage of 95.1%, range 28.8–100%; see Fig. 4) and Kp52.145 pII-like plasmids in *iro2*+*iuc2*+ genomes (mean plasmid coverage of 92.4%, range 87.2–100%; see Fig. 4). There were limited homologous regions shared between the two plasmids (Fig. 2), including the *iro*, *iuc*, *rmpA* and *fec* loci, and the IncFIB$_K$ replicon (Additional file 12). These shared regions were largely conserved across all isolates carrying *iuc/iro* lineages 1 or 2; the remaining regions unique to either pK2044 or Kp52.145 pII were largely conserved amongst

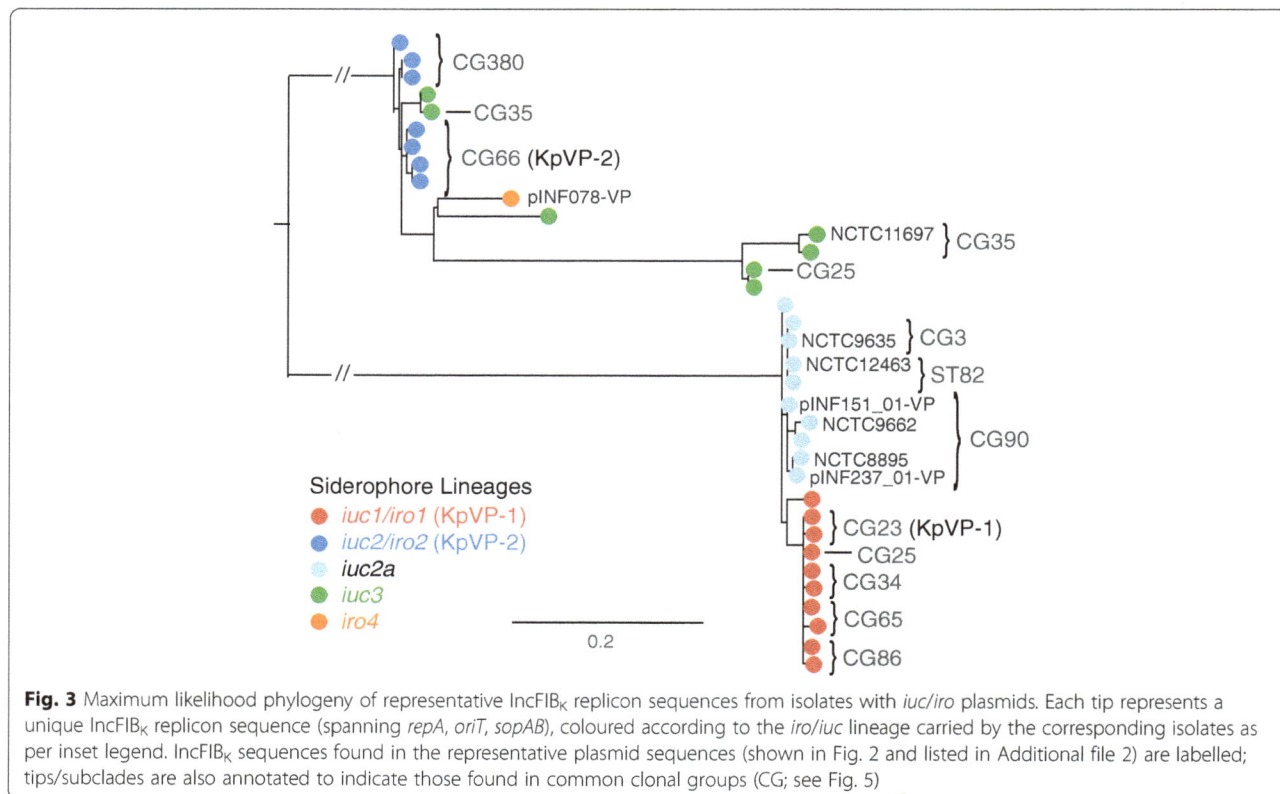

Fig. 3 Maximum likelihood phylogeny of representative IncFIB$_K$ replicon sequences from isolates with *iuc/iro* plasmids. Each tip represents a unique IncFIB$_K$ replicon sequence (spanning *repA*, *oriT*, *sopAB*), coloured according to the *iro/iuc* lineage carried by the corresponding isolates as per inset legend. IncFIB$_K$ sequences found in the representative plasmid sequences (shown in Fig. 2 and listed in Additional file 2) are labelled; tips/subclades are also annotated to indicate those found in common clonal groups (CG; see Fig. 5)

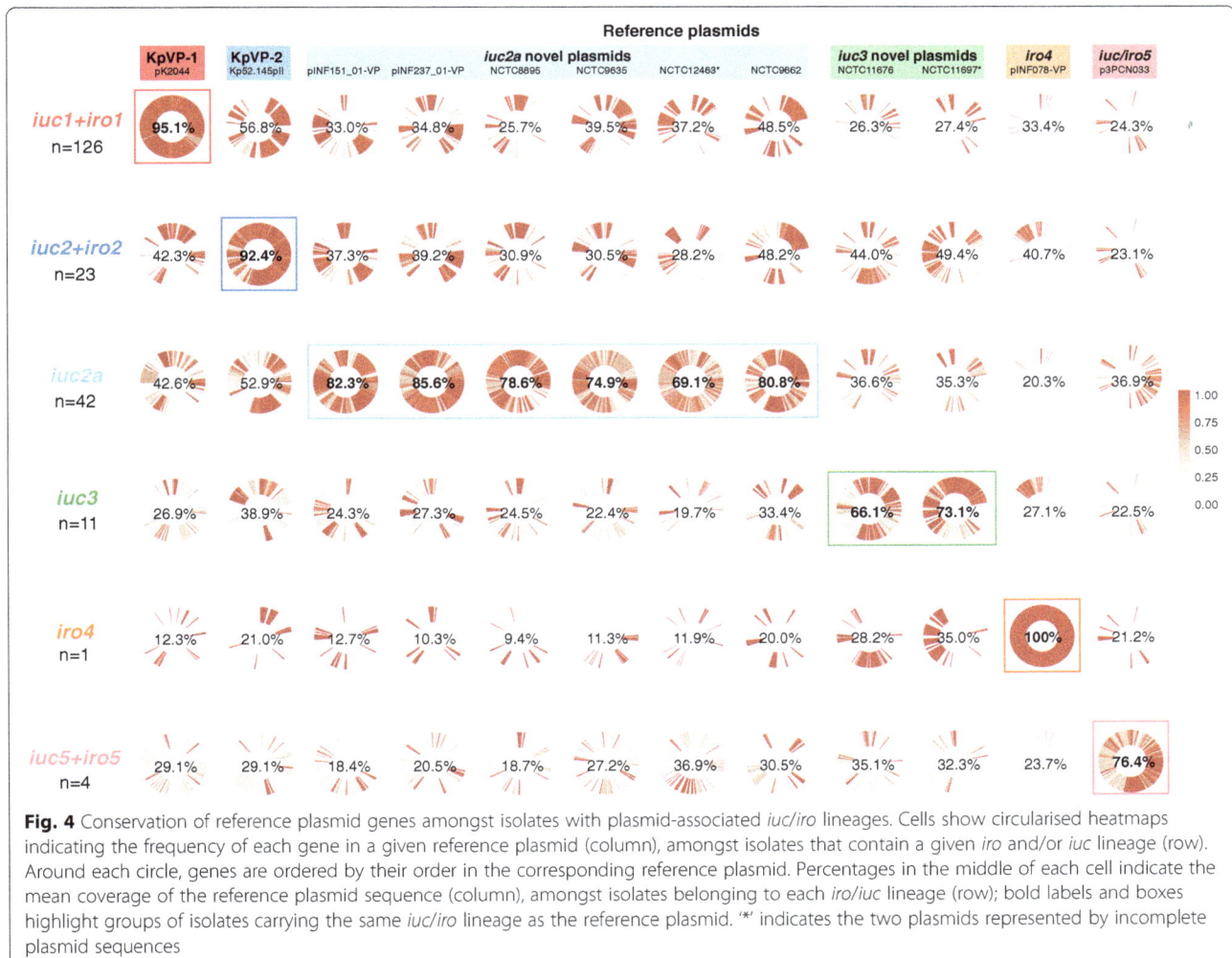

Fig. 4 Conservation of reference plasmid genes amongst isolates with plasmid-associated *iuc/iro* lineages. Cells show circularised heatmaps indicating the frequency of each gene in a given reference plasmid (column), amongst isolates that contain a given *iro* and/or *iuc* lineage (row). Around each circle, genes are ordered by their order in the corresponding reference plasmid. Percentages in the middle of each cell indicate the mean coverage of the reference plasmid sequence (column), amongst isolates belonging to each *iro/iuc* lineage (row); bold labels and boxes highlight groups of isolates carrying the same *iuc/iro* lineage as the reference plasmid. '*' indicates the two plasmids represented by incomplete plasmid sequences

the isolates that carried lineage 1 or 2 loci, respectively (Fig. 4). Notably, the loci encoding heavy metal resistances against copper (*pbr-pco*), silver (*sil*) and tellurite (*terXYW* and *terZABCDEF*) were highly conserved amongst lineage 1 isolates but not present in any of the lineage 2 isolates (Additional file 12). As noted above, *iuc/iro* lineages 1 and 2 were also each associated with a distinct variant of the IncFIB$_K$ replicon sequence (Fig. 3). Hence, we define pK2044-like plasmids carrying *iuc1* and *iro1* loci as *K. pneumoniae* virulence plasmid type 1 (KpVP-1), with reference plasmid pK2044, and Kp52.145 pII-like plasmids carrying *iuc2* and *iro2* loci as *K. pneumoniae* virulence plasmid type 2 (KpVP-2). Both plasmid types typically carry at least one copy of *rmpA*; neither one carries genes associated with conjugation; hence, we assume they are not self-transmissible.

KpVP-1 and KpVP-2 showed distinct distributions within the *K. pneumoniae* population. KpVP-1 was present in 5.0% of all isolates and accounted for 74% of *iuc+iro+* isolates. The KpVP-1 reference plasmid pK2044 originated

from an ST23 isolate (CG23), and KpVP-1 was strongly associated with this and two other well-known hypervirulent clones CG65 and CG86, in which it was present at high prevalence (ranging from 79.0 to 96.4%, see Fig. 5). KpVP-1 was also detected at low frequencies in other clones, including CG34, CG111, CG113 and CG25, suggesting it is mobile within the *K. pneumoniae* population (Fig. 5). KpVP-2 was present in 0.96% of all isolates and accounted for 14% of *iuc+iro+* isolates. The KpVP-2 reference plasmid Kp52.145 pII originated from an ST66 isolate, and KpVP-2 was present in all isolates of the associated clonal group CG66 ($n = 11$) and also all isolates of CG380 ($n = 12$) (Fig. 5).

An *iuc* lineage 2 variant (*iuc2a*) is associated with diverse plasmids with a KpVP-1-like IncFIB$_K$ replicon

Iuc2a was identified in 43 isolates largely belonging to three clonal groups (ST3, $n = 4$; CG90, $n = 19$; ST82, $n = 19$; ST382, $n = 1$; see Fig. 5), with the majority ($n = 38$, 88.4%) from the historical NCTC or Murray collections

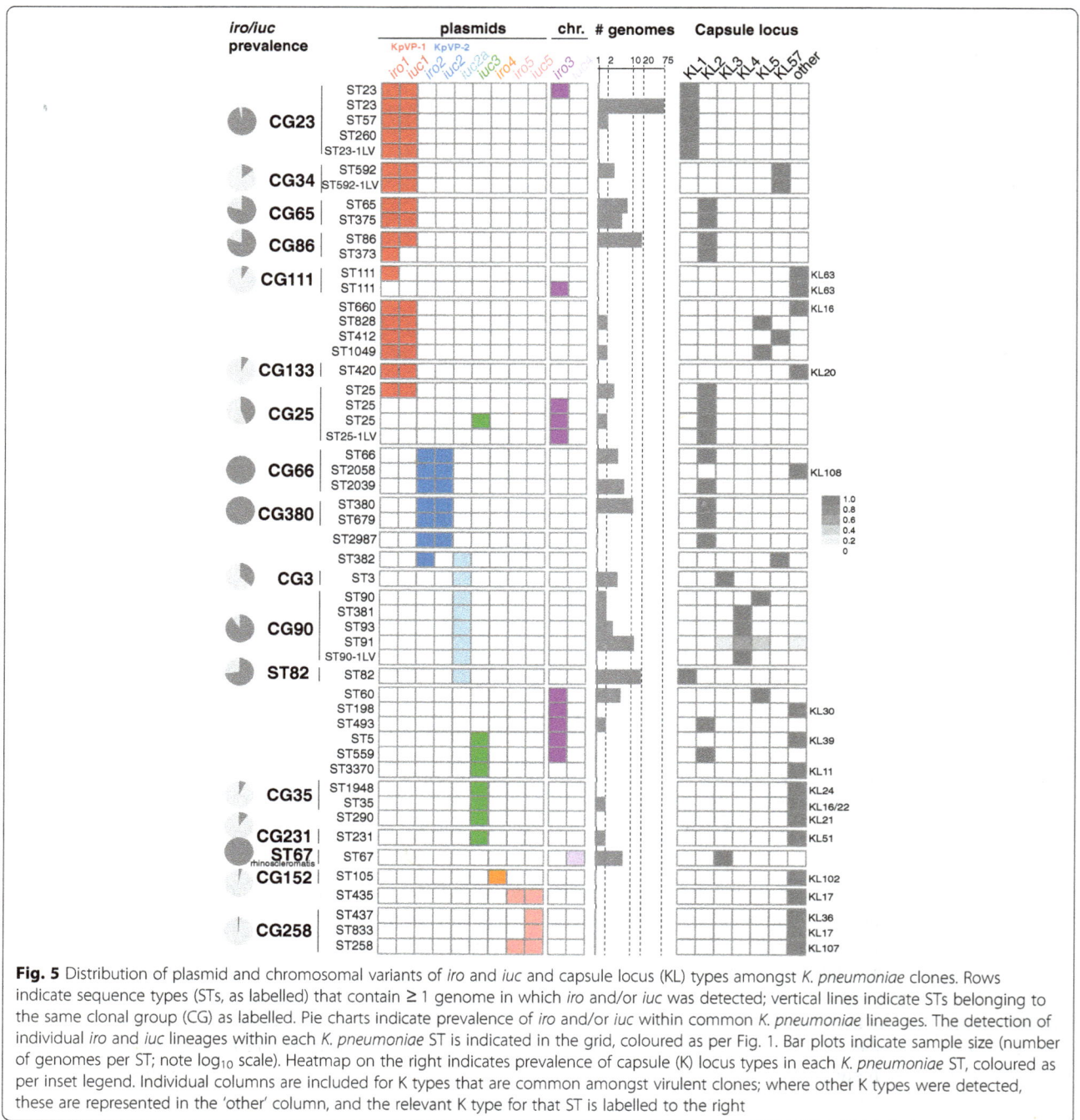

Fig. 5 Distribution of plasmid and chromosomal variants of *iro* and *iuc* and capsule locus (KL) types amongst *K. pneumoniae* clones. Rows indicate sequence types (STs, as labelled) that contain ≥ 1 genome in which *iro* and/or *iuc* was detected; vertical lines indicate STs belonging to the same clonal group (CG) as labelled. Pie charts indicate prevalence of *iro* and/or *iuc* within common *K. pneumoniae* lineages. The detection of individual *iro* and *iuc* lineages within each *K. pneumoniae* ST is indicated in the grid, coloured as per Fig. 1. Bar plots indicate sample size (number of genomes per ST; note $\log_{10}$ scale). Heatmap on the right indicates prevalence of capsule (K) locus types in each *K. pneumoniae* ST, coloured as per inset legend. Individual columns are included for K types that are common amongst virulent clones; where other K types were detected, these are represented in the 'other' column, and the relevant K type for that ST is labelled to the right

and isolated between 1932 and 1960 (Additional file 1). One of these isolates also carried *iro2* in addition to *iuc2a*, which in all other instances was only observed with *iuc2* on KpVP-2. Provenance information was available for only 12 of the *iuc2a+* isolates (1 ST3, 9 CG90, 2 ST82); all of which originated from the human respiratory tract (3 nose, 1 throat, 7 sputum and 2 NCTC isolates recorded only as a respiratory tract). We used long-read sequencing to resolve plasmids in two novel *iuc2a+* isolates from our

own collection, INF151and INF237, which were both CG90 Australian hospital sputum isolates (summarised in Additional file 3). This yielded IncFIB$_K$ plasmids in each genome, of size 138.1 kbp and 133.7 kbp, respectively (accessions: pINF151_01-VP, QWFT01000004; pINF237_01-VP, CP032834). Both plasmids carried *iuc2a* and one *rmpA* gene, but they differed slightly from one another in structure and gene content and differed substantially from the three complete *iuc2a+* plasmid sequences available from NCTC isolates (ST3 and CG90; see Figs. 2 and 4). Only one of these plasmids (from NCTC 12463; incomplete) carried a conjugative transfer region (IncFII); hence, we predict most are not self-transmissible. Mapping of *iuc2a+* genomes to each of the five representative *iuc2a+* plasmid sequences indicated a degree of conservation between plasmids in isolates belonging to the same *K. pneumoniae* clone, but none particularly well conserved across all *iuc2a+* isolates (Fig. 4, Additional file 13). However, all *iuc2a+* isolates formed a tight monophyletic cluster in the IncFIB$_K$ replicon tree (Fig. 3), consistent with recent shared plasmid ancestry followed by frequent structural and gene content changes. Notably, the *iuc2a*-associated IncFIB$_K$ replicon sequences were closely related to those of KpVP-1 and distant from those of KpVP-2; hence, we hypothesise that *iuc2a* plasmids share an ancestor that was a mosaic including *iuc2*-related sequences from KpVP-2 and IncFIB$_K$ replicon sequences from KpVP-1.

luc lineage 3 is mobilised by diverse plasmids carrying the IncFII$_K$ conjugative transfer region

Lineage *iuc3* was detected in 11 isolates from diverse sources and chromosomal STs (Fig. 5) and was associated with three related variants of the IncFIB$_K$ replicon (Fig. 3). We identified one complete and one near-complete *iuc3* plasmid sequences: a complete 189.8 kb plasmid from NCTC 11676 (isolated 1979, ST290) and a 155.4 kb contig from NCTC 11697 (isolated 1984, ST3370) (Fig. 2). The plasmids share around half of their gene content (96 kbp), including the IncFII$_K$ *tra-trb* conjugative transfer machinery, a fimbrial protein and the *fec* iron acquisition system in addition to *iuc3* (Figs. 2 and 4, Additional file 2). Mapping to these sequences showed all *iuc3+* isolates carried related plasmids with an IncFII$_K$ *tra-trb* transfer region (Fig. 4, Additional file 12).

Complete sequence of an *iro4* plasmid

Lineage *iro4* was identified in a single hospital UTI isolate INF078 (ST105) from Australia, whose genome sequence we completed using long reads (replicons summarised in Additional file 3). Hybrid assembly using short and long reads resolved a 399,913 kbp plasmid, pINF078-VP (accession CP032832) which carried multiple copies of *iro4*, the IncFIB$_K$ replicon (similar to the KpVP-2 variant, see Fig. 5) and the IncFII$_K$ replicon and *tra-trb* transfer region (Fig. 2). As noted above, the *iro4* locus is more closely related to *Enterobacter iro* than to other *K. pneumoniae iro* in terms of both structure (including the *iroE* gene; see Fig. 1b, Additional file 14) and sequence (Additional file 10), suggesting it has been transferred from *Enterobacter* into a *K. pneumoniae* IncFIB$_K$/FII$_K$ plasmid backbone. pINF078-VP harboured multiple tandem copies of a 17,129 bp region containing

iroBCDEN and 12 other genes of unknown function (Additional file 14). Long-read sequences (up to 70 kbp) spanning the non-repeat and repeat region of pINF078-VP confirmed at least $n = 3$ copies of the 17 kbp repeated sequence, whose mean read depth in the Illumina sequence data was 13.3 times that of the rest of the plasmid sequence, suggesting approximately 13 tandem copies.

luc/iro lineage 5 loci are associated with plasmids originating from *E. coli*

Four *K. pneumoniae* isolates carried the *E. coli* variant *iuc5*; two of these also carried the *E. coli* variant *iro5* (see species trees in Additional file 10). Three *iuc5+* isolates (including one with *iro5*) belonged to the globally disseminated, carbapenemase-producing *K. pneumoniae* CG258 (ST258, KPC+; ST437, KPC+; ST833, KPC−) and carried several AMR genes. Unfortunately, all four *iuc5+* genomes were sourced from public databases and were available in draft form only, and the complete plasmid sequences could not be resolved. However, the *iuc5+* contig sequences from *K. pneumoniae* share close homology with *iuc5+iro5+* IncFII conjugative plasmids from *E. coli* that also carry AMR genes (e.g. p3PCN033, CP006635.1; D3 plasmid A, CP010141.1). Notably, all *iuc5* contigs from *K. pneumoniae* shared > 75% coverage and 98.19–99.95% identity to the p3PCN033 reference plasmid.

Discussion

This study reveals significant genetic diversity underlying the biosynthesis of aerobactin and salmochelin in *K. pneumoniae* but shows the distribution of *iuc* and *iro* locus variants is highly structured within the population. Our data indicate that most of the burden of these hypervirulence-associated siderophores in the *K. pneumoniae* population is associated with two dominant virulence plasmids, which we define here as KpVP-1 and KpVP-2, that differ in terms of gene content (Fig. 2) and are each associated with co-segregating sequences of the non-self-transmissible IncFIB$_K$ replicon, *iuc* and *iro* loci (Figs. 1 and 3). These dominant virulence plasmid types are each represented by one of the previously characterised *K. pneumoniae* virulence plasmids [18, 20], pK2044 (KpVP-1, encoding *iro1* and *iuc1*) and Kp152.145pII (KpVP-2, encoding *iro2* and *iuc2*); both also carry hypermucoidy determinants, and together, they account for 74% and 14% of the *iuc+iro+ K. pneumoniae* genomes analysed. Importantly, our data indicate that each of these common virulence plasmid variants is maintained at high prevalence in a small number of known hypervirulent clones: KpVP-1 in CG23 (96%, including pK2044 [18]), CG86 (80%, including pLVPK [19]) and CG65 (79%); KpVP-2 in CG66 (100%, including Kp152.145pII) and CG380 (100%) (Fig. 5). This suggests that both plasmid types can persist for long periods within a host bacterial lineage as it undergoes clonal expansion; indeed, our recent study of the evolutionary history of CG23 indicates that KpVP-1 has been maintained in this clonally expanding lineage for at least a century [22]. The lack of conjugation machinery is likely an important variable contributing to clonal expansion being the primary mode of dispersal over horizontal gene trasfer, although notably, we also detected KpVP-1 at low prevalence in numerous other *K. pneumoniae* lineages and KpVP-2 at low prevalence in one other lineage, suggesting the possibility of wider dissemination of both plasmid types by occasional transfer to new lineages (Fig. 5). Given the stability of the plasmids observed in several clonal groups, we speculate that some of these transfer events will result in the emergence of novel hypervirulent strains that can stably maintain the plasmid into the future. In contrast, the non-plasmid form of *iro* (*iro3*, occasionally integrated into the chromosomes of *K. pneumoniae* via ICE*Kp1*) was found at low prevalence (< 0.5%) and included just 1 of the 79 ST23 isolates analysed (NTUH-K2044, in which ICE*Kp1* was first described), 1/1 ST5, 1/21 ST111 (13%), 1/2 ST198, 2/15 CG25, 2/2 ST493 and 5/5 ST60. Hence, while ICE*Kp1* is somewhat dispersed in the *K. pneumoniae* population, it shows little evidence of stability within lineages, consistent with our previous observations regarding ICE*Kp* in general [8].

We also detected several novel *iuc+* or *iro+* plasmid types, the most common being the group of *iuc2a* plasmids (21% of all *iuc+* isolates) that were detected in respiratory isolates from CG3, CG82 and CG90 and mostly originated from historical collections [51]. Interestingly, these combine an *iuc* sequence closely related to that of KpVP-2 (Fig. 1) with an IncFIB$_K$ replicon sequence very close to that of KpVP-1 (Fig. 3) and showed substantial mosaicism and gene content variation (Figs. 2 and 4). The *iuc3* lineage was also quite common amongst the novel plasmid types (5.3% of all *iuc+* isolates) and associated with a variety of diverse plasmids, most of which carried the IncFII *tra-trb* conjugative transfer region and thus are likely self-transmissible (Figs. 2 and 4). It is notable that *iuc2a* and *iuc3* plasmids were not only relatively rare in the bacterial population but also showed less evidence of stable maintenance within *K. pneumoniae* lineages (Fig. 5) and lower stability of gene content (Fig. 2) than the dominant KpVP-1 and KpVP-2 plasmids (Fig. 4). The position of *iuc2a* and *iuc3* in the *iuc* trees (Fig. 1, Additional file 10) suggests that both are derive from other *K. pneumoniae* loci; hence, we speculate it is the properties of the plasmids mobilising these loci, and not the siderophore biosynthesis loci themselves, that makes these variants less widespread in the *K. pneumoniae* population. This variation in gene content may be a consequence of self-transmissibility, exposing the plasmids to a wider gene pool of host bacteria and providing opportunities for gene content diversification, which could potentially include AMR genes. Notably, the *iuc3* plasmids carry an arsenal of additional virulence loci involved in iron metabolism and resistance to heavy metals, reminiscent of KpVP-1 (Fig. 2).

The other novel plasmids appear to derive from outside *K. pneumoniae* (Fig. 1, Additional file 10). Most concerning are the four *E. coli*-derived plasmids we detected carrying *iuc5* (and occasionally *iro5*) in the USA and Brazil, three of which were found in the MDR hospital outbreak-associated clone CG258. Whether these aerobactin plasmids harbour AMR genes as they do in *E. coli* is not currently resolvable; however, it seems that conjugative *E. coli* plasmids such as D3 plasmid A do have the potential to deliver hypervirulence and multi-drug resistance to *K. pneumoniae* strains in a single step. A recent study of *K. pneumoniae* submitted to Public Health England used PCR to screen for isolates carrying both carbapenemase genes and *rmpA*, as a marker of the virulence plasmid, and identified a plasmid harbouring *iuc*, *rmpA*, *rmpA2* and the AMR genes *sul1*, *sul2*, *armA*, *dfrA5*, *mph(A)* and *aph(3′)-VIb* [28]. To our knowledge, this is the first report of a complete sequence of a *K. pneumoniae* plasmid harbouring both AMR and virulence genes. The isolate (ST147) was not included in our original screen; however, subsequent analysis using *Kleborate* plus manual inspection of the plasmid sequence reveals it carries *iuc1* (AbST63, a novel single locus variant of AbST1 which is typical of hypervirulent clones CG23, CG65 and CG86) and appears to be a mosaic carrying sequences from KpVP-1 (40% coverage), an IncFII *tra-trb* conjugative transfer region and transposons carrying AMR genes.

The presence of aerobactin synthesis loci in the *iuc5+* *K. pneumoniae* isolates we identified here was not reported in the original studies [52, 53], and thus, it is not known whether they actually produce aerobactin or show enhanced virulence. This highlights the need to raise awareness of the *iuc* and *iro* loci as potentially clinically relevant hypervirulence factors and to screen for them in isolates and genome data. The latter, we aim to facilitate via the genotyping schemes established here, which can be used to easily screen new genome assemblies using Kleborate (https://github.com/katholt/Kleborate/) or BIGSdb-*Kp* (http://bigsdb.pasteur.fr/klebsiella/klebsiella.html), or new short-read data sets using SRST2 (https://github.com/katholt/srst2). PCR primers suitable for screening for *iro* and *iuc* can be found in Lee et al. [54]. Notably, many studies rely on the hypermucoidy phenotype to identify hypervirulent strains; however, this is dependent on growth conditions [55], and recent studies indicate that aerobactin synthesis is a more important virulence determinant [13, 14, 16]. Our data suggest that hypermucoidy screening would typically pick up most of the common aerobactin plasmids KpVP-1, KpVP-2 and *iuc2a+* plasmids, but not those carrying *iuc3* or the *iuc5* plasmids from *E. coli*. Additionally, it is important not to conflate the presence of the core chromosomal receptor gene *iutA* with the ability to synthesise aerobactin, which is encoded in the *iuc* locus [6]. False-positive detection of the aerobactin locus version of *iutA* can be avoided by using an identity threshold of < 20% divergence. Tellurite resistance has also been suggested as a phenotypic screen to identify hypervirulent isolates of CG23, CG65 and CG86 [56]; our data confirm this is a good marker for KpVP-1 (92.6% carry *ter*) but not for other aerobactin plasmid types (Additional file 12).

Conclusions

Our results illuminate that distinct virulence plasmid variants are associated with the various hypervirulent *K. pneumoniae* lineages but also highlight that these alongside other plasmids and MGEs can shuttle aerobactin and salmochelin synthesis loci to other lineages, threatening the emergence of novel hypervirulent strains. Indeed, reports of MDR clones acquiring *iuc* plasmids appear to be increasing in incidence, particularly in China [27, 29, 57–59] and have been associated with increased morbidity and mortality. The AbST and SmST typing schemes developed in this study provide an important resource to identify and monitor the movement of *iro* and *iuc* loci and associated MGEs in *K. pneumoniae* genomes; which will be important to detect and contain these emerging threats. Genotyping with our tools reveals the *iuc* plasmid identified in the recently reported fatal hospital outbreak of carbapenemase-producing ST11 in Beijing is a variant of KpVP-1 that carries *iuc1* (AbST1) and a single copy of *rmpA* but lacks the *iro* locus [27]. In this strain, the aerobactin plasmid does not carry any AMR determinants; the carbapenemase gene *bla*KPC and several other AMR genes were located on other plasmids. Concerningly, the ability for the virulence plasmids to be maintained in *K. pneumoniae* lineages suggests that once established in the MDR hospital outbreak-associated clones, they may become quite stable. The initial report of *iuc+* KPC+ ST11 in China prompted multiple other groups to report the detection of the same strain in their hospitals [60–62], suggesting this strain may indeed be emerging as a persistently hypervirulent and MDR form of *K. pneumoniae*. Genomic surveillance and control of the spread of such 'dual-risk' strains, or indeed even plasmids combining both characteristics of MDR and hypervirulence, clearly needs to be reinforced; the present work will bolster efforts to understand and limit the emergence of infections caused by *K. pneumoniae* strains carrying the high virulence determinants aerobactin and salmochelin.

Additional files

Additional file 1: Strain information for genomes included in this study.

Additional file 2: General features of reference plasmids or incomplete plasmid sequences carrying *iro* and/or *iuc*.

Additional file 3: Summary of replicon sequences from isolates INF151, INF237 and INF078.

Additional file 4: Aerobactin sequence types (AbSTs) and corresponding alleles.

Additional file 5: Salmochelin sequence types (SmSTs) and corresponding alleles.

Additional file 6: Representative Enterobacterales genome sequences included in *iro* and *iuc* phylogenetic analysis.

Additional file 7: Phylogenetic relationships between the predicted amino acid sequences encoded by aerobactin (*iuc*) and salmochelin (*iro*) locus sequence types. Each tip represents a translated amino acid sequence for an aerobactin sequence type (AbST, in a) or salmochelin sequence type (SmST, in b). Lineages defined from nucleotide sequences (see tree in Fig. 1) are highlighted and labelled.

Additional file 8: Single nucleotide variants and nucleotide divergence (%) observed within (shaded in grey) and between the aerobactin-encoding *iuc* lineages.

Additional file 9: Single nucleotide variants and nucleotide divergence (%) observed within (shaded in grey) and between the salmochelin-encoding *iro* lineages.

Additional file 10: Phylogenetic trees for salmochelin and aerobactin encoding *iuc* locus in *K. pneumoniae* and other Enterobacterales bacteria. Trees represent show a midpoint-rooted maximum likelihood phylogeny for representative sequences identified in various Enterobacterales species (listed in Additional file 6). Tip colours indicate the genetic context of the locus: black = plasmid, red = chromosome. *K. pneumoniae iro* lineages defined in Fig. 1 are coloured; other species-specific clades are highlighted in grey; individually labelled tips within highlighted clades indicate exceptions to the species label of the clade. Salmochelin trees were inferred using the *iroB* gene alone (panel a), which show a highly divergent form in *Salmonella*. Panel (b) shows a tree inferred from all four genes of the typical *K. pneumoniae iro* locus (*iroBCDN*), excluding the distantly related *Salmonella* variant, to increase resolution within the group containing *Klebsiella*. Similarly, aerobactin trees were inferred using the *iucB* gene alone (panel c) to show the overall structure, and separately for the full set of genes in the *K. pneumoniae* locus (*iucABCD, iutA*) to provide greater resolution within the group containing *Klebsiella* (panel d).

Additional file 11: Summary of aerobactin-encoding *iuc* and salmochelin-encoding *iro* loci BLAST hit.

Additional file 12: Prevalence of virulence loci and plasmid replication loci amongst isolates with virulence plasmids.

Additional file 13: Conservation of coding sequences from KpVP-2 and *iuc2a+* reference plasmids amongst isolates carrying plasmid-encoded *iuc2* or *iuc2a* loci. Cells show circularised heatmaps indicating the frequency of each gene in a given reference plasmid (column), amongst isolates of a given chromosomal sequence type (ST) or clonal group (CG) (rows) that carry either *iuc2* (CG66, CG380) or *iuc2a* (others). Around each circle, genes are ordered by their order in the corresponding reference plasmid.

Additional file 14: Genetic structure of 17 kbp repeat region in plasmid pINF078-VP and the chromosomally-encoded *E. cloacae iro* region. Shaded area indicates a homologous region of 95% nucleotide identity shared between the two sequences. Coding sequences are represented by the arrows and coloured according to the closest Enterobacteriaceae species match as indicated in the legend.

Abbreviations
AbST: Aerobactin sequence type; AMR: Antimicrobial resistance; CA: Community-associated; CG: Clonal group; CI: Confidence interval; Ent: Enterobactin; HA: Healthcare-associated; HGT: Horizontal gene transfer;

ICEs: Integrative and conjugative elements; Iro: Salmochelin; Iuc: Aerobactin; MDR: Multidrug-resistant; MGEs: Mobile genetic elements; MLST: Multi-locus sequence typing; OR: Odds ratio; SmST: Salmochelin sequence type; ST: Sequence type; Ybt: Yersiniabactin

Acknowledgements

We thank the team of the curators of the Institut Pasteur MLST system (Paris, France) for importing novel alleles, profiles and/or isolates at http://bigsdb.pasteur.fr.

Funding

This work was funded by the National Health and Medical Research Council (NHMRC) of Australia (project #1043822), a Senior Medical Research Fellowship from the Viertel Foundation of Australia and the Bill and Melinda Gates Foundation of Seattle, USA.

Authors' contributions

MMCL performed the majority of data analyses and wrote the paper together with KEH. RRW, KLW, SB and KEH contributed additional data analysis, visualisation and interpretation. SB incorporated the novel MLST schemes into the BIGSdb. RRW and KEH wrote the code. AJ contributed clinical isolates, data and interpretations. LMJ performed the DNA extraction and nanopore sequencing. All authors edited and approved the final paper.

Competing interests

The authors declare that they have no competing interests.

Author details

[1]Department of Biochemistry and Molecular Biology, Bio21 Molecular Science and Biotechnology Institute, University of Melbourne, Parkville, Victoria 3010, Australia. [2]Biodiversity and Epidemiology of Bacterial Pathogens, Institut Pasteur, 75015 Paris, France. [3]Department of Infectious Diseases and Microbiology Unit, The Alfred Hospital, Melbourne, Victoria 3004, Australia. [4]London School of Hygiene & Tropical Medicine, London WC1E 7HT, UK.

References

1. Podschun R, Ullmann U. Klebsiella spp. as nosocomial pathogens: epidemiology, taxonomy, typing methods, and pathogenicity factors. Clin Microbiol Rev. 1998;11(4):589–603.
2. Martin RM, Bachman MA. Colonization, infection, and the accessory genome of Klebsiella pneumoniae. Front Cell Infect Microbiol. 2018;8(4). https://doi.org/10.3389/fcimb.2018.00004.
3. Holt KE, Wertheim H, Zadoks RN, Baker S, Whitehouse CA, Dance D, et al. Genomic analysis of diversity, population structure, virulence, and antimicrobial resistance in Klebsiella pneumoniae, an urgent threat to public health. Proc Natl Acad Sci U S A. 2015;112(27):E3574–81.
4. Ramirez MS, Traglia GM, Lin DL, Tran T, Tolmasky ME. Plasmid-mediated antibiotic resistance and virulence in gram-negatives: the Klebsiella pneumoniae paradigm. Microbiol Spectr. 2014;2(5):1–15.
5. Gorrie CL, Mirceta M, Wick RR, Edwards DJ, Strugnell RA, Pratt N, et al. Gastrointestinal carriage is a major reservoir of K. pneumoniae infection in intensive care patients. Clin Infect Dis. 2017;65(2):208–15.
6. Runcharoen C, Moradigaravand D, Blane B, Paksanont S, Thammachote J, Anun S, et al. Whole genome sequencing reveals high-resolution epidemiological links between clinical and environmental Klebsiella pneumoniae. Genome Med. 2017;9(1):6. https://doi.org/10.1186/s13073-017-0397-1.
7. Lin TL, Lee CZ, Hsieh PF, Tsai SF, Wang JT. Characterization of integrative and conjugative element ICEKp1-associated genomic heterogeneity in a Klebsiella pneumoniae strain isolated from a primary liver abscess. J Bacteriol. 2008;190(2):515–26.
8. Lam MMC, Wick RR, Wyres KL, Gorrie C, Judd LM, Jenney A, et al. Genetic diversity, mobilisation and spread of the yersiniabactin-encoding mobile element ICEKp in Klebsiella pneumoniae populations. Microb Genom. 2018; 4(9). https://doi.org/10.1099/mgen.0.000196.
9. Nassif X, Sansonetti PJ. Correlation of the virulence of Klebsiella pneumoniae K1 and K2 with the presence of a plasmid encoding aerobactin. Infect Immun. 1986;54(3):603–8.
10. Müller S, Valdebenito M, Hantke K. Salmochelin, the long-overlooked catecholate siderophore of Salmonella. Biometals. 2009;22(4):691–5.
11. Goetz DH, Holmes MA, Borregaard N, Bluhm ME, Raymond KN, Strong RK. The neutrophil lipocalin NGAL is a bacteriostatic agent that interferes with siderophore-mediated iron acquisition. Mol Cell. 2002;10(5):1033–43.
12. Fischbach MA, Lin H, Zhou L, Yu Y, Abergel RJ, Liu DR, et al. The pathogen-associated iroA gene cluster mediates bacterial evasion of lipocalin 2. Proc Natl Acad Sci U S A. 2006;103(44):16502–7.
13. Russo TA, Olson R, Macdonald U, Beanan J, Davidson BA. Aerobactin, but not yersiniabactin, salmochelin, or enterobactin, enables the growth/survival of hypervirulent (hypermucoviscous) Klebsiella pneumoniae ex vivo and in vivo. Infect Immun. 2015;83(8):3325–33.
14. Russo TA, Olson R, Macdonald U, Metzger D, Maltese LM, Drake EJ. Aerobactin mediates virulence and accounts for increased siderophore production under iron-limiting conditions by hypervirulent (hypermucoviscous) Klebsiella pneumoniae. Infect Immun. 2014;82(6):2356–67.
15. Konopka K, Bindereif A, Neilands J. Aerobactin-mediated utilization of transferrin iron. Biochemistry. 1982;21(25):6503–8.
16. Russo TA, Olson R, Fang C-T, Stoesser N, Miller M, Hutson A, et al. Identification of biomarkers for the differentiation of hypervirulent Klebsiella pneumoniae from classical K. pneumoniae. J Clin Microbiol. 2018. https://doi.org/10.1128/JCM.00776-18.
17. Putze J, Hennequin C, Nougayrède JP, Zhang W, Homburg S, Karch H, et al. Genetic structure and distribution of the colibactin genomic island among members of the family Enterobacteriaceae. Infect Immun. 2009;77(11):4696–703.
18. Wu KM, Li NH, Yan JJ, Tsao N, Liao TL, Tsai HC, et al. Genome sequencing and comparative analysis of Klebsiella pneumoniae NTUH-K2044, a strain causing liver abscess and meningitis. J Bacteriol. 2009; 191(14):4492–501.
19. Chen Y, Chang H, Lai Y, Pan C, Tsai S. Sequencing and analysis of the large virulence plasmid pLVPK of Klebsiella pneumoniae CG43. Gene. 2004;337: 189–98.
20. Lery LM, Frangeul L, Tomas A, Passet V, Almeida AS, Bialek-Davenet S, et al. Comparative analysis of Klebsiella pneumoniae genomes identifies a phospholipase D family protein as a novel virulence factor. BMC Biol. 2014; 12(1):41.
21. Nassif X, Fournier J, Arondel J, Sansonetti PJ. Mucoid phenotype of Klebsiella pneumoniae is a plasmid-encoded virulence factor. Infect Immun. 1989; 57(2):546–52.
22. Lam MM, Wyres KL, Duchêne S, Wick RR, Judd LM, Gan Y, et al. Population genomics of hypervirulent Klebsiella pneumoniae clonal-group 23 reveals early emergence and rapid global dissemination. Nat Comms. 2018. https://doi.org/10.1101/225359.
23. Struve C, Roe CC, Stegger M, Stahlhut SG, Hansen DS, Engelthaler DM, et al. Mapping the evolution of hypervirulent Klebsiella pneumoniae. MBio. 2015;6(4):1–12.

24. Peng H, Wang P, Wu J, Chiu C, Chang H. Molecular epidemiology of *Klebsiella pneumoniae*. Zhonghua Min Guo Wei Sheng Wu Ji Mian Yi Xue Za Zhi. 1991;24:264–71.

25. Bialek-davenet S, Criscuolo A, Ailloud F, Passet V, Jones L, Garin B, et al. Genomic definition of hypervirulent and multidrug-resistant *Klebsiella pneumoniae* clonal groups. Emerg Infect Dis. 2014;20(11):1812–20.

26. Shon AS, Russo TA. Hypervirulent *Klebsiella pneumoniae*: the next superbug? Future Microbiol. 2012;7(6):669–71.

27. Gu D, Dong N, Zheng Z, Lin D, Huang M, Wang L, et al. A fatal outbreak of ST11 carbapenem-resistant hypervirulent *Klebsiella pneumoniae* in a Chinese hospital: a molecular epidemiological study. Lancet Infect Dis. 2018. https://doi.org/10.1016/S1473-3099(17)30489-9.

28. Turton JF, Payne Z, Coward A, Hopkins K, Turton J, Doumith M, et al. Virulence genes in isolates of *Klebsiella pneumoniae* from the UK during 2016, including among carbapenemase gene-positive hypervirulent K1-ST23 and "non-hypervirulent" types ST147, ST15 and ST383. J Med Microbiol. 2018;67(1):118–28.

29. Chen L, Kreiswirth BN. Convergence of carbapenem-resistance and hypervirulence in *Klebsiella pneumoniae*. Lancet Infect Dis. 2018. https://doi.org/10.1016/S1473-3099(17)30517-0.

30. Cheong HS, Chung DR, Lee C, Kim SH, Kang C, Peck KR. Emergence of serotype K1 *Klebsiella pneumoniae* ST23 strains co-producing the DHA-1 and an extended-spectrum beta-lactamase in Korea. Antimicrob Resist Infect Control. 2016. https://doi.org/10.1186/s13756-016-0151-2.

31. Shin J, Ko KS. Single origin of three plasmids bearing bla CTX-M-15 from different *Klebsiella pneumoniae* clones. J Antimicrob Chemother. 2014;69:969–72.

32. Wyres KL, Wick RR, Gorrie C, Jenney A, Follador R, Thomson NR, et al. Identification of *Klebsiella* capsule synthesis loci from whole genome data. Microb Genom. 2016. https://doi.org/10.1099/mgen.0.000102.

33. Wick RR, Judd LM, Gorrie C, Holt KE. Unicycler: resolving bacterial genome assemblies from short and long sequencing reads. PLoS Comput Biol. 2017;13(6):e1005595.

34. Bankevich A, Nurk S, Antipov D, Gurevich AA, Dvorkin M, Kulikov AS, et al. SPAdes: a new genome assembly algorithm and its applications to single-cell sequencing. J Comp Biol. 2012;19(5):455–77.

35. Seemann T. Prokka: rapid prokaryotic genome annotation. Bioinformatics. 2014;30(14):2068–9.

36. Wick RR, Judd LM, Gorrie CL, Holt KE. Completing bacterial genome assemblies with multiplex MinION sequencing. Microb Genom. 2017;3:1–7.

37. Diancourt L, Passet V, Verhoef J, Grimont PAD, Brisse S. Multilocus sequence typing of *Klebsiella pneumoniae* nosocomial isolates. J Clin Microbiol. 2005;43(8):4178–82.

38. Inouye M, Dashnow H, Raven L-A, Schultz MB, Pope BJ, Tomita T, et al. SRST2: rapid genomic surveillance for public health and hospital microbiology labs. Genome Med. 2014;6(11):90.

39. Wick RR, Heinz E, Holt KE, Wyres KL. Kaptive web: user-friendly capsule and lipopolysaccharide serotype prediction for *Klebsiella* genomes. J Clin Microbiol. 2018. https://doi.org/10.1128/JCM.00197-18.

40. Carattoli A, Zankari E, García-fernández A, Larsen V, Lund O, Villa L, et al. In silico detection and typing of plasmids using PlasmidFinder and plasmid multilocus sequence typing. Antimicrob Agents Chemother. 2014;58(7):3895–903.

41. Wick RR, Schultz MB, Zobel J, Holt KE. Bandage: interactive visualization of de novo genome assemblies. Bioinformatics. 2015;31:3350–2.

42. Edgar RC. MUSCLE: multiple sequence alignment with high accuracy and high throughput. Nucleic Acids Res. 2004;32(5):1792–7.

43. Stamatakis A. RAxML-VI-HPC: maximum likelihood-based phylogenetic analyses with thousands of taxa and mixed models. Bioinformatics. 2006;22(21):2688–90.

44. Carattoli A. Resistance plasmid families in *Enterobacteriaceae*. Antimicrob Agents Chemother. 2009;53(6):2227–38.

45. Yi H, Xi Y, Liu J, Wang J, Wu J, Xu T, et al. Sequence analysis of pKF3-70 in *Klebsiella pneumoniae*: probable origin from R100-like plasmid of *Escherichia coli*. PLoS One. 2010;5(1):e8601.

46. Darling ACE, Mau B, Blattner FR, Perna NT. Mauve: multiple alignment of conserved genomic sequence with rearrangements. Methods. 2004;14:1394–403.

47. Guy L, Kultima J, Andersson S. genoPlotR: comparative gene and genome visualization in R. Bioinformatics. 2010;26(18):2334–5.

48. Langmead B, Saizberg SL. Fast gapped-read alignment with Bowtie 2. Nat Methods. 2012;9:357–9.

49. Liu C, Zheng H, Yang M, Xu Z, Wang X, Wei L, et al. Genome analysis and in vivo virulence of porcine extraintestinal pathogenic *Escherichia coli* strain PCN033. BMC Genomics. 2015. https://doi.org/10.1186/s12864-015-1890-9.

50. Capone A, Giannella M, Fortini D, Giordano A, Meledandri M, Ballardini M, et al. High rate of colistin resistance among patients with carbapenem-resistant *Klebsiella pneumoniae* infection accounts for an excess of mortality. Clin Microbiol Infect. 2012. https://doi.org/10.1111/1469-0691.12070.

51. Wand ME, Baker KS, Benthall G, McGregor H, McCowen JWI, Deheer-Graham A, et al. Characterization of pre-antibiotic era *Klebsiella pneumoniae* isolates with respect to antibiotic/disinfectant susceptibility and virulence in *Galleria mellonella*. Antimicrob Agents Chemother. 2015;59(7):3966–72.

52. Bowers JR, Kitchel B, Driebe EM, MacCannell DR, Roe C, Lemmer D, et al. Genomic analysis of the emergence and rapid global dissemination of the clonal group 258 *Klebsiella pneumoniae* pandemic. PLoS One. 2015;10(7):1–24.

53. Davis GS, Waits K, Nordstrom L, Weaver B, Aziz M, Gauld L, et al. Intermingled *Klebsiella pneumoniae* populations between retail meats and human urinary tract infections. Clin Infect Dis. 2015;61:892–9.

54. Lee IR, Molton JS, Wyres KL, Gorrie C, Wong J, Hoh CH, et al. Differential host susceptibility and bacterial virulence factors driving *Klebsiella* liver abscess in an ethnically diverse population. Sci Rep. 2016. https://doi.org/10.1038/srep29316.

55. Catalán-Nájera JC, Garza-Ramos U, Barrios-Camacho H. Hypervirulence and hypermucoviscosity: two different but complementary *Klebsiella spp.* phenotypes? Virulence. 2017; doi: https://doi.org/10.1080/21505594.2017.1317412

56. Passet V, Brisse S. Association of tellurite resistance with hypervirulent clonal groups of *Klebsiella pneumoniae*. J Clin Microbiol. 2015;53(4):1380–2.

57. Zhan L, Wang S, Guo Y, Jin Y, Duan J, Hao Z, et al. Outbreak by hypermucoviscous *Klebsiella pneumoniae* ST11 isolates with carbapenem resistance in a tertiary Hospital in China. Front Cell Infect Microbiol. 2017. https://doi.org/10.3389/fcimb.2017.00182.

58. Zhang Y, Zeng J, Liu W, Zhao F, Hu Z, Zhao C, et al. Emergence of a hypervirulent carbapenem-resistant *Klebsiella pneumoniae* isolate from clinical infections in China. J Inf Secur. 2015. https://doi.org/10.1016/j.jinf.2015.07.010.

59. Araújo BF, Ferreira ML, De Campos PA, Royer S, Gonçalves IR, Fernandes MR, et al. Hypervirulence and biofilm production in KPC-2-producing *Klebsiella pneumoniae* CG258 isolated in Brazil. J Med Microbiol. 2018;67:523–8.

60. Du P, Zhang Y, Chen C. Emergence of carbapenem-resistant hypervirulent *Klebsiella pneumoniae*. Lancet Infect Dis. 2018. https://doi.org/10.1016/S1473-3099(17)30625-4.

61. Yao H, Qin S, Chen S, Shen J, Du X-D. Emergence of carbapenem-resistant hypervirulent *Klebsiella pneumoniae*. Lancet Infect Dis. 2018. https://doi.org/10.1016/S1473-3099(17)30628-X.

62. Wong MH, Shum H-P, Chen JH, Man M-Y, Wu A, Chan EW, et al. Emergence of carbapenem-resistant hypervirulent *Klebsiella pneumoniae*. Lancet Infect Dis. 2018. https://doi.org/10.1016/S1473-3099(17)30629-1.

10

Integrative analysis reveals functional and regulatory roles of H3K79me2 in mediating alternative splicing

Tianbao Li[1,2†], Qi Liu[2†], Nick Garza[2,3], Steven Kornblau[4] and Victor X. Jin[2*]

Abstract

Background: Accumulating evidence suggests alternative splicing (AS) is a co-transcriptional splicing process not only controlled by RNA-binding splicing factors, but also mediated by epigenetic regulators, such as chromatin structure, nucleosome density, and histone modification. Aberrant AS plays an important role in regulating various diseases, including cancers.

Methods: In this study, we integrated AS events derived from RNA-seq with H3K79me2 ChIP-seq data across 34 different normal and cancer cell types and found the higher enrichment of H3K79me2 in two AS types, skipping exon (SE) and alternative 3′ splice site (A3SS).

Results: Interestingly, by applying self-organizing map (SOM) clustering, we unveiled two clusters mainly comprised of blood cancer cell types with a strong correlation between H3K79me2 and SE. Remarkably, the expression of transcripts associated with SE was not significantly different from that of those not associated with SE, indicating the involvement of H3K79me2 in splicing has little impact on full mRNA transcription. We further showed that the deletion of DOT1L1, the sole H3K79 methyltransferase, impeded leukemia cell proliferation as well as switched exon skipping to the inclusion isoform in two MLL-rearranged acute myeloid leukemia cell lines. Our data demonstrate H3K79me2 was involved in mediating SE processing, which might in turn influence transformation and disease progression in leukemias.

Conclusions: Collectively, our work for the first time reveals that H3K79me2 plays functional and regulatory roles through a co-transcriptional splicing mechanism.

Keywords: Alternative Splicing, H3K79me2, DOT1L, AML

Background

Alternative splicing (AS) is a pre-mRNA process mainly controlled by post-transcriptional regulation involving 90% of human multi-exonic coding genes in a variety of tissues and cell types [1–3]. Many studies have highlighted the key role of AS in regulating cellular development and differentiation, and aberrant AS events lead to disease states such as muscular dystrophies and cancers [4–6]. Accumulating evidence further supports a new paradigm that AS is a co-transcriptional splicing process mutually coordinated by transcription and splicing [7–9]. Recent studies further illustrate that splicing is also regulated by epigenetic regulators, including chromatin structure, histone modifications, and CTCF [10, 11]. Dysregulation of some epigenetic components may alter the splicing process, resulting in various types of human diseases [12–15]. For instance, a recent study reported that a mutation of the histone methyl transferase SEDT2 alters AS of several key WNT signaling regulatory genes, resulting in colorectal cancer [16].

Recent genome-wide studies revealed histone marks such as H3K36me3 and H3K79me2 as well as nucleosome positioning were highly enriched within intragenic regions, implicating their regulatory roles in the RNA polymerase II elongation process and exon definition [17–20]. Further studies demonstrated the enrichment

* Correspondence: JinV@uthscsa.edu
†Equal contributors
2Department of Molecular Medicine, University of Texas Health, 8403 Floyd Curl, San Antonio, TX 78229, USA
Full list of author information is available at the end of the article

levels of histone modifications were correlated not only with transcriptional activity, but also with AS [21–23]. Despite these de novo genome-wide findings, knowledge on the causal and functional roles of histone modifications in AS is limited. In addition, little work has been done on aberrant AS processing in diseases caused by epigenetic defects.

H3K79, located in the globular domain of histone H3, is exposed on the nucleosome surface and then methylated by the sole enzyme DOT1-like histone lysine methyltransferase (DOT1L), a member of the lysine methyltransferase family [24]. This histone methylation typically functions in transcriptional regulation [25, 26], telomeric silencing [27, 28], cell-cycle regulation [29], and DNA damage repair [30–32]. Recent studies revealed a new role for it in regulating AS [33–35]. For example, H3K79me2 is able to recruit chromodomain-containing protein MRG15 and splicing factor PTB1 to influence AS outcomes [36, 37]. In particular, new findings demonstrated its crucial role in transformation as well as disease progression in leukemias [38–40]. DOT1L is frequently involved in chromosomal translocations, with numerous genes creating fusion genes that interfere with its interaction with the elongation complexes, resulting in a loss of function. This is common in the mixed-lineage leukemia (MLL) gene, resulting in aggressive leukemia [41], including 5–10% of adult acute leukemias [42] and 60–80% of infant acute leukemias [43]. These findings have established a foundation for disease-specific epigenetic therapies against acute leukemias.

In a previous study, we found a correlation between H3K79me2 enrichment level and an exon skipping event in GM12878 and K562 cells [20]. However, the common and cell type-specific genomic patterns and correlations between H3K79me2 and various types of splicing events across diverse cell types have not been fully explored. In this study, we integrated AS events derived from RNA-seq with H3K79me2 ChIP-seq data across 34 different normal and cancer cell types, and examine the enrichment of H3K79me2 in five major types of AS events, skipping exon (SE), mutual exclusive exon (MXE), retained intron (RI), alternative 5′-end splice site (A5SS), and alternative 3′-end splice site (A3SS). We attempt to elucidate functional and regulatory roles of H3K79me2 in mediating AS, particularly in MLL-rearranged (MLL-r) acute myeloid leukemia (AML) cells.

Methods

Raw data processing

H3K79me2 ChIP-seq and RNA-seq data for a total of 34 various normal and cancer cell lines were collected from the Gene Expression Omnibus (GEO) repository and ENCODE Consortia (Additional file 1: Table S1). Raw

sequence reads were aligned against the human genomic sequence (GRCh37) using bowtie2 for ChIP-seq data [44] and TopHat (version 2.0.14) for RNA-seq data [45]. Only uniquely mapped reads were used for further downstream analysis.

Identification of AS events and H3K79me2 enrichment and peaks

Unique reads from RNA-seq data in bam format are used as input for MISO (The Mixture of Isoforms), which detected AS events based on Bayes factors, filtering criteria, Psi values (Ψ) and confidence intervals [46]. Sashimi plots were generated to illustrate all five types of AS events for visualization. The enrichment of H3K79me2/kb is calculated as the number of reads from H3K79me2 ChIP-seq data in exon skipping gene regions (the exon part of an exon skipping gene plus 50 bp upstream and downstream around exons) per kilobase pair (the length of the exon skipping gene region) normalized by the total number of reads of each dataset. The H3K79me2 peaks were identified by Model-based Analysis of ChIP-Seq version 2 (MACS2) with a q value (minimum false discovery rate (FDR)) of 0.01 [47].

Self-organizing map clustering

We used self-organizing map (SOM) clustering for dimension reduction for feature extraction associated with exon skipping sites. SOM is a model of two-layer artificial neural networks that maps high dimensional input datasets to a set of nodes arranged in lattice. SOM has two steps: (i) determining a winner node and (ii) updating weighted vectors associated with the winner node and some of its neighboring nodes. According to the enrichment of H3K79me2 for each SE site, the SOM algorithm maps multi-dimensional input vectors to two-dimensional neurons, helping to understand the high-dimensional SE data; the most enriched cluster for each cell is assigned to their cell type. The SOM training was performed using the R package "kohonen". SOM training parameters and node number optimization were defined on the basis of Xie et al. [48]. Node grouping was based on a hierarchical clustering approach using the hclust function of the "Stats" package of R. The number of clusters was chosen based on homogeneity analyses.

Cell culture and reagents

Human cell lines MV-4-11, K562, and OCI-LY7 were cultured in Iscove's modified Dulbecco's medium (Thermo Fisher Scientific) and GM12878, MM.1S, and MOLM-14 cell lines were cultured in RPMI-1640/10% fetal bovine serum (FBS; Invitrogen, Carlsbad, CA, USA) at 37 °C in 5% CO_2. MOLM-14 and OCI-LY7 cells were purchased from the DSMZ (Deutsche Sammlung von Mikroorganismen und Zellkulturen, Braunschweig,

Germany), and GM12878, K562, MM.1S, and MV-4-11 cells were purchased from ATCC (American Type Culture Collection).

Co-transfection and cell viability assay

siRNAs of DOT1L were purchased from Thermo Fisher Scientific Silencer® Select siRNAs. For transfection of siRNA oligos, cells were seeded in six-cell plates with Lipofectamine® RNAiMAX Transfection Reagent for 48 h.

The Cell Counting Kit-8 method was used to measure cell viability. Cells were seeded in 96-well plates at a density of 3×10^3 cells/ml. The viability of cells was assessed using the CCK8 reagent (Dojindo Laboratories, Japan) according to the manufacturer's protocols. The absorbance at 450 nm was recorded on a microplate reader.

RT-PCR and ChIP-qPCR

Total RNAs from cells were extracted using Quick-RNA™ MiniPrep kit (Zymo Research). Then cDNA was prepared using a RevertAid H Minus First Strand cDNA Synthesis Kit (Thermo Fisher Scientific). The PCR primers for amplifying cDNA fragments between the upstream exon and downstream exon of five exon-skipping event sites are described in Additional file 1: Table S2. PCR was performed with NEBNext® High-Fidelity 2X PCR Master Mix (New England Biolabs, UK), and the cycling conditions were 98 °C for 1 min, then 30 cycles of 98 °C for 10 s, 58 °C for 20 s, 72 °C for 30 s. PCR products were visualized on 3% agarose gels.

ChIP-qPCR was performed as described in Zhu et al. [49]. Briefly, crosslinking was performed with 1% formalin and the cells were lysed in SDS buffer. DNA was fragmented by sonication with a Covaris S220. Chromatin immunoprecipitation (ChIP) was performed using an antibody to the H3K79me2 modification (Abcam, ab3594). Quantification of ChIP-DNA analysis was performed with the LightCycler® 480 SYBR Green I Masteron and LightCycler® 480 System Sequence Detection System (Roche Applied Science) using GAPDH for normalization with primers listed in Additional file 1: Table S3.

Results

Identification of the AS events across 34 normal and cancer cell types

We obtained both RNA-seq and H3K79me2 ChIP-seq data for a total of 34 different cell types with 18 normal and 16 cancer cell types from the GEO repository and EN-CODE Consortia (Additional file 1: Table S1). Using the MISO tool and an annotated AS database [46], we first identified exon junction reads, calculated the ψ-value (Psi, percent splice in) for the number of reads aligned to splice junctions vs target exons (Additional file 2: Figure S1), and finally determined the specific predominant isoform for each of five major types of AS events: SE, MXE, RI,

A5SS, A3SS (Fig. 1a). As demonstrated in Fig. 1b for the ψ-value distribution, ψ-value ≤ 0.2 was used to determine the predominant splicing isoform for SE and A3SS, but ψ-value ≥ 0.8 was used for RI and A5SS; however, either ψ-value was used for MXE. Consequently, we identified a total of 41,840 SE, 5228 MXE, 3909 RI, 7386 A3SS, and 7303 A5SS events for all 34 cell types (Fig. 1c), with SE clearly the major splicing event. We applied unsupervised clustering on all AS events to illustrate the difference among samples. Among the three types of cell clusters, most normal cell types, such as fibroblast, myotube, GM12878, and others, showed distinct AS event patterns compared with cancer or blood cancer cell types (Fig. 1d). The numbers of identified AS events were quite diverse in terms of genomic locations and among different cell types, 330–3035 for SE, 0–290 for MXE, 0–249 for RI, 112–301 for A5SS, and 0–345 for A3SS events, respectively (Additional file 2: Figure S2 and Additional file 1: Table S4).

Characterization of H3K79me2 enrichment around splice sites

Our previous data integration revealed strong enrichment of H3K79me2 at exon skipping sites in GM12878 and K562 cells [20]. To extend this observation, we set out to comprehensively characterize H3K79me2 enrichment with each of the five types of AS events. We first examined the average H3K79me2 enrichment for each AS event for the combined set of all 34 cell types. We were particularly interested in understanding the enrichment at the alternative and junction sites of four discrete genomic regions, including 50 bp around the 5′-end of the splice site, 50 bp around the 3′-end of the splice site, 50 bp around the 3′-end of the upstream exon, and 50 bp around the 5′-end of the downstream exon. We also selected a set of non-AS sites randomly from exons and genes without any AS events as a control. Interestingly, we found only two AS event types, SE and A3SS, were highly enriched with H3K79me2 in comparison to non-splice sites (Fig. 2a). For SE, skipping and junction sites exhibited 118 and 64% higher levels of H3K79me2, respectively, than these random non-skipping sites, and for A3SS, alternative 3′ splice sites and the 3′-end of the upstream exon showed dramatic 187 and 367% increases in enrichment, respectively, but only a 21.5% increase for the 5′-end of the downstream exon. We noted that we did not observe any enrichment of H3K79me2 in the other three splicing events (Additional file 2: Figure S3). A close examination of the distribution of H3K79me2 at SE sites showed a diversity of its enrichment levels in each individual cell type (Additional file 2: Figure S4). Further, we identified 33,765 (80.7%) of 41,840 SE sites with higher H3K79me2 enrichment, 10.3% with no significant difference, and 9.0% with decreased enrichment

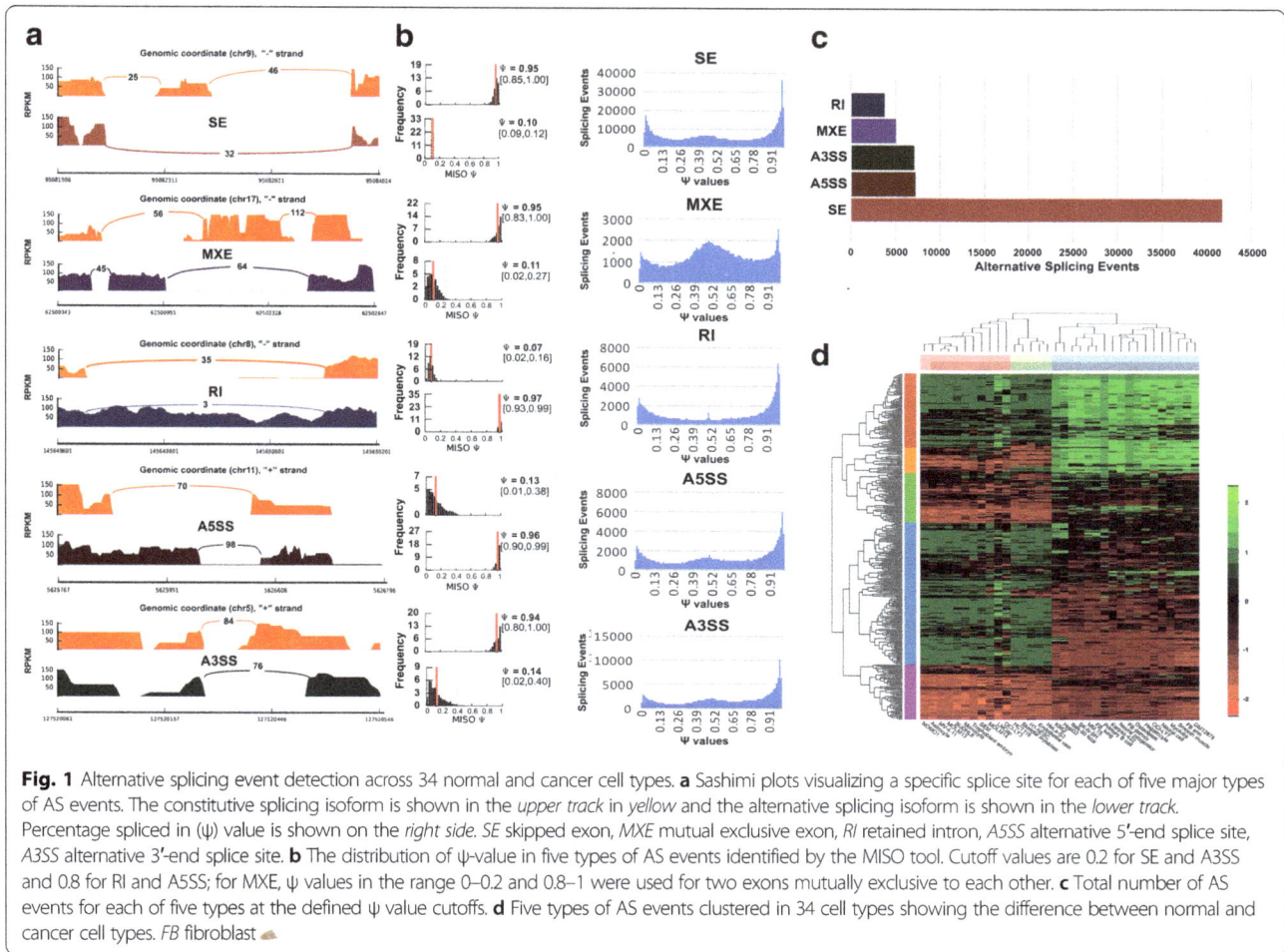

Fig. 1 Alternative splicing event detection across 34 normal and cancer cell types. **a** Sashimi plots visualizing a specific splice site for each of five major types of AS events. The constitutive splicing isoform is shown in the *upper track* in *yellow* and the alternative splicing isoform is shown in the *lower track*. Percentage spliced in (ψ) value is shown on the *right side*. *SE* skipped exon, *MXE* mutal exclusive exon, *RI* retained intron, *A5SS* alternative 5'-end splice site, *A3SS* alternative 3'-end splice site. **b** The distribution of ψ-value in five types of AS events identified by the MISO tool. Cutoff values are 0.2 for SE and A3SS and 0.8 for RI and A5SS; for MXE, ψ values in the range 0–0.2 and 0.8–1 were used for two exons mutually exclusive to each other. **c** Total number of AS events for each of five types at the defined ψ value cutoffs. **d** Five types of AS events clustered in 34 cell types showing the difference between normal and cancer cell types. *FB* fibroblast

relative to the average H3K79me2 enrichment at non-ES sites. Remarkably, 35.2% of these have an enriched H3K79me2 peak called by MACS2. For A3SS, the numbers were 56.7% (4141 of 7303), 33.0%, and 10.3% with higher, the same, and lower levels of H3K79me2 enrichment compared to non-A3SS sites (Fig. 2b and Additional file 2: Figure S3). We further looked into the AS events with H3K79me2 peaks around the skipped exons and A3SS event start sites. The density plot of the raw read enrichment for each event by z-score normalization within a range of 200 bp upstream and 400 bp downstream showed clear H3K79me2 enrichment around exon junction sites toward the skipped exon in SE events and higher H3K79me2 enrichment around the A3SS event start sites (Fig. 2c). We visually illustrate two examples of RNA-seq and H3K79me2 ChIP-seq data in Fig. 2d, a specific SE event in the ZNF512 gene in GM12878 cells vs non-SE in primary B cells and a A3SS event in the MATR3 gene in skeletal muscle myoblast cells vs non-A3SS in arm fibroblast cells.

SOM clustering for SE sites across 34 different cell types

Since SE is the predominant splicing event and is highly enriched for the H3K79me2 mark, we sought to further characterize the genes or transcripts associated with SE sites to dissect their relationship with cancer cell type specificity. We ranked cell type by H3K79me2 enrichment/kb (see the definition in "Methods") based on the H3K79me2 enrichment level for a total of 7017 genes associated with ES sites in all 34 cell types. Interestingly, we found that two blood cancer cell lines, MV-4-11 and OCI-LY3, have the highest levels. We then performed SOM clustering on the data with at least 100 iterations and obtained optimized parameters that enabled the assignment of all genes into a 40×25 hexagon matrix and definition of six clusters, A to F (Fig. 3a and Additional file 2: Figure S5). Each of the 34 cell types was able to be assigned into one of the six clusters. We strikingly identified two clusters, A and F, which consisted predominately of cell lines derived from hematological malignancies: cluster A included AML lines MOLM14, MV-4-11, NOMO1, and OCI-LY3 and the chronic

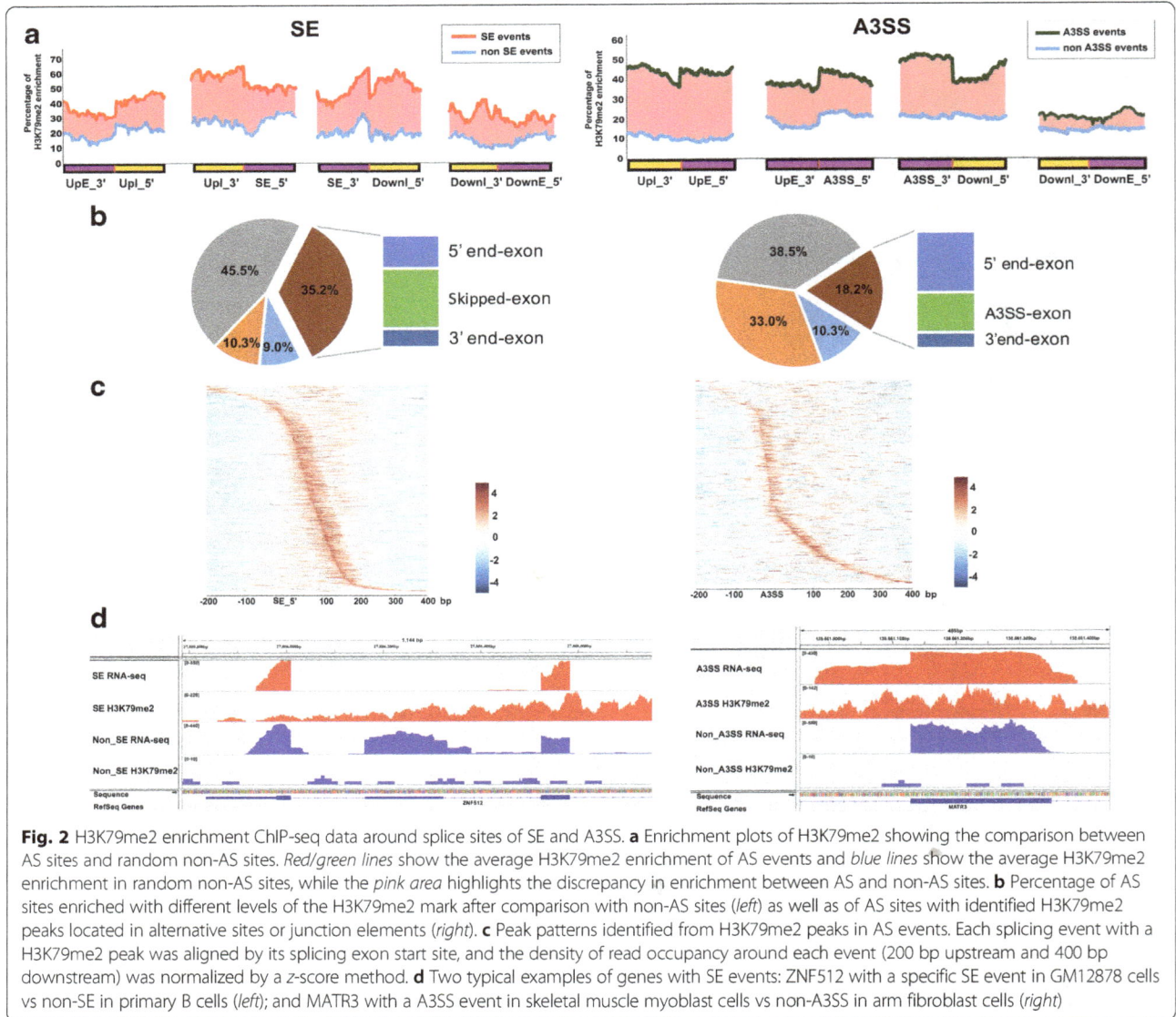

Fig. 2 H3K79me2 enrichment ChIP-seq data around splice sites of SE and A3SS. **a** Enrichment plots of H3K79me2 showing the comparison between AS sites and random non-AS sites. *Red/green lines* show the average H3K79me2 enrichment of AS events and *blue lines* show the average H3K79me2 enrichment in random non-AS sites, while the *pink area* highlights the discrepancy in enrichment between AS and non-AS sites. **b** Percentage of AS sites enriched with different levels of the H3K79me2 mark after comparison with non-AS sites (*left*) as well as of AS sites with identified H3K79me2 peaks located in alternative sites or junction elements (*right*). **c** Peak patterns identified from H3K79me2 peaks in AS events. Each splicing event with a H3K79me2 peak was aligned by its splicing exon start site, and the density of read occupancy around each event (200 bp upstream and 400 bp downstream) was normalized by a *z*-score method. **d** Two typical examples of genes with SE events: ZNF512 with a specific SE event in GM12878 cells vs non-SE in primary B cells (*left*); and MATR3 with a A3SS event in skeletal muscle myoblast cells vs non-A3SS in arm fibroblast cells (*right*)

myeloid leukemia (CML) line K562; and cluster F included the B-cell non-Hodgkin lymphoma line Karpas-422, multiple myeloma line MM.1S, diffuse large B-cell lymphoma line OCI-LY7, acute lymphoblastic leukemia line SEM, and lymphoblastoid line GM12878 (Fig. 3b). We also found that clusters C and D were mainly composed of various normal cell types. Further, we examined the enrichment of H3K79me2 between SE sites and non-SE sites in each of the six clusters. Remarkably, we found cluster A had the most significant enrichment difference (1.792 log2 fold change, *p* value < 0.001) and cluster F the second-most (1.671 log2 fold change and *p* value < 0.01) (Fig. 3c and Additional file 2: Figure S6). Our results clearly demonstrate that H3K79me2 enrichment within splice sites was highly correlated with blood cell types, especially for AML and B-cell lymphoma. In particular, we noticed that

the cell types in cluster A are mainly MLL-r cell types (MOLM14 and NOMO1 are MLL-AF9 and MV-4-11 is MLL-AF4). However, only SEM in cluster F is of the MLL-r cell type. Interestingly, several recent studies have demonstrated the functional role of DOT1L in the development and progression in MLL-r type leukemia [39, 50]. Together, our data reveal the potential regulatory or functional contribution of epigenetic-mediated splicing events to progression of this particular disease.

Gene expression, Gene Ontology, and motif analyses of SE-associated genes

To further examine the expression level of transcripts associated with SE sites, we compared transcripts associated with SE sites with a random set of non-SE genes in each of six clusters and didn't observe any significant

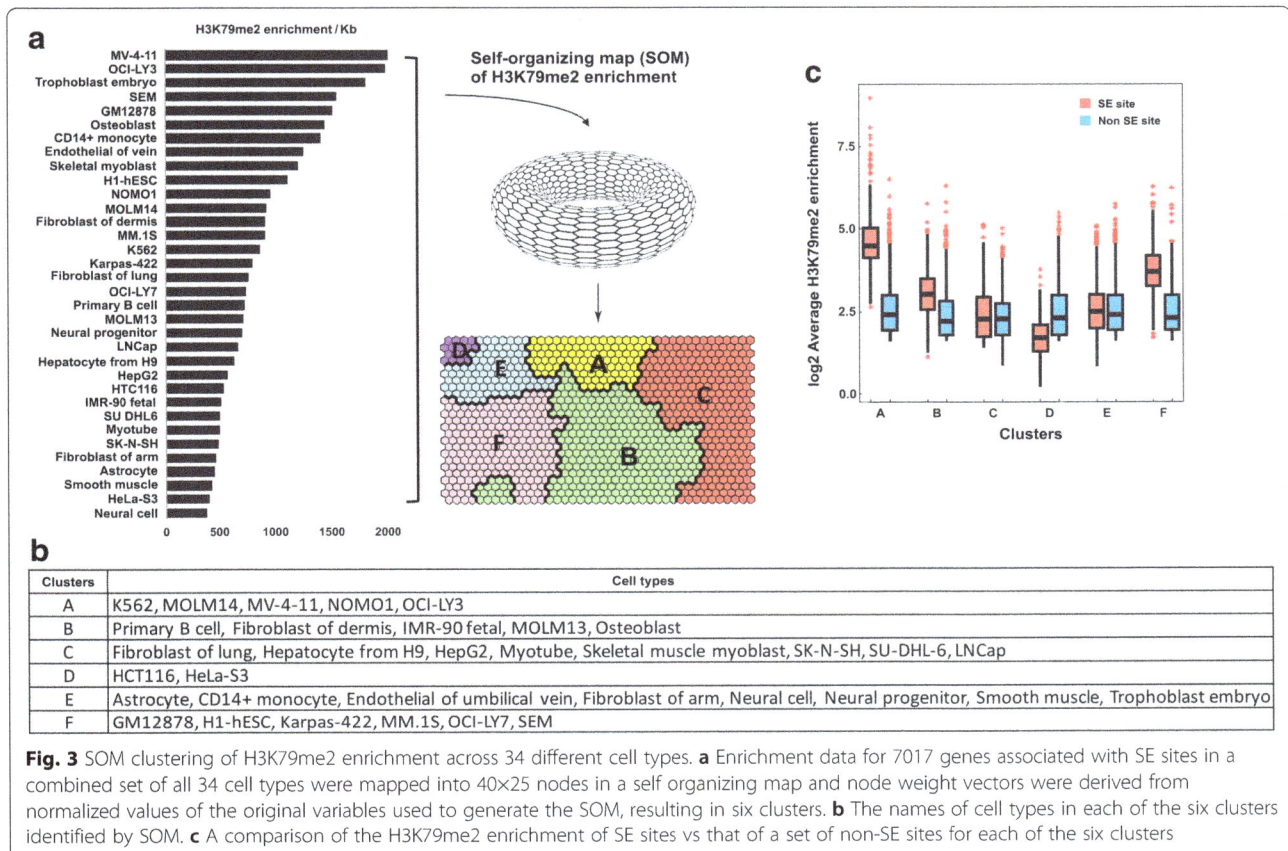

Fig. 3 SOM clustering of H3K79me2 enrichment across 34 different cell types. **a** Enrichment data for 7017 genes associated with SE sites in a combined set of all 34 cell types were mapped into 40×25 nodes in a self organizing map and node weight vectors were derived from normalized values of the original variables used to generate the SOM, resulting in six clusters. **b** The names of cell types in each of the six clusters identified by SOM. **c** A comparison of the H3K79me2 enrichment of SE sites vs that of a set of non-SE sites for each of the six clusters

difference between any two sets in any of the six clusters (Fig. 4a). This result is not so surprising given SE sites' known role in the precursor mRNA (pre-mRNA) regulatory stage as opposed to full mRNA translation [51]. However, it does indicate that the involvement of H3K79me2 in splicing might not impact full mRNA expression. Furthermore, we carried out Gene Ontology (GO) term enrichment analysis using EnrichR [52, 53]. We found that genes in clusters A and F were involved in mRNA splicing via spliceosome with a p value < 0.001, as were genes in cluster B (p value 0.026). However, genes in clusters C, D, and E were not associated with any splicing events (Additional file 2: Figure S7). To further examine the pathway analysis, we overlaid 912 SE genes in cluster A and 726 in cluster F and compared these with a public data set of 114 MLL-r target genes enriched with H3K79me2 [54]. Consequently, we identified 767 unique SE genes in cluster A, 583 in cluster F, and 139 overlapping between clusters A and F, as well as 24 genes common to all three data sets (Fig. 4b). We then carried out KEGG pathway analysis for the unique and overlapping genes in clusters A and F. Interestingly, cancer pathways, transcriptional misregulation, spliceosome, AML, and CML were among the top significantly enriched (p value < 0.01) pathways in the overlapping genes between clusters A and F (Fig. 4c).

The *trans*-acting RNA-binding proteins, often called splicing factors (SFs), play central roles in promoting or suppressing the use of a particular splice site. Thus, we searched for SF or RBP motifs in the sequences spanning skipping sites, 50 bp extending into the exon and intron, using the RBPmaptool, a tool designed to map SF binding sites in human genomic regions using the COS(WR) algorithm [55]. We compared the frequency of predicted SF motifs (SFMs) in the four defined genomic regions immediately adjacent to skipping sites versus non-skipping locations. As shown in Fig. 4d, for the common genes in clusters A and F, the top 30 highly enriched SFMs showed a strong tendency towards being within 50 bp of a skipping exon start site, which are highly involved in the exon junction process. In contrast, for the unique genes identified in clusters A or F, the top enriched SFMs were towards the end of the skipped exon. Interestingly, we found that two enriched motifs, SRSF2 and U2AF2, were previously reported to be highly involved in AML progression through aberrant splicing regulation [56] and another motif, PTBP1, was shown to play an important role in breast and colorectal cancers [57, 58]. Taken together, our in silico analyses unveil a potential mechanistic or functional link between H3K79me2-mediated skipping exon processing, splicing factors, and disease progression.

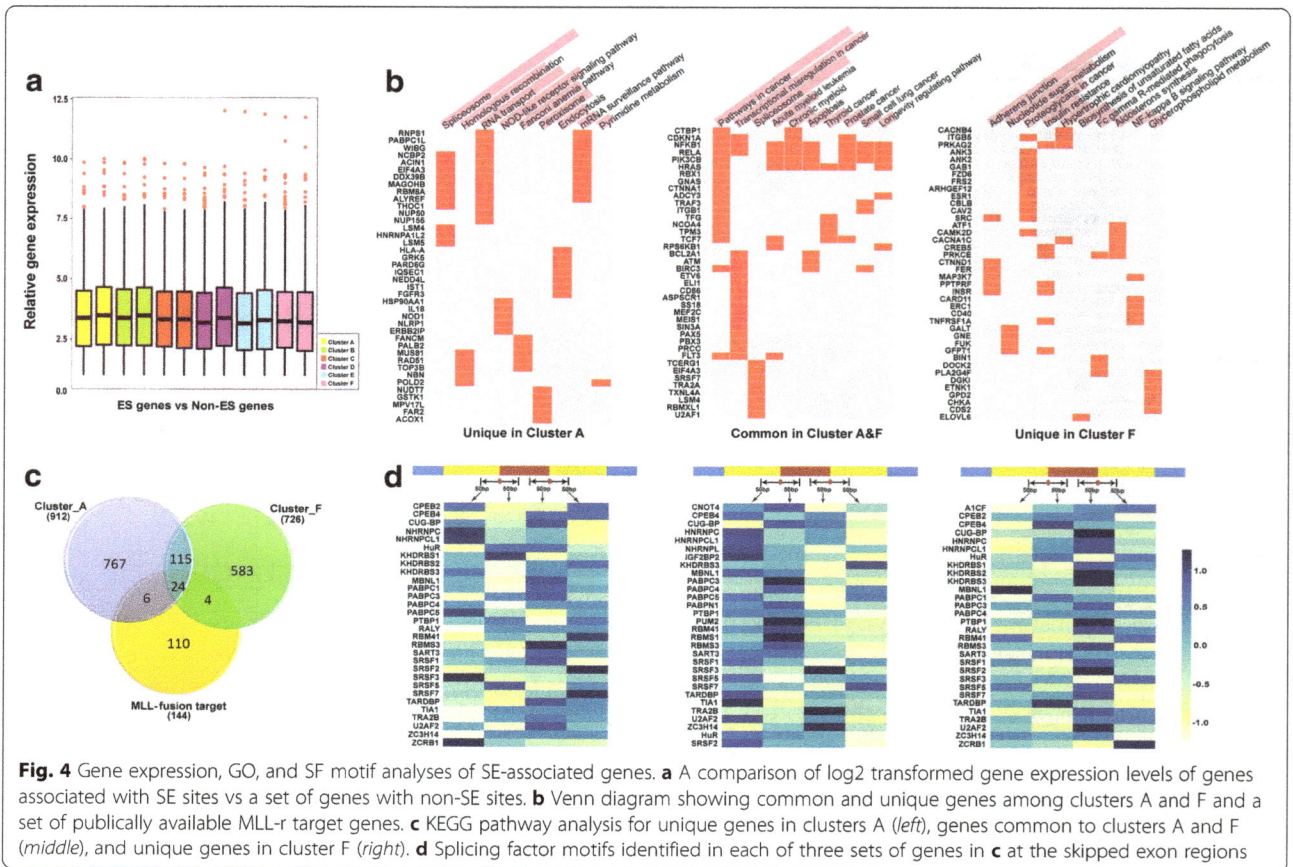

Fig. 4 Gene expression, GO, and SF motif analyses of SE-associated genes. **a** A comparison of log2 transformed gene expression levels of genes associated with SE sites vs a set of genes with non-SE sites. **b** Venn diagram showing common and unique genes among clusters A and F and a set of publically available MLL-r target genes. **c** KEGG pathway analysis for unique genes in clusters A (*left*), genes common to clusters A and F (*middle*), and unique genes in cluster F (*right*). **d** Splicing factor motifs identified in each of three sets of genes in **c** at the skipped exon regions

Functional characterization of DOT1L-mediated SE in MLL-r AML cells

Recent studies have demonstrated that knockdown of DOT1L effectively reduced the H3K79 methylation level in AML cell lines [29, 59] and impeded leukemia cell proliferation [60]. Since DOT1L is the sole K79me methyltransferase, we reasoned that DOT1L is the major regulator in mediating SE in MLL-r AML progression. To functionally characterize the role of H3K79me2 or DOT1L in mediating SE sites in AML, we conducted several functional assays in two selected MLL-r AML cell lines, MV-4-11 (MLL-AF4) and MOLM14 (MLL-AF9), and a lymphoblastoid cell line, GM12878. DOT1L knockdown by siDOT1L clearly reduced the DOT1L protein level in all three cell lines (Fig. 5a) as well as in another three cell lines, K562, MM.1S, and OCI-LY7 (Additional file 2: Figure S8). This depletion dramatically impeded proliferation in both AML cell lines ($P < 0.05$ vs control, one-way ANOVA), but not in GM12878 cells ($P > 0.05$) (Fig. 5b and Additional file 2: Figure S9). We further tested if this depletion of DOT1L would decrease the enrichment level of H3K79me2. To do this, we selected five genes with exon skipping events, MAGOHB, CTBP1, MEIS1, RELA, and THOC1, from the

overlapped genes between clusters A and F and unique genes in cluster A. Indeed, the enrichment of H3K79me2 level at ~ 100 bp around the SE start site was decreased at all five sites in three cell lines after DOT1L knockdown (Fig. 5c). These five genes showed SE events in MOLM14, MV-4-11, K562, MM.1S, and GM12878 cell lines but not in the OCI-LY7 cell line. Strikingly, we found that the exon skipped sites were able to switch to exon inclusion in both DOT1L knockdown AML cell lines, suggesting H3K79me2 is involved in the exon skipping process (Fig. 5d and Additional file 2: Figure S10). Although MEIS1 was previously shown to drive MLL-r leukemogenesis through altering DOT1L activity and hypermethylation at H3K79 [39], our data further suggest that DOT1L-mediated splicing drives this leukemogenesis. In addition, we also validated our assertion by re-analyzing public genome-wide datasets. Interestingly, we observed changes in exon usage from SE to non-SE after DOT1L treatment at three concentrations, 58 genes at 0.5 µM, 60 genes at 1 µM, and 73 genes at 2 µM, with an overlap of 14 genes for all treatments (Additional file 2: Figure S11) [59]. Collectively, our results support novel regulatory and functional roles of H3K79me2 in mediating AS.

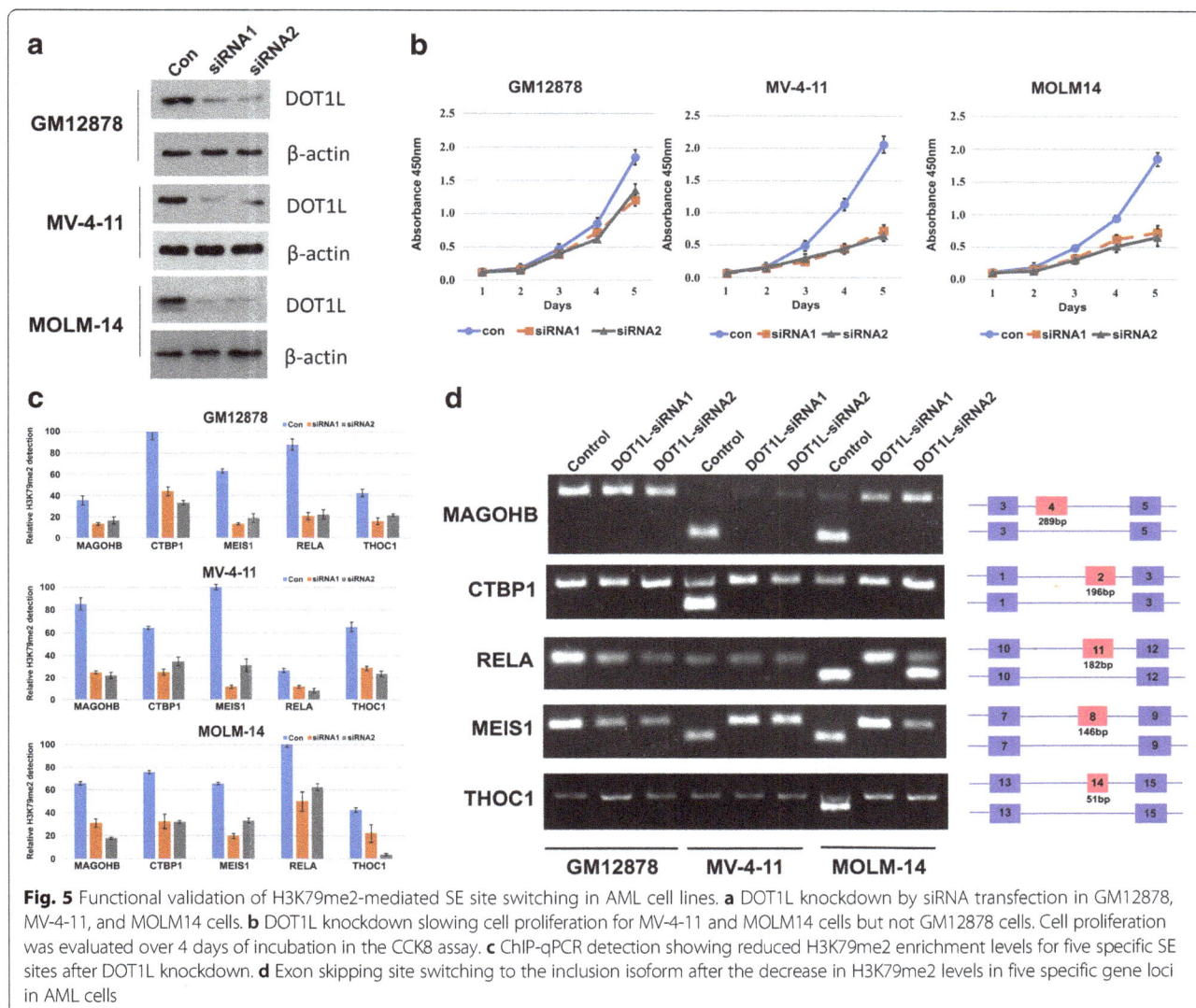

Fig. 5 Functional validation of H3K79me2-mediated SE site switching in AML cell lines. **a** DOT1L knockdown by siRNA transfection in GM12878, MV-4-11, and MOLM14 cells. **b** DOT1L knockdown slowing cell proliferation for MV-4-11 and MOLM14 cells but not GM12878 cells. Cell proliferation was evaluated over 4 days of incubation in the CCK8 assay. **c** ChIP-qPCR detection showing reduced H3K79me2 enrichment levels for five specific SE sites after DOT1L knockdown. **d** Exon skipping site switching to the inclusion isoform after the decrease in H3K79me2 levels in five specific gene loci in AML cells

Discussion

The current paradigm of pre-mRNA splicing centers on a post-transcriptional process mediated by the spliceosome machinery [61]. However, accumulating evidence suggests that AS is a co-transcriptional splicing process not only controlled by RNA-binding splicing factors, but also mediated by epigenetic regulators, such as chromatin structure, nucleosome density, and histone modification [62]. Many recent genome-wide studies, including ours, have revealed the regulatory roles of H3K36me3, H3K79me2, and nucleosome positioning in the RNA polymerase II elongation process and exon definition [18–20]. To further extend our previous study in which we observed a high enrichment of H3K79me2 at skipped exon sites in GM12878 and K562 cells, we conducted an integrative analysis of RNA-seq and H3K79me2 ChIP-seq data across 34 normal and cancer cell types. Intriguingly, we not only confirmed high enrichment of H3K79me2 in SE type splicing events, but also uncovered its enrichment in A3SS events (Fig. 2a). Further, a large proportion of SE sites are characterized by computationally defined H3K79me2 peaks (Fig. 2b), reflecting the high confidence of regulatory activity of H3K79me2 on the exon skipping process.

One novel finding in this study is the identification of six clusters of cell type-specific enrichment of H3K79me2 at skipping exons among 34 cell types. In particular, we discovered that a pattern of histone marks that promote exon skipping was a common feature in cell lines derived from hematological malignancies, in particular MLL-r AML cell types (Fig. 3b). Indeed, when closely examining this in each individual cell type, we observed a clear separation of enrichment of H3K79me2 in a majority of blood-related cell types (Additional file 2: Figure S3). Our data highlight the importance of H3K79me2 in AS events across different cell types, but most noticeably in blood cells. Previous studies showed that, for specific gene expression, inactivation of DOT1L led to the downregulation of direct MLL-AF9 targets and an MLL translocation-associated gene expression signature [59, 63]. However, in our study, due to a lack of data for DOT1L inhibition for all 34 cell types, we examined the expression level of transcripts associated with SE sites against a random set of non-SE genes in each cell type and did not observe any significant difference in gene expression between these two sets (Fig. 4a), indicating the correlation of H3K79me2 and SE may be independent of gene expression and such correlation might be through a co-transcriptional pre-RNA splicing mechanism. To our knowledge, this is the first comprehensive study to integrate all available matched RNA-seq and H3K79me2 ChIP-seq data in the same cell type. In a broader aspect, such an integrative strategy may provide a general approach for dissecting the relationship of other histone marks or epigenetic factors with the splicing process and further uncover their novel functionalities associated with various diseases or cancer types, providing a rationale to further explore the underlying mechanism for AML patients without mutations or independent of gene expression.

The gene enrichment and pathway analyses further revealed that H3K79me2-mediated exon skipping-associated genes were highly involved in acute or chronic myeloid leukemia cell types, underscoring their functional relevance to blood cancer progression. Indeed, the various functional assays in this study confirmed that such exon skipping events were highly coordinated by the H3K79me2 or DOT1L activities with DOT1L siRNA treatment in two MLL-r AML cell lines (Fig. 5), providing a new line of evidence of a co-transcriptional splicing process involved in AML. Other studies have shown that higher levels of H3K79me2 are associated with poorer prognosis in MLL-r leukemias [63], and the fusion of DOT1L and MLL partners, AF4, AF9, ENL, and AF10, leads to misregulation of DOT1L targets, resulting in aberrant H3K79me2 activity followed by leukemic transformation [64, 65]. However, our results further unveiled new regulatory and functional roles of H3K79me2 in determining transcript isoforms, providing a mechanistic link between H3K79me2 or DOT1L and splicing events in this particular disease progression.

Our findings may provide a new avenue and opportunity to develop novel combinatorial therapeutic drugs targeting both epigenetic mechanisms and splicing processes. EPZ-5676, a small-molecule inhibitor of DOT1L, is currently under clinical investigation for acute leukemias harboring rearrangements of the MLL gene. Although the agent effectively targets the DOT1L molecule in vitro, the results of a phase 1 clinical trial were disappointing due to low bioavailability and frequent adverse events [39]. In light of this finding, we may consider in future studies testing a co-treatment model which adds the inhibition of a splicing factor as a second synergistic agent, which may enhance efficacy for treating this deadly disease.

Conclusions

Our study identifies for the first time at a genome-wide scale cell type-specific correlation between H3K79me2 enrichment and skipped exons. This correlation is further utilized to classify the diverse cell types into six distinct clusters. Experimental assays confirm H3K79me2's functional and regulatory roles in AML disease progression. Our work provides more insights into underlying epigenetic regulatory mechanisms in the co-transcriptional AS process in normal or disease conditions.

Abbreviations

A3SS: Alternative 3′ splice site; A5SS: Alternative 5′-end splice site; AML: Acute myeloid leukemia; AS: Alternative splicing; DOT1L: DOT1-like histone lysine methyltransferase; MISO: Mixture of isoforms; MLL-r: MLL-rearranged; MXE: Mutually exclusive exon; RI: Retained intron; SE: Skipping exon; SFMs: Splicing factor motifs; SFs: Splicing factors; SOM: Self-organizing map

Acknowledgements

We are grateful to all members of the Jin laboratories for valuable discussion.

Funding

This study is partially supported by NIH R01GM114142 and U54CA217297, as well as Owens foundation. Funding for open access charge: NIH. The authors gratefully acknowledge financial support from Scholarship of Jilin University.

Authors' contributions

TL and VXJ conceived the project. TL and QL performed the computational analysis with help from NG and performed experiments. TL and VXJ wrote the manuscript with input from SK and all other authors. All authors read and approved the final manuscript.

Competing interests

The authors declare that they have no competing interests.

Author details

[1]College of Life Science, Jilin University, Changchun 130012, China. [2]Department of Molecular Medicine, University of Texas Health, 8403 Floyd Curl, San Antonio, TX 78229, USA. [3]Department of Biomedical Engineering, Johns Hopkins University, Baltimore, MD 21218, USA. [4]Department of Leukemia, UT MD Anderson Cancer Center, Houston, TX 77030, USA.

References

1. Pan Q, Shai O, Lee LJ, Frey BJ, Blencowe BJ. Deep surveying of alternative splicing complexity in the human transcriptome by high-throughput sequencing. Nat Genet. 2008;40(12):1413–5.
2. Nilsen TW, Graveley BR. Expansion of the eukaryotic proteome by alternative splicing. Nature. 2010;463(7280):457–63.
3. da Costa PJ MJ, Romão L. The role of alternative splicing coupled to nonsense-mediated mRNA decay in human disease. Int J Biochem Cell Biol. 2017;91(Pt B):168–75.
4. Liu J, Lee W, Jiang Z, Chen Z, Jhunjhunwala S, Haverty PM, et al. Genome and transcriptome sequencing of lung cancers reveal diverse mutational and splicing events. Genome Res. 2012;22(12):2315–27.
5. Santoro M, Masciullo M, Bonvissuto D, Bianchi ML, Michetti F, Silvestri G. Alternative splicing of human insulin receptor gene (INSR) in type I and type II skeletal muscle fibers of patients with myotonic dystrophy type 1 and type 2. Mol Cell Biochem. 2013;380(1-2):259–65.
6. Walter KR, Goodman ML, Singhal H, Hall JA, Li T, Holloran SM, et al. Interferon-Stimulated Genes Are Transcriptionally Repressed by PR in Breast Cancer. Mol Cancer Res. 2017;15(10):1331–40.
7. Roberts GC, Gooding C, Mak HY, Proudfoot NJ, Smith CW. Co-transcriptional commitment to alternative splice site selection. Nucleic Acids Res. 1998; 26(24):5568–72.
8. Listerman I, Sapra AK, Neugebauer KM. Cotranscriptional coupling of splicing factor recruitment and precursor messenger RNA splicing in mammalian cells. Nat Struct Mol Biol. 2006;13(9):815–22.
9. Luco RF, Allo M, Schor IE, Kornblihtt AR, Misteli T. Epigenetics in alternative pre-mRNA splicing. Cell. 2011;144(1):16–26.
10. Trincado JL, Sebestyén E, Pagés A, Eyras E. The prognostic potential of alternative transcript isoforms across human tumors. Genome Med. 2016;8(1):85.
11. Agirre E, Bellora N, Alló M, Pagès A, Bertucci P, Kornblihtt AR, et al. A chromatin code for alternative splicing involving a putative association between CTCF and HP1α proteins. BMC Biol. 2015;13:31.
12. Zhu L, Wang X, Li XL, Towers A, Cao X, Wang P, et al. Epigenetic dysregulation of SHANK3 in brain tissues from individuals with autism spectrum disorders. Hum Mol Genet. 2014;23(6):1563–78.
13. Verma A, Jiang Y, Du W, Fairchild L, Melnick A, Elemento O. Transcriptome sequencing reveals thousands of novel long non-coding RNAs in B cell lymphoma. Genome Med. 2015;7:110.
14. Li T, Xu X, Li J, Xing S, Zhang L, Li W, et al. Association of ACP1 gene polymorphisms and coronary artery disease in northeast Chinese population. J Genet. 2015;94(1):125–8.
15. Ntziachristos P, Abdel-Wahab O, Aifantis I. Emerging concepts of epigenetic dysregulation in hematological malignancies. Nat Immunol. 2016;17(9):1016–24.
16. Yuan H, Li N, Fu D, Ren J, Hui J, Peng J, et al. Histone methyltransferase SETD2 modulates alternative splicing to inhibit intestinal tumorigenesis. J Clin Invest. 2017;127(9):3375–91.
17. Kolasinska-Zwierz P, Down T, Latorre I, Liu T, Liu XS, Ahringer J. Differential chromatin marking of introns and expressed exons by H3K36me3. Nat Genet. 2009;41(3):376–81.
18. Andersson R, Enroth S, Rada-Iglesias A, Wadelius C, Komorowski J. Nucleosomes are well positioned in exons and carry characteristic histone modifications. Genome Res. 2009;19(10):1732–41.
19. Sveen A, Agesen TH, Nesbakken A, Rognum TO, Lothe RA, Skotheim RI. Transcriptome instability in colorectal cancer identified by exon microarray analyses: Associations with splicing factor expression levels and patient survival. Genome Med. 2011;3(5):32.
20. Ye Z, Chen Z, Lan X, Hara S, Sunkel B, Huang TH, et al. Computational analysis reveals a correlation of exon-skipping events with splicing, transcription and epigenetic factors. Nucleic Acids Res. 2014;42(5):2856–69.
21. Spies N, Nielsen CB, Padgett RA, Burge CB. Biased chromatin signatures around polyadenylation sites and exons. Mol Cell. 2009;36(2):245–54.
22. de Almeida SF, Grosso AR, Koch F, Fenouil R, Carvalho S, Andrade J, et al. Splicing enhances recruitment of methyltransferase HYPB/Setd2 and methylation of histone H3 Lys36. Nat Struct Mol Biol. 2011;18(9):977–83.
23. Zhang X, Zhao D, Xiong X, He Z, Li H. Multifaceted histone H3 methylation and phosphorylation readout by the plant homeodomain finger of human nuclear antigen Sp100C. J Biol Chem. 2016;291(24):12786–98.
24. Feng Q, Wang H, Ng HH, Erdjument-Bromage H, Tempst P, Struhl K, et al. Methylation of H3-lysine 79 is mediated by a new family of HMTases without a SET domain. Curr Biol. 2002;12(12):1052–8.
25. Steger DJ, Lefterova MI, Ying L, Stonestrom AJ, Schupp M, Zhuo D, et al. DOT1L/KMT4 recruitment and H3K79 methylation are ubiquitously coupled with gene transcription in mammalian cells. Mol Cell Biol. 2008;28(8):2825–39.
26. Wang Z, Zang C, Rosenfeld JA, Schones DE, Barski A, Cuddapah S, et al. Combinatorial patterns of histone acetylations and methylations in the human genome. Nat Genet. 2008;40(7):897–903.
27. Kimura A, Umehara T, Horikoshi M. Chromosomal gradient of histone acetylation established by Sas2p and Sir2p functions as a shield against gene silencing. Nat Genet. 2002;32(3):370–7.
28. Suka N, Luo K, Grunstein M. Sir2p and Sas2p opposingly regulate acetylation of yeast histone H4 lysine16 and spreading of heterochromatin. Nat Genet. 2002;32(3):378–83.
29. Kim W, Kim R, Park G, Park JW, Kim JE. Deficiency of H3K79 histone methyltransferase Dot1-like protein (DOT1L) inhibits cell proliferation. J Biol Chem. 2012;287(8):5588–99.
30. Huyen Y, Zgheib O, Ditullio RA, Gorgoulis VG, Zacharatos P, Petty TJ, et al. Methylated lysine 79 of histone H3 targets 53BP1 to DNA double-strand breaks. Nature. 2004;432(7015):406–11.
31. Wysocki R, Javaheri A, Allard S, Sha F, Côté J, Kron SJ. Role of Dot1-dependent histone H3 methylation in G1 and S phase DNA damage checkpoint functions of Rad9. Mol Cell Biol. 2005;25(19):8430–43.
32. Li J, Liu X, Chu H, Fu X, Li T, Hu L, et al. Specific dephosphorylation of Janus Kinase 2 by protein tyrosine phosphatases. Proteomics. 2015;15(1):68–76.
33. Zhou HL, Hinman MN, Barron VA, Geng C, Zhou G, Luo G, et al. Hu proteins regulate alternative splicing by inducing localized histone hyperacetylation in an RNA-dependent manner. Proc Natl Acad Sci U S A. 2011;108(36):E627–35.
34. Long L, Thelen JP, Furgason M, Haj-Yahya M, Brik A, Cheng D, et al. The U4/U6 recycling factor SART3 has histone chaperone activity and associates with USP15 to regulate H2B deubiquitination. J Biol Chem. 2014;289(13):8916–30.
35. Liu Q, Bonneville R, Li T, Jin VX. Transcription factor-associated combinatorial epigenetic pattern reveals higher transcriptional activity of TCF7L2-regulated intragenic enhancers. BMC Genomics. 2017;18(1):375.
36. Singh NN, Lawler MN, Ottesen EW, Upreti D, Kaczynski JR, Singh RN. An intronic structure enabled by a long-distance interaction serves as a novel target for splicing correction in spinal muscular atrophy. Nucleic Acids Res. 2013;41(17):8144–65.
37. Xu Y, Gan ES, Zhou J, Wee WY, Zhang X, Ito T. Arabidopsis MRG domain proteins bridge two histone modifications to elevate expression of flowering genes. Nucleic Acids Res. 2014;42(17):10960–74.
38. Nguyen AT, Zhang Y. The diverse functions of Dot1 and H3K79 methylation. Genes Dev. 2011;25(13):1345–58.
39. Daigle SR, Olhava EJ, Therkelsen CA, Basavapathruni A, Jin L, Boriack-Sjodin PA, et al. Potent inhibition of DOT1L as treatment of MLL-fusion leukemia. Blood. 2013;122(6):1017–25.
40. Deshpande AJ, Deshpande A, Sinha AU, Chen L, Chang J, Cihan A, et al. AF10 regulates progressive H3K79 methylation and HOX gene expression in diverse AML subtypes. Cancer Cell. 2014;26(6):896–908.
41. Ayton PM, Cleary ML. Molecular mechanisms of leukemogenesis mediated by MLL fusion proteins. Oncogene. 2001;20(40):5695–707.
42. Daser A, Rabbitts TH. Extending the repertoire of the mixed-lineage leukemia gene MLL in leukemogenesis. Genes Dev. 2004;18(9):965–74.
43. Krivtsov AV, Armstrong SA. MLL translocations, histone modifications and leukaemia stem-cell development. Nat Rev Cancer. 2007;7(11):823–33.
44. Langmead B, Salzberg SL. Fast gapped-read alignment with Bowtie 2. Nat Methods. 2012;9(4):357–9.
45. Kim D, Pertea G, Trapnell C, Pimentel H, Kelley R, Salzberg SL. TopHat2: accurate alignment of transcriptomes in the presence of insertions, deletions and gene fusions. Genome Biol. 2013;14(4):R36.
46. Katz Y, Wang ET, Airoldi EM, Burge CB. Analysis and design of RNA sequencing experiments for identifying isoform regulation. Nat Methods. 2010;7(12):1009–15.
47. Zhang Y, Liu T, Meyer CA, Eeckhoute J, Johnson DS, Bernstein BE, et al. Model-based analysis of ChIP-Seq (MACS). Genome Biol. 2008;9(9):R137.
48. Xie D, Boyle AP, Wu L, Zhai J, Kawli T, Snyder M. Dynamic trans-acting factor colocalization in human cells. Cell. 2013;155(3):713–24.
49. Zhu J, Sammons MA, Donahue G, Dou Z, Vedadi M, Getlik M, et al. Gain-of-function p53 mutants co-opt chromatin pathways to drive cancer growth. Nature. 2015;525(7568):206–11.

50. Chen CW, Koche RP, Sinha AU, Deshpande AJ, Zhu N, Eng R, et al. DOT1L inhibits SIRT1-mediated epigenetic silencing to maintain leukemic gene expression in MLL-rearranged leukemia. Nat Med. 2015;21(4):335–43.

51. Keren H, Lev-Maor G, Ast G. Alternative splicing and evolution: diversification, exon definition and function. Nat Rev Genet. 2010;11(5):345–55.

52. Chen EY, Tan CM, Kou Y, Duan Q, Wang Z, Meirelles GV, et al. Enrichr: interactive and collaborative HTML5 gene list enrichment analysis tool. BMC Bioinformatics. 2013;14:128.

53. Kuleshov MV, Jones MR, Rouillard AD, Fernandez NF, Duan Q, Wang Z, et al. Enrichr: a comprehensive gene set enrichment analysis web server 2016 update. Nucleic Acids Res. 2016;44(W1):W90–7.

54. Wang QF, Wu G, Mi S, He F, Wu J, Dong J, et al. MLL fusion proteins preferentially regulate a subset of wild-type MLL target genes in the leukemic genome. Blood. 2011;117(25):6895–905.

55. Paz I, Kosti I, Ares M, Cline M, Mandel-Gutfreund Y. RBPmap: a web server for mapping binding sites of RNA-binding proteins. Nucleic Acids Res. 2014; 42(Web Server issue):W361–7.

56. Landau DA, Wu CJ. Chronic lymphocytic leukemia: molecular heterogeneity revealed by high-throughput genomics. Genome Med. 2013;5(5):47.

57. He X, Arslan AD, Ho TT, Yuan C, Stampfer MR, Beck WT. Involvement of polypyrimidine tract-binding protein (PTBP1) in maintaining breast cancer cell growth and malignant properties. Oncogene. 2014;3:e84.

58. Takahashi H, Nishimura J, Kagawa Y, Kano Y, Takahashi Y, Wu X, et al. Significance of polypyrimidine tract-binding protein 1 expression in colorectal cancer. Mol Cancer Ther. 2015;14(7):1705–16.

59. Kerry J, Godfrey L, Repapi E, Tapia M, Blackledge NP, Ma H, et al. MLL-AF4 spreading identifies binding sites that are distinct from super-enhancers and that govern sensitivity to DOT1L inhibition in leukemia. Cell Rep. 2017; 18(2):482–95.

60. Riedel SS, Haladyna JN, Bezzant M, Stevens B, Pollyea DA, Sinha AU, et al. MLL1 and DOT1L cooperate with meningioma-1 to induce acute myeloid leukemia. J Clin Invest. 2016;126(4):1438–50.

61. Ilagan JO, Ramakrishnan A, Hayes B, Murphy ME, Zebari AS, Bradley P, et al. U2AF1 mutations alter splice site recognition in hematological malignancies. Genome Res. 2015;25(1):14–26.

62. Braunschweig U, Barbosa-Morais NL, Pan Q, Nachman EN, Alipanahi B, Gonatopoulos-Pournatzis T, et al. Widespread intron retention in mammals functionally tunes transcriptomes. Genome Res. 2014;24(11):1774–86.

63. Bernt KM, Zhu N, Sinha AU, Vempati S, Faber J, Krivtsov AV, et al. MLL-rearranged leukemia is dependent on aberrant H3K79 methylation by DOT1L. Cancer Cell. 2011;20(1):66–78.

64. Mueller D, Bach C, Zeisig D, Garcia-Cuellar MP, Monroe S, Sreekumar A, et al. A role for the MLL fusion partner ENL in transcriptional elongation and chromatin modification. Blood. 2007;110(13):4445–54.

65. Mohan M, Herz HM, Takahashi YH, Lin C, Lai KC, Zhang Y, et al. Linking H3K79 trimethylation to Wnt signaling through a novel Dot1-containing complex (DotCom). Genes Dev. 2010;24(6):574–89.

11

BALDR: a computational pipeline for paired heavy and light chain immunoglobulin reconstruction in single-cell RNA-seq data

Amit A. Upadhyay[1], Robert C. Kauffman[2], Amber N. Wolabaugh[1], Alice Cho[2], Nirav B. Patel[3], Samantha M. Reiss[4,5], Colin Havenar-Daughton[4,5], Reem A. Dawoud[1], Gregory K. Tharp[3], Iñaki Sanz[2,6], Bali Pulendran[7,8,9], Shane Crotty[4,5,10], F. Eun-Hyung Lee[2,11], Jens Wrammert[2] and Steven E. Bosinger[1,3,12]*

Abstract

B cells play a critical role in the immune response by producing antibodies, which display remarkable diversity. Here we describe a bioinformatic pipeline, *BALDR* (**B**CR **A**ssignment of **L**ineage using *De novo* **R**econstruction) that accurately reconstructs the paired heavy and light chain immunoglobulin gene sequences from Illumina single-cell RNA-seq data. BALDR was accurate for clonotype identification in human and rhesus macaque influenza vaccine and simian immunodeficiency virus vaccine induced vaccine-induced plasmablasts and naïve and antigen-specific memory B cells. BALDR enables matching of clonotype identity with single-cell transcriptional information in B cell lineages and will have broad application in the fields of vaccines, human immunodeficiency virus broadly neutralizing antibody development, and cancer.

Background

B cells comprise a major component of the immune system, and they function primarily by secreting antibodies that bind and neutralize discrete protein moieties on pathogens. Antibodies, also referred to as immunoglobulins (Ig) or B cell antigen receptors (BCRs), are produced by the paired expression of a "heavy chain" (IgH) immunoglobulin gene and a "light chain" (IgL) immunoglobulin gene. The unique combination of heavy and light chain genes defines the immunological activity of a B cell and also its identity, also referred to as its clonotype. In order to deal with the near infinite array of pathogenic structures that may face the immune system, B cells exhibit an incredible level of clonotypic diversity, principally achieved by recombination at the DNA level of multiple gene segments, referred to as V (variable), D (diversity), and J (joining) segments for heavy chains, and V and J segments for light chains [1]. With approximately 38–46 V, 23 J, and 6 D functional gene

segments for the heavy chains and 63–71 V and 9–10 J light chain gene segments in the human genome [2, 3], the number of possible clonotypic variants is estimated to be approximately 10^{14} [4]. Given the functional importance of clonotypic diversity to immune function, the ability to investigate transcriptional information at the clonotype level would provide valuable insight into the regulatory mechanisms that regulate antibody breadth, evolution of the B cell immune repertoires, and other immunological determinants of B cell immunity.

The advent of next generation sequencing (NGS) technology has spurred the development of several tools to broadly sequence antigen receptor genes in B lymphocytes [5–7]. The earliest tools used deep sequencing of the immunoglobulin heavy or light chains, by polymerase chain reaction (PCR) amplification of the variable region, followed by MiSeq-based sequencing of the resultant amplicon. While the achievable depth of these amplicon-based approaches provided remarkable resolution (10^5–10^6 chains in a single experiment) [8], a significant limitation of this technology for functional studies of the immune system is that it only sequences a single chain and cannot provide information on

* Correspondence: sbosing@emory.edu
[1]Division of Microbiology and Immunology, Yerkes National Primate Research Center, Atlanta, GA, USA
[3]Yerkes NHP Genomics Core Laboratory, Yerkes National Primate Research Center, 954 Gatewood Rd, Atlanta, GA 30329, USA
Full list of author information is available at the end of the article

endogenous pairing of IgH/IgL genes to definitively identify a B cell clonotype. Recently, a novel, ultra high-throughput method to identify millions of paired IgH + IgL genes was developed by Georgiou, DeKosky, and colleagues [9]. This method uses an upfront capture of individual B cells into droplets, after which an elegant in-drop PCR ligation strategy creates a single DNA amplicon containing both IgH and IgL chains for *en masse* Illumina sequencing [9]. Additionally, others have developed "medium-throughput" techniques to sequence the paired IgH and IgL repertoire; each involved single-cell sorting followed by multiplex PCR amplification in individual wells [10] or emulsions [11] yielding sequences of 1000–2000 IgH/IgL pairs. The ability to generate deep sequence data of IgH + IgL pairings constitutes a significant advance over single-chain profiling; however, it does not provide functional or transcriptional information.

Medium-scale methodologies to obtain paired T cell or B cell receptor clonotypes alongside shallow transcriptional data have recently emerged. Han, Davis, and colleagues reported the sequencing of paired T cell α/β chains along with 17 immune genes using a PCR-barcoding/MiSeq strategy in experiments that obtained data for ~150–300 cells [12]. Similarly, Robinson and colleagues developed a methodology for barcoding of PCR-amplified paired IgH and IgL chains from single cells that can be combined with the query of a limited set of co-expressed functional genes [13–15]. The common strategy in these techniques involved single-cell sorting into 96-well plates followed by PCR-based amplification of the paired antigen-specific receptors with a multiplex set of primers for V gene sequences and a finite set of additional genes of interest.

Recently, several groups have demonstrated that it is possible to reconstruct clonotype sequences of the paired α and β chains of T cells (TCRs) from single-cell RNA-seq data. Stubbington and Teichmann developed the TraCeR pipeline, which uses *de novo* assembly after a pre-filtering step against a custom database containing *in silico* combinations for all known human V and J gene segments/alleles in the International Immunogenetics Information System (IMGT) repository [16]. Another pipeline, VDJPuzzle [17], filters in reads by mapping to TCR genes followed by Trinity-based assembly; the total reads are then mapped back to the assemblies in order to retrieve reads missed in the initial mapping step, followed by another round of assembly with Trinity [18].

In this study, we demonstrate the utility of *de novo* assembly for the reconstruction of paired IgH and IgL of the B cell antigen receptor from single-cell RNA-seq data. We also report the development of *BALDR* (**B**CR **A**ssignment of **L**ineage using *De novo* **R**econstruction), an optimized bioinformatics pipeline that recovers BCR

sequences from single-cell RNA-seq data. The accuracy of paired IgH + IgL gene identification using the BALDR pipeline was validated using primary human plasmablasts obtained after seasonal influenza vaccination, and it had a clonotype identification accuracy rate of 98%. We generated a validation dataset containing 255 samples with matched NGS and reverse transcription (RT)-PCR IgH/IgL Sanger sequence data [19] and determined (1) the accuracy, recovery rate, and efficiency of four different bioinformatic immunoglobulin filtering strategies and (2) optimal sequencing parameters to minimize sequencing cost and computing time while preserving accuracy. Lastly, we applied BALDR to analyze several B lymphocyte subsets from rhesus macaques receiving novel vaccine formulations and demonstrated that, even in species with relatively poor annotation of the Ig loci, our pipeline faithfully recreates paired antibody sequences.

Methods

Single-cell isolation of human plasmablast and B cell subsets

Plasmablasts for single-cell RNA sequencing (sc-RNA-seq) were isolated by flow cytometric sorting from 20×10^6 freshly isolated peripheral blood mononuclear cells (PBMCs) 7 days after vaccination with the seasonal 2016–2017 quadrivalent Fluarix influenza vaccine (GlaxoSmithKline (GSK), Brentford, UK), as previously described [20]. Plasmablasts were defined as CD3– CD19+ CD27hi CD38hi CD20– lymphocytes; these markers have been previously validated to specifically phenotype human plasmablasts [20]. PBMCs were stained with the following titrated mAbs at the specified concentrations in a volume of 3.5 mL phosphate-buffered saline (PBS) with 2% fetal bovine serum (FBS): CD19-FITC (6:100; Cat# 340719 RRID:AB_400118; BD Biosciences, San Jose, CA, USA), CD3-PacificBlue (3:100; Cat# 558124 RRID:AB_397044, BD Biosciences), CD38-PE (3:100; Cat# 347687 RRID:AB_400341, BD Biosciences), CD20-PECy7 (1.5:100; Cat# 560735 RRID:AB_1727450, BD Biosciences), IgD-PECy7 (3:100; Cat# 561314 RRID:AB_10642457, BD Biosciences), and CD27-APC (3:100; Cat# 17–0271-82 RRID:AB_469370, Thermo Fisher Scientific). Plasmablasts were single-cell sorted into 96-well PCR plates (Bio-Rad, Waltham, MA, USA) containing 10 µL 10 mM Tris pH 8.0 hypotonic catch buffer supplemented with RNasin at 1 U/µL (Promega, Madison, WI, USA) using a FACSAria II instrument, and were frozen immediately on dry ice, as previously described [20]. In some cases, as described in the text, plasmablasts were sorted into 10 µL of RLT buffer (QIAGEN, Hilden, Germany). Sorted samples were stored at −80 °C for long-term storage. Conventional blood B cells were defined as

(CD3– CD19+ CD14– CD16–) and were sorted into 10 µL QIAGEN RLT buffer using a FACSAria II, and then immediately placed on dry ice prior to storage at –80 °C. The antibodies used for B cell staining were CD3-AlexaFluora700 (Cat# 557917 RRID:AB_396938, BD Biosciences), CD14-ECD (Cat# IM2707U RRID:AB_130853, Beckman Coulter, Pasadena, CA, USA), CD16-BrilliantViolet421 (Cat# 302037 RRID:AB_10898112, BioLegend, San Diego, CA, USA), and CD19-PC5.5 (Clone: 3–119, Cat# A66328, Beckman Coulter).

Enzyme-Linked ImmunoSpot (ELISPOT) assay

ELISPOT was performed to enumerate influenza-specific plasmablasts present in PBMC samples. We coated 96-well ELISPOT assay mixed cellulose ester filter plates (Millipore) overnight with either the 2016/2017 Fluarix quadrivalent influenza (GlaxoSmithKline) at 1:20 in PBS or polyvalent goat anti-human Ig (Jackson ImmunoResearch, West Grove, PA, USA) at 10 µg/mL in PBS. The plates were washed and blocked by incubation with R10 media (RPMI-1640 supplemented with 10% FBS, penicillin, streptomycin, and L-glutamine) at 37 °C for 2 h. Freshly isolated PBMCs were added to the plates in a dilution series starting at 5×10^5 cells and incubated overnight at 37 °C in R10 media. The plates were washed with PBS, followed by PBS/0.05% Tween, and then incubated with biotinylated anti-human IgG, IgA, or IgM antibody (Invitrogen) at room temperature for 90 min. After washing, the plates were incubated with avidin D-horseradish peroxidase conjugate (Vector Laboratories) and developed using 3-amino-9-ethylcarbazole substrate (Sigma-Aldrich). Plates were scanned and analyzed using an automated ELISPOT counter (Cellular Technology Limited (CTL)).

Single-cell isolation of rhesus macaque plasmablast and B cell subsets

Plasmablasts were obtained by single-cell sorting from a PBMC sample obtained from a rhesus macaque 4 days after vaccination with an experimental HIV vaccine as described in [21] using the flow cytometry panel described in [22]. Single antigen-specific B cells and germinal center B cells were obtained from rhesus macaques after immunization. Single peripheral blood antigen-specific memory B cells were obtained from cryopreserved PBMCs and stained with biotin-labeled antigen-specific probes, and were further defined as CD20+ and CD4–. Splenic germinal center B cells were obtained by single-cell sorting from a cryopreserved sample and were defined without an antigen-specific probe as live, CD20+ CD38– CD71+.

Single-cell RT-PCR amplification of immunoglobulin variable domain sequences

Single-cell sorted plasmablasts in 10 µL of hypotonic catch buffer (10 mM Tris pH 8.0, 1 U/uL RNasin (Promega)) were thawed on ice. We used 1 µL of well-mixed single-cell sorted cell lysate to generate complementary DNA (cDNA) using Sensiscript cDNA synthesis reagents (QIAGEN) according to the manufacturer's recommended reaction conditions. The remaining 9 µL of lysate was used to generate the RNA-seq library as described below. The 1 µL of cell lysate was added to 7.5 µL of reaction mixture containing water, gene-specific primers, and 0.85 µL of 10X reaction buffer. This reaction was incubated at 72 °C for 5 min, 50 °C for 1 min, and 4 °C for 30 s, and then immediately transferred to ice. Afterwards, the reaction was brought to a final volume of 10 µL by adding 1.5 µL of a reaction master mix containing deoxynucleotides (dNTPs), 2 units of Sensiscript RT, 4 units of RNasin (Promega), and 0.15 µL of 10X reaction buffer. The reaction mixtures were then incubated at 25 °C for 10 min, 37 °C for 1 h, and 95 °C for 5 min. cDNA was stored at –20 °C prior to PCR amplification. cDNA synthesis reactions were primed using a cocktail of oligonucleotides specific for the human IgG, IgA, and IgM heavy chain constant domains and the κ and λ light chain constant domains at a final concentration of 1 µM per primer. Constant domain-specific primers were the same as those used for first round PCR amplification. Ig heavy chain and light chain (κ/λ) variable domain sequences were subsequently amplified by nested PCR using chain-specific primer cocktails encompassing all variable (V) gene families and the constant domain. PCRs were performed as previously described [19] using 2 µL of cDNA template. PCR amplicons were purified using a PCR cleanup column (QIAGEN) and sequenced by Sanger sequencing (Eurofins, North Kingstown, RI, USA) as previously described [19].

The PCRs for rhesus macaque single cells were performed as previously described [22] using an amplified SMART-Seq messenger RNA (mRNA) library (1:10 diluted).

Single-cell RNA-seq

RNA-seq analysis was conducted at the Yerkes Nonhuman Primate Genomics Core Laboratory (http://www.yerkes.emory.edu/nhp_genomics_core). Single cells were sorted by flow cytometry into 10 µL of QIAGEN RLT buffer or hypotonic catch buffer as indicated in the text. RNA was purified using RNACleanXP Solid Phase Reversible Immobilization (SPRI) beads (Beckman Coulter). The beads with bound RNA were re-suspended in Clontech buffers for mRNA amplification using 5′ template switching PCR with the Clontech SMART-Seq v4 Ultra Low Input RNA kit according to the manufacturer's instructions. Amplified cDNA was fragmented and appended with dual-indexed barcodes using Illumina Nextera XT DNA Library Prep kits. Libraries were validated on an Agilent 4200

TapeStation, pooled, and sequenced on an Illumina HiSeq 3000. The sequencing conditions and read depth are indicated in Additional file 1: Table S1. For the VH dataset comprising human 36 CD19+ Lin− cells, the sequencing was carried out on an Illumina MiSeq. Out of the 36 B cells, 6 were sequenced using the Clontech SMART-Seq v4. The remaining 30 were sequenced with a modified protocol where instead of using the Clontech SMART-Seq v4 kit, the cDNA was synthesized using Clontech buffers and enzymes (SMARTer method), while the template switching oligos (TSOs) were ordered from Exiqon (Woburn, MA, USA) for full-length cDNA synthesis and the primers for cDNA synthesis were ordered from Integrated DNA Technologies (Skokie, IL, USA). The libraries for the human AW1 and the rhesus BL6.1 and BL6.2 datasets were sequenced on the Illumina HiSeq 3000 twice in order to obtain greater read depth. The combined sequences from both runs for each sample were pooled prior to analysis. For the VH dataset, PCR for Sanger sequencing was performed as described above using a 1:10 dilution of 1 μL of sequencing library after the SMART-Seq amplification stage, similar to methods described for single T cells [16].

BALDR pipeline for immunoglobulin reconstruction of human BCRs
Assembly
Adapter sequences were removed from fastq files using Trimmomatic-0.32 [23]. After trimming, the unfiltered or filtered reads were used as input for assembly with Trinity v2.3.2 [18] without normalization except where indicated.

Ig transcript filtering methods

IG_mapped and IG_mapped+Unmapped The reads were mapped to the human reference genome (Ensembl GRCh38 release 86 primary assembly [24]) using STAR v2.5.2b [25]. In order to avoid missing any Ig reads due to incomplete annotation, we chose to use the coordinates for the complete loci instead of individual genes. The coordinates for the Ig loci (IGH 14:105586437−106,879,844, IGK 2:88857361−90,235,368, IGL 22:22026076−22,922,913) were obtained from the National Center for Biotechnology Information (NCBI) Gene database. Reads mapping to these coordinates were extracted from the bam file using SAMtools 0.1.19 [26] and seqtk-1.2 (https://github.com/lh3/seqtk). The resultant reads that were enriched for Ig transcripts were then used for assembly with Trinity. In addition, the Unmapped reads that were obtained from STAR were combined with these IG_mapped reads for the IG_mapped+Unmapped method prior to assembly.

IMGT_mapped The human V, J, and C sequences (F + ORF+in-frame P) were obtained from the IMGT database

[3]. The V, J, and C sequences were combined into a single file separately for heavy and light chains. A bowtie index was created, and the reads mapping to the IMGT sequences were obtained using bowtie2−2.9 [27] (AW2) and bowtie2−2.3.0 (AW1 and VH samples) with the following parameters: -no-unal -k 1 −local.

Recombinome_mapped We designed an *in silico* database containing all possible combinations of V, J, and C sequences. This "Ig recombinome" was created using a design similar to that of a previous study detailing creation of a T cell receptor recombinome [16]. A database of all possible recombined sequences from human V, J, and C alleles obtained from IMGT was constructed. Twenty N bases were added in the beginning of the sequence for alignment with the leader sequence, and the D gene was replaced with 10 N bases. The resulting database comprised 250,250 IGH (350 V, 13 J, 55 C), 11,830 IGL (91 V, 10 J, 13 C), and 4860 IGK (108 V, 9 J, 5 C). A bowtie index was created for the heavy and light chain recombined sequences separately using bowtie2. The reads mapping to the recombined Ig sequences were obtained using bowtie2−2.9 (AW2) and bowtie2−2.3.0 (AW1 and VH samples) with the parameters −no-unal -k 1 −np 0 −rdg 1,1 −rfg 1,1.

Post-assembly and Ig transcript model selection
After assembly of unfiltered and filtered reads (IG_mapped, IG_mapped+Unmapped, IMGT_mapped, and Recombinome_mapped), IgBLAST v1.6.1 [28] was used for annotation of reconstructed Ig chains with the IMGT V, D, J, and C sequences as germline databases, the imgt domain system, and an e-value threshold of 0.001. The top hit was used for annotation of V, D, J, and C genes. In order to select the best model, reads used for assembly were mapped back to the reconstructed Ig sequence using bowtie2−2.3.0 (-no-unal −no-hd −no-discordant −gbar 1000 −end-to-end -a). The models were ranked according to the number of reads mapped. The models that were predicted as unproductive and models that had the same V(D)J gene annotations along with the CDR3 nucleotide sequence as a higher ranking model were filtered out. The top ranking Ig model was selected from the remaining set. The analysis was run on Amazon Web Services Elastic Compute Cloud (EC2) m4.16xlarge instances (Intel Xeon E5-2676 v3, 64 cores and 256 GB RAM) by running 8 simultaneous processes with 8 threads each.

Processing of Sanger sequences for the validation dataset
Sanger sequences obtained from RT-PCR were manually trimmed using Seqman Pro software in the DNASTAR Lasergene package v14.0.0.86 to remove low-quality reads at the ends. The trimmed reads were annotated with IgBLAST, and productive RT-PCR sequences were

selected for validation. The reconstructed Ig chains were aligned with the PCR sequences using ncbi blastn v2.6.0 [29]. Accuracy of reconstruction was determined by comparing the V(D)J gene annotations and the CDR3 nucleotide sequence.

Somatic hypermutation and clonality analysis

The somatic hypermutation (SHM) levels were determined by depositing the Ig sequences reconstructed using Unfiltered method to the IMGT/HighV-QUEST web server [30]. The SHM levels were also determined for PCR sequences using the IMGT/HighV-QUEST web server. The number of mutations used does not include those resulting from N diversity.

The single cells were assigned to clonal families on the basis of shared V gene, J gene, and the CDR3 length for both heavy and light chains.

Immunoglobulin transcript reconstruction pipeline for rhesus macaque

Ig reconstruction in rhesus macaques (*Macaca mulatta*) was carried out using four approaches: (1) Unfiltered, (2) Filter-Non-IG, (3) IG_mapped, and (4) IG_mapped+Unmapped. After trimming, the unfiltered or filtered reads were used for assembly with Trinity v2.3.2 without normalization. The Trinity assemblies were run on a local PowerEdge R630 Server (Intel Xeon E5-2620 v4, 16 cores/32 threads, 196 GB RAM) by executing 4 jobs, each with 8 threads and 32 GB RAM. The MacaM v7 genome reference was used to map the rhesus Ig loci and to remove conventional protein coding genes prior to assembly [31]. Since the Ig loci are not well annotated in rhesus macaques, the V, D, J, and C sequences from Sundling et al., 2012 [32] (available in IgBLAST), Ramesh et al., 2017 [33], and the IMGT database were aligned to the MacaM genome fasta file with blastn with an e-value threshold of 1e-5. The alignment positions were used to generate a bed file, and the coordinates were merged using BEDTools v2.26.0 [34]. The coordinates used for retrieving Ig reads were chr02a:90333086–9 1,387,066; chr02a:108598746–108,953,331; chr05:2485043 5–24,889,290; chr09:31850493–31,851,761; chr14:3378413 0–33,784,611; chr14:168090141–169,063,206; chr14:169167 858–169,720,918; chr15:58889859–58,901,394; chr15:6238 7209–62,387,505; chr15:63455638–64,109,298; chr15:64226 628–64,285,171; chr15:64411063–64,745,369; chr15:6544 0882–65,445,469; chr15:66221918–66,222,233. The reads were mapped to the MacaM reference using STAR, and Ig reads were retrieved with SAMtools and seqtk as done for human samples. The Unmapped reads were obtained from STAR and merged with IG_mapped reads and then assembled. For the Filter-Non-IG method, reads that mapped to annotated genes (non-Ig) in the rhesus genome were filtered out, and the assembly was run with the remaining reads.

The post-assembly analysis was similar to that for the human analysis pipeline. For annotation, we used the sequences available from IgBLAST (original source [32]).

Results
Experimental design

The goal of this study was to design and test a method for reconstructing accurate nucleotide sequences of rearranged immunoglobulin heavy and light chain genes from single-cell RNA-seq data. Plasmablasts are a class of B cell that is present at low frequencies in blood under steady-state conditions, but these cells undergo a rapid, transient expansion approximately 4–7 days after vaccination. To obtain a suitable population of plasmablasts enriched for vaccine-specific cells, plasmablasts were sorted as previously described [19] from blood collected from healthy human donors at day 7 after vaccination with the 2016/2017 Fluarix quadrivalent vaccine during the 2016 autumn flu season (Fig. 1a). Plasmablasts are a particularly useful population to query emergent B cell responses, as they are highly enriched for antigen-specific cells, and they allow for unbiased interrogation of relevant, vaccine-induced B cells without using fluorescently labeled antigenic probes or other technologies. Consistent with previous data [19, 35, 36], plasmablasts were massively expanded at 7 days post-vaccination, and were nearly 100% antigen-specific (Fig. 1b). We generated a dataset of sc-RNA-seq transcriptomes from 176 plasmablasts (Additional file 1: Table S1), obtained by flow cytometric sorting single B cells into 10 μL of lysis buffer of 96-well plates. We used 9 μL of the 10 μL cell lysate as input material into SMART-Seq mRNA amplification library preparation (Fig. 1a). After cDNA amplification of single plasmablasts, prominent peaks representing the IgH and IgL mRNA were readily apparent by microcapillary electrophoresis (Fig. 1c). The remaining 1 μL of lysate was used for conventional RT-PCR and Sanger sequencing of the heavy and light chain genes (Fig. 1a). In total, we generated a dataset of 255 Ig chains (115 heavy and 140 light chains) from Sanger sequencing with which to test the accuracy of our pipeline. Out of the 176 cells, 159 cells had at least one Ig chain represented in this dataset, while 96 cells had both the heavy and light chains (Additional file 1: Table S1).

Pipeline to reconstruct paired immunoglobulin sequences

An overview of the bioinformatics pipeline is shown in Fig. 2. The pipeline comprises the following major stages: (1) adapter trimming, (2) filtering of reads to enrich immunoglobulin transcripts, (3) *de novo* assembly of contiguous reads using the Trinity assembler, (4)

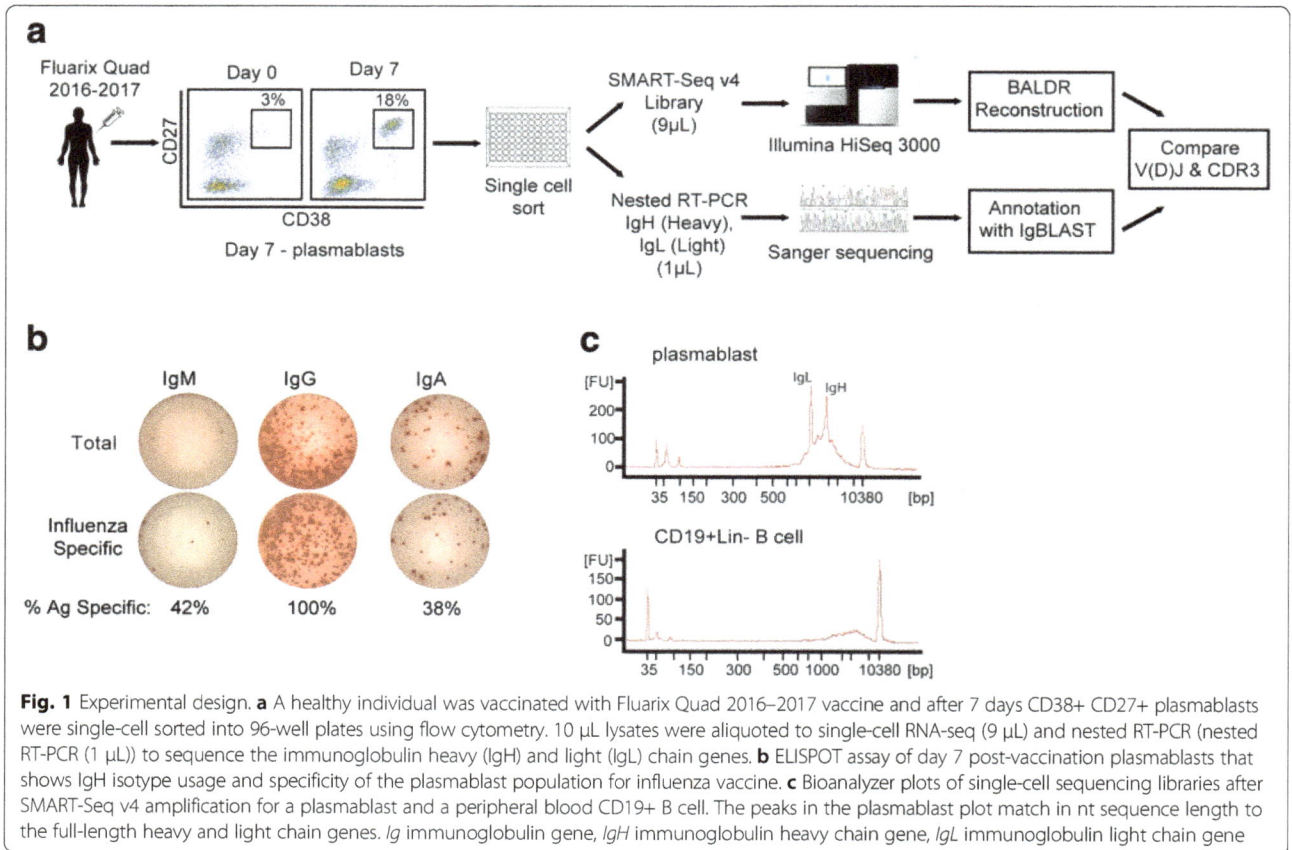

Fig. 1 Experimental design. **a** A healthy individual was vaccinated with Fluarix Quad 2016–2017 vaccine and after 7 days CD38+ CD27+ plasmablasts were single-cell sorted into 96-well plates using flow cytometry. 10 μL lysates were aliquoted to single-cell RNA-seq (9 μL) and nested RT-PCR (nested RT-PCR (1 μL)) to sequence the immunoglobulin heavy (IgH) and light (IgL) chain genes. **b** ELISPOT assay of day 7 post-vaccination plasmablasts that shows IgH isotype usage and specificity of the plasmablast population for influenza vaccine. **c** Bioanalyzer plots of single-cell sequencing libraries after SMART-Seq v4 amplification for a plasmablast and a peripheral blood CD19+ B cell. The peaks in the plasmablast plot match in nt sequence length to the full-length heavy and light chain genes. *Ig* immunoglobulin gene, *IgH* immunoglobulin heavy chain gene, *IgL* immunoglobulin light chain gene

annotation of Ig transcript models with IgBLAST, (5) read quantification, and (6) filtering of non-productive or redundant Ig transcript models. Models were then selected based on having the highest number of mapped reads, and validated with the Sanger sequencing data.

Adapter sequences used for library preparation were trimmed from the sequenced reads using Trimmomatic [23]. Trimmed reads were then assembled using Trinity. *De novo* assembly is a highly computationally intensive task, and scalability becomes a significant limitation in single-cell studies that involve analysis of hundreds or thousands of cells. In order to overcome this bottleneck, four different filtering strategies were evaluated for selecting Ig-specific reads. The first filtering strategy (termed IG_mapped) involved mapping of reads to the Ig loci in the human reference genome (GRCh38) using the STAR aligner [25]. Reads mapping to the three major Ig loci (IGH chr14, IGK chr2, and IGL chr22) were selected and assembled with Trinity. Due to the highly divergent nature of Ig sequences, it is possible that some reads may not map to the Ig loci in the reference genome. As a result, we also tested a filtering strategy that included unmapped reads (reads not mapping to the GRCh38 reference genome) in addition to the reads mapping to the major Ig loci (IG_mapped

+Unmapped). The third filtering strategy involved creating an *in silico* "Ig recombinome" database of all possible combinations of human V, J, and C genes from IMGT, similar to a previously described strategy for T cells [16]. Sequencing reads that mapped to the recombined sequences were retained for assembly (Recombinome_mapped). Lastly, in our fourth strategy, (IMGT_mapped) reads were mapped to the IMGT database [3] of human V, D, and J sequences and extracted for assembly. We also tested assembly of all reads without filtering (Unfiltered). After running Trinity assembly to build contig models of the remaining transcripts, IgBLAST [28] was used on assembled Ig sequences for V(D)J gene annotation, prediction of the CDR3 sequence, and to determine whether the Ig chain was productive. We observed that assembly of RNA-seq reads can result in several Ig transcript models (Fig. 3). For selecting the most representative model, all reads used for assembly were mapped to each Ig model. Ig transcript models were ranked according to the number of reads mapped and then filtered to remove (1) models predicted to be unproductive and (2) models having the same V(D)J genes and the CDR3 sequence as a higher ranked model. The top ranking model that remained after filtering was then selected for validation with nested RT-PCR-derived sequences.

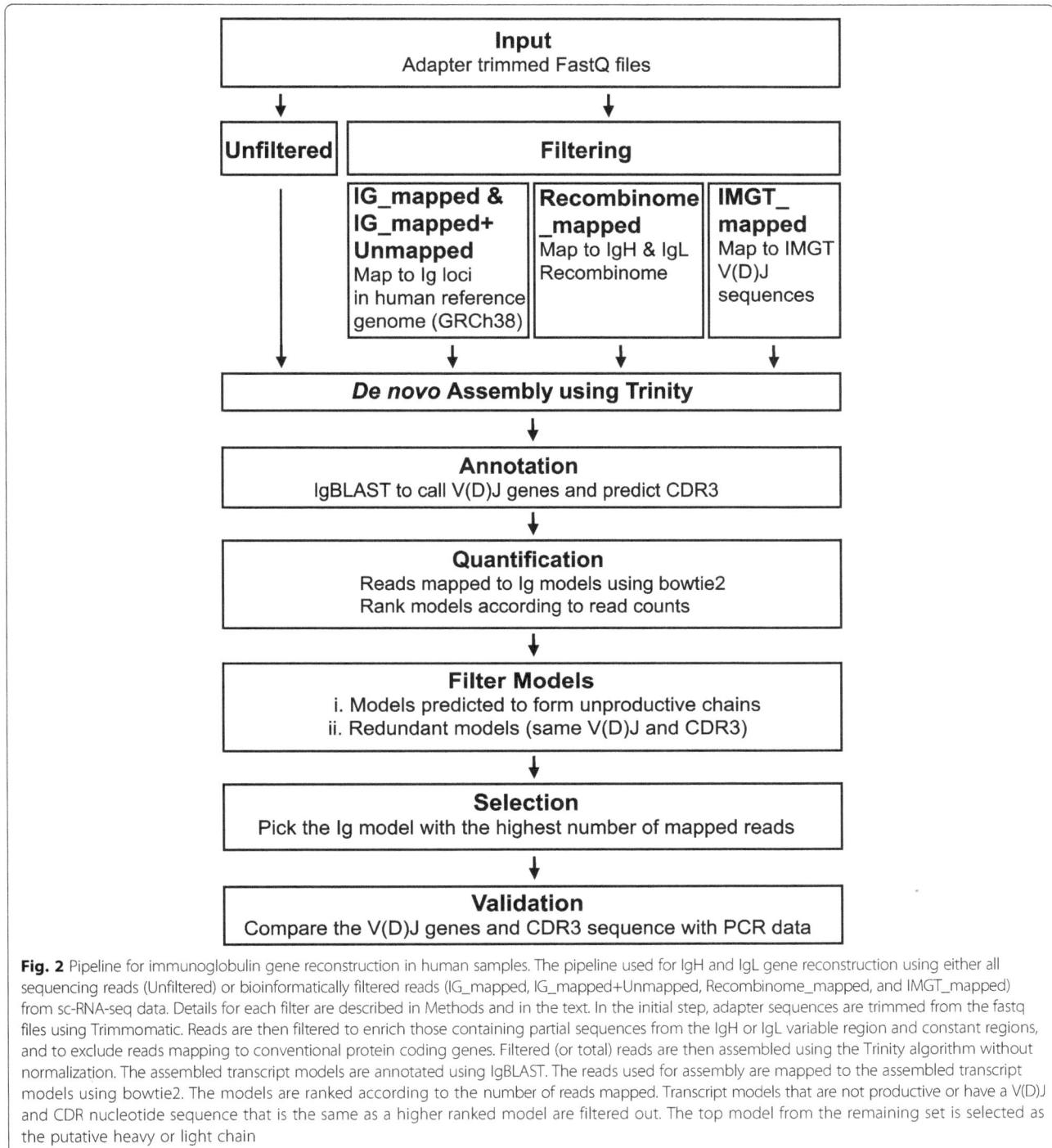

Fig. 2 Pipeline for immunoglobulin gene reconstruction in human samples. The pipeline used for IgH and IgL gene reconstruction using either all sequencing reads (Unfiltered) or bioinformatically filtered reads (IG_mapped, IG_mapped+Unmapped, Recombinome_mapped, and IMGT_mapped) from sc-RNA-seq data. Details for each filter are described in Methods and in the text. In the initial step, adapter sequences are trimmed from the fastq files using Trimmomatic. Reads are then filtered to enrich those containing partial sequences from the IgH or IgL variable region and constant regions, and to exclude reads mapping to conventional protein coding genes. Filtered (or total) reads are then assembled using the Trinity algorithm without normalization. The assembled transcript models are annotated using IgBLAST. The reads used for assembly are mapped to the assembled transcript models using bowtie2. The models are ranked according to the number of reads mapped. Transcript models that are not productive or have a V(D)J and CDR nucleotide sequence that is the same as a higher ranked model are filtered out. The top model from the remaining set is selected as the putative heavy or light chain

De novo assembly of plasmablast sc-RNA-seq data yields a single dominant assembly model of IgH and IgL transcripts

As discussed above, assembly of RNA-seq reads results in multiple putative assembly models for Ig transcripts. However, we observed that each cell was found to have a dominant heavy and light chain model with all the evaluated methods, regardless of filtering approach (Fig. 3 and Additional file 1: Figure S1). The median number of reads mapping to the first and second most prevalent reconstructed heavy chain assembly models from our preferred filtering method, IG_mapped+Unmapped, was 334,090 and 937, respectively (Fig. 3a). Similarly, the median read count for the top and the

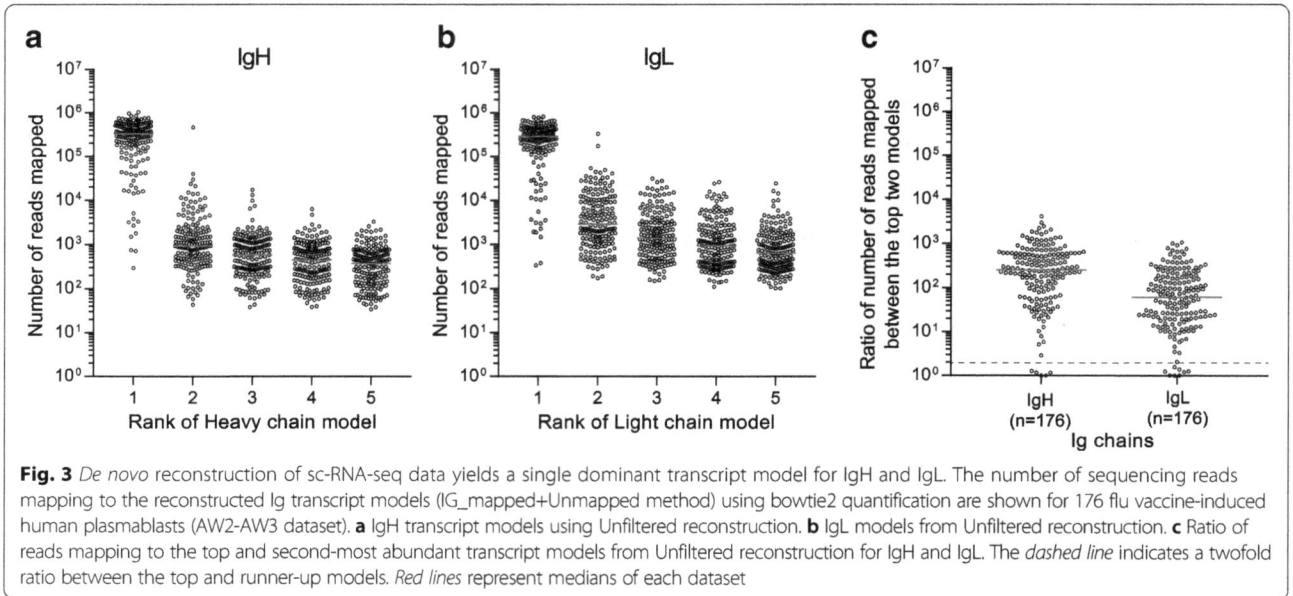

Fig. 3 *De novo* reconstruction of sc-RNA-seq data yields a single dominant transcript model for IgH and IgL. The number of sequencing reads mapping to the reconstructed Ig transcript models (IG_mapped+Unmapped method) using bowtie2 quantification are shown for 176 flu vaccine-induced human plasmablasts (AW2-AW3 dataset). **a** IgH transcript models using Unfiltered reconstruction. **b** IgL models from Unfiltered reconstruction. **c** Ratio of reads mapping to the top and second-most abundant transcript models from Unfiltered reconstruction for IgH and IgL. The *dashed line* indicates a twofold ratio between the top and runner-up models. *Red lines* represent medians of each dataset

second most abundant assembly models for light chains was 289,539 and 2896, respectively (Fig. 3b). The median ratio of mapped reads for the top model relative to the runner-up model was 250-fold and 61-fold for heavy and light chains, respectively (Fig. 3c). Of note, we observed that of the 176 cells, five had a ratio of the top model:runner-up of less than two-fold for IgH (Fig. 3c), and eight had ratios of less than two-fold for IgL. Collectively, these data indicate that *de novo* assembly, with or without filtering, is able to provide an unambiguous transcript model for the IgH and IgL chains in 93–98% and 95–97% of cells, respectively.

Immunoglobulin reconstruction accuracy is near 100% at the clonotype and nt levels

We next assessed the accuracy of each method to reconstruct IgH and IgL chains from single-cell NGS data by comparing the reconstructed sequences to matched sequences obtained by conventional nested RT-PCR/Sanger sequencing [19]. We defined overall accuracy as the fraction of IgH and IgL chains in which reconstruction correctly called the V(D)J gene usage and CDR3 sequence relative to the RT-PCR/Sanger matched reference sequences in the 115 samples with matched NGS + PCR heavy chain sequences and 140 samples with matched light chain sequences (Fig. 4a). A high recovery of reconstruction was observed, regardless of filtering method, for IgH chains, as all methods successfully reconstructed a productive chain in all samples, with the exception of IG_mapped filtering, which had 98% recovery of IgH chains (Additional file 1: Figure S2A and Table S2). Out of the 176 plasmablasts sequenced, all filtering methods were able to yield productive IgL chains

for 100% of samples (Additional file 1: Figure S2A and Table S2). Reconstructions using the Unfiltered approach showed the highest concordance (115/115 IgH (100%) and 139/140 IgL (99.3%)) with RT-PCR results (Fig. 4a, Additional file 2). Using the best filtering method (IG_mapped+Unmapped), the accuracy for IgH was 99.1% (114/115 chains) and for IgL was 99.3% (139/140 chains) (Fig. 4a). Recombinome_mapped filtering showed 111 IgH (96.5%) and 139 IgL (99.3%), and filtering against IMGT_mapped 109 IgH (94.7%) and 139 IgL (99.3%) (Fig. 4a, Additional file 1: Table S2, Additional file 2). A significant dropoff in accuracy in clonotype determination for the heavy chain was observed for the IG_mapped filtering method (103 IgH (89.5%) and 139 IgL (99.3%)) (Fig. 4a, Additional file 2). In general, the accuracy of reconstruction was higher for the less diverse light chains compared to the heavy chains. Evaluation of BALDR's accuracy rate for yielding paired clonotype information showed that it was able to get accurate reconstructions for both IgH + IgL chains in 98.9% of the 96 cells where we had paired IgH-IgL sequences from RT-PCR with the Unfiltered method. IG_mapped+Unmapped showed the next best accuracy with accurate reconstructions in 94 out of the 96 cells (97.9%), followed by Recombinome_mapped (94.8%) and IMGT_mapped (92.7%), and again, a substantial dropoff was seen for the IG_mapped method (88.5%) (Additional file 1: Table S2). Collectively, these data demonstrate that our Ig chain reconstruction pipeline can efficiently and accurately determine the clonotype usage of plasmablasts from sc-RNA-seq data.

To assess if our accuracy estimates could be biased by clonotypes that were overrepresented in the

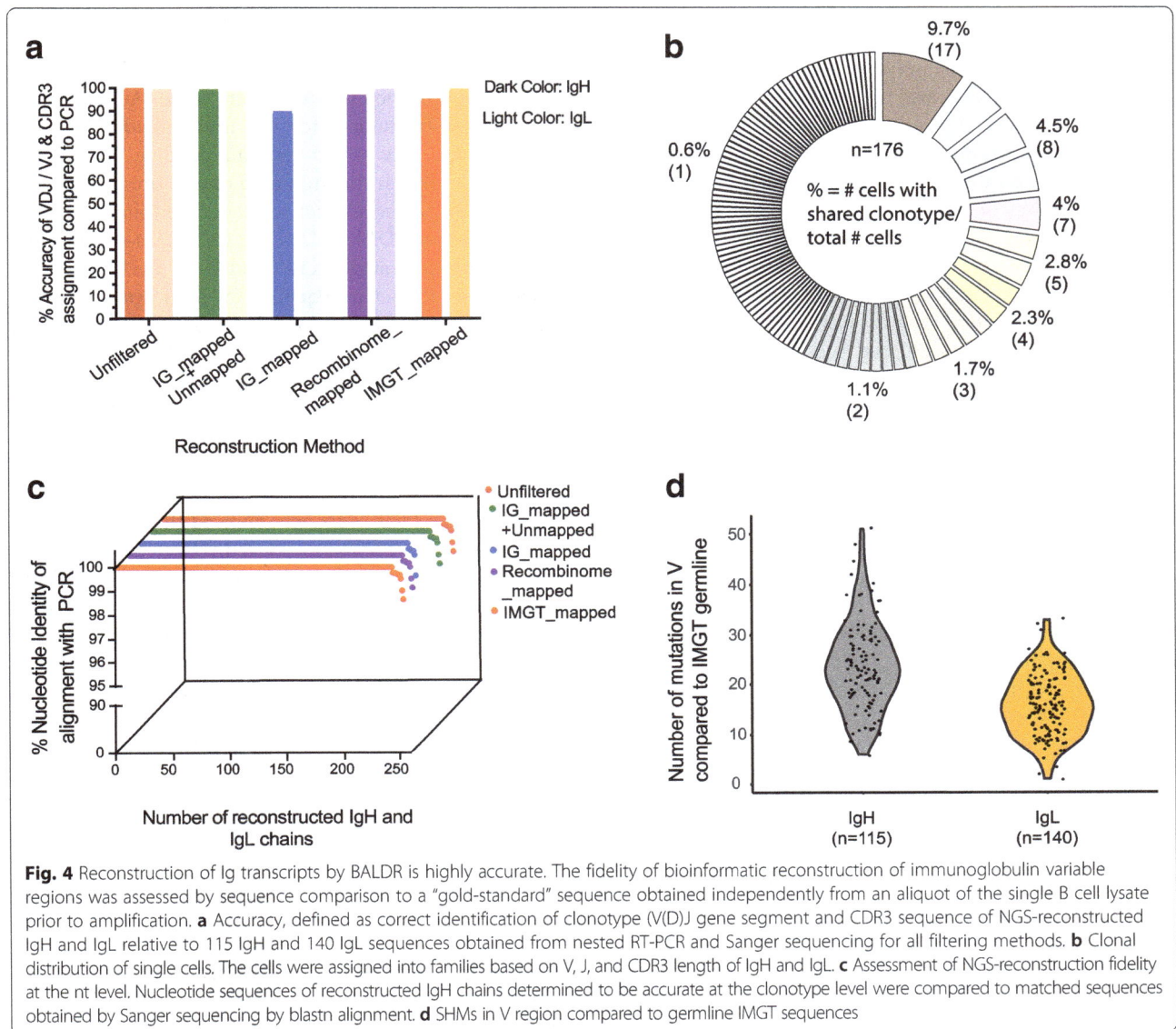

Fig. 4 Reconstruction of Ig transcripts by BALDR is highly accurate. The fidelity of bioinformatic reconstruction of immunoglobulin variable regions was assessed by sequence comparison to a "gold-standard" sequence obtained independently from an aliquot of the single B cell lysate prior to amplification. **a** Accuracy, defined as correct identification of clonotype (V(D)J gene segment and CDR3 sequence of NGS-reconstructed IgH and IgL relative to 115 IgH and 140 IgL sequences obtained from nested RT-PCR and Sanger sequencing for all filtering methods. **b** Clonal distribution of single cells. The cells were assigned into families based on V, J, and CDR3 length of IgH and IgL. **c** Assessment of NGS-reconstruction fidelity at the nt level. Nucleotide sequences of reconstructed IgH chains determined to be accurate at the clonotype level were compared to matched sequences obtained by Sanger sequencing by blastn alignment. **d** SHMs in V region compared to germline IMGT sequences

dataset, we calculated the degree of clonality (Fig. 4b). We found that the 176 plasmablasts exhibited high clonality (Fig. 4b, Additional file 3) with the largest clonal family comprising 9.7% of the cells. We recalculated the accuracy considering the clonotype and found that the accuracy for Unfiltered method remained high at 100% for IgH, 98.8% for IgL, and 98.3% for paired IgH-IgL as well as the IG_mapped +Unmapped method (98.5% for IgH, 98.8% for IgL, and 96.6% for paired IgH-IgL) (Additional file 1: Table S3). Investigation into the reason for the loss of accuracy using the IG_mapped filtering method, which relies on retaining reads that map to the GRCh38 genome reference, revealed that for cells that had yielded incorrect IgH assembly models, these models had a substantially lower number of reads

mapping when compared to the correct model yielded by the Unfiltered method (Additional file 4). In the majority of cases, we found that the "correct" V gene was incorporated into models with high read count, but these models were non-productive and filtered out (data not shown). The inclusion of unmapped reads (i.e., using the IG_mapped+Unmapped method) rescued these IgH models. This difference in accuracy between a method that relies solely on mapping to a reference (IG_mapped) compared to one that adds unmapped reads (IG_mapped+Unmapped) demonstrates the value in retaining unmapped reads, which helps to retain reads that may be otherwise lost due to incompleteness of a reference, allelic diversity or SHM.

Having determined the accuracy of clonotype assignment, we next examined the fidelity of reconstruction at the nucleotide level. The nucleotide sequences of reconstructed Ig chains were compared to the 255 RT-PCR generated sequences using blastn (Fig. 4c, Additional file 1: Figure S2B). In the vast majority of cells, the reconstructed sequences showed 100% nucleotide identity to the PCR-derived sequences (Fig. 4c). We observed that 96.5% of the reconstructed heavy and light chains had zero mismatches or gaps across all methods (Additional file 1: Figure S2). Of the remaining sequences that were not an exact match, the nucleotide identity exceeded 98.6% (Additional file 1: Figure S2). To ensure that our estimates of nucleotide identity were not biased by short alignments, we also considered the degree of sequence coverage in the reconstructed chain compared to the RT-PCR data. Out of the 255 chains, the sequence coverage was greater than 97% for 254 chains with Unfiltered and IG_mapped+Unmapped methods, 252 with Recombinome_mapped and IMGT_mapped, and 246 for IG_mapped (Additional file 1: Figure S2). Of note, we calculated the degree of SHM in the 176 plasmablasts and found it to be relatively high (median 23 nt changes from germline for IgH, 16 for IgL) (Fig. 4d, Additional file 5). Overall, these data demonstrate that our reconstruction pipeline faithfully reconstructs Ig transcript nucleotide sequences and has the ability to detect nucleotide changes induced by junctional diversity and SHM between individual cells in a clonal lineage.

De novo reconstruction of NGS data typically involves substantial computational resources, and a significant practical consideration of our pipeline is the computing time needed for assembly of each sample. We tested the computation times needed for each filtering method for Trinity assembly (Additional file 1: Figure S3). The median assembly time for a plasmablast cell was 2831 s (47 min) for the Unfiltered method, 310 s (5.2 min) for IG_mapped+Unmapped, 211 s (3.5 min) for IG_mapped, 317 s (5.3 min) for Recombinome_mapped, and 316 s (5.3 min) for the IMGT_mapped filtering methods. The time taken for assembly of Unfiltered reads was more than ninefold higher compared to filtering methods for enriching Ig transcripts. Taken together with the accuracy rates, these data demonstrate that Ig-transcript filtering significantly reduces the computational burden for assembly, with a negligible impact on accuracy.

The most recent version of the Trinity assembly software provides a feature for in silico normalization of reads to reduce the computation time for assembly. We found that running Trinity with the normalization feature resulted in reduced accuracy for Ig reconstruction in most cases (Additional file 1: Figure S4, Additional file 2). However, for the Recombinome_mapped and IMGT_mapped methods, normalization was found to slightly improve the accuracy by 2% and 3%, respectively.

BALDR reconstructs paired Ig chains in conventional B cells

Plasmablasts are a unique cell population in that approximately 5–50% of the mRNA transcriptome (Additional file 6) comprises transcripts for the immunoglobulin heavy and light chain genes. To test our pipeline on a B cell population in which the immunoglobulin transcripts were less abundant, we sorted conventional, peripheral blood B cells (defined as CD19+ CD3− CD16− CD14−) cells from a healthy donor as single cells (Additional file 1: Table S1). At least one productive sequence for each heavy and light chain was reconstructed for all 36 B cells. Due to the lower amount of Ig RNA, nested RT-PCR was carried out from the amplified SMART-Seq mRNA library, rather than from a portion of the single-cell lysate. Thirty-one IgH and 31 IgL high-quality Ig sequences were obtained from Sanger sequencing of nested RT-PCR Ig chains. Comparison of the V(D)J genes and the CDR3 sequence with the 62 RT-PCR sequences showed that Ig chains can be reconstructed accurately even in B cells with much lower levels of Ig transcripts (Fig. 5a, Additional file 2). All methods showed 100% (31/31 chains) accuracy for light chain reconstruction. The accuracy for the heavy chain ranged from 90.3% (28/31 chains) to 96.8% (30/31 chains) with Unfiltered and IG_mapped+Unmapped having the highest accuracy. A dominant heavy and light chain model was also observed in all B cells similar to plasmablasts (Additional file 1: Figure S5 and Table S4). In contrast to plasmablasts, where ~ 39% of all RNA-seq reads were Ig, the percentage of Ig reads in B cells ranged from 0.2 to 7.9% with a median of 2.2% (Additional file 6), and the majority of B cells had low or absent levels of SHM (Fig. 5b).

BALDR maintains accuracy across a broad array of sequencing parameters

The 176 plasmablast cells described thus far were sequenced using single-ended 151-base reads (SE 151). However, sc-RNA-seq data can be generated with varying configurations of read length and/or single vs paired ends. To test the effect of these sequencing parameters, we generated a new sc-RNA-seq dataset of 101-base paired-end reads using 86 plasmablasts from another healthy individual obtained 7 days after influenza vaccination. We also generated a new matched dataset of IgH and IgL sequences from RT-PCR in which the starting material was 1 μL of unamplified lysate. We were able to get high-quality sequences for 34 IgH chains and 41 IgL chains with RT-PCR. To test the effect of sequencing parameters on clonotype assignment accuracy, we generated datasets simulating alternate sequencing parameters by truncating the 101-base reads to 75-base and 50-base reads in silico, and by omitting the second read of the mate pair. As above, the accuracy of the reconstructed

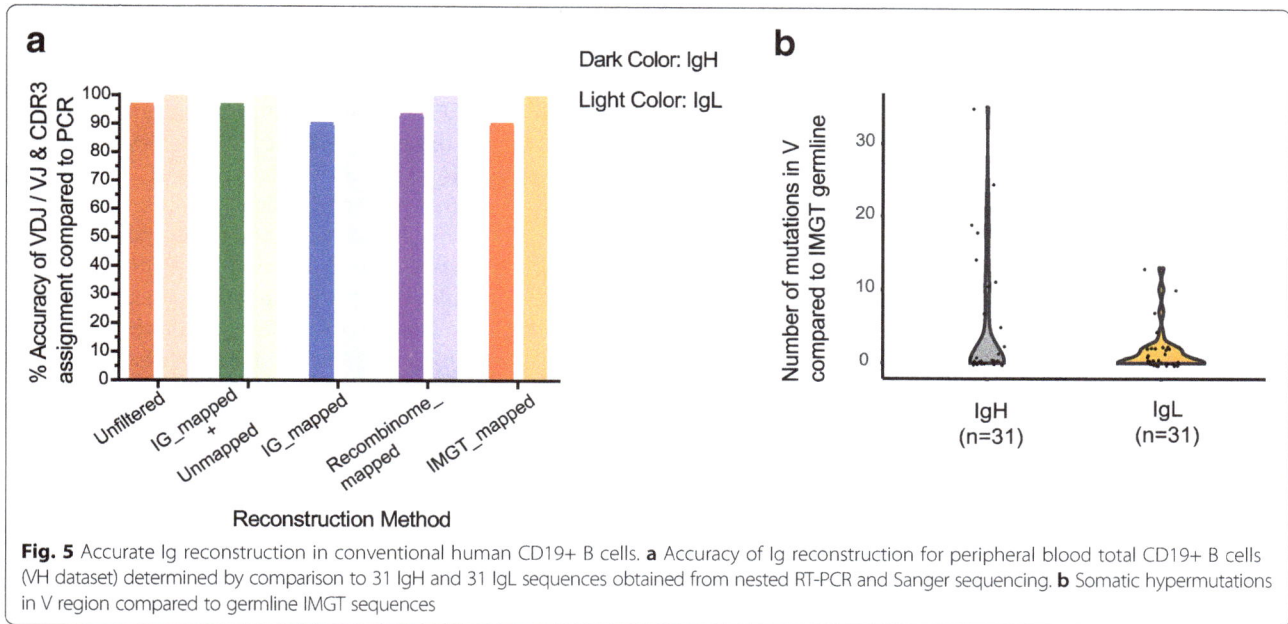

Fig. 5 Accurate Ig reconstruction in conventional human CD19+ B cells. **a** Accuracy of Ig reconstruction for peripheral blood total CD19+ B cells (VH dataset) determined by comparison to 31 IgH and 31 IgL sequences obtained from nested RT-PCR and Sanger sequencing. **b** Somatic hypermutations in V region compared to germline IMGT sequences

Ig chains was determined by comparing the V(D)J gene annotation and the CDR3 sequence with the RT-PCR sequences.

The Unfiltered and the IG_mapped+Unmapped methods showed the same accuracy, 100% for IgH chains and 97% for IgL chains (Fig. 6, Additional file 1: Table S5, and Additional file 2). The IgL chain did not match the reconstructed sequences for only one sequence out of 41. These methods showed the same accuracies across all the sequencing conditions tested. Comparatively, the accuracy derived from data filtered with the IG_mapped, Recombinome_mapped, and IMGT_mapped methods were much more sensitive to reductions in read length. Mapping-based approaches showed a decline in accuracy with decreasing read length, and the decline was much higher for heavy chains compared to the light chains (Fig. 6). IG_mapped and Recombinome_mapped also showed better accuracies for paired-end sequencing. For IMGT, using paired-end sequencing showed less accuracy, since concordantly mapping reads may not be obtained with the small J sequences. Collectively, these data demonstrate

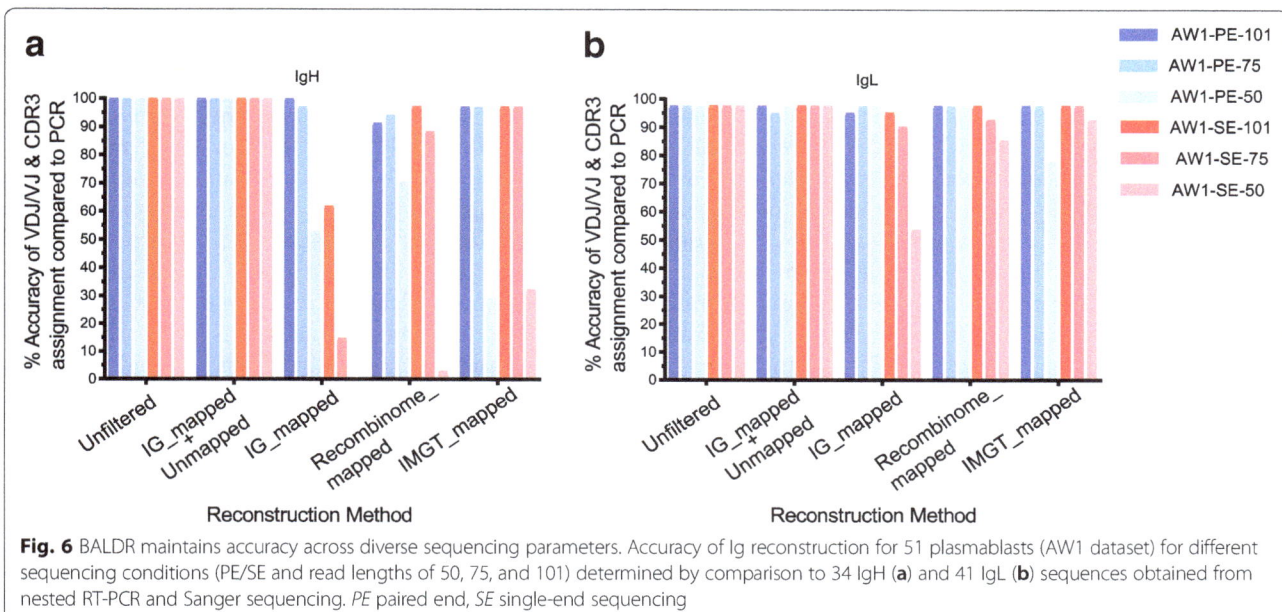

Fig. 6 BALDR maintains accuracy across diverse sequencing parameters. Accuracy of Ig reconstruction for 51 plasmablasts (AW1 dataset) for different sequencing conditions (PE/SE and read lengths of 50, 75, and 101) determined by comparison to 34 IgH (**a**) and 41 IgL (**b**) sequences obtained from nested RT-PCR and Sanger sequencing. *PE* paired end, *SE* single-end sequencing

that the Unfiltered and IG_mapped+Unmapped filtering methods, in addition to having the highest overall accuracy rates, are also the most flexible in terms of maintaining accuracy over differing sequencing parameters.

Comparison of BALDR to alternate methods

A semi-*de novo* pipeline called BCR assembly from single cells (BASIC) has been recently developed for reconstructing Ig chains from single cells [37]. BASIC reconstructs the Ig sequence by anchoring reads to the V and the C genes and then extends the sequence by progressively stitching overlapping reads to the anchor sequence. We compared the performance of BASIC with BALDR on three B cell datasets and at varying sequencing parameters. When run using default values and hg19 reference, we obtained productive chains for 59% heavy (104/176) and 57% light (100/176) chains for the AW2-AW3 dataset using SE 151 base reads. The concordance of productive chains with RT-PCR-derived sequences based on the comparison of V(D)J genes and CDR3 sequence was 53% (61/115) for the heavy and 54% (76/140) for the light chains (Additional file 1: Table S6, Additional file 2). These accuracies were much lower than reported in the original study. As the dataset used in the BASIC study used 50 base reads, we trimmed our AW2-AW3 reads to 50 bases, retaining only the proximal ends of the read. Using the trimmed reads, the accuracy of reconstruction for productive chains was 93% for heavy and 97% for light chains (Additional file 1: Table S6). For the same trimmed reads, the IG_mapped +Unmapped method showed an accuracy of 98% for heavy and 99% for light chains. We also tested BASIC for the CD19+ Lin− B cell dataset which made use of paired-end 76-base reads. The accuracies for heavy and light chains were 93.5% and 100% for BASIC, while those for IG_mapped+Unmapped were 96.8% and 100%, respectively (Additional file 1: Table S6). Furthermore, we also compared the accuracy of BASIC in reconstructing Ig chains on a set of 86 plasmablasts under different conditions of read lengths and single-end or paired-end sequencing. We found that the accuracy of BASIC varies with the sequencing condition, ranging from 73.5% to 97% for IgH and from 95.1% to 97.6% for IgL. Overall, the accuracy of obtaining paired chains ranged from 70.8 to 91.7% for the different conditions. In contrast, the recommended IG_mapped+Unmapped method in the BALDR pipeline consistently shows high accuracies of 100% for IgH, 95.1–97.6% for IgL, and 95.8% for accurately obtaining paired IgH-IgL under all conditions. Overall, the IG_mapped+Unmapped method shows higher accuracy than BASIC, with significantly higher accuracy with longer reads, and maintains accuracy over a greater range of sequencing parameters.

The BALDR pipeline accurately reconstructs Ig chains in rhesus macaques

The rhesus macaque model is critical to the development of an AIDS vaccine. Historically, the majority of vaccines that demonstrate efficacy and achieve licensure elicit high levels of antibodies capable of neutralizing infection by the pathogen. To date, development of an HIV vaccine capable of generating neutralizing antibodies has remained elusive due to the high level of diversity in circulating viral strains. Nevertheless, several of the most promising HIV vaccine candidates have been capable of eliciting antibodies that exhibit moderate levels of neutralizing antibodies [38]. Despite its inherently high research value, the Ig loci in the rhesus macaque remain poorly annotated. There are currently 224 V(D)J genes for the rhesus macaque in the IMGT database [3]; however, it has been estimated that as many as 50% or more of Ig gene segments may be missing [39]. To enable reconstruction of antibody sequences in rhesus macaques, we designed and tested three Ig transcript filtering transcript strategies, taking into account the current state of rhesus macaque genome references (Fig. 7). Similar to the strategy for humans, we tested filtering strategies in which reads mapping to the immunoglobulin loci (IG_mapped), or to the Ig loci and also to reads that did not map to annotated, non-Ig genes (IG_mapped+Unmapped) were retained for reconstruction. In order to determine the Ig loci in the macaque MacaM v7 reference genome, rhesus V, D, J, and constant region sequences from the IMGT database, and those reported by Sundling [32] and more recently by Ramesh [33] were aligned to the genome fasta files using blastn. Once defined, these loci (details in Methods) were then used for mapping to identify and retain reads containing immunoglobulin sequences in our single-cell data. We also tested another strategy (Filter-Non-IG) where we aligned reads to the MacaM (v7) reference genome, all reads mapping to an annotated, non-immunoglobulin gene were discarded, and the remaining reads were retained for assembly. For annotation, we used the sequences available from IgBLAST (original source [32]).

We sequenced 42 plasmablasts, 33 splenic germinal center (GC) B cells, and 33 memory B cells, the latter of which were purified based on their specificity for epitopes in the experimental vaccine. For the rhesus plasmablast dataset, 42/42 cells had both IgH and IgL genes for which annotation was available; for the rhesus splenic B cells high confidence annotations could be made for 24 cells for both IgH and IgL. A productive chain was reconstructed for all plasmablasts with each method (Additional file 1: Figure S6A and Table S7, Additional file 2). The reconstruction success was 84.8% for IgH and IgL for the GC B cells and 81.8% for IgH and 100% for IgL for antigen-specific memory B cells

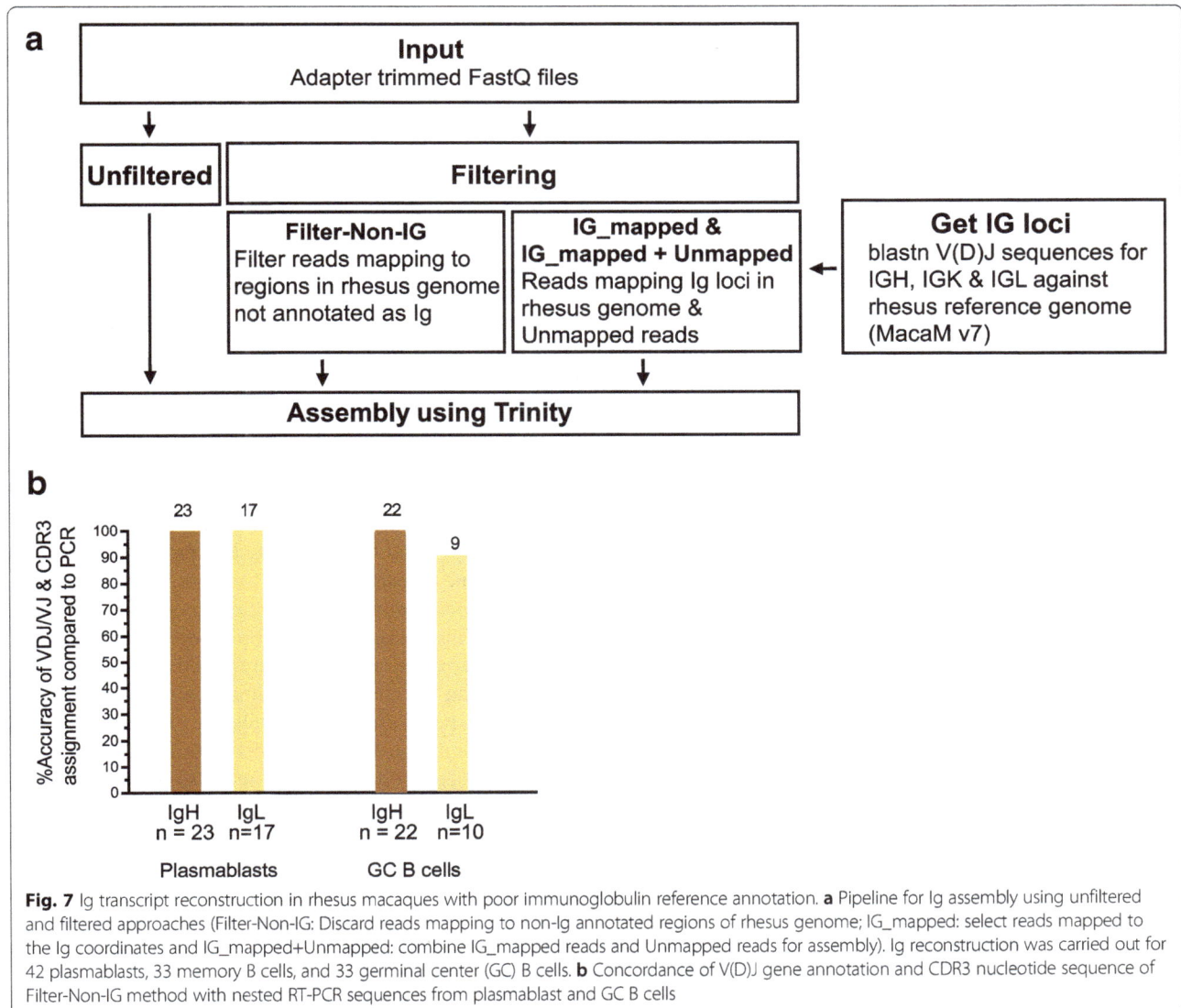

Fig. 7 Ig transcript reconstruction in rhesus macaques with poor immunoglobulin reference annotation. **a** Pipeline for Ig assembly using unfiltered and filtered approaches (Filter-Non-IG: Discard reads mapping to non-Ig annotated regions of rhesus genome; IG_mapped: select reads mapped to the Ig coordinates and IG_mapped+Unmapped: combine IG_mapped reads and Unmapped reads for assembly). Ig reconstruction was carried out for 42 plasmablasts, 33 memory B cells, and 33 germinal center (GC) B cells. **b** Concordance of V(D)J gene annotation and CDR3 nucleotide sequence of Filter-Non-IG method with nested RT-PCR sequences from plasmablast and GC B cells

using the Unfiltered method (Additional file 1: Table S7, Additional file 2). The Filter-Non-IG and the IG_mapped+Unmapped methods showed similar results, with Filter-Non-IG performing slightly better in the memory B cells. Lastly, the lowest number of productive reconstructions was obtained with the IG_mapped method (Additional file 1: Figure S6A and Table S7).

In order to determine the accuracy of reconstructions, we obtained the PCR sequence for the single cells. We were able to obtain high-quality PCR sequences for 23 IgH and 17 IgL from plasmablasts and 22 IgH and 10 IgL from GC B cells. Unfiltered, Filter-Non-IG, and IG_mapped+Unmapped showed the same high accuracy of 100% for IgH and IgL in plasmablasts and 100% for IgH and 90% for IgL (9/10) in GC B cells (Fig. 7b, Additional file 1: Figure S6B and Table S7). The

discordant reconstruction differed only in the J gene assignment with the PCR (Additional file 2). The IG_mapped method showed high accuracies with plasmablast but showed very low accuracy for IgH (40.9%) in GC B cells.

We also assessed the computational time for assembly of each filtering method. The median time for assembly using the Unfiltered method was 19,701 s (328 min), 8020 s (134 min), and 5863 s (98 min) for memory B cells, GC B cells, and plasmablasts, respectively (Additional file 1: Figure S6C). The Filter-Non-IG method is two to three times faster than the Unfiltered method, while IG_mapped+Unmapped is 4–30 times faster than the Unfiltered method. Collectively, these data demonstrate that the BALDR pipeline can accurately reconstruct paired immunoglobulin genes from scRNA-seq data generated from rhesus macaque B cells.

Discussion

In this study we report the utility of *de novo* assembly for the accurate reconstruction of the BCR heavy and light chain sequences from full-length single-cell RNA-seq data. We further tested the impact of various filtering methods and sequencing parameters on V(D)J sequence accuracy and recovery efficacy. Lastly, we present the optimal parameters for BCR reconstruction with a bioinformatics pipeline we refer to as BALDR (**B**CR **A**ssignment of **L**ineage using *De novo* **R**econstruction). It is important to note that we have developed and validated the BALDR methodology using primary human B cells, namely vaccine-induced plasmablasts, and primary peripheral blood CD19+ B cells. Further, we have demonstrated that BALDR accurately reconstructs paired IgH + IgL sequences from B cells from rhesus macaques.

The ability to efficiently extract paired antigen receptor information from primary human immune cells *ex vivo* and link it with single-cell transcriptome data opens the way for powerful new analyses with clinical samples that were previously only possible in murine models. One attractive application of this technology is to perform "lineage-tracing" studies that link the transcriptional data from individual B cell clonotypes at specified differentiation states and then follow the "fates" of individual clones by repertoire sequencing. The clonotype sequence provided by the BALDR pipeline also makes it possible to generate monoclonal antibodies and thus link transcriptional information with functional qualities (e.g., affinity, neutralization activity) of the antibody. Here, we have used BALDR to extract IgH + IgL clonotypic information in vaccine-induced B cells; this clonotype sequence information can be used to monitor vaccine recipients over time and identify individual B cell lineages capable of differentiating into long-lived antibody-secreting plasma cells or persistent memory B cells and link it to transcriptional information. An alternative use of this tool is to link transcriptional state with clonotype-specific properties of the antibody, such as the proclivity to undergo class switching, SHM, or post-translational modifications. Used in this way, the application of BALDR and sc-RNA-seq to primary B cells induced in human vaccination studies also provides a novel analytic tool to the emerging field of "systems vaccinology" in which high-throughput technologies are used to identify factors predicting vaccine efficacy [40].

We evaluated different filtering strategies and found that the most accurate strategy was to retain reads that (1) mapped to the three defined immunoglobulin loci in the GRCh38 genome and (2) did not map to an annotated gene. This method, IG_mapped+Unmapped, identified the correct clonotype in 99.2% (253/255) of paired chains and correctly paired IgH + IgL information in

96.9% (93/96) cells. The accuracy of our pipeline compares favorably with recent reports using similar approaches for T cells where the accuracies ranged from 77.5% (14/20 α chain and 17/20 β chain) [17] to 78.4% [16]. In both the human and rhesus datasets, the inclusion of unmapped reads for Ig reconstruction improved the recovery rate and accuracy rate of the reconstructed chains compared to strategies that relied on inclusion of reads mapping to a reference. This advantage becomes increasingly important when analyzing human populations or models with poor representation of alleles in IMGT, or as we demonstrated, for B cell populations with high levels of SHM. Indeed, inclusion of the unmapped reads also provides more flexibility with respect to the read length used as input data, since shorter reads may not map to highly variable regions of Ig chains during the pre-filtering stage. The IG_mapped+Unmapped method involves mapping the reads to the reference genome with STAR, which allows us to simultaneously obtain the transcript quantification needed for pairing of the transcriptome information. For the rhesus, where the Ig loci are not well annotated in the genome, using this strategy of the Filter-Non-IG method provides nearly identical results to using all reads (Unfiltered method), at the same time reducing the computation time to almost half.

We have not looked specifically at the effect of sequencing depth on the Ig reconstruction. However, our datasets ranged from ~ 400,000 reads to 4 million reads, and we were able to get a high rate of reconstruction in most samples. For analyzing the transcriptome, a sequencing depth of 1 million reads per cell has been recommended for saturated gene detection [41] in sc-RNA-seq. When analyzing plasmablasts, where 5–50% of the mRNA transcripts can be immunoglobulins, a secondary consideration is achieving sufficient depth for the remaining transcriptional analysis, and we typically target for ~ 1.5 to 2 million reads per single plasmablast. For conventional B cells, we observed reads attributed to immunoglobulin to be less than 8%, and a sequencing depth of 1–1.5 million reads is adequate to capture the transcriptome along with Ig reconstruction.

All filtering methods described in the current study are made available in the BALDR pipeline. We recommend using IG_mapped+Unmapped for human cells and the Filter-Non-IG method for rhesus macaques. The transcript quantification that is obtained simultaneously with these methods can be used to carry out gene expression analysis. Further improvements in the pipeline will involve adapting the Unfiltered method towards organisms with low-quality/missing reference genomes. Additionally, improving the Ig annotations for rhesus will result in higher accuracy for the IG_mapped+Unmapped method while reducing the computation time significantly.

One of the key strengths of the BALDR pipeline is its ability to generate accurate Ig transcript reconstructions for samples in which genomic references of immunoglobulin gene sequences are lacking. We demonstrated this activity by reconstructing Ig transcripts from single B cells obtained from rhesus macaques after vaccination with experimental vaccines. Currently, resources for Ig annotation in the rhesus macaque are underdeveloped. For example, the IMGT database contains 19 immunoglobulin heavy chain variable (IGHV) genes, despite estimates that up to 60 genes are present in the rhesus immunoglobulin IgH loci [3, 39]. Efforts to improve genomic resources of the Indian rhesus macaque immunoglobulin loci are currently underway, and a high density map of the rhesus immunoglobulin loci has recently been published [33] and will be an important advance for AIDS vaccine development. However, it will be some time before the allelic diversity of the immunoglobulin genes is characterized for the North American captive rhesus macaque population. The BALDR pipeline maintains high accuracy of Ig transcript reconstruction when input data are from a species with scant annotation of the Ig loci, such as currently exist for the rhesus macaque, and thus confident analysis of sc-RNA-seq data can be applied to current ongoing studies in the macaque model.

The independence of the BALDR pipeline from high-quality Ig reference sequences may also have added utility for human vaccine studies, particularly in populations in Africa and Asia, where allelic diversity is relatively uncharacterized. In a recent study by Morris and colleagues, analysis of 28 HIV-infected women in South Africa characterized approximately 130 IGHV alleles that were not represented in the IMGT database [42]. In these scenarios, bioinformatic tools that rely on mapping to an Ig reference are likely to have higher rates of incorrect or abortive clonotype reconstructions. In these populations, the BALDR pipeline can be particularly useful for sc-RNA-seq studies of HIV-specific B cells or to enhance the recovery of paired IgH + IgL sequences and accelerate discovery of novel antibodies capable of neutralization breadth against HIV.

The BALDR pipeline requires sequence information across the entirety of the BCR variable region. This requirement necessitates that the NGS library be prepared separately for each cell, so that sequence fragments across the full length of transcripts can be barcoded. These whole-transcript methods (e.g., SMART-Seq) have been extensively used for sc-RNA-seq in the literature, but they have the drawback of being relatively expensive. Recently, several novel technologies for obtaining large numbers of single-cell transcriptomes at low cost have been reported including the use of nanowells (ICELL8) [43] and emulsion droplets (Drop-seq [44], inDrop [45], 10X Genomics [46]). These methods are able to drastically reduce the cost per transcriptome by incorporating cell barcodes during reverse transcription, eliminating the need for library preparation on each cell. One consequence to these approaches, however, is that only 3′ sequence information is retained and they are unable to capture sequence across the 5′ variable region of Ig transcripts. However, while SMART-Seq (as used in this study) and other well-based techniques are capable of generating high-quality transcriptome data with accurate clonotype information, the cost and low throughput are significant limitations. Ongoing improvements in automation and reduction in sequencing costs have mitigated these factors somewhat, and studies including > 5000 SMART-Seq transcriptomes have been published [47]. For most labs, however, datasets comprising a few hundred cells are practical, and are best suited for populations where the clonotypes of interest are enriched (e.g., antigen-specific cells), rather than for large-scale screening of paired repertoires.

One potential alternate use for the BALDR pipeline is for antibody cloning. Existing methodology uses primers specific for the V region followed by extensive PCR to obtain antibody sequences from plasmablasts [19, 48]. On a technical level, sc-RNA-seq combined with BALDR Ig reconstruction offers some advantages over traditional cloning. (1) The recovery of IgH + IgL sequences is highly efficient, at near 100% for plasmablasts and total B cells, and > 80% for antigen-specific memory B cells. Whereas this difference is marginal for reported cloning efficiencies for human plasmablasts (~ 70–80%) [19], it differs more significantly for non-plasmablast B cells with lower levels of immunoglobulin transcripts, and for plasma cells from rhesus macaques, where efficiencies are < 50% [22]. (2) Because BALDR has the ability to quantitate reconstructed Ig chains and select the most abundant chains, it is relatively resistant to interwell contamination. (3) Lastly, the use of template switching rather than multiplex priming at the 5′ end of the Ig transcript provides greater utility for recovery of antibodies in populations or animal models with poorly characterized V genes. Despite these advantages, sc-RNA-seq is about twice the cost per recovered Ig pair compared to conventional cloning, and it requires access to bioinformatics expertise; thus, the utility of BALDR for antibody cloning may be limited to unique circumstances (such as cloning from rhesus macaques). However, the continuing decline of sc-RNA-seq costs may lead to a more general use of sc-RNA-seq for antibody recovery.

Conclusions

Here, we have developed and validated a novel bioinformatics pipeline capable of accurate reconstruction of antibody gene sequences in humans and other animal models from sc-RNA-seq data, which offers flexibility in the sequencing format requirements of input data. The BALDR pipeline allows linking of sc-RNA-seq transcriptome data of individual B cells with antibody clonotype information and will likely have broad utility for dissecting antibody responses in vaccine studies and for longitudinal "lineage-tracing" studies in which clonotype data tracked over time can be mapped back to early B cell transcriptome information.

To enable open access to our method by researchers analyzing B cells using sc-RNA-seq, we have made all necessary scripts and supporting documentation to run the BALDR tool freely available for download (https://github.com/BosingerLab/BALDR). Additionally, to enable further advancement and refinement of bioinformatic strategies to reconstruct antibody genes, we have made available the validation dataset containing paired NGS + Sanger sequence data. The ability to link clonal dynamics, antibody specificity, and transcriptional information of antigen-specific B cells is likely to be of widespread use for multiple fields of immunology and genomics and to provide novel molecular insight into multiple aspects of B lymphocyte biology.

Additional files

Additional file 1; Supplementary figures and tables. (PDF 8130 kb)

Additional file 2: Results of Ig reconstruction using BALDR. The V(D)J gene annotations, CDR3 sequences, the number of reads mapping to the Ig chain using bowtie2, whether the chain is productive, and the complete sequences are shown for the Ig chains reconstructed using BALDR pipeline for all the human datasets (AW2-AW3 (SE151) plasmablast dataset with and without *in silico* read normalization, plasmablast AW1 (PE101, PE75, PE50, SE101, SE75, and SE50), the VH (PE76) CD19+ Lin– B cell dataset, and the AW2-AW3 (SE50) for IG_mapped+Unmapped method) and the rhesus macaque datasets (BL8, BL6.1, and BL6.2). When the RT-PCR sequence is available, the V(D)J genes and the CDR3 sequence are also shown for the corresponding chains, and concordance between the BALDR reconstructed chains and the RT-PCR sequence is indicated. The results for Ig reconstruction using the BASIC method are also shown along with matching RT-PCR for AW2-AW3 (SE101 and SE50), VH (PE76), and AW1 (PE101, PE75, PE50, SE101, SE75, and SE50) datasets.

Additional file 3: Clonal assignments for human single-cell datasets. The single cells were assigned to clonal families based on the V, J and CDR length for paired IGH and IgL chains.

Additional file 4: Discordant reconstructions for AW2_AW3 dataset IgH chains. The V, D, J genes, CDR3 sequences, and complete reconstructed sequence are shown for discordant IgH reconstructions along with annotations for Ig reconstruction with Unfiltered methods and the PCR sequence. Also included are models that were filtered in the BALDR pipeline, as they were not predicted to be productive.

Additional file 5: Somatic hypermutations in human single-cell datasets. The number of somatic hypermutations for AW2_AW3 plasmablast and VH CD19+ Lin– single cells compared to the IMGT germline sequences.

Additional file 6: Percentage of immunoglobulin reads in human plasmablasts and CD19+ Lin– B cells. The percentage of Ig reads is calculated by dividing the number of reads mapping to the top model

to the total number of reads for AW2-AW3 plasmablast dataset and VH CD19+ Lin– B cell dataset.

Additional file 7: Sequences from nested RT-PCR. The Ig chains obtained from Sanger sequencing of nested RT-PCR.

Abbreviations

BALDR: BCR Assignment of Lineage by De novo Reconstruction; D: Diversity gene segments; HIV: Human immunodeficiency virus; Ig: Immunoglobulin(s); IGH: Immunoglobulin heavy chain; IgH: Immunoglobulin heavy chain; IGK: Immunoglobulin kappa light chain; IGL: Immunoglobulin lambda light chain; IgL: Immunoglobulin light chain; J: Joining gene segments; NGS: Next generation sequencing; PBMC: Peripheral blood mononuclear cell; RT-PCR: Reverse transcription polymerase chain reaction; sc-RNA-seq: Single-cell RNA-seq; SIV: Simian immunodeficiency virus; TCR: T-cell receptor; V: Variable gene segments

Acknowledgements

We thank Robert Karaffa at the Emory School of Medicine flow cytometry core, as well as Aaron Rae at Emory Pediatric's flow cytometry core for their technical assistance with the cell sorting experiments. The authors are grateful to Hinel Patel at Emory University for conducting phlebotomy on vaccine recipients and to Jane Lawson for arranging the healthy blood donor cohort. We also thank Guido Silvestri, Diane Carnathan, Traci Legere, and the Yerkes Veterinary Staff at the Yerkes National Primate Research Center at Emory University for conducting NHP studies and providing samples. Sudhir Kasturi provided insightful discussion and ideas, and Rama Amara, R. Paul Johnson, John Altman, Carl Davis, and Rafi Ahmed provided critical advice on study direction. Lastly, we wish to acknowledge the contributions of the study volunteers and of the animals that provided samples.

Funding

This study was funded by grant U24 AI120134 (NIAID/NIH) to S.E.B, and UM1 AI124436 (NIAID/NIH) to S.E.B. and J.W.

Authors' contributions

AAU designed the study, developed the pipeline, performed bioinformatics analysis, analyzed data, and wrote the manuscript. RCK performed nested RT-PCR and Sanger sequencing. ANW and NBP carried out single-cell sequencing. AC sorted single-cell plasmablasts for human and rhesus macaques. SMR conducted single-cell center sorting of activated splenic germinal center B cells from rhesus macaques. CHD performed experiments to identify and sort Ag-specific memory B cells. RD sorted human CD19+ Lin– single cells. GKT developed the pipeline and analyzed data. BP designed the study and analyzed data. SC designed the study, analyzed data, and wrote the manuscript.

EHL and IS designed the study, oversaw the Institutional Review Board (IRB) of human studies, and provided flu vaccine samples. JW designed the study, analyzed data, and wrote the manuscript. SEB designed the study, developed the pipeline, analyzed data, and wrote the manuscript. All authors read and approved the final manuscript.

Ethics approval and consent to participate

Two healthy individuals were vaccinated with the 2016 Fluarix quadrivalent seasonal influenza vaccine. Vaccinated individuals who participated in this study provided informed consent in writing in accordance with the protocols approved by the IRB of Emory University IRB#00089789, entitled "sc-RNA-seq for clinical samples." Peripheral blood CD19+ B cells were obtained from a healthy, unvaccinated individual who provided informed consent and was recruited under the auspices of Emory IRB#00045821, entitled "Phlebotomy of healthy adults for the purpose of evaluation and validation of immune response assays." These protocols adhere to international guidelines established in the Declaration of Helsinki by the World Medical Association.

All rhesus macaque samples were obtained from animals undergoing vaccine studies housed at the Yerkes National Primate Research Center, which is accredited by the American Association of Accreditation of Laboratory Animal Care. This study was performed in strict accordance with the recommendations in the Guide for the Care and Use of Laboratory Animals of the National Institutes of Health, a national set of guidelines in the USA, and also to international recommendations detailed in the Weatherall Report (2006). This work received prior approval by the Institutional Animal Care and Use Committees (IACUC) of Emory University (IACUC protocol #YER-2002353-061916GA, entitled Center for HIV/AIDS Vaccine Immunology and Immunogen Discovery-Parent Project, and #2000936, entitled B-cell Biology of Mucosal Immune Protection from SIV Challenge. Appropriate procedures were performed to ensure that potential distress, pain, discomfort, and/or injury were limited to that unavoidable in the conduct of the research plan. The sedative ketamine (10 mg/kg) and/or tiletamine/zolazepam (Telazol, 4 mg/kg) was applied as necessary for blood draws, and analgesics were used when determined appropriate by veterinary medical staff.

Competing interests

The authors declare that they have no competing interests.

Author details

[1]Division of Microbiology and Immunology, Yerkes National Primate Research Center, Atlanta, GA, USA. [2]Department of Pediatrics, School of Medicine, Emory University, Atlanta, GA, USA. [3]Yerkes NHP Genomics Core Laboratory, Yerkes National Primate Research Center, 954 Gatewood Rd, Atlanta, GA 30329, USA. [4]Division of Vaccine Discovery, La Jolla Institute for Allergy and Immunology, La Jolla, CA, USA. [5]Scripps Center for HIV/AIDS Vaccine Immunology and Immunogen Discovery (CHAVI-ID), La Jolla, CA, USA. [6]Division of Rheumatology, School of Medicine, Emory University, Atlanta, GA, USA. [7]Institute for Immunity, Transplantation and Infection, Stanford University School of Medicine, Stanford, CA, USA. [8]Department of Pathology, Stanford University School of Medicine, Stanford, CA, USA. [9]Department of Microbiology and Immunology, Stanford University School of Medicine, Stanford, CA, USA. [10]Division of Infectious Diseases, Department of Medicine, University of California, San Diego, La Jolla, CA, USA. [11]Divisions of Pulmonary, Allergy and Critical Care Medicine, Emory University, Atlanta, GA, USA. [12]Department of Pathology & Laboratory Medicine, School of Medicine, Emory University, Atlanta, GA, USA.

References

1. Teng G, Papavasiliou FN. Immunoglobulin somatic hypermutation. Annu Rev Genet. 2007;41:107–20.

2. Lefranc M-P, Lefranc G. The immunoglobulin factsbook. London: Academic Press; 2001.

3. Lefranc M. IMGT® databases, web resources and tools for immunoglobulin and T cell receptor sequence analysis. Leukemia. 2003;17:260.

4. Yaari G, Kleinstein SH. Practical guidelines for B-cell receptor repertoire sequencing analysis. Genome Med. 2015;7:121.

5. Newell EW, Davis MM. Beyond model antigens: high-dimensional methods for the analysis of antigen-specific T cells. Nat Biotechnol. 2014;32:149–57.

6. Georgiou G, Ippolito GC, Beausang J, Busse CE, Wardemann H, Quake SR. The promise and challenge of high-throughput sequencing of the antibody repertoire. Nat Biotechnol. 2014;32:158–68.

7. Calis JJ, Rosenberg BR. Characterizing immune repertoires by high throughput sequencing: strategies and applications. Trends Immunol. 2014; 8:00155–0.

8. Turchaninova MA, Davydov A, Britanova OV, Shugay M, Bikos V, Egorov ES, Kirgizova VI, Merzlyak EM, Staroverov DB, Bolotin DA, et al. High-quality full-length immunoglobulin profiling with unique molecular barcoding. Nat Protoc. 2016;11:1599–616.

9. DeKosky BJ, Kojima T, Rodin A, Charab W, Ippolito GC, Ellington AD, Georgiou G. In-depth determination and analysis of the human paired heavy-and light-chain antibody repertoire. Nat Med. 2015;21:86–91.

10. Busse CE, Czogiel I, Braun P, Arndt PF, Wardemann H. Single-cell based high-throughput sequencing of full-length immunoglobulin heavy and light chain genes. Eur J Immunol. 2014;44:597–603. https://doi.org/10.1002/eji.201343917.

11. DeKosky BJ, Ippolito GC, Deschner RP, Lavinder JJ, Wine Y, Rawlings BM, Varadarajan N, Giesecke C, Dorner T, Andrews SF, et al. High-throughput sequencing of the paired human immunoglobulin heavy and light chain repertoire. Nat Biotechnol. 2013;31:166–9. https://doi.org/10.1038/nbt.2492.

12. Han A, Glanville J, Hansmann L, Davis MM. Linking T-cell receptor sequence to functional phenotype at the single-cell level. Nat Biotechnol. 2014;32:684–92. https://doi.org/10.1038/nbt.2938.

13. Tan YC, Kongpachith S, Blum LK, Ju CH, Lahey LJ, Lu DR, Cai X, Wagner CA, Lindstrom TM, Sokolove J. Barcode-enabled sequencing of plasmablast antibody repertoires in rheumatoid arthritis. Arthritis Rheumatol. 2014;66:2706–15.

14. Tan Y-C, Blum LK, Kongpachith S, Ju C-H, Cai X, Lindstrom TM, Sokolove J, Robinson WH. High-throughput sequencing of natively paired antibody chains provides evidence for original antigenic sin shaping the antibody response to influenza vaccination. Clin Immunol. 2014;151:55–65.

15. Robinson WH. Sequencing the functional antibody repertoire—diagnostic and therapeutic discovery. Nat Rev Rheumatol. 2015;11:171–82.

16. Stubbington MJT, Lonnberg T, Proserpio V, Clare S, Speak AO, Dougan G, Teichmann SA. T cell fate and clonality inference from single-cell transcriptomes. Nat Methods. 2016;13:329–32.

17. Eltahla AA, Rizzetto S, Pirozyan MR, Betz-Stablein BD, Venturi V, Kedzierska K, Lloyd AR, Bull RA, Luciani F. Linking the T cell receptor to the single cell transcriptome in antigen-specific human T cells. Immunol Cell Biol. 2016;94:604–11.

18. Grabherr MG, Haas BJ, Yassour M, Levin JZ, Thompson DA, Amit I, Adiconis X, Fan L, Raychowdhury R, Zeng Q. Trinity: reconstructing a full-length transcriptome without a genome from RNA-Seq data. Nat Biotechnol. 2011; 29:644.

19. Wrammert J, Smith K, Miller J, Langley WA, Kokko K, Larsen C, Zheng NY, Mays I, Garman L, Helms C, et al. Rapid cloning of high-affinity human monoclonal antibodies against influenza virus. Nature. 2008;453:667–71. https://doi.org/10.1038/nature06890.

20. Smith K, Garman L, Wrammert J, Zheng N-Y, Capra JD, Ahmed R, Wilson PC. Rapid generation of fully human monoclonal antibodies specific to a vaccinating antigen. Nat Protoc. 2009;4:372.

21. Kasturi SP, Kozlowski PA, Nakaya HI, Burger MC, Russo P, Pham M, Kovalenkov Y, Silveira EL, Havenar-Daughton C, Burton SL, et al. Adjuvanting a simian immunodeficiency virus vaccine with Toll-like receptor ligands encapsulated in nanoparticles induces persistent antibody responses and enhanced protection in TRIM5α restrictive macaques. J Virol. 2017;91:e01844–16.

22. Silveira EL, Kasturi SP, Kovalenkov Y, Rasheed AU, Yeiser P, Jinnah ZS, Legere TH, Pulendran B, Villinger F, Wrammert J. Vaccine-induced plasmablast responses in rhesus macaques: phenotypic characterization and a source for generating antigen-specific monoclonal antibodies. J Immunol Methods. 2015;416:69–83.

23. Bolger AM, Lohse M, Usadel B. Trimmomatic: a flexible trimmer for Illumina sequence data. Bioinformatics. 2014;30:2114–20.

24. Cunningham F, Amode MR, Barrell D, Beal K, Billis K, Brent S, Carvalho-Silva D, Clapham P, Coates G, Fitzgerald S, et al. Ensembl 2015. Nucleic Acids Res. 2015;43:D662–9.

25. Dobin A, Davis CA, Schlesinger F, Drenkow J, Zaleski C, Jha S, Batut P, Chaisson M, Gingeras TR. STAR: ultrafast universal RNA-seq aligner. Bioinformatics. 2013; 29:15–21.

26. Li H, Handsaker B, Wysoker A, Fennell T, Ruan J, Homer N, Marth G, Abecasis G, Durbin R. The sequence alignment/map format and SAMtools. Bioinformatics. 2009;25:2078–9.

27. Langmead B, Salzberg SL. Fast gapped-read alignment with Bowtie 2. Nat Methods. 2012;9:357–9.

28. Ye J, Ma N, Madden TL, Ostell JM. IgBLAST: an immunoglobulin variable domain sequence analysis tool. Nucleic Acids Res. 2013;41:W34–40.

29. Camacho C, Coulouris G, Avagyan V, Ma N, Papadopoulos J, Bealer K, Madden TL. BLAST+: architecture and applications. BMC Bioinformatics. 2009;10:421.

30. Alamyar E, Giudicelli V, Li S, Duroux P, Lefranc M-P. IMGT/HighV-QUEST: the IMGT® web portal for immunoglobulin (IG) or antibody and T cell receptor (TR) analysis from NGS high throughput and deep sequencing. Immunome Res. 2012;8:26.

31. Zimin AV, Cornish AS, Maudhoo MD, Gibbs RM, Zhang X, Pandey S, Meehan DT, Wipfler K, Bosinger SE, Johnson ZP, et al. A new rhesus macaque assembly and annotation for next-generation sequencing analyses. Biol Direct. 2014;9:20.

32. Sundling C, Phad G, Douagi I, Navis M, Karlsson Hedestam GB. Isolation of antibody V(D)J sequences from single cell sorted rhesus macaque B cells. J Immunol Methods. 2012;386:85–93.

33. Ramesh A, Darko S, Hua A, Overman G, Ransier A, Francica JR, Trama A, Tomaras GD, Haynes BF, Douek DC, Kepler TB. Structure and diversity of the rhesus macaque immunoglobulin loci through multiple de novo genome assemblies. Front Immunol. 2017;8:1407.

34. Quinlan AR, Hall IM. BEDTools: a flexible suite of utilities for comparing genomic features. Bioinformatics. 2010;26:841–2.

35. Ellebedy AH, Jackson KJ, Kissick HT, Nakaya HI, Davis CW, Roskin KM, McElroy AK, Oshansky CM, Elbein R, Thomas S, et al. Defining antigen-specific plasmablast and memory B cell subsets in human blood after viral infection or vaccination. Nat Immunol. 2016;17:1226–34.

36. Wrammert J, Koutsonanos D, Li GM, Edupuganti S, Sui J, Morrissey M, McCausland M, Skountzou I, Hornig M, Lipkin WI, et al. Broadly cross-reactive antibodies dominate the human B cell response against 2009 pandemic H1N1 influenza virus infection. J Exp Med. 2011;208:181–93.

37. Canzar S, Neu KE, Tang Q, Wilson PC, Khan AA. BASIC: BCR assembly from single cells. Bioinformatics. 2017;33:425–7.

38. Kelsoe G, Haynes BF. Host controls of HIV broadly neutralizing antibody development. Immunol Rev. 2017;275:79–88.

39. Sundling C, Zhang Z, Phad GE, Sheng Z, Wang Y, Mascola JR, Li Y, Wyatt RT, Shapiro L, Karlsson Hedestam GB. Single-cell and deep sequencing of IgG-switched macaque B cells reveal a diverse Ig repertoire following immunization. J Immunol. 2014;192:3637–44.

40. Hagan T, Pulendran B. Will systems biology deliver its promise and contribute to the development of new or improved vaccines? From data to understanding through systems biology. Cold Spring Harb Perspect Biol. 2017; https://doi.org/10.1101/cshperspect.a028894.

41. Svensson V, Natarajan KN, Ly LH, Miragaia RJ, Labalette C, Macaulay IC, Cvejic A, Teichmann SA. Power analysis of single-cell RNA-sequencing experiments. Nat Methods. 2017;14:381–7.

42. Scheepers C, Shrestha RK, Lambson BE, Jackson KJ, Wright IA, Naicker D, Goosen M, Berrie L, Ismail A, Garrett N, et al. Ability to develop broadly neutralizing HIV-1 antibodies is not restricted by the germline Ig gene repertoire. J Immunol. 2015;194:4371–8.

43. Goldstein LD, Chen YJ, Dunne J, Mir A, Hubschle H, Guillory J, Yuan W, Zhang J, Stinson J, Jaiswal B, et al. Massively parallel nanowell-based single-cell gene expression profiling. BMC Genomics. 2017;18:519.

44. Macosko EZ, Basu A, Satija R, Nemesh J, Shekhar K, Goldman M, Tirosh I, Bialas AR, Kamitaki N, Martersteck EM. Highly parallel genome-wide expression profiling of individual cells using nanoliter droplets. Cell. 2015; 161:1202–14.

45. Klein AM, Mazutis L, Akartuna I, Tallapragada N, Veres A, Li V, Peshkin L, Weitz DA, Kirschner MW. Droplet barcoding for single-cell transcriptomics applied to embryonic stem cells. Cell. 2015;161:1187–201.

46. Zheng GX, Terry JM, Belgrader P, Ryvkin P, Bent ZW, Wilson R, Ziraldo SB, Wheeler TD, McDermott GP, Zhu J, et al. Massively parallel digital transcriptional profiling of single cells. Nat Commun. 2017;8:14049.

47. Puram SV, Tirosh I, Parikh AS, Patel AP, Yizhak K, Gillespie S, Rodman C, Luo CL, Mroz EA, Emerick KS. Single-cell transcriptomic analysis of primary and metastatic tumor ecosystems in head and neck cancer. Cell. 2017;171:1611-24.

48. Liao HX, Levesque MC, Nagel A, Dixon A, Zhang R, Walter E, Parks R, Whitesides J, Marshall DJ, Hwang KK, et al. High-throughput isolation of immunoglobulin genes from single human B cells and expression as monoclonal antibodies. J Virol Methods. 2009;158:171–9.

12

Landscape of genomic alterations in high-grade serous ovarian cancer from exceptional long- and short-term survivors

S. Y. Cindy Yang[1,2], Stephanie Lheureux[1,3], Katherine Karakasis[1], Julia V. Burnier[1], Jeffery P. Bruce[1],
Derek L. Clouthier[1], Arnavaz Danesh[1], Rene Quevedo[1,2], Mark Dowar[1], Youstina Hanna[1], Tiantian Li[1], Lin Lu[1],
Wei Xu[1], Blaise A. Clarke[4,5], Pamela S. Ohashi[1,2,6], Patricia A. Shaw[4,5], Trevor J. Pugh[1,2,7]* and Amit M. Oza[1,3]*

Abstract

Background: Patients diagnosed with high-grade serous ovarian cancer (HGSOC) who received initial debulking surgery followed by platinum-based chemotherapy can experience highly variable clinical responses. A small percentage of women experience exceptional long-term survival (long term (LT), 10+ years), while others develop primary resistance to therapy and succumb to disease in less than 2 years (short term (ST)). To improve clinical management of HGSOC, there is a need to better characterize clinical and molecular profiles to identify factors that underpin these disparate survival responses.

Methods: To identify clinical and tumor molecular biomarkers associated with exceptional clinical response or resistance, we conducted an integrated clinical, exome, and transcriptome analysis of 41 primary tumors from LT ($n = 20$) and ST ($n = 21$) HGSOC patients.

Results: Younger age at diagnosis, no residual disease post debulking surgery and low CA125 levels following surgery and chemotherapy were clinical characteristics of LT. Tumors from LT survivors had increased somatic mutation burden (median 1.62 vs. 1.22 non-synonymous mutations/Mbp), frequent BRCA1/2 biallelic inactivation through mutation and loss of heterozygosity, and enrichment of activated CD4+, CD8+ T cells, and effector memory CD4+ T cells. Characteristics of ST survival included focal copy number gain of *CCNE1*, lack of *BRCA* mutation signature, low homologous recombination deficiency scores, and the presence of *ESR1-CCDC170* gene fusion.

Conclusions: Our findings suggest that exceptional long- or short-term survival is determined by a concert of clinical, molecular, and microenvironment factors.

Keywords: Ovarian cancer, Immuno-genomics, Tumor microenvironment

Background

High-grade serous ovarian cancer (HGSOC) is the most lethal gynecologic malignancy, accounting for 70–80% of ovarian cancer deaths worldwide [1]. Despite promising results with cytoreductive surgery and platinum-based chemotherapy, more than 75% of women with HGSOC will relapse after completion of first-line therapy [2]. The window of opportunity to tailor therapeutic interventions to control progressive disease is limited due to the inherent cellular heterogeneity and genomic instability of HGSOC. While platinum chemotherapy is the cornerstone of contemporary treatment, ultimately, the majority of women with epithelial ovarian cancer (EOC) will develop chemotherapy resistance and succumb to their disease within 5 years of diagnosis (46.2% 5-year survival) [3]. However, 16% of patients with serous histology experience overall survival greater than 10 years [4]. In contrast, other patients diagnosed at the same disease stage and treated with similar therapeutic approaches will experience rapid disease

* Correspondence: trevor.pugh@utoronto.ca; amit.oza@uhn.ca
S Y Cindy Yang and Stephanie Lheureux are joint first authors.
Trevor J Pugh and Amit M Oza are joint senior authors.
[1]Princess Margaret Cancer Centre, University Health Network, 610 University Avenue, Toronto, Ontario M5G 2M9, Canada
Full list of author information is available at the end of the article

progression. Current clinical algorithms cannot discern these patient survival outcomes at the time of diagnosis and therefore patients are given similar treatment.

In many ovarian cancer studies, age at diagnosis, disease stage, grade, histology, residual disease post-surgery, and disease recurrence have been identified and validated to have prognostic value [4, 5]. Molecular characteristics such as *BRCA1/2* mutations [6, 7] and homologous repair deficiency in HGSOC have been demonstrated and validated as predictive of response to platinum therapy and poly-ADP polymerase (PARP) inhibitors [7–9]. In addition, recent publications have demonstrated that immune cell populations infiltrating ovarian tumor tissue may be prognostic [10–14]. However, without complete long-term follow-up information to accompany patient and tumor molecular profiles, clinical and molecular factors that contribute to long-term (LT) and short-term (ST) survival in HGSOC remain elusive.

In this pilot study, we sought to identify clinical and molecular factors that distinguish HGSOC patients who share similar clinical characteristics and pathology at diagnosis with exceptional survival outcomes, either LT or ST, through integrated analysis of clinical features, germline variants, somatic genomic alterations, and tumor immune microenvironment.

Methods

Sample inclusion criteria

We identified patients from the Princess Margaret Cancer Registry diagnosed with HGSOC who underwent primary debulking surgery. To obtain a clinically homogeneous population at diagnosis, we selected patients with the following criteria: (1) diagnosis of advanced HGSOC confirmed by an expert gynecologic pathologist and stage III according to the FIGO classification; (2) primary debulking surgery followed by at least 6 cycles of platinum-based chemotherapy; and (3) availability of chemotherapy-naïve tumor and matched normal tissue of sufficient quantity and quality for molecular analysis. Patient cohorts representing extreme tails of the HGSOC overall survival distribution were selected for comparison in this study. Short-term survival patients were defined as patients with (1) overall survival between 6 months and 2 years, (2) primary platinum resistance, and (3) documented disease progression within 6 months from completing platinum-based chemotherapy. Patients with LT survival had durable platinum sensitivity and were identified based on OS greater than 10 years following HGSOC diagnosis (Additional file 1: Figures S1, S2A). The presence of residual disease post debulking surgery was collected from the original surgical notes.

Patient tissues processing

Treatment-naïve frozen or formalin-fixed paraffin-embedded (FFPE) preserved primary HGSOC tumors and matched normal tissues from these patients were obtained from the University Health Network Biobank with Research Ethics Board approval. DNA and RNA were co-isolated from available tissues using Qiagen AllPrep DNA/RNA/miRNA Universal kit or the Qiagen AllPrep DNA/RNA FFPE kit following the manufacturer's protocol.

TCGA data

TCGA data for HGSOC was downloaded from Broad GDAC Firebrowse (http://firebrowse.org/?cohort=OV/). RNA-seq V2 FASTQ files for each TCGA OV sample was downloaded from Genomic Data Commons Data Portal (https://portal.gdc.cancer.gov).

Exome and RNA sequencing

Exome libraries were constructed from 200ng starting genomic DNA using the Agilent SureSelect Human All Exon V5+UTRs kit. One hundred base pair paired-end reads were sequenced using Illumina HiSeq 2000 or 2500 instruments to 250X target read depth for tumor and 50X for normal tissue libraries. Tumor RNA libraries were prepared from 200ng of RNA using the Illumina TruSeq Stranded Total RNA kit with Ribo-Zero Gold. Libraries were sequenced with pair-end 100 cycles V3 using Illumina HiSeq 2000 to achieve a minimum of ~ 80 million reads per sample. Whole exome FASTQ files were aligned to reference human genome hg19 using BWA [15] and pre-processed following GATK Best Practices Protocol [16, 17]. RNA-seq FASTQ files were aligned to human genome version hg19 and transcript annotation GENCODE v19 (Additional file 2).

Mutational profiling

Germline variants were called using GATK HaplotypeCaller (version 1.130) from normal tissue BAM files with default settings. Somatic mutations were called from tumor/normal BAM file pairs using muTect (version 1.1.4) [18], Varscan2 (version 2.4.2) [19], and Strelka (version 1.0.14)) [20] for single nucleotide variations (SNVs) and small insertions and deletions (Indels) on paired normal and tumor tissue BAM files. Mutations were annotated using Oncotator (version 1.5.3) [21]. Deep sequencing of all coding exons of *TP53* was performed on all tumors lacking detectable *TP53* mutation in exome data using custom hybrid-capture probes (Additional file 2).

CNV profiling

Sequencing depth ratios for each tumor and normal exome pair were collected using GATK mpileup (version 3.3.0) using paired sample mode. Varscan2 (version 2.4.2) [19] was used to identify contiguous segments of DNA with similar depth ratio and variant allele frequencies. Given DNA copy segments and SNPs, and tumor cellularity estimate from *TP53* mutation allele fraction, Sequenza (version 2.1.2) [22] was used to estimate the tumor ploidy and allele-specific copy number for each DNA segment. GISTIC2 (version 2.0.22) [23] was used to identify recurrent somatic copy number alterations (SCNAs) across the cohort and within each survival group. For copy number analysis of specific genes such as *TP53*, *BRCA1*, *BRCA2*, and *CCNE1*, segment files containing total and allele-specific copy numbers were annotated using a custom R script. We defined a focally amplified gene (defined as < 3 Mb according to Krijgsman et al. [24]) as having a copy number greater than the estimated sample ploidy plus 2. We selected a purity-corrected absolute copy number of 2 above background ploidy (i.e., ploidy = 4 for largely diploid genomes) as this is the threshold commonly used for reporting clinical cytogenetic alterations in cancer. We also selected this relatively high threshold to avoid reporting false-positive variants from arm-level chromosomal alterations inherent to the highly complex genomes found in ovarian cancer, as well as the varying tumor content levels encountered in clinical specimens such as those used in our study. As shown in Additional file 3, this approach ensures that we are focused on clearly focally amplified regions that stand out from a highly aneuploid background. Loss of heterozygosity (LOH) was defined as the lack of the alternate allele (B allele copy number = 0). A focal gene deletion was defined as copy number less than the global ploidy minus 1 and lacking the alternate allele. The HRD-LOH score, the number of large (> 15 Mbp, less than a chromosome arm) LOH genomic segments, was determined for each tumor CNV profile.

Immune enrichment analysis

We used single sample gene set enrichment analysis (ssGSEA) [25] to assess the gene set activation score of each tumor specimen (LT (n = 13), ST (n = 16)). Immune-reactive HGSOC subtype [26] and ESTIMATE immune score [27] gene sets were used to infer overall immune infiltration by ssGSEA. Gene sets describing specific immune cell types (activated CD8$^+$ T, activated CD4$^+$ T, T cells, effector memory CD8$^+$ T, effector memory CD4$^+$ T, NK cells, macrophages, T-regs, and activated B cells) are used to infer cell-type-specific infiltration levels [28]. GSVA R-package (version 1.22) [29] implementation of ssGSEA was used to calculate sample scores. For each gene set, z-score normalization of ssGSEA scores centered at medians was applied across all samples.

Fusion gene detection

Tophat fusion (tophat2 version 2.0.8b) [30] with default parameters was used to nominate potential fusion transcripts from RNA-seq data. Fusion candidates were filtered and prioritized based on total number of junction spanning reads (> 10), read pairs spanning fusion gene partners (> 2), and read pairs containing a read that partially span the fusion junction (> 0).

Statistical methods

To compare continuous variables such as mutation frequency, gene-expression, HDR-LOH score, and gene-set enrichment scores between two groups, two-sided non-parametric Wilcoxon Rank Sum tests were used to assess statistical significance. Two-sided Fisher's exact tests were used for comparisons of discrete or dichotomized variables such as *BRCA* mutation enrichment, *TP53* mutation enrichment, *CCNE1* amplification enrichment, HRD-LOH scores, and HRD mutation signature enrichment. Given two categorical variables, Fisher's exact test was applied to assess whether the proportions of one categorical variable are independent of the other one. Wilcoxon Rank Sum tests were conducted to test whether the medians of the distributions of a continuous variable in stratified groups are the same. Spearman correlation was conducted to test the monotonic relationship between two continuous variables. Two-sided tests were conducted with significance level at 0.05. All data consolidation, statistical testing, and data visualization were performed using SAS 9.4 and R-scripts in the R (version 3.3.1) [31] statistical environment. Power analysis is provided in Additional file 2.

Results

Clinical description of the study cohort

From 829 patients with HGSOC entered in the Princess Margaret (PM) Cancer Registry from 2000 to 2013, we selected two cohorts of patients with exceptionally ST (< 2 years, 20 patients) and LT OS (≥ 10 years, 21 patients) (Table 1, Additional file 1: Figures S1, S2A). On average, patients with LT survival were younger than ST (56 vs. 61 years mean age at diagnosis) and were less likely to have residual disease post-surgery (35% versus 76%). Disease recurred in all ST patients and 3 (3/20, 15%) LT patients. Cancer antigen 125 (CA125) levels in the blood serum at diagnosis did not correlate with survival; however, LT survivors had significantly lower CA125 levels post-surgery and at the end of chemotherapy (Table 1) ($p < 0.001$).

As independent validation of our observation, we identified patients with similar clinical data made available through a study of serous ovarian cancer by The Cancer Genome Atlas (TCGA) [32]. From data accessed on November 1, 2016, we found 214 of 603 patients with stage III HGSOC and completed overall survival data. Applying the same selection criteria used to filter the PM cohort, we identified 60 of 288 patients had primary platinum resistance and OS between 6 months and 2 years (28%),

Table 1 Clinical characteristics of patients diagnosed with stage III, grade III, serous ovarian epithelial cancer at Princess Margaret by length of survival

Covariate	Full Sample (n = 41)	LT (n = 20)	ST (n = 21)	p value
Number of patients	41	20	21	
Stage III, HGSOC	41 (100)	20 (49)	21 (51)	
Overall Survival				< 0.001
< 6 months	0 (0)	0 (0)	0 (0)	
6–12 months	2 (5)	0 (0)	4 (19)	
12–24 months	19 (46)	0 (0)	17 (81)	
> 24 months	20 (49)	20 (100)	0 (0)	
Age at diagnosis				0.024
Mean (sd)	59 (9.3)	56.1 (9.4)	61.7 (8.7)	0.024
Median (min,max)	57 (40,84)	55.5 (40,84)	59 (47,76)	
Residual disease				0.012
No	18 (44)	13 (65)	5 (24)	
Yes	23 (56)	7 (35)	16 (76)	
Disease recurrence				< 0.001
No	17 (41)	17 (85)	0 (0)	
Yes	24 (59)	3 (15)	21 (100)	
Number of disease recurrence				< 0.001
0	17 (41)	17 (85)	0 (0)	
1	15 (37)	1 (5)	14 (67)	
2	7 (17)	1 (5)	6 (29)	
> 2	2 (5)	1 (5)	1 (5)	
CA125 at diagnosis				0.39
Mean (sd)	1207 (1781.6)	870.4 (863.1)	1491 (2277.9)	
Median (min,max)	475 (67,9162)	585 (67,2700)	399 (184,9162)	
Missing	**6**	**4**	**2**	
CA125 at diagnosis rate				0.41
Unknown	6 (15)	4 (20)	2 (10)	
0–35 U/mL	0 (0)	0 (0)	0 (0)	
> 35 U/mL	35 (85)	16 (80)	19 (90)	
CA125 post-surgery				< 0.001
Mean (sd)	421 (932.4)	63.9 (74.8)	799.1 (1243.4)	
Median (min,max)	121 (7,4712)	33 (7299)	296 (53,4712)	
Missing	**6**	**2**	**4**	
CA125 post-surgery rate				< 0.001
Unknown	6 (15)	2 (10)	4 (19)	
0–35 U/mL	9 (22)	9 (45)	0 (0)	
> 35 U/mL	26 (63)	9 (45)	17 (81)	
CA125 post chemotherapy				< 0.001
Mean (sd)	656.4 (3772.9)	4.6 (2.1)	1308 (5325.7)	
Median (min,max)	6.5 (2,23,290)	4 (2,10)	18 (4, 23,287)	
Missing	**3**	**1**	**2**	

Table 1 Clinical characteristics of patients diagnosed with stage III, grade III, serous ovarian epithelial cancer at Princess Margaret by length of survival *(Continued)*

Covariate	Full Sample (*n* = 41)	LT (*n* = 20)	ST (*n* = 21)	*p* value
CA125 post chemotherapy rate				*0.0063*
Unknown	3 (7)	1 (5)	2 (10)	
0–35 U/mL	31 (76)	19 (95)	12 (57)	
> 35 U/mL	7 (17)	0 (0)	7 (33)	

and 10 patients (5%) with extended platinum sensitivity and OS ≥ 10 years (Additional file 1: Figure S2B). Consistent with the PM cohort, the median age of diagnosis was lower for LT compared to ST patients (60.5 vs. 67 years median age at diagnosis). While CA125 levels were not available in the TCGA cohort clinical data, > 85% of ST survivors had measurable tumor burden post-surgery and 40% (4/10) LT patients had residual disease.

High somatic mutation burden is associated with long-term survival in HGSOC

To identify genomic features associated with LT survival, we conducted exome and transcriptome analysis of 39 tumors at diagnosis and matched normal material from patients registered at PM (19 ST and 20 LT; 2 ST tumors from the clinical analysis were not included due to low-quality genomic data; Additional file 4: Tables S1, S2). Exomes were sequenced to median coverage 235× in tumors and 67× normal. Tumor transcriptomes were sequenced using a median 208 million reads. This analysis uncovered a median mutation frequency of 1.49 non-synonymous mutations per megabase (Fig. 1a) (range 0.678–6.740) consistent with TCGA report (Fig. 1b). In our cohort, and in the TCGA data, we found that mutation frequency was higher in LT versus ST samples ($p = 0.022$, median 1.62 vs. 1.22 non-synonymous mutations/Mbp). The tumor with the highest mutation burden was a carrier of a pathogenic *BRCA1* variant (p.Asn1236Phefs) and harbored two-hit somatic inactivation of *MLH1* through a truncating mutation (p.Ser170-Argfs*20) coupled with loss of heterozygosity of chromosome 3p22.2 (Fig. 2), consistent with hypermutation seen in other cancers [33]. Increased mutation rate has been associated with enhanced immunogenicity in other tumors [34] and may explain increased survival in HGSOC. A long-term survivor patient in the TCGA cohort also carried a somatic *MLH1* mutation (p.Arg100Ter).

Consistent with genome landscape studies of HGSOC [32, 35, 36], *TP53* (38/39, 97%), *BRCA1* (7/39, 18%), and *BRCA2* (6/39, 15%) were the most frequently mutated genes in our cohort (Fig. 2). Genes mutated at lower frequencies in HGSOC (*CDK12*, *KRAS*, *PTEN*, *RB1*, *EFEMP1*, and *NF1*)

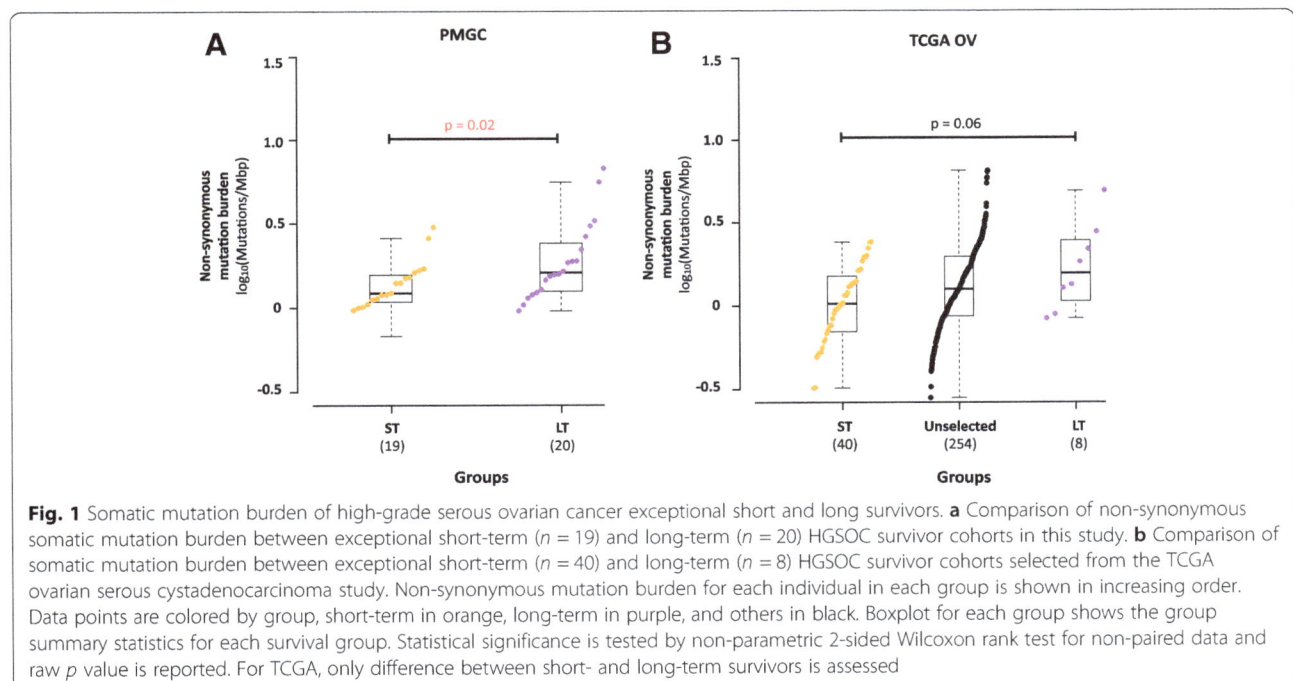

Fig. 1 Somatic mutation burden of high-grade serous ovarian cancer exceptional short and long survivors. **a** Comparison of non-synonymous somatic mutation burden between exceptional short-term (*n* = 19) and long-term (*n* = 20) HGSOC survivor cohorts in this study. **b** Comparison of somatic mutation burden between exceptional short-term (*n* = 40) and long-term (*n* = 8) HGSOC survivor cohorts selected from the TCGA ovarian serous cystadenocarcinoma study. Non-synonymous mutation burden for each individual in each group is shown in increasing order. Data points are colored by group, short-term in orange, long-term in purple, and others in black. Boxplot for each group shows the group summary statistics for each survival group. Statistical significance is tested by non-parametric 2-sided Wilcoxon rank test for non-paired data and raw *p* value is reported. For TCGA, only difference between short- and long-term survivors is assessed

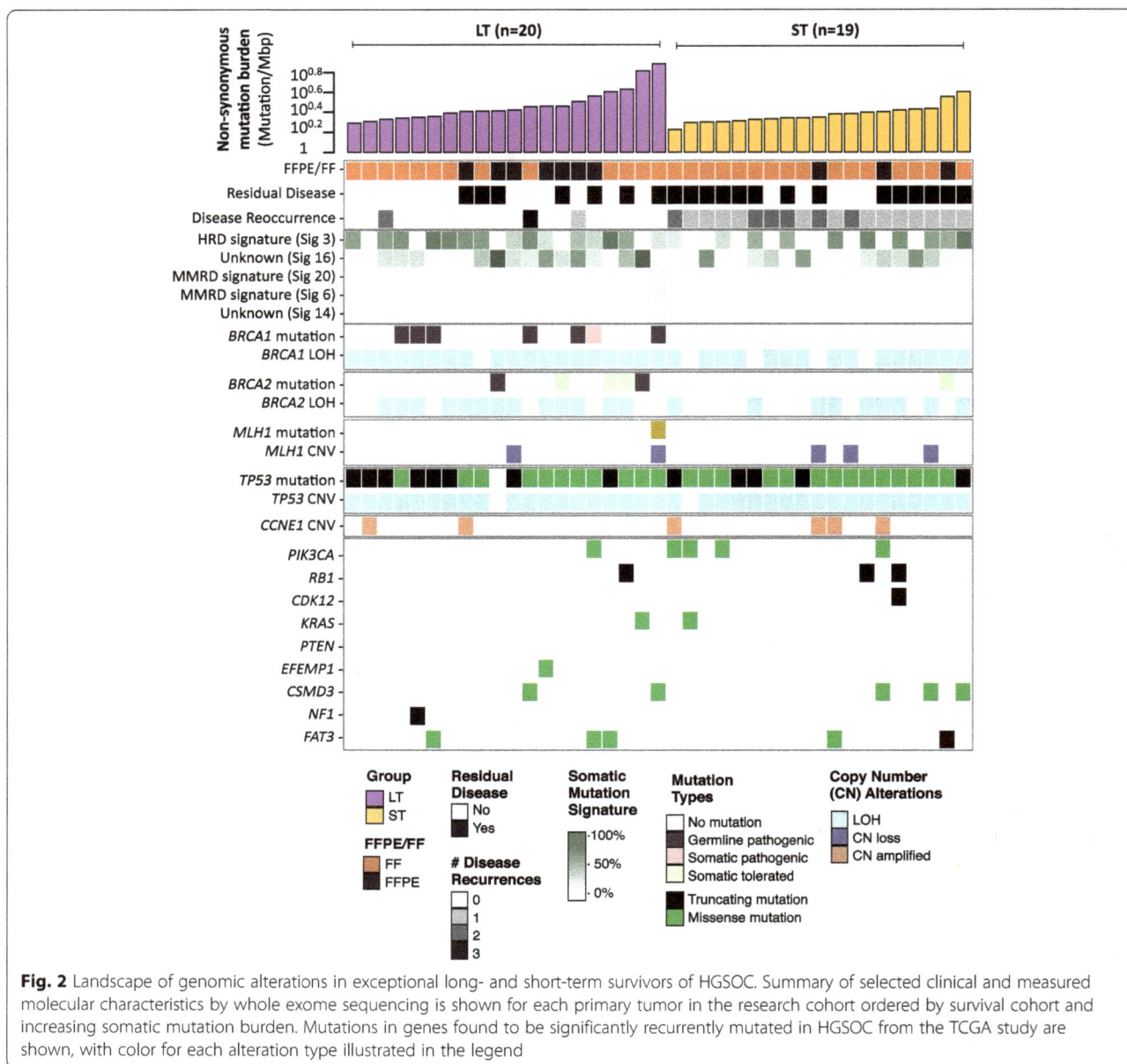

Fig. 2 Landscape of genomic alterations in exceptional long- and short-term survivors of HGSOC. Summary of selected clinical and measured molecular characteristics by whole exome sequencing is shown for each primary tumor in the research cohort ordered by survival cohort and increasing somatic mutation burden. Mutations in genes found to be significantly recurrently mutated in HGSOC from the TCGA study are shown, with color for each alteration type illustrated in the legend

were mutated in < 10% of our cohort, consistent with the TCGA data.

Loss of BRCA1 or BRCA2 function is a molecular characteristic of long-term survival

We observed an enrichment of *BRCA1* and *BRCA2* mutations in the LT compared to the ST group (LT = 12/20, ST = 1/19, Fisher's exact p = 0.0004) (Table 2). Pathogenic germline mutations in *BRCA1* and *BRCA2* are identified exclusively in the long-term survivors (*BRCA1* = 6, *BRCA2* = 2). Of the 5 somatic mutations identified in *BRCA1* and *BRCA2*, only 2 were truncation mutations that could result in loss of *BRCA1/2* function (*BRCA1* p.Trp1712Ter and *BRCA2* p.ThrAsp1867fs). All

somatic mutations detected are also coupled with loss of heterozygosity (LOH) in the corresponding gene locus. One tumor from a ST patient had a somatic missense mutation in *BRCA2* (p.Pro2257Ser, MAF = 0.15) that is classified as tolerated and benign by SIFT (score = 0.12) and PolyPhen2 (score = 0.047), and therefore considered as non-pathogenic. This mutation has also never been reported in other tumors within the COSMIC database.

Overall, tumors with loss of function *BRCA1/2* mutations had a trend towards higher mutation frequency compared to tumors with intact *BRCA1/2* (p = 0.059) (Fig. 3a), with *BRCA2*-mutated tumors having the highest mutation burden, suggesting that defects in DNA

Table 2 Germline and somatic mutations in *BRCA1* and *BRCA2*

Patient ID	Group	Germline/somatic	Gene	Protein Change	MAF (normal)	MAF (tumor)	Pathogenic/Tolerated	LOH	COSMIC
LTS-004	LT	Germline	BRCA1	p.Q1111fs	0.42	0.75	Pathogenic	yes	
LTS-012	LT	Germline	BRCA1	p.V299fs	0.55	0.65	Pathogenic	yes	
LTS-017	LT	Germline	BRCA1	p.NIP1236fs	0.49	0.9	Pathogenic	yes	
LTS-019	LT	Germline	BRCA1	p.W1815*	0.45	0.85	Pathogenic	yes	
LTS-022	LT	Somatic	BRCA1	p.W1712*	0	0.5	Pathogenic	yes	
LTS-025	LT	Germline	BRCA1	p.S267fs	0.43	0.87	Pathogenic	yes	
LTS-029	LT	Germline	BRCA1	p.Q1756fs	0.46	0.91	Pathogenic	yes	
LTS-007	LT	Germline	BRCA2	p.V2527fs	0.32	0.43	Pathogenic	no	
LTS-013	LT	Somatic	BRCA2	p.TD1867fs	0	0.59	Pathogenic	yes	
LTS-021	LT	Somatic	BRCA2	p.N991D	0	0.74	Tolerated	yes	yes
LTS-023	LT	Somatic	BRCA2	p.S2835P	0	0.81	Tolerated	yes	yes
LTS-031	LT	Germline	BRCA2	p.D2242fs	0.65	0.68	Pathogenic	yes	
LTS-038	ST	Somatic	BRCA2	p.P2257S	0	0.15	Tolerated	no	no

homologous recombination repair may render the genome vulnerable to accumulating sequence mutations. We also observed a similar trend in the TCGA dataset (Fig. 3b).

While LOH in *BRCA1* was present in 88% (36/41) of all subjects (LT and ST) and frequently coupled with DNA copy loss (72%, 26/36), we did not observe significant loss or decrease of *BRCA1* gene expression in these samples as compared to samples without *BRCA1* copy loss (Additional file 1: Figure S3A). This observation could be confounded by wild-type *BRCA1* gene expression from contaminating normal tissue in the tumor specimen. Despite higher frequency of *BRCA1* loss of

function mutations in the samples from LT cohort, no difference was seen in *BRCA1* transcript expression between the two survival groups. Similarly, *BRCA2* was most often affected by LOH (58%, 24/41 of all patients) and DNA copy loss across both survival groups (92%, 22/24) with no differences in gene expression between LT and ST groups (Additional file 1: Figure S3B).

Spectrum and frequency of TP53 somatic mutations in LT and ST HGSOC

TP53 mutations were prevalent across all HGSOC tumor samples (38/39, 97%, Table 3, Additional file 1: Figure S4A),

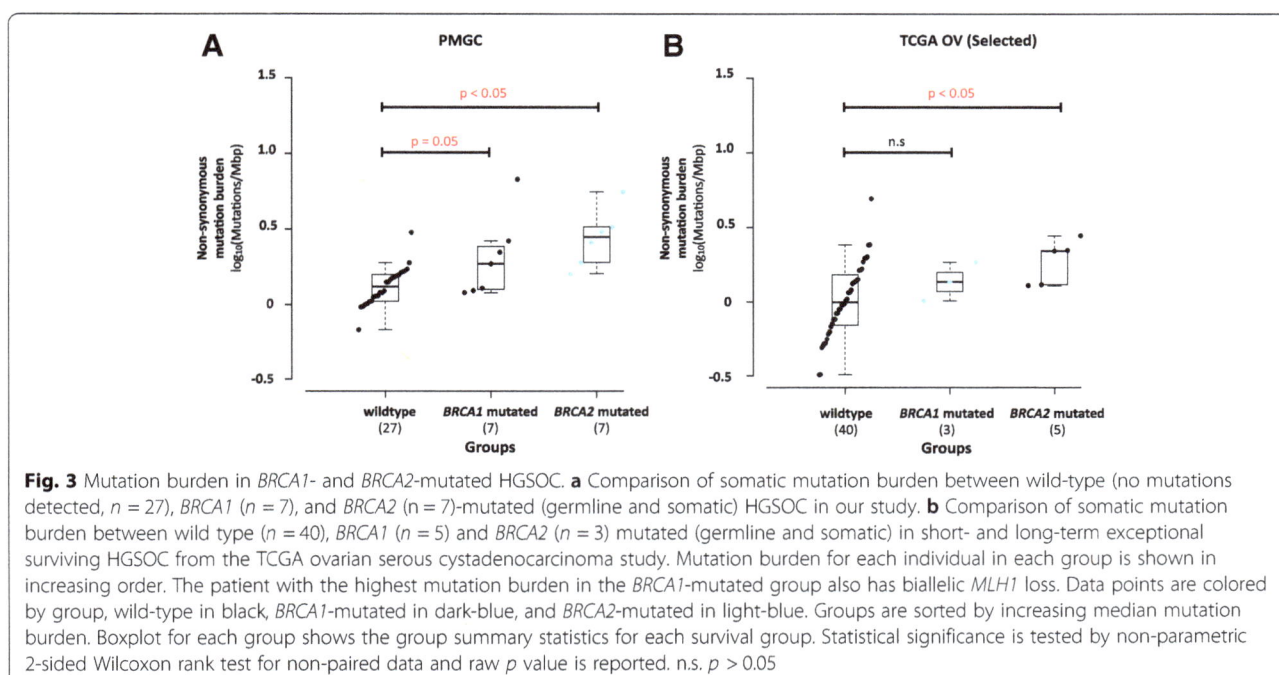

Fig. 3 Mutation burden in *BRCA1*- and *BRCA2*-mutated HGSOC. **a** Comparison of somatic mutation burden between wild-type (no mutations detected, *n* = 27), *BRCA1* (*n* = 7), and *BRCA2* (*n* = 7)-mutated (germline and somatic) HGSOC in our study. **b** Comparison of somatic mutation burden between wild type (*n* = 40), *BRCA1* (*n* = 5) and *BRCA2* (*n* = 3) mutated (germline and somatic) in short- and long-term exceptional surviving HGSOC from the TCGA ovarian serous cystadenocarcinoma study. Mutation burden for each individual in each group is shown in increasing order. The patient with the highest mutation burden in the *BRCA1*-mutated group also has biallelic *MLH1* loss. Data points are colored by group, wild-type in black, *BRCA1*-mutated in dark-blue, and *BRCA2*-mutated in light-blue. Groups are sorted by increasing median mutation burden. Boxplot for each group shows the group summary statistics for each survival group. Statistical significance is tested by non-parametric 2-sided Wilcoxon rank test for non-paired data and raw *p* value is reported. n.s. *p* > 0.05

Table 3 *TP53* Mutations in Study Cohort

Patient ID	Group	Variant type	Mutation protein change	Mutant allele fraction	Function affected	Oncomorphic?	Detection method
LTS-001	LT	Nonsense	p.S183*	0.47		no	Mutect
LTS-002	ST	Missense	p.E224D	0.27		no	Mutect
LTS-003	ST	Missense	p.R175H	0.83	Structural Change	yes	Mutect
LTS-004	LT	Frame Shift Del	p.P223fs	0.45		no	Strelka
LTS-005	ST	Missense	p.D281E	0.75		no	Mutect
LTS-006	ST	Missense	p.Y220C	0.46	Structural Change	yes	Mutect
LTS-007	LT	Missense	p.I195T	0.15		no	Strelka SNV/None by targeted seq
LTS-008	ST	Missense	p.C242F	0.64		no	Mutect
LTS-009	ST	Missense	p.M237I	0.57		no	Mutect
LTS-010	ST	Missense	p.Y220C	0.89	Structural Change	yes	Mutect
LTS-011	LT	Missense	p.R248Q	0.51	Structural Change	yes	Mutect
LTS-012	LT	Missense	p.R248Q	0.76	Structural Change	yes	Mutect
LTS-013	LT	Frame Shift Del	p.A70fs	0.57		no	Varscan2/Targeted Sequencing
LTS-014	LT	Splice Site	c.e7+1	0.89		no	Strelka SNV/Targeted Sequencing (g.chr17:7577498C > A)
LTS-015	ST	Splice Site	c.e8+1	0.74		no	Mutect/Strelka SNV
LTS-016	LT	Missense	p.R248Q	0.82	Structural Change	yes	Mutect
LTS-017	LT	Missense	p.I195T	0.7		no	Mutect
LTS-018	ST	Missense	p.G266E	0.73		no	Mutect
LTS-019	LT	Missense/Frame shift Ins	p.K139Q/ p.V143fs	0.72		no	Mutect/Strelka
LTS-020	LT	Splice Site	p.Q331Q	0.62		no	Mutect
LTS-021	LT	Missense	p.R248W	0.39	DNA binding	yes	Mutect
LTS-022	LT	Missense	p.G245S	0.72	Structural Change	no	Mutect
LTS-023	LT	Missense	p.T125P	1		no	Exome & Targeted sequencing
LTS-024	ST	Missense	p.R282W	0.6	Structural Change	no	Mutect
LTS-025	LT	Missense	p.R273H	0.91	DNA binding	yes	Targeted Sequencing
LTS-026	ST	Nonsense	p.E349*	0.46		no	Mutect
LTS-027	LT	Nonsense	p.R196*	0.56		no	Mutect
LTS-028	ST	Nonsense	p.G266*	0.93		no	Mutect
LTS-029	LT	Missense	p.Y163H	0.73		no	Mutect
LTS-030	LT	Missense	p.R273C	0.67	DNA binding	yes	Mutect
LTS-031	LT	Not detected	Not detected	–		no	None detected by WES on all callers/poor RNAseq
LTS-032	LT	Nonsense	p.W146*	0.86		no	Mutect
LTS-033	ST	Missense	p.R175H	0.4	Structural Change	yes	Mutect
LTS-034	ST	Missense	p.R273L	0.8		yes	Also found in normal (transformed adjacent normal)
LTS-035	ST	In Frame Insertion	p.266_267insLG	0.18	DNA binding	no	Strelka Exome & RNAseq
LTS-037	ST	Frame Shift Del	p.P87fs	0.77		no	Strelka

Table 3 *TP53* Mutations in Study Cohort *(Continued)*

Patient ID	Group	Variant type	Mutation protein change	Mutant allele fraction	Function affected	Oncomorphic?	Detection method
LTS-038	ST	Missense	p.R175H	0.63	Structural Change	yes	Mutect
LTS-039	ST	Missense	p.F270S	0.68		no	Strelka SNV
LTS-040	ST	Nonsense	p.E204*	0.51		no	Mutect

and 39/41 tumors show loss of heterozygosity at the *TP53* locus. Through a combination of exome and deep-targeted sequencing, we detected 25 missense, 6 nonsense, 3 frame-shift deletion, 1 in-frame insertion, and 3 splice site mutations (Fig. 2 and Additional file 1: Figure S4A). A mutation in *TP53* was not detected in 1 LT patient, possibly due to a combination of low tumor cellularity (predicted 26% from Sequenza) and poor DNA quality from FFPE preservation. No differences in the frequencies of mutation types were observed between LT and ST. To assess the prognostic potential of *TP53* mutations, we categorized all mutations into 3 major categories as described by Brachova et al. [37]: 12/38 (32%) oncomorphic, 10/38 (26%) loss of function (LOF), and 16/38 (42%) unclassified *TP53* mutations. There was no statistical significant difference in the frequency of oncomorphic mutations between LT and ST cohorts (ST: 6/19, LT: 6/20, $p = 0.72$), although both cohorts harbored a significant fraction of unclassified mutations (ST: 9/19, LT: 7/20) (Additional file 1: Figure S4C). Therefore, further characterization of *TP53* mutations in LT and ST cohorts is needed to establish the function of these mutations.

Consistent with known mutation spectra in *TP53*, 30 of 38 mutations were located within the p53 DNA-binding domain with oncomorphic p.Arg248 having the highest mutation frequency (4/29, 3 Arg > Gln, 1 Arg > Trp) (Additional file 1: Figure S3A). While p.Arg248 mutations occurred exclusively in tumors from LT survivors in our cohort, these mutations occurred exclusively in 4 ST patients in the TCGA cohort (Additional file 1: Figure S3B). Between the three categories of *TP53* mutations, we observed that tumors containing oncomorphic *TP53* mutations have the highest *TP53* mRNA expression (two-sided Wilcoxon Rank Sum: oncomorphic vs LOF (median expression log2(TPM + 1): 4.34 vs. 2.18, $p = 0.008$); oncomorphic vs unclassified (median expression log2(TPM + 1): 4.34 vs. 3.73, $p = 0.22$) (Additional file 1: Figure S4D). We observed a broad range of *TP53* mRNA expression in tumors with unclassified mutations. This observation further suggests that the unclassified set of *TP53* missense mutations may contain additional oncomorphic mutations that may come to light with further functional characterization of these variants.

Short-term survivors lack BRCAness

Alexandrov et al. [38] described 20 distinct mutational signatures based on the frequency of somatic base substitution events and the flanking sequence context. To better understand the underlying mutational processes in our cohort, we determined the composition of mutational signatures by applying non-negative matrix factorization from the catalog of somatic mutations identified in each tumor. Signature 3 (BRCA signature), associated with inactivating *BRCA1* or *BRCA2* mutations in breast and pancreatic cancers and prevalent in ovarian cancer [35], is present in 27/39 samples. However, not all LT tumors are positive for signature 3. This observation suggests that presence of a BRCA-associated signature alone is not prognostic in HGSOC (Fig. 2). The BRCA signature occurs less frequently in short-term survivors (ST vs LT, 10/19 vs 17/20, fisher's exact test $p = 0.04$), suggesting that lack of BRCAness [39] may be associated with poor survival in HGSOC (Additional file 1: Figure S6). Signature 16, possibly associated with active DNA repair by transcription-coupled nucleotide excision repair, is the dominant signature in tumors that have germline *BRCA2* mutations. Mutation signature associated with DNA mismatch repair deficiency and high mutation frequency (Signatures 20, 6, and 14) was only evident in the high mutation burden tumor with both *BRCA1* and *MLH*1 inactivation.

HRD-LOH in short- and long-term survivors

All tumors exhibit highly altered karyotype with evidence of genome doubling (average estimated ploidy of 2.5 and 2.8, respectively for long- and short-survival) with frequent chromosome alterations characteristic of HGSOC including arm-level gains in 1p, 3q, 6p, and 20q, and losses in 4p, 4q, 6q 8p, 8q, 9q, 11p, 11q, 13q, 16p, 16q, 17p, 17q, 18q, 19q, 21q, and 22q (Additional file 1: Figures S7 and S8). All of the frequently detected arm-level events in our cohort were previously reported by the TCGA. Two hundred fifteen and 156 unique genes within focal amplification regions were found in long- and short-term samples, respectively using GISTIC2.0 algorithm [23] (Additional file 1: Figure S9). One of these genes, *CCNE1*, is focally amplified in 4/19 ST and 2/20 LT survivor tumors. The increased frequency of *CCNE1* gain in patients with short survival time is consistent with its known association with poor prognosis in ovarian cancer [40]. However, *CCNE1* amplification has also been observed in long-term survivors within the TCGA cohort at a 10% (1/10) frequency.

We also compared frequencies of copy number alterations in 5 genomic regions (19q12 amplification, 14q32.33 amplification, 3q29 amplification, 20q13.21-q13.32 amplification, and 20q13.2 amplification) previously associated with ovarian cancer survival [41–43]. In this analysis, only amplification of 19q12 (containing *CCNE1*) was frequently altered in ST and not in LT.

To evaluate reported prognostic value of DNA homologous repair deficiency in HGSOC [44, 45], we compared homologous recombination deficiency-loss of heterozygosity (HRD-LOH) score between LT and ST tumors. While we did not observe significant difference between the estimated tumor cellularity of LT and ST groups (Fig. 4a), we have observed lower sensitivity of CNA detection in tumors with low cellularity. To mitigate the effects of tumor cellularity, we only selected tumors with > 50% (LT n = 14, ST n = 13) cellularity for the HRD-LOH comparison. While more ST tumors have lower HRD-LOH score, no significant difference is observed between LT and ST groups (Fig. 4b). A larger range of HRD-LOH score is seen in the ST group (0–24) as compared to LT (8–23). This suggests the existence of other uncharacterized mechanisms that contribute to genomic instability and survival in HGSOC beyond *BRCA1/2* disruption.

Increased tumor immune-reactivity and immune cell infiltration are features of LT HGSOC

To assess relationships of immune cell infiltration with survival, we assessed enrichment of four published gene expression subtypes (including an immunoreactive subtype, IMR) [26] as well as a total immune cell infiltration score (ESTIMATE algorithm) [27] in 29 tumors with available RNA-seq data (13 LT and 16 ST). Consistent with previous reports, all tumors showed enrichment in more than one gene expression subtype (Fig. 5a). Through unsupervised hierarchical clustering of each tumor by the gene-expression subtype score profiles, it was evident that a group of 4 *BRCA1/2* mutated tumors, characterized by high immunoreactive subtype score, formed a unique cluster. We also observed a cluster of tumors characterized by strong mesenchymal expression subtype signature containing almost exclusively of short-term ST survivors (n = 4/5) with the exception of one long-term survivor that also exhibited strong immunoreactive signature. The remaining 4 clusters contain various proportion of LT and ST members, illustrating the complexity of the underlying molecular pathology of HGSOC.

While we did not observe a statistically significant difference in immune scores between LT and ST tumors across the cohort (two-sided Wilcoxon Rank Sum, n = 13 vs 16, mean = 1.6 vs 1.5, p = 0.170) (Fig. 5b), more LTs than STs were amongst the top 25% of tumors with the highest ESTIMATE Immune score (fisher's exact test p = 0.027). Focusing on *BRCA1/2*-mutated tumors, we found higher immune enrichment scores compared to tumors with wild-type *BRCA1/2* (two-sided Wilcoxon Rank Sum, n = 7 vs 22, mean = 1.7 vs 1.5, q = 0.09) (Fig. 5).

As specific immune cell types in the tumor microenvironment may underlie LT survival, we also assessed the role of 8 immune cell populations previously

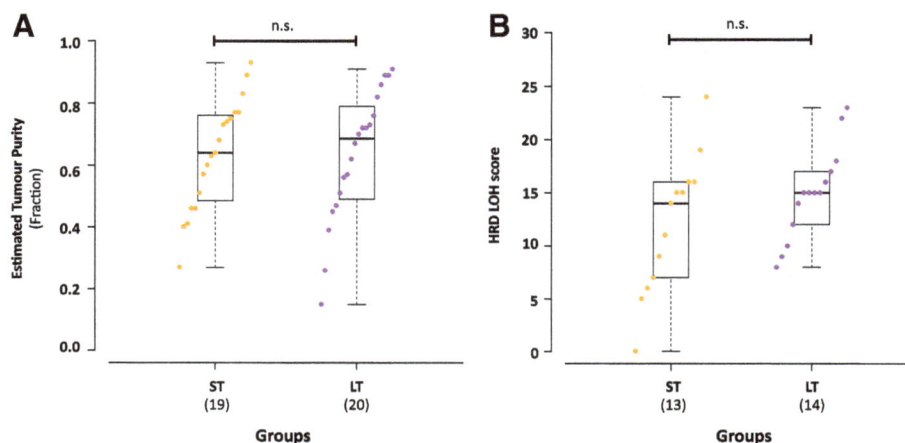

Fig. 4 Homologous recombination deficiency in exceptional short- and long-term HGSOC survivors. **a** Comparison of estimated tumor cell cellularity in the sequenced tumor tissue between long- (n = 20) and short- (n = 19) term HGSOC in this study. **b** Comparison of whole exome sequencing data derived HRD-LOH scores from tumors with greater than 50% tumor cellularity between exceptional survivor groups (long-term = 14, short-term 13). Individual data points in each group is shown in increasing order. Data points are colored by group, short-term in orange and long-term in purple. Boxplot for each group shows the group summary statistics for each survival group. Statistical significance is tested by non-parametric 2-sided Wilcoxon rank test for non-paired data and raw p values are reported. n.s. p > 0.05

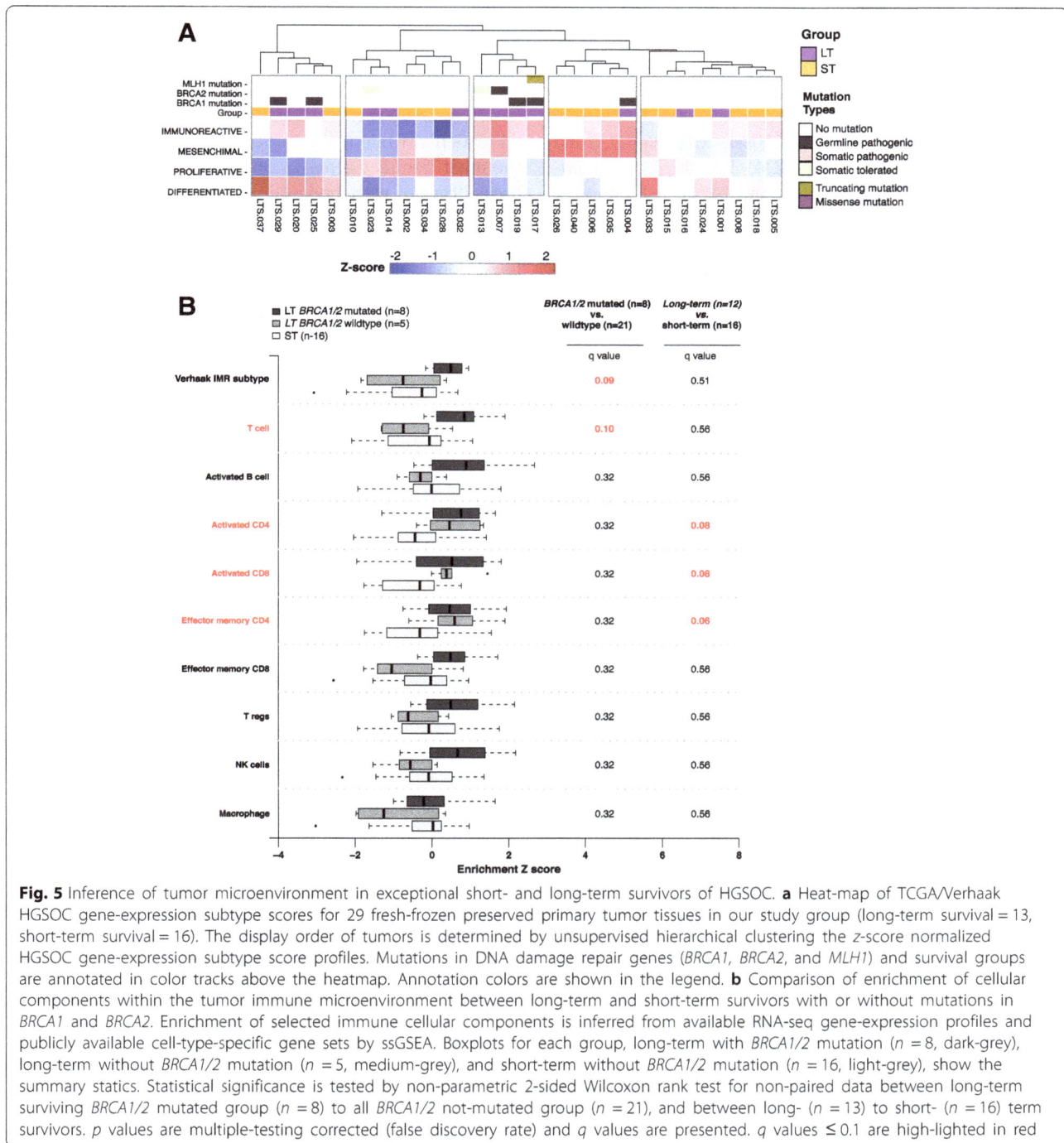

Fig. 5 Inference of tumor microenvironment in exceptional short- and long-term survivors of HGSOC. **a** Heat-map of TCGA/Verhaak HGSOC gene-expression subtype scores for 29 fresh-frozen preserved primary tumor tissues in our study group (long-term survival = 13, short-term survival = 16). The display order of tumors is determined by unsupervised hierarchical clustering the z-score normalized HGSOC gene-expression subtype score profiles. Mutations in DNA damage repair genes (*BRCA1*, *BRCA2*, and *MLH1*) and survival groups are annotated in color tracks above the heatmap. Annotation colors are shown in the legend. **b** Comparison of enrichment of cellular components within the tumor immune microenvironment between long-term and short-term survivors with or without mutations in *BRCA1* and *BRCA2*. Enrichment of selected immune cellular components is inferred from available RNA-seq gene-expression profiles and publicly available cell-type-specific gene sets by ssGSEA. Boxplots for each group, long-term with *BRCA1/2* mutation (*n* = 8, dark-grey), long-term without *BRCA1/2* mutation (*n* = 5, medium-grey), and short-term without *BRCA1/2* mutation (*n* = 16, light-grey), show the summary statics. Statistical significance is tested by non-parametric 2-sided Wilcoxon rank test for non-paired data between long-term surviving *BRCA1/2* mutated group (*n* = 8) to all *BRCA1/2* not-mutated group (*n* = 21), and between long- (*n* = 13) to short- (*n* = 16) term survivors. *p* values are multiple-testing corrected (false discovery rate) and *q* values are presented. *q* values ≤ 0.1 are high-lighted in red

associated with survival outcome in various cancer types, including HGSOC [12, 13, 28, 46]. Using ssGSEA [25], we found LT tumors were enriched for activated CD8$^+$ T (q = 0.08), activated CD4$^+$ T (q = 0.08), and effector memory CD4$^+$ T cells (q = 0.06) (Fig. 5b). To further illustrate the independence of cell-type specific infiltration from total immune enrichment, we found enrichment

scores of activated CD8$^+$ T cells, activated CD4$^+$ T cells, and effector memory CD4$^+$ T cells were not correlated with total immune or immune reactivity scores (Pearson correlation < 0.5, p > 0.05, Additional file 1: Figure S10C, D, E). LT and ST showed no difference in enrichment of effector memory CD8$^+$, regulatory T cells, activated B cells, macrophages, and NK cells (Fig. 5b), although this may be due to a lack of adequate reference gene sets or low frequency in the tumor microenvironment for these cell types.

From the TCGA ovarian cancer cohort, we identified 8 LT and 32 ST tumors that matched the survival selection criteria of our cohort. Here, we observed a similar trend of increased activated CD8+ T, CD4+ T, and effector memory CD4+ T cell gene-set enrichment between LT and ST tumors. This observation provided additional support to suggest that increased activated CD8+ and CD4+T lymphocytes in the tumor microenvironment may play an important role in improved LT survival outcome in HGSOC (Additional file 1: Figure S11). We also confirmed no difference in enrichment of macrophages, effector memory CD8+ T cells, NK cells, or regulatory T cells between LT versus ST TCGA tumors (Additional file 1: Figure S11).

ESR1-CCDC170 is a novel recurrent gene fusion in HGSOC with short survival

Fusion gene RNA transcripts were predicted for 13 LT and 16 ST HGSOC from the RNAseq data. Of the 125 total potential fusions involving different gene partner pairs identified, 4 candidate fusions (*ESR1-CCDC170*, *DLEU1-DLEU7*, *KMT2E-LHFPL3*, and *LOC101928103-A-BAC12*) were recurrent (occurred in two or more tumors) (Additional file 4: Table S3). *ESR1-CCDC170*, present in 2 ST patients, while has never been reported in HGSOC, is the most frequent gene-fusion (6–8%) found in luminal B breast cancer with poor clinical prognosis [47] (Fig. 6). *DLEU1-DLEU7*, present in 2 LT and 1 ST patient, has not been previously reported in HGSOC or other cancer types (Additional file 1: Figures S12-S14). However, increased *DLEU1* expression has been shown to sequester the tumor suppressor function of miR-290-3p and increase growth and invasiveness of ovarian cancer cell lines in vitro [48]. This fusion product lacks the predicted miR-290-3p binding sequence and therefore may provide a new mechanism to control HGSOC aggressiveness in vivo.

Discussion

With limited number of approved treatments for managing HGSOC, long-term survival is strongly dependent

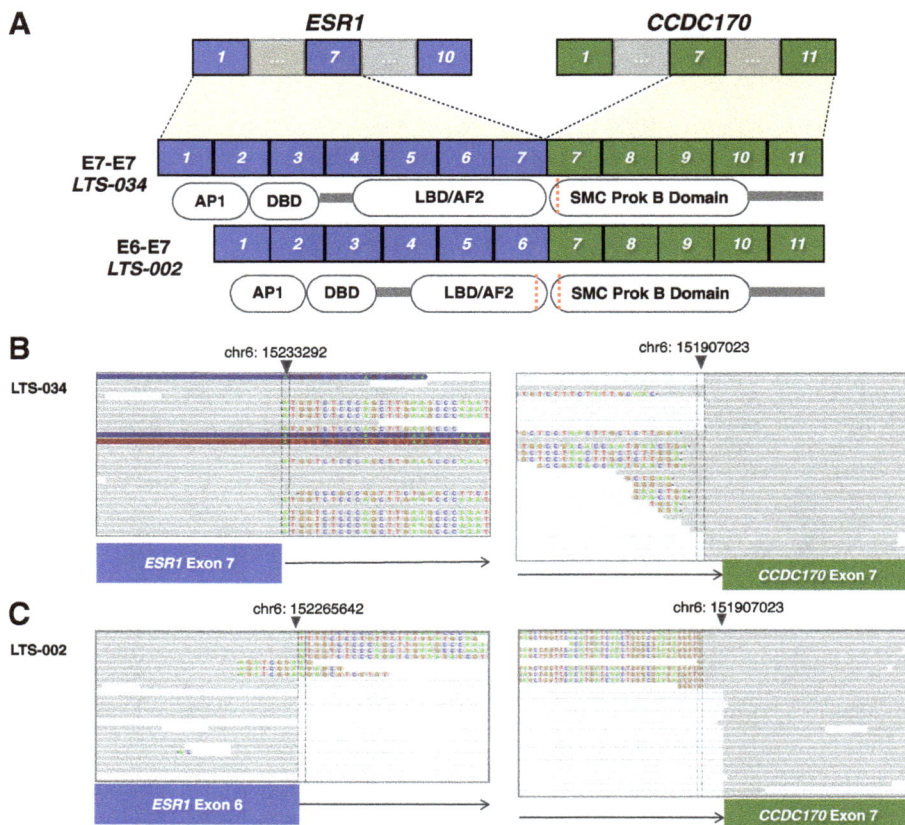

Fig. 6 Recurrent *ESR1-CCDC170* gene fusion in exceptional short-term surviving HGSOC. **a** Schematic diagram of the exons from *ESR1* and *CCDC170* included within the detected gene-fusion mRNA by RNA-seq in the two HGSOC primary tumor tissues from exceptionally short-term surviving patients. Diagram of protein domains encoded by the retained exons is shown for each fusion. **b** RNA-seq reads supporting the *ESR1-CCDC170* fusion mRNA in patient LTS-034. **c** RNA-seq reads supporting the *ESR1-CCDC170* fusion mRNA in patient LTS-002. Portions of the junction-spanning reads that align to the reference sequence of *ESR1* and *CCDC170* are colored in grey and the mismatched bases are shown in color

on the extent and duration of chemosensitivity in the cancer cells. Beyond *BRCA1/2* mutation status, no other biomarker enables up-front and precise identification of patients with platinum sensitive or resistant disease. As such, initial treatment plans are not informed by the underlying disease biology. Given the high rate of relapse following initial treatment in HGSOC, several trials are on-going to add anti-angiogenics, PARP and/or PDL-1 inhibitors to standard chemotherapy in the hope to increase the progression free and overall survivals. However, identification of mechanisms of inherent platinum resistance and platinum sensitivity will enable the discovery of biomarkers that may be further validated in this new trials approach. By comparing molecular characteristics of primary advanced HGSOC from patients who experienced prolonged chemosensitivity (OS > 10 years) to patients with primary chemoresistance (OS < 2 years), we sought to uncover factors that may be used for treatment decision in HGSOC. Currently, the strongest predictors of LT survival remain the disease stage and no residual disease post-surgery [49]. Consistent with this finding, the majority of our LT patients had complete disease resection (Table 1, Fig. 2). While initial tumor burden measured by CA125 serum levels did not predict exceptional survival, low serum CA125 levels post-treatment (surgery and chemotherapy) are associated with long-term survival. Specifically, CA125 levels for all long-term responders fell to less than 10 units/mL post-chemotherapy, suggesting that these tumors are highly sensitive to standard of care treatment. This finding provides additional evidence that CA125 kinetics may have predictive value and may be used as a tool in drug response assessment [50, 51].

Previous studies in HGSOC have focused on describing mutational processes that contribute to tumorigenesis, molecular signatures that correlate to survival and mechanisms of chemoresistance. However, most of these studies rely on limited survival data with less than 5 years of patient follow-up. Our cohort with greater than 10 years of follow-up confirms that biallelic inactivation of *BRCA1* or *BRCA2*, through either germline or somatic mutation, coupled with loss of heterozygosity, is associated with extended long survival (Fig. 2, Table 2). The association of *BRCA1/2* mutations with improved OS and progression-free survival has been previously reported in ovarian cancers [9]. Biallelic inactivation of *BRCA1* was reported as a potential mechanism of long-term response to Olaparib, a PARP inhibitor, in a HGSOC patient with > 7 years response [51]. Interestingly, the only *BRCA2* somatic mutation detected in the short-term survivor patient had low mutant allele frequency (MAF = 0.15) and retained the wildtype allele. The intact wildtype *BRCA2* allele may provide material for somatic *BRCA*1/2 recovery by copy number gain or upregulation to facilitate chemotherapy resistance and disease

progression. Additionally, while there exists an enrichment of *BRCA1/2* abnormalities in the LT patients, not all LT patients harbor *BRCA1/2* mutations, suggesting alternate mechanisms conferring prolonged chemosensitivity are present in these tumors [6].

BRCAness is a term coined to describe tumors exhibiting phenotypes that are similar to those with loss of *BRCA1/2* function in the absence of a *BRCA1/2* mutation [39]. With the success of PARP inhibitors for patients with *BRCA1/2* mutation-positive ovarian cancers [7, 8, 52], the focus is now on identifying other molecular abnormalities that may confer "BRCAness" to tumors without apparent *BRCA* mutations. We hypothesize that LT tumors, regardless of *BRCA* mutation status, exhibit more characteristics of homologous repair deficiency as compared to the ST patients. We measured features of BRCAness by overall mutation burden, identifying mutations in other genes involved in DNA homologous recombination repair, inferring *BRCA* mutational signature and the homologous recombination deficiency loss of heterozygosity (HRD-LOH) score for each tumor from exome profiles [44, 45]. We identified higher number of non-synonymous mutations in LT compared to ST, consistent with higher mutation burden in *BRCA1/2* deficient tumors. Unlike previous reports, we did not identify an enrichment of loss of function mutations in other HR genes in our study cohort [35], probably given the small size of our study cohort and the low frequency of non-*BRCA* HR gene mutations in HGSOC. However, a mutational signature associated with BRCA inactivation is prevalent in both LT and ST groups (total 28/39 tumors). Although both survival groups have high percentage of *BRCA* mutation signatures, the tumors from short-term survivors are enriched within the tumors lacking this signature. In addition, tumors with low HRD-LOH scores are enriched with ST patients. Together, findings suggest absence of BRCAness may be a prognostic characteristic of poor survival in HGSOC.

Given the prevalence of *TP53* mutations in HGSOC, it was suggested that some non-synonymous mutations may provide survival advantage to tumor cells and associated with poor patient survival [37]. By over-expressing specific *TP53* mutations in *TP53*–/– ovarian cancer cell lines in vitro or by measuring tumorigenesis in mouse and rat models, studies have demonstrated a subset of mutations that increase chemo-resistance and promote cancer cell growth [37]. Our analysis of this subset of oncomorphic mutations did not uncover enrichment in LT versus ST tumors. However, both cohorts contained a substantial number of unclassified variants expressed at differing levels, suggesting further characterization of these mutations is warranted.

Increased lymphocytic infiltration in the tumor microenvironment is a histological phenotype observed in

BRCA1/2-mutated ovarian tumor [53]. The association of infiltrating immune cells and patient survival is strongly dependent on quantity and the composition of cell types present [10, 12]. As such, B cells, CD4$^+$, and CD8$^+$ T cells have been associated with improved clinical outcomes whereas regulatory cell types, such as regulatory T cells and neutrophils, have been associated with poor outcome in ovarian, breast, lung, and colon cancers [54–57]. Therapeutic strategies to increase the quantities of infiltrating immune cells with tumor-killing abilities such as immune-checkpoint inhibition and adoptive cell transfer therapies have been at the forefront of clinical trials and research in recent years. Using whole transcriptome analysis and publically available gene sets, we inferred the enrichment of lymphocytic infiltration as a whole, as well as of individual subtypes of immune cells for each tumor specimen. Using this method, we confirmed that the immune-reactive subtype of HGSOC is correlated with the immune score measure from ESTIMATE and both are higher in LT tumors. We also observed an increase in immune score in *BRCA1/2*-mutated tumors compared to *BRCA1/2* wild-type tumors. This trend is consistent when comparing LT to ST groups, in which activated CD4$^+$, CD8$^+$, and effector CD4$^+$ T lymphocytes were enriched in LT tumors; however, these gene set scores did not correlate directly with bulk immune scores. This observation suggests that the presence of specific cells in the microenvironment may contribute directly to eliminating tumor cells or increasing chemosensitivity, with or without the involvement of *BRCA* inactivation by mutation. In addition, we observed a small group of ST tumors with high mesenchymal gene-expression subtype scores. The mesenchymal subtype was described by Tothill et al. who showed that HGSOCs within this molecular subgroup had poorer overall survival as compared with those defined by other molecular subtypes [58]. A recent study showed that HGSOC tumors with mesenchymal gene-expression subtype are associated with disseminated intraperitoneal disease and lower rates of complete tumor resection [59]. Together, these studies further suggest that mesenchymal HGSOCs have poor clinical outcomes. A recent retrospective analysis showed that mesenchymal HGSOC tumors may respond favorably to anti-angiogenic treatment, providing an option for targeted therapy in this specific subgroup [60].

While clinical and molecular factors contributing to chemo-resistance in HGSOC have been described, recurrent gene-fusions in HGSOC associated with therapeutic outcome have yet to be replicated across multiple studies [35]. Using RNA-seq in our small study cohort, we identified the *ESR1-CCDC170* fusion, previously reported in aggressive luminal B breast cancers, in 2/16 short-term survivors. In vitro experiments showed increases in cellular proliferation and migration when *ESR1-CCDC170*

fusions are expressed in the MCF10A breast epithelial cell-line. The presence of this variant within exceptionally short-term survivors with platinum resistance may point to a novel mechanism that contributes the aggressive oncogenic phenotype in these tumors. Further functional validations will have to be performed in other HGSOC cohorts in future investigations.

Conclusions

In this comprehensive analysis, we focused on comparing treatment-naïve primary HGSOC tumor from two groups of patients selected based on their extreme differences in OS. We have demonstrated that compared to primary chemoresistant HGSOC, LT survival in HGSOC can be characterized by elevated mutation burden, biallelic inactivation of *BRCA1* or *BRCA2*, and increased CD4$^+$ and CD8$^+$ lymphocytic infiltration in the tumor microenvironment. We are also the first to report the *ESR1-CCDC170* gene fusion in tumors from two HGSOC patients with extremely short survival. Identifying mechanisms involved in the response or resistance to treatment is essential to devising precision treatment plans, and future strategies will likely rely on multiple clinical and immunogenomic factors. With only a small group of patients, this study is exploratory and hypothesis generating in nature and will require validation by future studies. However, this analysis of exceptional responders in HGSOC has the potential to contribute to our understanding of the biology of ovarian cancer, with the goal of improving the survival of patients [61, 62]. Given the molecular heterogeneity that exists within HGSOC, we suggest that optimal patient care should be provided through a multidisciplinary longitudinal approach that integrates expertise from meaningful tumor characterizations such as *BRCA1/2* mutation status, mutation burden, HR deficiency, and tumor microenvironment immune composition at the time of diagnosis and relapse [7, 8, 63].

Additional files

Additional file 1: Supplementary figures for the manuscript.

Additional file 2: Supplementary methods for the manuscript.

Additional file 3: CNV segment size as distribution per sample. Distribution of CNV segment size as percentage of chromosome arm in each sequenced tumor sample. Sequenza estimated sample ploidy and the threshold used for determining copy number amplification is shown for each sample as colored horizontal lines.

Additional file 4: Supplementary tables for the manuscript.

Additional file 5: All Strelka indels. All Indels called by Strelka and annotated by Oncotator.

Additional file 6: All CNV segs annotated. All CNV segs generated by Sequenza and annotated by Oncotator.

Additional file 7 All Mutect mutations 1. SNV mutations called by Mutect and annotated by Oncotator for samples LTS-001_T, LTS-002_T, LTS-003_T, LTS-004_T, LTS-005_T, LTS-006_T.

Additional file 8: All Mutect mutations 2. All SNV mutations called by Mutect and annotated by Oncotator for samples LTS-007_T in chromosomes 1 to 10.

Additional file 9: All Mutect mutations 3. All SNV mutations called by Mutect and annotated by Oncotator for samples LTS-007_T in chromosomes 11 to 22, M, X, and Y.

Additional file 10: All Mutect mutations 4. All SNV mutations called by Mutect and annotated by Oncotator for samples LTS-008_T, LTS-009_T, LTS-010_T, LTS-011_T, LTS-012_T, LTS-013_T, LTS-014_T, LTS-015_T, LTS-016_T.

Additional file 11: All Mutect mutations 5. All SNV mutations called by Mutect and annotated by Oncotator for samples LTS-017_T, LTS-018_T, LTS-021_T.

Additional file 12 All Mutect mutations 6. All SNV mutations called by Mutect and annotated by Oncotator for samples LTS-019_T, LTS-020_T, LTS-022_T, LTS-023_T, LTS-024_T, LTS-025_T, LTS-026_T, LTS-027_T, LTS-028_T.

Additional file 13: All Mutect mutations 7. All SNV mutations called by Mutect and annotated by Oncotator for samples LTS-029_T, LTS-030_T, LTS-031_T.

Additional file 14: All Mutect mutations 8. All SNV mutations called by Mutect and annotated by Oncotator for samples LTS-032_T, LTS-033_T, LTS-034_T, LTS-035_T, LTS-037_T, LTS-038_T, LTS-039_T, LTS-040_T.

Abbreviations
ABAC12: ATP-binding cassette, subfamily A, member 12; BRCA1: Breast Cancer Gene 1; BRCA2: Breast Cancer Gene 2; CA125: Cancer Antigen 125; CCDC170: Coiled-coil domain containing 170; CCNE1: Cyclin E 1; CD4: Cluster of differentiation 4; CD8: Cluster of differentiation 8; CDK12: Cyclin dependent kinase 12; CNV: Copy number variation; DLEU1: Deleted in lymphocytic leukemia 1; DLEU7: Deleted in lymphocytic leukemia 7; DNA: Deoxyribose nucleic acid; EFEMP1: EGF containing fibulin-like extracellular matrix protein 1; EOC: Epithelial ovarian cancer; ESR1: Estogen receptor 1; FDR: False discovery rate; FF: Fresh frozen; FFPE: Formalin-fixed paraffin embedded; FIGO: International Federation of Gynecology and Obstetrics; GATK: Genome analysis toolkit; HGSOC: High-grade serous ovarian cancer; HR: Homologous recombination; HRD: Homologous recombination deficiency; IMR: Immunoreactive; KMT2E: Lysine methyltransferase 2E; KRAS: Kristen rat sarcoma viral oncogene homolog; LHFPL3: Lipoma HMGIC fusion partner-like 4; LOH: Loss of heterozygosity; LT: Long term; MAF: Mutant allele frequency; Mbp: Million base pairs; miRNA: MicroRNA; MLH1: MutL homolog 1; NF1: Neurofibromin 1; NK: Natural killer; OS: Overall survival; PARP: Poly-ADP polimerase; PM: Princess Margaret; PTEN: Phosphatase and tensin homolog; RB1: Retinoblastoma 1; RNA: Ribose nucleic acid; SCNA: Somatic copy number alteration; SNV: Single nucleotide variant; ssGSEA: Single sample geneset enrichment analysis; ST: Short term; TCGA: The Cancer Genome Atlas; TP53: Tumor protein 53; TPM: Transcripts per million; Tregs: Regulatory T cells; VAF: Variant allele frequency; WES: Whole exome sequencing

Acknowledgements
We thank the staff of the Princess Margaret Genomics Centre (Neil Winegarden, Julissa Tsao, and Nick Khuu) and Bioinformatics Services (Carl Virtanen, Zhibin Lu, and Natalie Stickle) for their expertise in generating the sequencing data used in this study (www.pmgenomics.ca). We would also like to thank Dr. Robert Rottapel and Dr. Paul Boutros for their scientific input and expertise throughout this project.

Funding
This study was funded by the Princess Margaret Cancer Foundation and Terry Fox Translational Cancer Research Program for The Immunotherapy Network (iTNT): Targeting Ovarian Cancer. TJP was supported by Canada Foundation for Innovation, Leaders Opportunity Fund, CFI #32383, Ontario Ministry of Research and Innovation, Ontario Research Fund Small Infrastructure Program, and the Canada Research Chairs Program. SYCY was funded by the Ontario Graduate Scholarship and the University of Toronto Department of Medical Biophysics Program Excellence Awards.

Authors' contributions
SYCY and SL contributed equally as joint first authors. SYCY processed the tumor samples and consolidated, analyzed, and interpreted the genomics data. SL gathered, analyzed, and interpreted the patient clinical data. KK and JVB provided support for patient data collection. JPB, AD, RQ, provided bioinformatics support. MD, YH, and TL provided wet-lab support to process tumor samples for sequencing experiments. LL and WX provided the statistical and power analysis for the clinical and genomics data. PAS and BAC performed pathological reviews and selected the patient tumor tissues for this study. DLC and PSO provided input for interpretation of immune infiltration data. TJP and AMO contributed equally as joint senior authors. All authors read and approved the final manuscript.

Competing interests
DLC is currently an employee of Pfizer Canada Inc.. PSO has received compensation as a consultant or advisor for Venus, Symphogen, and Providence. The remaining authors declare that they have no competing interests.

Author details
[1]Princess Margaret Cancer Centre, University Health Network, 610 University Avenue, Toronto, Ontario M5G 2M9, Canada. [2]Department of Medical Biophysics, University of Toronto, Toronto, Ontario, Canada. [3]Department of Medicine, University of Toronto, Toronto, Canada. [4]Department of Laboratory Medicine and Pathobiology, University of Toronto, Toronto, Canada. [5]Department of Pathology, University Health Network, Toronto, Canada. [6]Department of Immunology, University of Toronto, Toronto, Canada. [7]Ontario Institute for Cancer Research, Toronto, Canada.

References
1. Bowtell DD, Böhm S, Ahmed AA, Aspuria P-J, Bast RC Jr, et al. Rethinking ovarian cancer II: reducing mortality from high-grade serous ovarian cancer. Nat Rev Cancer. 2015;15:668 [cited 2017 Jun 18]. Available from: https://www.ncbi.nlm.nih.gov/pmc/articles/PMC4892184/.
2. Lheureux S, Karakasis K, Kohn EC, Oza AM. Ovarian cancer treatment: the end of empiricism? Cancer. 2015;121:3203–11.
3. Howlander N, Noone A, Krapcho M, Miller D, Bishop K, Kosary C, et al. Cancer Statistics Review, 1975–2014 - SEER Statistics. [cited 2017 Apr 10]. Available from: https://seer.cancer.gov/csr/1975_2014/.
4. Cress RD, Chen YS, Morris CR, Petersen M, Leiserowitz GS. Characteristics of long-term survivors of epithelial ovarian cancer. Obstet Gynecol. 2015;126: 491 [cited 2017 Jun 19]. Available from: https://www.ncbi.nlm.nih.gov/pmc/articles/PMC4545401/.

5.   Dao F, Schlappe BA, Tseng J, Lester J, Nick AM, Lutgendorf SK, et al. Characteristics of 10-year survivors of high-grade serous ovarian carcinoma. Gynecol Oncol. 2016;141:260–3.

6.   McLaughlin JR, Rosen B, Moody J, Pal T, Fan I, Shaw PA, et al. Long-term ovarian cancer survival associated with mutation in BRCA1 or BRCA2. J Natl Cancer Inst. 2013;105:141–8.

7.   Ledermann J, Harter P, Gourley C, Friedlander M, Vergote I, Rustin G, et al. Olaparib maintenance therapy in patients with platinum-sensitive relapsed serous ovarian cancer: a preplanned retrospective analysis of outcomes by BRCA status in a randomised phase 2 trial. Lancet Oncol. 2014;15:852–61.

8.   De Picciotto N, Cacheux W, Roth A, Chappuis PO, Labidi-Galy SI. Ovarian cancer: status of homologous recombination pathway as a predictor of drug response. Crit Rev Oncol Hematol. 2016;101:50–9.

9.   Gorodnova TV, Sokolenko AP, Ivantsov AO, Iyevleva AG, Suspitsin EN, Aleksakhina SN, et al. High response rates to neoadjuvant platinum-based therapy in ovarian cancer patients carrying germ-line BRCA mutation. Cancer Lett. 2015;369:363–7.

10. Sato E, Olson SH, Ahn J, Bundy B, Nishikawa H, Qian F, et al. Intraepithelial CD8+ tumor-infiltrating lymphocytes and a high CD8+/regulatory T cell ratio are associated with favorable prognosis in ovarian cancer. Proc Natl Acad Sci U S A. 2005;102:18538–43.

11. Webb JR, Milne K, Watson P, Deleeuw RJ, Nelson BH. Tumor-infiltrating lymphocytes expressing the tissue resident memory marker CD103 are associated with increased survival in high-grade serous ovarian cancer. Clin Cancer Res. 2014;20:434–44.

12. Wouters MCA, Komdeur FL, Workel HH, Klip HG, Plat A, Kooi NM, et al. Treatment regimen, surgical outcome, and T-cell differentiation influence prognostic benefit of tumor-infiltrating lymphocytes in high-grade serous ovarian cancer. Clin Cancer Res. 2016;22:714–24.

13. Montfort A, Pearce O, Maniati E, Vincent BG, Bixby L, Böhm S, et al. A strong B-cell response is part of the immune landscape in human high-grade serous ovarian metastases. Clin Cancer Res. 2017;23:250–62.

14. Kroeger DR, Milne K, Nelson BH. Tumor-infiltrating plasma cells are associated with tertiary lymphoid structures, cytolytic T-cell responses, and superior prognosis in ovarian Cancer. Clin Cancer Res. 2016;22:3005–15.

15. Li H, Durbin R. Fast and accurate long-read alignment with Burrows-Wheeler transform. Bioinformatics. 2010;26:589–95.

16. Van der Auwera GA, Carneiro MO, Hartl C, Poplin R, Del Angel G, Levy-Moonshine A, et al. From FastQ data to high confidence variant calls: the Genome Analysis Toolkit best practices pipeline. Curr Protoc Bioinformatics. 2013;43:11.10.1–33.

17. DePristo MA, Banks E, Poplin R, Garimella KV, Maguire JR, Hartl C, et al. A framework for variation discovery and genotyping using next-generation DNA sequencing data. Nat Genet. 2011;43:491–8.

18. Lawrence MS, Stojanov P, Polak P, Kryukov GV, Cibulskis K, Sivachenko A, et al. Mutational heterogeneity in cancer and the search for new cancer-associated genes. Nature. 2013;499:214–8.

19. Koboldt DC, Zhang Q, Larson DE, Shen D, McLellan MD, Lin L, et al. VarScan 2: somatic mutation and copy number alteration discovery in cancer by exome sequencing. Genome Res. 2012;22:568–76.

20. Saunders CT, Wong WSW, Swamy S, Becq J, Murray LJ, Cheetham RK. Strelka: accurate somatic small-variant calling from sequenced tumor-normal sample pairs. Bioinformatics. 2012;28:1811–7.

21. Ramos AH, Lichtenstein L, Gupta M, Lawrence MS, Pugh TJ, Saksena G, et al. Oncotator: cancer variant annotation tool. Hum Mutat. 2015;36:E2423–9.

22. Favero F, Joshi T, Marquard AM, Birkbak NJ, Krzystanek M, Li Q, et al. Sequenza: allele-specific copy number and mutation profiles from tumor sequencing data. Ann Oncol. 2015;26:64–70.

23. Mermel CH, Schumacher SE, Hill B, Meyerson ML, Beroukhim R, Getz G. GISTIC2.0 facilitates sensitive and confident localization of the targets of focal somatic copy-number alteration in human cancers. Genome Biol. 2011;12:R41.

24. Krijgsman O, Carvalho B, Meijer GA, Steenbergen RDM, Ylstra B. Focal chromosomal copy number aberrations in cancer-needles in a genome haystack. Biochim Biophys Acta. 1843;2014:2698–704.

25. Barbie DA, Tamayo P, Boehm JS, Kim SY, Moody SE, Dunn IF, et al. Systematic RNA interference reveals that oncogenic KRAS-driven cancers require TBK1. Nature. 2009;462:108–12.

26. Verhaak RGW, Tamayo P, Yang J-Y, Hubbard D, Zhang H, Creighton CJ, et al. Prognostically relevant gene signatures of high-grade serous ovarian carcinoma. J Clin Invest. 2013;123:517–25.

27. Yoshihara K, Shahmoradgoli M, Martínez E, Vegesna R, Kim H, Torres-Garcia W, et al. Inferring tumour purity and stromal and immune cell admixture from expression data. Nat Commun. 2013;4:2612.

28. Angelova M, Charoentong P, Hackl H, Fischer ML, Snajder R, Krogsdam AM, et al. Characterization of the immunophenotypes and antigenomes of colorectal cancers reveals distinct tumor escape mechanisms and novel targets for immunotherapy. Genome Biol. 2015;16:64.

29. Hänzelmann S, Castelo R, Guinney J. GSVA: gene set variation analysis for microarray and RNA-seq data. BMC Bioinformatics. 2013;14:7.

30. Kim D, Salzberg SL. TopHat-Fusion: an algorithm for discovery of novel fusion transcripts. Genome Biol. 2011;12:R72 [cited 2018 Feb 6]. Available from: http://genomebiology.biomedcentral.com/articles/10.1186/gb-2011-12-8-r72.

31. R Development Core Team. R: a language and environment for statistical computing. Vienna: the R Foundation for Statistical Computing; 2015. [cited 2017 Jun 19]. Available from: http://www.R-project.org/

32. Network TCGAR. Integrated genomic analyses of ovarian carcinoma. Nature. 2011;474:609–15 [cited 2017 Jun 19]. Available from: https://www.nature.com/nature/journal/v474/n7353/full/nature10166.html.

33. Pugh TJ, Morozova O, Attiyeh EF, Asgharzadeh S, Wei JS, Auclair D, et al. The genetic landscape of high-risk neuroblastoma. Nat Genet. 2013;45:279–84.

34. Rizvi NA, Hellmann MD, Snyder A, Kvistborg P, Makarov V, Havel JJ, et al. Cancer immunology. Mutational landscape determines sensitivity to PD-1 blockade in non-small cell lung cancer. Science. 2015;348:124–8.

35. Patch A-M, Christie EL, Etemadmoghadam D, Garsed DW, George J, Fereday S, et al. Whole-genome characterization of chemoresistant ovarian cancer. Nature. 2015;521:489–94.

36. Kanchi KL, Johnson KJ, Lu C, McLellan MD, Leiserson MDM, Wendl MC, et al. Integrated analysis of germline and somatic variants in ovarian cancer. Nat Commun. 2014;5:3156.

37. Brachova P, Mueting SR, Carlson MJ, Goodheart MJ, Button AM, Mott SL, et al. TP53 oncomorphic mutations predict resistance to platinum- and taxane-based standard chemotherapy in patients diagnosed with advanced serous ovarian carcinoma. Int J Oncol. 2015;46:607–18.

38. Alexandrov LB, Nik-Zainal S, Wedge DC, Aparicio SAJR, Behjati S, Biankin AV, et al. Signatures of mutational processes in human cancer. Nature. 2013;500:415–21 [cited 2017 Jun 19]. Available from: https://www.nature.com/nature/journal/v500/n7463/full/nature12477.html.

39. Lord CJ, Ashworth A. BRCAness revisited. Nat Rev Cancer. 2016;16:110–20.

40. Nakayama N, Nakayama K, Shamima Y, Ishikawa M, Katagiri A, Iida K, et al. Gene amplification CCNE1 is related to poor survival and potential therapeutic target in ovarian cancer. Cancer. 2010;116:2621–34.

41. Etemadmoghadam D, deFazio A, Beroukhim R, Mermel C, George J, Getz G, et al. Integrated genome-wide DNA copy number and expression analysis identifies distinct mechanisms of primary chemoresistance in ovarian carcinomas. Clin Cancer Res. 2009;15:1417–27.

42. Despierre E, Moisse M, Yesilyurt B, Sehouli J, Braicu I, Mahner S, et al. Somatic copy number alterations predict response to platinum therapy in epithelial ovarian cancer. Gynecol Oncol. 2014;135:415–22.

43. Gorringe KL, George J, Anglesio MS, Ramakrishna M, Etemadmoghadam D, Cowin P, et al. Copy number analysis identifies novel interactions between genomic loci in ovarian cancer. PLoS One. 2010;5(9). https://doi.org/10.1371/journal.pone.0011408.

44. Abkevich V, Timms KM, Hennessy BT, Potter J, Carey MS, Meyer LA, et al. Patterns of genomic loss of heterozygosity predict homologous recombination repair defects in epithelial ovarian cancer. Br J Cancer. 2012;107:1776–82.

45. Isakoff SJ, Mayer EL, He L, Traina TA, Carey LA, Krag KJ, et al. TBCRC009: a multicenter phase II clinical trial of platinum monotherapy with biomarker assessment in metastatic triple-negative breast cancer. J Clin Oncol. 2015;33:1902–9.

46. Lundgren S, Berntsson J, Nodin B, Micke P, Jirström K. Prognostic impact of tumour-associated B cells and plasma cells in epithelial ovarian cancer. J Ovarian Res. 2016;9:21.

47. Veeraraghavan J, Tan Y, Cao X-X, Kim JA, Wang X, Chamness GC, et al. Recurrent ESR1–CCDC170 rearrangements in an aggressive subset of oestrogen receptor-positive breast cancers. Nat Commun. 2014;5 Available from: http://www.nature.com/doifinder/10.1038/ncomms5577.

48. Wang L-L, Sun K-X, Wu D-D, Xiu Y-L, Chen X, Chen S, et al. DLEU1 contributes to ovarian carcinoma tumourigenesis and development by interacting with miR-490-3p and altering CDK1 expression. J Cell Mol Med. 2017;21:3055–65 [cited 2018 Feb 6]. Available from: http://doi.wiley.com/10.1111/jcmm.13217.

Landscape of genomic alterations in high-grade serous ovarian cancer from exceptional...

175

49. Du Bois A, Reuss A, Pujade-Lauraine E, Harter P, Ray-Coquard I, Pfisterer J. Role of surgical outcome as prognostic factor in advanced epithelial ovarian cancer: a combined exploratory analysis of 3 prospectively randomized phase 3 multicenter trials: by the Arbeitsgemeinschaft Gynaekologische Onkologie Studiengruppe Ovarialkarzinom (AGO-OVAR) and the Groupe d'Investigateurs Nationaux Pour les Etudes des Cancers de l'Ovaire (GINECO). Cancer. 2009;115:1234–44.

50. Wilbaux M, Hénin E, Oza A, Colomban O, Pujade-Lauraine E, Freyer G, et al. Dynamic modeling in ovarian cancer: an original approach linking early changes in modeled longitudinal CA-125 kinetics and survival to help decisions in early drug development. Gynecol Oncol. 2014;133:460–6.

51. You B, Colomban O, Heywood M, Lee C, Davy M, Reed N, et al. The strong prognostic value of KELIM, a model-based parameter from CA 125 kinetics in ovarian cancer: data from CALYPSO trial (a GINECO-GCIG study). Gynecol Oncol. 2013;130:289–94.

52. Oza AM, Cibula D, Benzaquen AO, Poole C, Mathijssen RHJ, Sonke GS, et al. Olaparib combined with chemotherapy for recurrent platinum-sensitive ovarian cancer: a randomised phase 2 trial. Lancet Oncol. 2015;16:87–97.

53. McAlpine JN, Porter H, Köbel M, Nelson BH, Prentice LM, Kalloger SE, et al. BRCA1 and BRCA2 mutations correlate with TP53 abnormalities and presence of immune cell infiltrates in ovarian high-grade serous carcinoma. Mod Pathol. 2012;25:740–50.

54. Clarke B, Tinker AV, Lee C-H, Subramanian S, van de Rijn M, Turbin D, et al. Intraepithelial T cells and prognosis in ovarian carcinoma: novel associations with stage, tumor type and BRCA1 loss. Mod Pathol. 2009;22:393–402 [cited 2018 Feb 9]. Available from: http://www.nature.com/articles/modpathol2008191.

55. Salgado R, Denkert C, Demaria S, Sirtaine N, Klauschen F, Pruneri G, et al. The evaluation of tumor-infiltrating lymphocytes (TILs) in breast cancer: recommendations by an International TILs Working Group 2014. Ann Oncol. 2015;26:259–71 [cited 2018 Feb 9]. Available from: http://academic.oup.com/annonc/article/26/2/259/2800585/The-evaluation-of-tumorinfiltrating-lymphocytes.

56. Petersen RP, Campa MJ, Sperlazza J, Conlon D, Joshi M-B, Harpole DH, et al. Tumor infiltrating Foxp3+ regulatory T-cells are associated with recurrence in pathologic stage I NSCLC patients. Cancer. 2006;107:2866–72 [cited 2018 Feb 9]. Available from: http://doi.wiley.com/10.1002/cncr.22282.

57. Clarke SL, Betts GJ, Plant A, Wright KL, El-Shanawany TM, Harrop R, et al. CD4+CD25+FOXP3+ regulatory T cells suppress anti-tumor immune responses in patients with colorectal cancer. PLoS One. 2006;1:e129 [cited 2018 Feb 9]. Available from: http://dx.plos.org/10.1371/journal.pone.0000129. Arendt C, editor.

58. Tothill RW, Tinker AV, George J, Brown R, Fox SB, Lade S, et al. Novel molecular subtypes of serous and endometrioid ovarian cancer linked to clinical outcome. Clin Cancer Res. 2008;14:5198–208.

59. Torres D, Wang C, Kumar A, Bakkum-Gamez JN, Weaver AL, McGree ME, et al. Factors that influence survival in high-grade serous ovarian cancer: a complex relationship between molecular subtype, disease dissemination, and operability. Gynecol Oncol. 2018;150(2):227–32. https://doi.org/10.1016/j.ygyno.2018.06.002.

60. Kommoss S, Winterhoff B, Oberg AL, Konecny GE, Wang C, Riska SM, et al. Bevacizumab may differentially improve ovarian cancer outcome in patients with proliferative and mesenchymal molecular subtypes. Clin Cancer Res. 2017;23:3794–801.

61. Mehra N, Lorente D, de Bono JS. What have we learned from exceptional tumour responses?: review and perspectives. Curr Opin Oncol. 2015;27:267–75.

62. Hoppenot C, Eckert MA, Tienda SM, Lengyel E. Who are the long-term survivors of high grade serous ovarian cancer? Gynecol Oncol. 2018;148:204–12.

63. Lheureux S, Bruce JP, Burnier JV, Karakasis K, Shaw PA, Clarke BA, et al. Somatic BRCA1/2 recovery as a resistance mechanism after exceptional response to poly (ADP-ribose) polymerase inhibition. J Clin Oncol Off J Am Soc Clin Oncol. 2017;35:1240–9.

13

A computational tool to detect DNA alterations tailored to formalin-fixed paraffin-embedded samples in cancer clinical sequencing

Mamoru Kato[1]* iD, Hiromi Nakamura[2], Momoko Nagai[1], Takashi Kubo[3], Asmaa Elzawahry[1], Yasushi Totoki[2], Yuko Tanabe[4], Eisaku Furukawa[1], Joe Miyamoto[1], Hiromi Sakamoto[5], Shingo Matsumoto[6], Kuniko Sunami[7], Yasuhito Arai[2], Yutaka Suzuki[8], Teruhiko Yoshida[5], Katsuya Tsuchihara[6], Kenji Tamura[4], Noboru Yamamoto[4], Hitoshi Ichikawa[3], Takashi Kohno[7] and Tatsuhiro Shibata[2,9]

Abstract

Advanced cancer genomics technologies are now being employed in clinical sequencing, where next-generation sequencers are used to simultaneously identify multiple types of DNA alterations for prescription of molecularly targeted drugs. However, no computational tool is available to accurately detect DNA alterations in formalin-fixed paraffin-embedded (FFPE) samples commonly used in hospitals. Here, we developed a computational tool tailored to the detection of single nucleotide variations, indels, fusions, and copy number alterations in FFPE samples. Elaborated multilayer noise filters reduced the inherent noise while maintaining high sensitivity, as evaluated in tumor-unmatched normal samples using orthogonal technologies. This tool, cisCall, should facilitate clinical sequencing in everyday diagnostics.

Background

In recent years, large-scale cancer genome projects such as the International Cancer Genome Consortium [1–3] (ICGC) and The Cancer Genome Atlas (TCGA) have greatly expanded the available knowledge on genomic alterations in cancer. Along with this increasing knowledge, the number of investigational and approved drugs that target aberrant gene products continues to grow [4]. Genomics technologies that have matured through research are now being translated to the clinical setting. In cancer clinical sequencing, next-generation sequencing (NGS) is applied to identify genetic alterations in biopsy or surgical specimens [4–6]. The detected variants are used as targets for molecularly targeted drugs. The advantage of NGS technologies is that they allow the simultaneous detection of various types of aberrations, i.e., single nucleotide variations (SNVs), indels, copy number alterations (CNAs), and gene fusions, in a multitude of genes.

A practical application of clinical sequencing is the identification of DNA alterations in the exons of hundreds of genes in formalin-fixed paraffin-embedded (FFPE) samples, as reported by Frampton et al. [6]. FFPE samples are the first choice for clinical sequencing because such archival samples are needed for mandatory pathological examination, and their storage at room temperature is substantially less costly than that of fresh frozen tissues. One critical issue is the accurate calling of DNA alterations from FFPE-based sequencing data. Chemical processing damages and fragments genomic DNA, resulting in increased error rates and artificial base substitution bias [6–8]. Moreover, low tumor purity [6] and the non-availability of matched normal samples and panels of normal (PON) samples [9] are frequent problems peculiar to clinical sequencing that arise owing to practical and ethical reasons.

Most current computational tools [9–21] for calling cancer DNA alterations have been developed for

* Correspondence:
[1]Department of Bioinformatics, National Cancer Center Research Institute, Chuo-ku, Tokyo 104-0045, Japan
Full list of author information is available at the end of the article

exploratory research, mostly assuming the use of fresh frozen samples with relatively high tumor purity for Illumina exome/genome sequencing. Some tools for SNVs assume low tumor content but high read depth [22, 23]. Clearly, these tools are not optimal for FFPE sequencing. One successful variant caller for FPPE samples has been reported by a private company [6]; however, the software is not publicly available.

Here, we report the development of an accurate caller termed "clinical sequencing caller" (cisCall), specialized for identifying DNA alterations from FFPE samples. cisCall is composed of cisMuton, cisFusion, and cisCton, which respectively call SNVs/indels, DNA gene fusions, and CNAs. We show that this computational tool exhibits high performance under a variety of experimental conditions. In this report, we focus on the bioinformatics research aspects of the present calling tool for FFPE samples. The regulatory or clinical testing standards, as well as the clinical significance and the validity of experimental processes (which have been discussed elsewhere [24]), are beyond the scope of this work.

Methods
Materials
Sequencing data were derived from cell lines (HCC78 and NCI-H2228), patient samples, and a commercial sample. HCC78 and NCI-H2228 were provided by Dr. John D. Minna of the UT Southwestern Medical Center. Snap-frozen tumor and normal tissues as well as FFPE archival samples that had been obtained at diagnosis were provided by the National Cancer Center (NCC) Biobank. A commercial synthetic human FFPE sample, HD200, was purchased from Horizon (Cambridge, United Kingdom). Twenty normal DNA samples were extracted from noncancerous lung tissues deposited in the NCC Biobank (the biobank did not collect control non-pathological FFPE samples). Half of the lung tissues were from smokers. From the mixture of the 20 normal DNA samples, an unmatched pooled sample was prepared and used as a background dataset in alteration calling. In total, 70 FFPE clinical samples were used as foreground datasets for SNV/indel analysis, and 75 FFPE clinical samples were used as foreground datasets for CNA analysis (five samples were increased because CNA analysis was performed later than SNV analysis). The details on samples are summarized in Additional file 1: Table S1. We validated alterations in 27 and 23 FFPE samples for SNV/indel and CNA analyses, respectively.

Genomic DNA from FFPE tissues was prepared with a QIAamp DNA FFPE tissue kit (Qiagen, Hilden, Germany) and quantified using a Qubit dsDNA BR assay kit (Thermo Fisher Scientific, Waltham, MA, USA) as well as quantitative PCR analysis. The ratio of PCR-amplifiable DNA to total dsDNA indicates DNA quality. When this quality value was ≥ 0.1, samples were retained for sequencing. We further selected FFPE samples with a pathologically measured tumor purity of $\geq 10\%$.

Targeted Illumina sequencing
We used custom gene panels for target capture sequencing: the NCC oncopanel v1 (all exons of 134 tumor-related genes and introns of three fusion genes) and v2 (all exons of 90 tumor-related genes and introns of 35 fusion genes; Additional file 2: Table S2) and the NCC Hospital East oncopanel (all exons of 121 tumor-related genes and introns of 12 fusion genes). The bait libraries were designed with SureDesign (Agilent Technologies, Santa Clara, CA, USA). Sequencing libraries were prepared using SureSelect XT reagent (Agilent Technologies), and paired-end read sequencing was performed on MiSeq or HiSeq sequencers (Illumina, San Diego, CA, USA).

Targeted Ion sequencing
We used custom gene panels for target capture sequencing: the NCC oncopanel v1 and the RET panel (37 fusion genes), the latter of which was specifically designed for genes fused with RET [25–28]. The bait libraries were designed with SureDesign, and the sequencing libraries were prepared using SureSelect XT reagent. For amplicon sequencing, we used the commercial Ion AmpliSeq Cancer Hotspot Panel v2 (hotspot regions of 50 genes; Thermo Fisher Scientific). The sequencing libraries were prepared using an Ion AmpliSeq Library Kit (Thermo Fisher). Single-end read sequencing was performed on Ion PGM or Proton sequencers (Thermo Fisher).

Validation of SNVs/indels by mass spectrometry
SNVs/indels were validated by iPLEX SNP genotyping using Sequenom MassARRAY, according to the manufacturer's instructions (Agena Bioscience, San Diego, CA, USA). PCR primers and an extended primer were designed using Assay Design Suite software (Agena Bioscience). After PCR amplification and single-nucleotide extension, data were collected on the MassARRAY Analyzer 4 system.

Validation of CNAs by qPCR
CNAs were validated by qPCR using TaqMan Fast Universal Master Mix and TaqMan probes (Additional file 3: Table S3) on an Applied Biosystems 7500 Fast Sequence Detection System according to the manufacturer's instructions (Applied Biosystems, Foster City, CA, USA). Samples were run in triplicate and standardized against endogenous RNase P with RNase P Detection Reagents Kit (Applied Biosystems).

cisMuton

cisMuton was developed for variation calling from Illumina sequencing data from FFPE samples and Illumina/Ion sequencing data from frozen tissues. cisMuton uses FASTQ and BAM file formats. The algorithm comprises prep filters, the variant extraction step, and eight and nine noise filters for Illumina and Ion sequencing data, respectively (Additional file 2: Figure S1). The prep filters filter out reads based on mapping and base qualities. The variant extraction step uses several statistics derived from Fisher's exact test to detect A/C/G/T and indels at each chromosomal position. The subsequent noise filter consists of three sets. The first set contains the misalignment filter, strand-bias filter, and others, for which we utilized as many statistical tests and internal controls as possible. Filters in the second set remove erroneous reads and trim erroneous read ends, followed by a second Fisher's exact test for the remaining reads. Filters in the third set remove errors that escaped the previous filters, utilizing statistical tests based on variant allele frequencies (VAFs). The algorithmic details are described in Additional file 2: Text S1.

cisFusion

cisFusion is a fusion caller applicable to single-end (Ion) and paired-end (Illumina) DNA sequence reads. cisFusion searches for a gene fusion of which at least one gene is indicated by a user. The algorithm consists of the "2map" and "VF" steps for the single-end mode, and further of the "paired-end" step for the paired-end mode (Additional file 2: Figure S2). The 2map step searches for reads that are mapped to two different genes on the right and left ends, with fusion breakpoints. The VF step saves reads that are missed by the 2map step because of too short alignment, using "virtual fusion" sequences constructed from reads found in the 2map step. The paired-end step searches for R1 and R2 reads between which a fusion breakpoint exists. The algorithmic details are described in Additional file 2: Text S1.

cisCton

cisCton first executes a GC-content correction, in which locally weighted scatterplot smoothing (LOWESS) regression between binned depths and GC content is performed to correct the depths. Then, it performs circular binary segmentation (CBS) with a non-parametric statistic (the Mann–Whitney U statistic) for $logR$ calculated from the GC-corrected depths. For a fast computation, cisCton splits a chromosome into windows of a specified size, within which it performs CBS to finally compile the CBS results to chromosome-size segments. It then executes the abortion process: it aborts a segment if the number of individual $logR$ values that deviate from the median $logR$ of a segment exceeds a threshold.

Finally, cisCton defines amplifications or deletions by a bootstrapping approach. The algorithmic details are described in Additional file 2: Text S1.

Performance evaluation

Details of the procedures for performance evaluation are presented in Additional file 2: Text S1.

Results

We evaluated cisCall using maximally 75 FFPE samples from a clinical study for entry into early-phase clinical trials at the National Cancer Center Japan [24]. In the study, all exons of 90 genes and reportedly translocated introns of 35 fusion genes (12 kinases and 23 partners) were captured by our original gene panel (NCC oncopanel v2; Additional file 2: Table S2). These exons and introns were sequenced for the detection of SNVs/indels, CNAs, and DNA gene fusions. Target capturing and sequencing were performed using Agilent SureSelect and Illumina MiSeq. Paired-end 150-base sequencing reads were obtained. Reads from a tumor sample and from a frozen sample mixed with noncancerous samples of 20 individuals were used as test (foreground) and control (background) datasets to call DNA alterations, respectively.

The FFPE samples were mostly from breast (31%), gastric (29%), and ovarian (14%) cancers; the histologically determined median tumor content was 40% (interquartile range of 25–65%). The median sequencing depth was 760× (interquartile range, 526–903×). The traceable storage time of all but one FFPE sample sequenced on the basis of the threshold of the FFPE sample quality (Methods) was less than 10 years. For more detailed information about the samples, please refer to Additional file 1: Table S1 and Additional file 2: Figure S3.

SNV/indel calling

Features of cisMuton

cisMuton detects SNVs/indels from targeted sequencing data. It extracts variants using a non-parametric test, Fisher's exact test [10], by statistically comparing the numbers of A/C/G/T and insertions/deletions of a tumor sample with those of a control sample at each chromosomal position. We chose this method because a non-parametric test makes fewer assumptions than model-based (likelihood or Bayesian) methods; no assumptions are made on Phred scores or error rates, for which the calibration and degrees may differ between FFPE and frozen samples and between different experimental conditions.

cisMuton is characterized by elaborate noise filters to manage the high level of noise in FFPE samples (Additional file 2: Figure S1). Variant extraction methods such as the frequency cutoff method [29] and likelihood or Bayesian methods [11–15, 22, 23] alone do not suffice to filter out noise that arises from errors correlated between different chromosomal positions, such as misalignment. Because we observed that FFPE samples produce many correlated errors, we focused on the improvement of noise filters by incorporating multiple, robust statistical tests and internal controls (e.g., error rates calculated from the data), resulting in a greater flexibility to handle data with different qualities.

We devised the following filters: 1) misalignment filter, 2) strand-bias filter, 3) within-long-homopolymer filter, 4) MQ0 filter, 5) read-end-call filter, 6) surrounded-by-dust filter, 7) abnormal-BQ-drop filter (for Ion-derived indels only), 8) second Fisher filter combined with mismatch filter and trim filter, and 9) VAF-lees filter.

For example, the VAF-lees filter removes "lees" of calls that show suspiciously low VAFs but are not filtered by the other filters for unknown reasons. The distribution of VAFs is regarded as a beta-mixture distribution and the component beta distributions are automatically detected by the expectation maximization algorithm [30]. The algorithm calculates the ICL-BIC criterion [31] to select the best model of all models with different numbers (ranging from 1 to 10) of beta components. The algorithm then searches for the beta component for which the distribution's average is within a range of low frequencies (e.g., 1–3%), which means that a peak of the VAFs is found at such a low value. It regards such a component as an error distribution, and performs a beta-binomial test for variant and depth counts in a tumor sample to remove lees. cisMuton itself does not have any hard cut-off for VAFs, though variants with low VAFs may be removed from a clinical viewpoint by the tumor board. The algorithmic details and illustrations of all filters are presented in Additional file 2: Text S1 and Additional file 2: Figure S1, respectively. The execution time of cisMuton is typically 1 h 50 min ± 22 (standard deviation (s.d.)) min on a 10-core 2.0 GHz CPU with 264 GB memory for FASTQ files with 7.9 ± 0.6 million reads (either R1 or R2 reads) with 150-bp length.

Performance evaluation of cisMuton

We evaluated the performance of cisMuton in comparison with Mutect [9], Shearwater [23], Varscan2 [10], and Strelka [11]. We first evaluated these tools using controlled negative/positive data. As negative data, the same tissue block was used to extract tumor FFPE samples for foreground data and tumor frozen samples for background data. Here, not FFPE but frozen samples were used as the background because we assumed unavailability of non-pathological FFPE samples in *actual* clinical sequencing. The extracted FFPE and frozen samples

theoretically have the same tumor mutations; therefore, any calls from these data should be false positives in the FFPE samples. cisMuton and Mutect yielded no calls (Fig. 1a). Shearwater and Varscan2 reported some (2 and 10 per 477 kb target size) calls, whereas Strelka generated ~ 1000 calls per 477-kb target size (Fig. 1a).

For the false-negative rate, we used semi-simulated data as positive data because it is difficult to know all variants in natural samples. We randomly mixed reads from a lung cancer cell line (100% tumor purity) with reads from an unmatched normal sample to mimic a wide range of tumor purity. The depth was 970 on average, where we aimed for a depth of 1000 because our power calculation suggested that this would be ideal. We used these mixed datasets and a different normal dataset as the fore- and background datasets for calling, respectively. Variants genotyped by SNP arrays in the pure cell-line sample were used as answers. cisMuton showed 100% sensitivity for cell line/normal sample ratios down to 10%, and nearly 80% sensitivity at a ratio of 5% (Fig. 1b). Strelka showed the same sensitivity, but the other tools performed less well. The specificity was almost the same (~ 1) among all the tools. Based on both the negative control and these positive control results, cisMuton demonstrated the best performance.

Next, we made calls for 70 FFPE samples (Additional file 2: Figure S4). For each tool, we counted the number of variants called, as well as those not called by the given tool but detected by all other tools, because we considered that such isolated calls would reflect the specific nature of each algorithm. cisMuton reported the least isolated SNVs and indels, indicating that it was the most balanced among all tools (Fig. 1c). For reference, the numbers of variants removed by the noise filters are shown in Additional file 2: Table S4. cisMuton's calls together with their VAFs and histologically determined tumor purity are shown in Additional file 2: Figure S5.

Variants with low VAFs (such as < 10%) are recommended to be filtered out in sequencing of FFPE samples [32]. Because our criterion in this clinical sequencing was to select FFPE samples with a pathologically measured tumor purity of ≥ 10%, we stratified the isolated calls at 5% VAFs (assuming the maximum major clone in the copy number neutral state). Even taking into account ≥ 5% VAFs, substantial numbers of isolated calls were found in all of the other tools for SNVs, and cisMuton was the most balanced (Fig. 1c). For indels, cisMuton was not the most balanced anymore; many (23 per 477 kb target size) indels were called only by cisMuton. Nevertheless, validation analysis, as described below, should be needed for such isolated calls, which may be false negatives for the other tools.

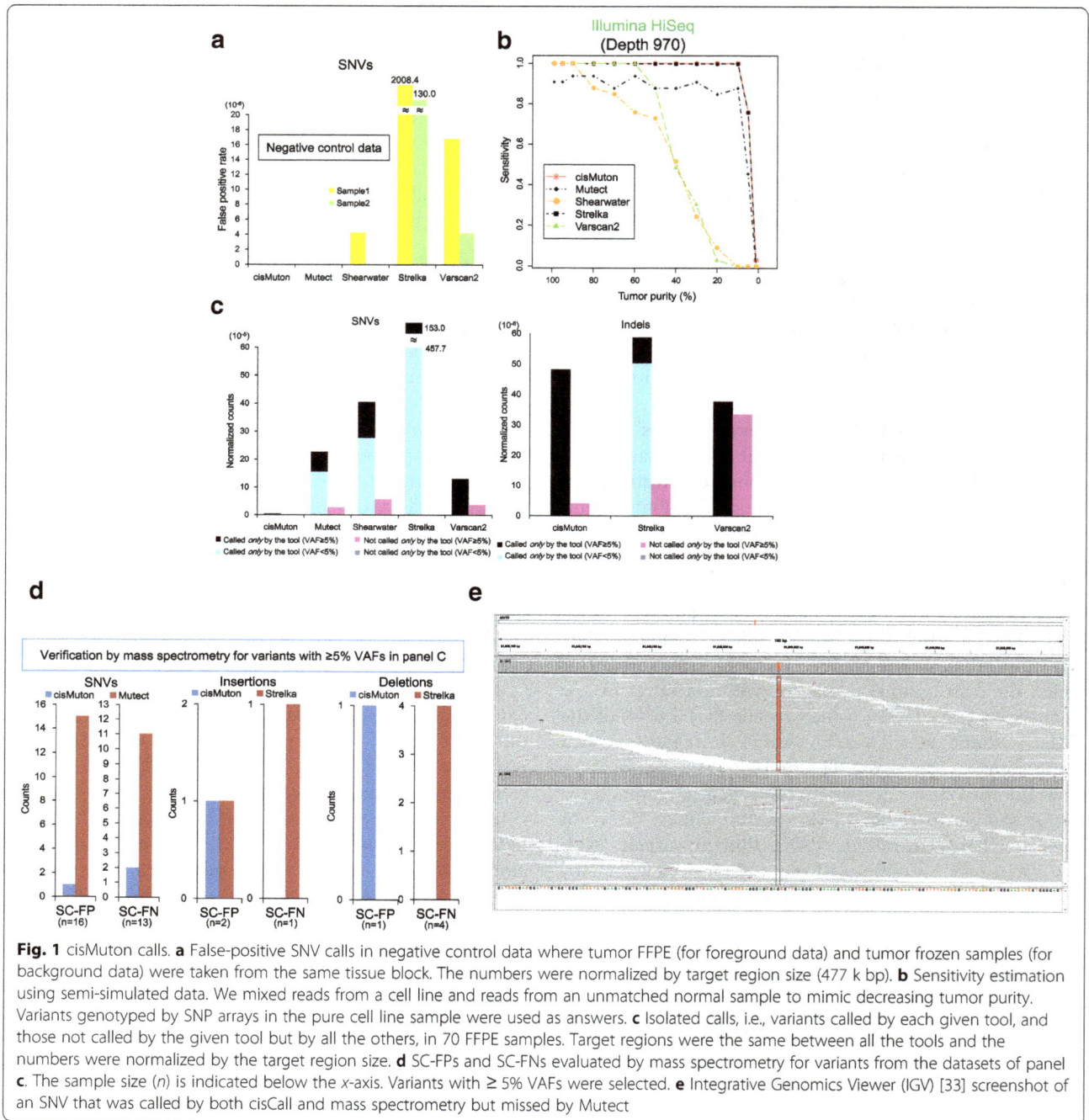

Fig. 1 cisMuton calls. **a** False-positive SNV calls in negative control data where tumor FFPE (for foreground data) and tumor frozen samples (for background data) were taken from the same tissue block. The numbers were normalized by target region size (477 k bp). **b** Sensitivity estimation using semi-simulated data. We mixed reads from a cell line and reads from an unmatched normal sample to mimic decreasing tumor purity. Variants genotyped by SNP arrays in the pure cell line sample were used as answers. **c** Isolated calls, i.e., variants called by each given tool, and those not called by the given tool but by all the others, in 70 FFPE samples. Target regions were the same between all the tools and the numbers were normalized by the target region size. **d** SC-FPs and SC-FNs evaluated by mass spectrometry for variants from the datasets of panel **c**. The sample size (n) is indicated below the x-axis. Variants with ≥ 5% VAFs were selected. **e** Integrative Genomics Viewer (IGV) [33] screenshot of an SNV that was called by both cisCall and mass spectrometry but missed by Mutect

We selected variants from isolated calls in Fig. 1c for validation by mass spectrometry (Sequenom MassAR-RAY), where calls with ≥ 5% VAFs were selected because of difficulty in detecting variants with lower VAFs by mass spectrometry, and because of our criterion to select FFPE samples with a tumor purity of ≥ 10%. We refer to false positives/negatives in this isolated-call validation as severe conditioned-false positives/negatives (SC-FPs and SC-FNs) because isolated calls were expected to be less validated than the other calls such as those called by multiple tools. We compared the performance of cisMuton with that of Mutect and Strelka for SNVs and indels, respectively. Whereas cisMuton yielded 1/16 SC-FPs and 2/13 SC-FNs, Mutect generated 15/16 SC-FPs and 11/13 SC-FNs (Fig. 1d). An Integrative Genomics Viewer [33] screenshot of mass spectrometry-validated SNVs that were called by cis-Call but missed by Mutect shows substantial noise *around* the SNV that was supposed to come from FFPE processes (Fig. 1e). For deletions, cisMuton yielded no SC-FNs, whereas Strelka generated 4/4 SC-FNs. Both tools did not greatly differ (one or zero counts) in SC-FP in deletions and SC-FP/FN in insertions.

We examined factors that may be associated with performance. 1) SC-FP and SC-FN variants seemed to be affected by depth and tumor purity. The effective depth, defined by the depth of each variant × pathologically measured tumor purity, was low for the SC-FP variants in cisCall (median 26.0, compared with 184.5 for the other variants) and in Mutect (29.7) (plotted in Additional file 2: Figure S6). The effective depth was low for the SC-FN variants in cisCall (53.1) and high for those of Mutect (503.1), probably due to excess filtering as shown above in Fig. 1e. 2) The FFPE storage time seemed to affect the performance. SC-FP tended to be found in older FFPE samples (median 53.0 and 55.0 months over samples with SC-FP variants for cisCall and Mutect, compared with 24.5 months over the other samples; Additional file 2: Figure S6). 3) Mutation load did not seem to be related to SC-FP and SC-FN (Additional file 2: Figure S6), although the range of the number of mutations was insufficient in this study (5–20 somatic mutations detected in 90% of the samples).

Fusion calling
Features of cisFusion
cisFusion detects gene fusions and their breakpoint positions in either single-end or paired-end targeted DNA sequencing reads. In contrast, most existing tools have been developed for RNA-seq or paired-end whole-genome sequencing [18]. As RNA is more prone to degradation than DNA, we used DNA for fusion calling from the FPPE samples. Because most gene fusions occur in intron regions [25], we designed capture regions to include such introns. cisFusion utilizes local alignment (BWA-SW [34]) to easily extract breakpoint positions; in contrast, many other callers primarily use global alignment, in which additional complex procedures such as splitting reads are usually required for extracting breakpoint positions. Please refer to the "Methods" and Additional file 2: Text S1 for the algorithmic details. cisFusion typically takes 1 h 52 min ± 35 min (s.d.) using the same settings described above in the cisMuton section.

Performance evaluation of cisFusion
Because the prevalence of fusion genes in actual clinical samples is very low [35], we used cell lines ($n = 5$), frozen tissue ($n = 4$), and FFPE tissue samples ($n = 5$) known to contain fusion genes (Additional file 1: Table S1). We compared cisFusion with FusionMap [16], which is also applicable to DNA target sequencing using single- and paired-end reads. In all 14 datasets, cisFusion ranked correct fusions as the top candidate, as indicated by signal-to-noise (S/N) ratios of more than one (Fig. 2a, b). cisFusion yielded no false positives in all but one case, as indicated by S/N ratios noted as infinity. In contrast, FusionMap ranked incorrect fusion candidates as the top candidate in 12 of the 14 samples, as indicated by S/N ratios of less than one. In two of the five FFPE samples (Fig. 2b), FusionMap did not even list correct fusions, as indicated by S/N ratios of zero. Fig. 2c shows an example of support reads of a fusion gene in an FFPE sample that was detected by cisFusion but not by FusionMap. Mismatch bases are substantially observed. The normalized support read count (Fig. 2a, b) indicates that cisFusion demonstrated better sensitivity than FusionMap in all cases except one. In particular, remarkable superiority in both the specificity (the S/N ratio) and sensitivity was observed in FFPE samples. Additionally, fusion breakpoints were correctly predicted in 9/9 frozen and 3/5 FFPE cases by cisFusion, and in 8/9 frozen and 1/5 FFPE cases by FusionMap (although with some differences in base pairs; Additional file 4: Table S5).

CNA calling
Features of cisCton
cisCton discovers CNAs in targeted sequencing data on the basis of the log ratio of the read depth of a tumor sample to that of a control sample. cisCton utilizes a non-parametric statistic in the circular binary segmentation (CBS) framework [36] and a process to abort detected segments with high fluctuations to manage the strong noise in FFPE data, as shown in Fig. 3a. Details of the algorithm are described in the Methods and Additional file 2: Text S1. cisCton typically takes 1 h 55 min ± 6 min (s.d.) using the same settings described above in the cisMuton section.

Performance evaluation of cisCton
We first evaluated false positives using the same negative control data as used in SNV/indel calling. Performance was compared with that of Varscan2 [10], ExomeCNV [19], and Control-FREEC [20], which can call somatic CNAs from targeted (or exome) sequencing data by the read-depth method [21]. For a fair comparison, we counted the number of amplified or deleted target-capture regions. In the negative control data, cisCton called no amplified regions and almost no (3 per 477-kb target size) deleted regions (Fig. 3b, c). The other tools called hundreds of false amplified and deleted regions per 477-kb target size (Fig. 3b, c).

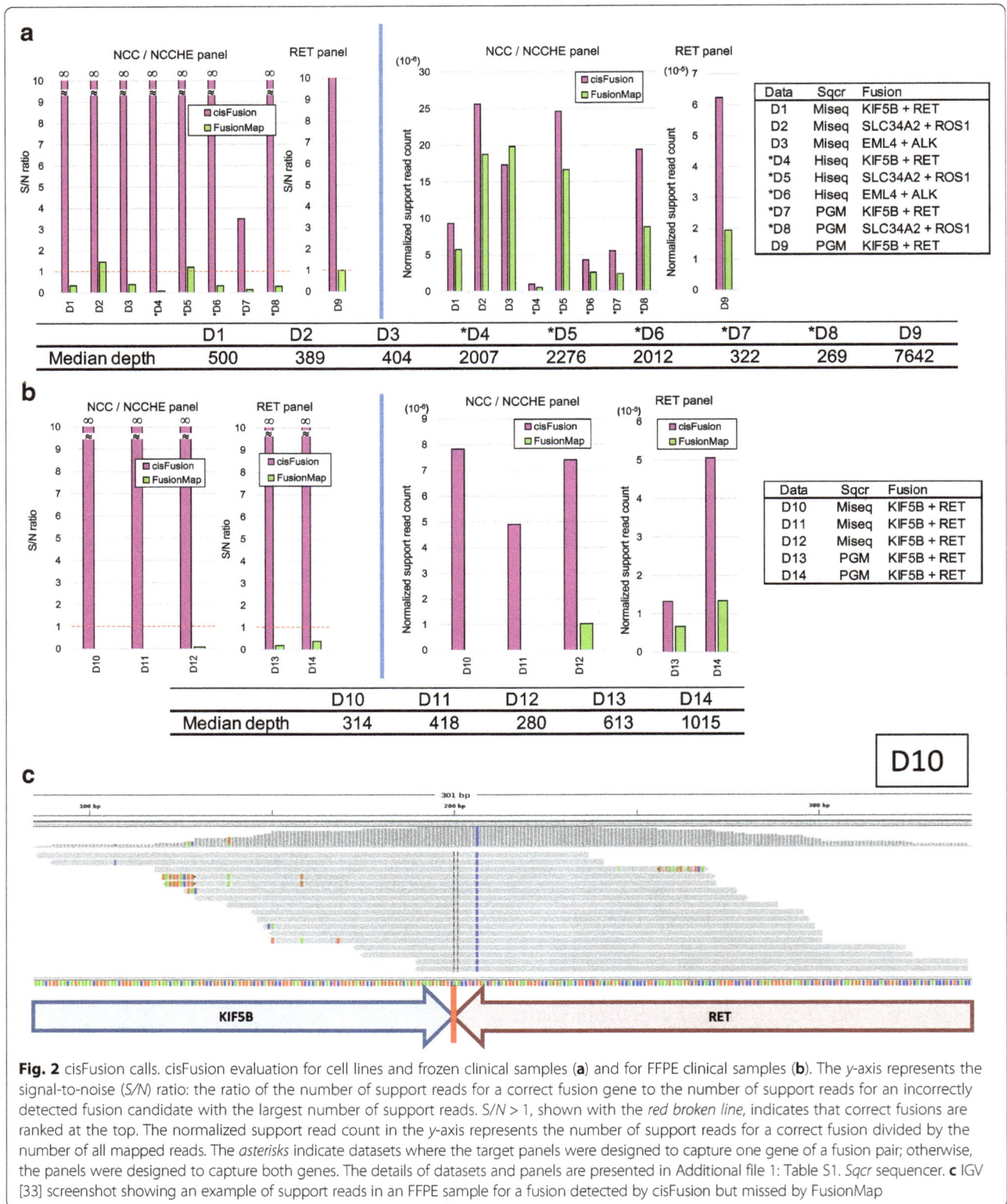

Fig. 2 cisFusion calls. cisFusion evaluation for cell lines and frozen clinical samples (**a**) and for FFPE clinical samples (**b**). The *y*-axis represents the signal-to-noise (*S/N*) ratio: the ratio of the number of support reads for a correct fusion gene to the number of support reads for an incorrectly detected fusion candidate with the largest number of support reads. *S/N* > 1, shown with the *red broken line*, indicates that correct fusions are ranked at the top. The normalized support read count in the *y*-axis represents the number of support reads for a correct fusion divided by the number of all mapped reads. The *asterisks* indicate datasets where the target panels were designed to capture one gene of a fusion pair; otherwise, the panels were designed to capture both genes. The details of datasets and panels are presented in Additional file 1: Table S1. *Sqcr* sequencer. **c** IGV [33] screenshot showing an example of support reads in an FFPE sample for a fusion detected by cisFusion but missed by FusionMap

Next, we ran the tools on the 75 FFPE samples. The Venn diagrams of the calls are shown in Additional file 2: Figure S7. In clinical sequencing, molecularly targeted drugs are usually applied to amplifications; thus, we focused on amplifications. For each tool, we counted isolated calls, i.e., amplified regions called by the given tool,

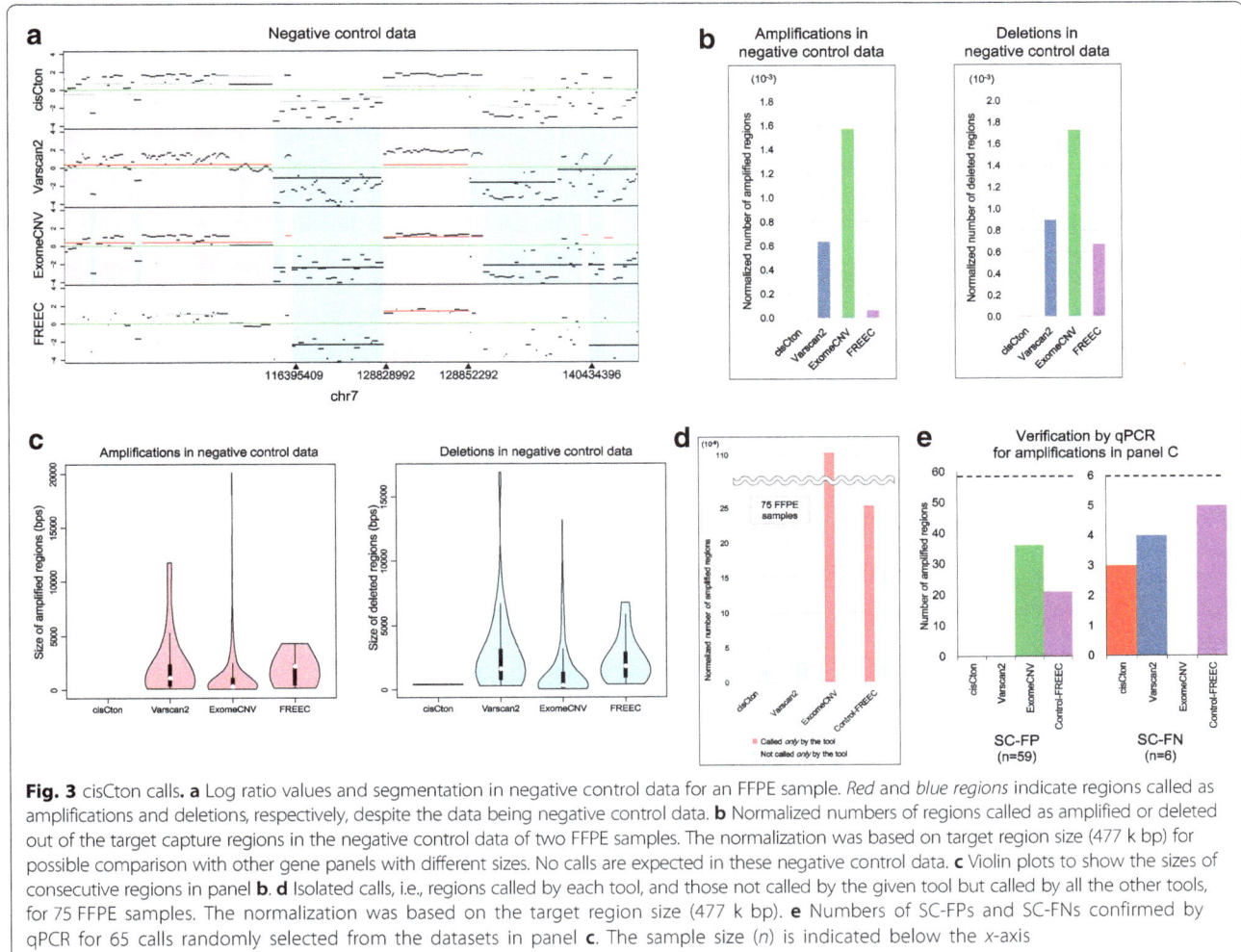

Fig. 3 cisCton calls. **a** Log ratio values and segmentation in negative control data for an FFPE sample. *Red* and *blue regions* indicate regions called as amplifications and deletions, respectively, despite the data being negative control data. **b** Normalized numbers of regions called as amplified or deleted out of the target capture regions in the negative control data of two FFPE samples. The normalization was based on target region size (477 k bp) for possible comparison with other gene panels with different sizes. No calls are expected in these negative control data. **c** Violin plots to show the sizes of consecutive regions in panel **b**. **d** Isolated calls, i.e., regions called by each tool, and those not called by the given tool but called by all the other tools, for 75 FFPE samples. The normalization was based on the target region size (477 k bp). **e** Numbers of SC-FPs and SC-FNs confirmed by qPCR for 65 calls randomly selected from the datasets in panel **c**. The sample size (*n*) is indicated below the *x*-axis

and those called by the other tools but not the given tool. cisCton had the lowest count of isolated calls, whereas ExomeCNV and Control-FREEC yielded approximately 100 isolated calls (Fig. 3d). From isolated calls made at the gene level, we randomly selected 65 calls for which qPCR probes were successfully designed. qPCR experiments revealed that cisCton was most balanced for SC-FPs (0/59) and SC-FNs (3/6) (Fig. 3e). ExomeCNV had many SC-FPs (36/59) but no SC-FNs (0/6). Control-FREEC yielded 21/59 SC-FPs and 5/6 SC-FNs. Varscan2 yielded the same number of SC-FPs (0/59) as cisCton but slightly more SC-FNs (4/6).

Discussion

We developed an SNV/indel/fusion/CNA calling tool specialized for data obtained from FFPE samples. cisCall was previously employed in clinical sequencing for a clinical study [24], in which a good validation rate of 128/129 for SNVs and 12/13 for indels in 70 samples

was confirmed by mass spectrometry. We also used a commercially available FFPE reference material and successfully detected all eight SNVs with > 5% VAFs, further obtaining a good concordance between expected and computed VAFs ($R = 0.99$; Additional file 2: Figure S8), although the specificity cannot be evaluated in this type of material because not all variants are known in advance. We conducted a rigorous tool comparison using SC-FPs and SC-FNs based on isolated calls; however, it is worth noting that these numbers would be inflated compared with the validation rate based on all calls. A more rigorous way to evaluate the performance would be to 1) prioritize samples, 2) call alterations by tools, 3) validate all alterations called by any of the tools based on orthogonal methods such as mass spectrometry and qPCR, and 4) calculate evaluation indices such as specificity, sensitivity, and F-measure. We demonstrated that cisCall outperformed currently available tools developed for exploratory research purposes, which generally assume the use of cell lines or fresh-frozen clinical samples. One caveat is that we used default parameters for the compared tools; we did not use LOD_T of > 50 for Mutect, which is recommended for FFPE samples [37].

We reason that our tool performed well because 1) we used non-parametric statistical methods wherever possible to absorb abrupt, unpredictable fluctuations stemming from FFPE errors, and 2) we elaborated noise filters for all types of mutations, such as the misalignment filter for SNVs/indels and the abortion filter for CNAs. We believe that this design concept also makes cisCall applicable to reads from Ion sequencers. When we evaluated the performance of cisMuton for Ion PGM data using semi-simulated data, it showed the highest (100%) sensitivity among all tested tools for cell line/normal mixtures down to 10% cell line ratios (Additional file 2: Figure S9; the specificity was ~ 1 for all tools).

Commercially developed algorithms for detecting SNVs/indels and CNAs from FFPE-based sequencing data have been reported [6]; however, the software is not publicly available. Moreover, regarding SNVs, the software performance was systematically evaluated mainly using cell lines, the sample features of which are more similar to frozen than to FPPE clinical samples, and based on germline, not tumor, variants [6]. In addition, the fusion algorithm was not systematically evaluated. Another research group reported an in-house SNV/indel-calling program fine-tuned for FFPE samples [38]; however, the detailed algorithm was not described, and the tools were not subjected to systematic comparison with other tools. In contrast, we evaluated all SNV/indel/CNA/fusion calling algorithms in FFPE samples. Our software tool is publicly available.

Although cisCall showed the best performance on SC-FN in CNA evaluation (Fig. 3), the SC-FN rate was relatively high. The reason for this was the discrepancy in the strength of GC-content correction between FFPE and frozen samples. Depth values fluctuated more in foreground FFPE samples than in the background frozen sample. Depth values in regions with high GC content in the FFPE samples scattered up to high values. Because there were only a few high GC content regions in our targeted regions, the LOWESS curve was easily pulled upward. GC-content correction was thus weaker in FFPE samples than in frozen samples for regions with high GC content, and hence amplification signals in FFPE samples were cancelled out. cisCall failed to call CNAs in high GC-content regions. It is necessary to improve the LOWESS procedure for regions with high GC content. Also, use of control FFPE samples will be another possibility to improve the baselines for CNA detection.

The limitations of our algorithms are: 1) large indels are not targeted, i.e., we assumed indels with BWA-mapped sizes (≤ 6 bps found in our cases); 2) we did not assume whole-exome or whole-genome sequencing; and 3) consequently, we cannot handle structural variations beyond targeted fusion genes. We are currently working on overcoming these limitations. For application to different experimental settings, such as whole-exome sequencing, elaborate parameter tuning will be necessary. Additionally, application to other gene panels should be tested and the algorithms and codes should be improved for faster computation.

Because matched normal samples were not available in this project, we evaluated our tool in tumor–mixed normal paired samples. To filter out germline SNPs, we removed mutations listed in SNP databases and those with 40–60% and > 96% VAFs. This simple approach can largely remove germline SNPs and a more sophisticated approach using machine learning may be possible [39]; however, it is desirable to use matched normal samples for precise filtering if such samples are available. It is in principle possible to apply our tool to tumor–matched normal paired samples and we are obtaining preliminary results in such samples, though further investigation should be needed. Off-target reads that mapped on non-target regions constituted more than 0.1× coverage (0.3–0.4× on average) genome-wide in our data; utilization of these reads may help identifying copy-number loss related to homologous recombination repair deficiency in non-target regions in FFPE samples [40, 41]. cisCall was developed for research purposes in clinical studies and is not intended for use in clinical tests regulated by the authorities, where analytical validity at the manufacturing level should be demonstrated. Nevertheless, these alteration-calling algorithms enable first steps in the translation of cancer clinical sequencing to everyday diagnostics.

Conclusions

Clinical sequencing requires an accurate computational tool to call multiple types of DNA alterations—SNVs/indels, fusion genes, and CNAs—from NGS data in FFPE samples. We developed such a tool and demonstrated that our tool outperformed seven other tools that have been developed for explanatory research purposes. This is because our tool uses robust non-parametric statistics to select alteration candidates and more than ten elaborated noise filters that maximally utilize internal control values automatically calculated from observed data as inputs for the tool's parameters so that the tool can efficiently remove inherent noise arising in FFPE samples that cannot be filtered out using other tools. Our tool allows us to accurately detect DNA alterations in multiple genes, which will promote more accurate and efficient cancer precision medicine.

Abbreviations

CBS: Circular binary segmentation; CNA: Copy number alteration; CNV: Copy number variation; FFPE: Formalin-fixed paraffin-embedded; ICGC: International Cancer Genome Consortium; IGV: Integrative Genomics Viewer; LOWESS: Locally weighted scatterplot smoothing; NCC: National Cancer Center; NGS: Next-generation sequencing; PON: Panels of normal; S/N: Signal-to-noise; SC-FN: Severe conditioned-false negative; SC-FP: Severe conditioned-false positive; SNV: Single nucleotide variation; TCGA: The Cancer Genome Atlas; VAF: Variant allele frequency

Acknowledgements

We thank Tatsuji Mizukami, Yuichi Shiraishi, and Masao Nagasaki for useful discussions, and Isao Kurosaka for providing technical assistance.

Funding

This work was supported by Takeda Science Foundation (to MK), Japan Agency for Medical Research and Development (15ck0106012h0002 to MK and TKo, 15ck0106117h0002 to MK), CREST-JST (14531766 to MK), and the National Cancer Center Research and Development Funds (24-A-1 to MK, TS, and TKo, 25-A-6 to MK and KTs, 26-A-3 to MK and TKo, and 27-A-1 to MK and TKo). These funding bodies played no role in the design of the study, the collection, analysis, and interpretation of the data, or in the writing of the manuscript.

Authors' contributions

MK developed the algorithms. HN, TS, YS, and YTo aided in algorithm development. AE, HN, JM, MK, and MN prepared the software. AE, EF, HN, MK, and MN analyzed the data. KS, KTa, NY, and YTa provided the samples. HI, HS, KTs, TKo, TKu, TY, SM, and YA provided the data. MK, HI, TKo, and TS wrote the manuscript. All authors read and approved the final manuscript.

Competing interests

NY received grants from Astellas, Bayer, Boehringer Ingelheim, Chugai, Daiichi-Sankyo, Eisai, Kyowa-Hakko Kirin, Lilly Japan, Novartis, Pfizer, Quintiles, Taiho, and Takeda, and honoraria from AstraZeneca, BMS, Chugai, Lilly Japan, Ono, and Pfizer. The remaining authors declare that they have no competing interests.

Author details

[1]Department of Bioinformatics, National Cancer Center Research Institute, Chuo-ku, Tokyo 104-0045, Japan. [2]Division of Cancer Genomics, National Cancer Center Research Institute, Chuo-ku, Tokyo 104-0045, Japan. [3]Department of Clinical Genomics, National Cancer Center Research Institute, Chuo-ku, Tokyo 104-0045, Japan. [4]Department of Experimental Therapeutics, National Cancer Center Hospital, Chuo-ku, Tokyo 104-0045, Japan. [5]Division of Genetics, National Cancer Center Research Institute, Chuo-ku, Tokyo 104-0045, Japan. [6]Division of Translational Genomics, Exploratory Oncology Research & Clinical Trial Center, National Cancer Center, Kashiwa, Chiba 277-8577, Japan. [7]Division of Genome Biology, National Cancer Center Research Institute, Chuo-ku, Tokyo 104-0045, Japan. [8]Department of Computational Biology and Medical Sciences, Graduate School of Frontier Sciences, The University of Tokyo, Kashiwa-shi, Chiba 277-8568, Japan. [9]Laboratory of Molecular Medicine, Human Genome Center, The Institute of Medical Science, The University of Tokyo, Minato-ku, Tokyo 108-8639, Japan.

References

1. International Cancer Genome C, Hudson TJ, Anderson W, Artez A, Barker AD, Bell C, Bernabe RR, Bhan MK, Calvo F, Eerola I, et al. International network of cancer genome projects. Nature. 2010;464:993–8.
2. Totoki Y, Tatsuno K, Covington KR, Ueda H, Creighton CJ, Kato M, Tsuji S, Donehower LA, Slagle BL, Nakamura H, et al. Trans-ancestry mutational landscape of hepatocellular carcinoma genomes. Nat Genet. 2014;46:1267–73.
3. Fujimoto A, Furuta M, Totoki Y, Tsunoda T, Kato M, Shiraishi Y, Tanaka H, Taniguchi H, Kawakami Y, Ueno M, et al. Whole-genome mutational landscape and characterization of noncoding and structural mutations in liver cancer. Nat Genet. 2016;48:500–9.
4. Simon R, Roychowdhury S. Implementing personalized cancer genomics in clinical trials. Nat Rev Drug Discov. 2013;12:358–69.
5. Roychowdhury S, Iyer MK, Robinson DR, Lonigro RJ, Wu YM, Cao X, Kalyana-Sundaram S, Sam L, Balbin OA, Quist MJ, et al. Personalized oncology through integrative high-throughput sequencing: a pilot study. Sci Transl Med. 2011;3:111ra121.
6. Frampton GM, Fichtenholtz A, Otto GA, Wang K, Downing SR, He J, Schnall-Levin M, White J, Sanford EM, An P, et al. Development and validation of a clinical cancer genomic profiling test based on massively parallel DNA sequencing. Nat Biotechnol. 2013;31:1023–31.
7. Yost SE, Smith EN, Schwab RB, Bao L, Jung H, Wang X, Voest E, Pierce JP, Messer K, Parker BA, et al. Identification of high-confidence somatic mutations in whole genome sequence of formalin-fixed breast cancer specimens. Nucleic Acids Res. 2012;40:e107.
8. Kerick M, Isau M, Timmermann B, Sultmann H, Herwig R, Krobitsch S, Schaefer G, Verdorfer I, Bartsch G, Klocker H, et al. Targeted high throughput sequencing in clinical cancer settings: formaldehyde fixed-paraffin embedded (FFPE) tumor tissues, input amount and tumor heterogeneity. BMC Med Genet. 2011;4:68.
9. Cibulskis K, Lawrence MS, Carter SL, Sivachenko A, Jaffe D, Sougnez C, Gabriel S, Meyerson M, Lander ES, Getz G. Sensitive detection of somatic point mutations in impure and heterogeneous cancer samples. Nat Biotechnol. 2013;31:213–9.
10. Koboldt DC, Zhang Q, Larson DE, Shen D, McLellan MD, Lin L, Miller CA, Mardis ER, Ding L, Wilson RK. VarScan 2: somatic mutation and copy number alteration discovery in cancer by exome sequencing. Genome Res. 2012;22:568–76.
11. Saunders CT, Wong WS, Swamy S, Becq J, Murray LJ, Cheetham RK. Strelka: accurate somatic small-variant calling from sequenced tumor-normal sample pairs. Bioinformatics. 2012;28:1811–7.
12. Roth A, Ding J, Morin R, Crisan A, Ha G, Giuliany R, Bashashati A, Hirst M, Turashvili G, Oloumi A, et al. JointSNVMix: a probabilistic model for accurate detection of somatic mutations in normal/tumour paired next-generation sequencing data. Bioinformatics. 2012;28:907–13.
13. Larson DE, Harris CC, Chen K, Koboldt DC, Abbott TE, Dooling DJ, Ley TJ, Mardis ER, Wilson RK, Ding L. SomaticSniper: identification of somatic point mutations in whole genome sequencing data. Bioinformatics. 2012;28:311–7.
14. Shiraishi Y, Sato Y, Chiba K, Okuno Y, Nagata Y, Yoshida K, Shiba N, Hayashi Y, Kume H, Homma Y, et al. An empirical Bayesian framework for somatic mutation detection from cancer genome sequencing data. Nucleic Acids Res. 2013;41:e89.

15. Albers CA, Lunter G, MacArthur DG, McVean G, Ouwehand WH, Durbin R. Dindel: accurate indel calls from short-read data. Genome Res. 2011;21: 961–73.

16. Ge H, Liu K, Juan T, Fang F, Newman M, Hoeck W. FusionMap: detecting fusion genes from next-generation sequencing data at base-pair resolution. Bioinformatics. 2011;27:1922–8.

17. Suzuki S, Yasuda T, Shiraishi Y, Miyano S, Nagasaki M. ClipCrop: a tool for detecting structural variations with single-base resolution using soft-clipping information. BMC Bioinformatics. 2011;12(Suppl 14):S7.

18. Wang Q, Xia J, Jia P, Pao W, Zhao Z. Application of next generation sequencing to human gene fusion detection: computational tools, features and perspectives. Brief Bioinform. 2013;14:506–19.

19. Sathirapongsasuti JF, Lee H, Horst BA, Brunner G, Cochran AJ, Binder S, Quackenbush J, Nelson SF. Exome sequencing-based copy-number variation and loss of heterozygosity detection: ExomeCNV. Bioinformatics. 2011;27:2648–54.

20. Boeva V, Zinovyev A, Bleakley K, Vert JP, Janoueix-Lerosey I, Delattre O, Barillot E. Control-free calling of copy number alterations in deep-sequencing data using GC-content normalization. Bioinformatics. 2011;27:268–9.

21. Liu B, Morrison CD, Johnson CS, Trump DL, Qin M, Conroy JC, Wang J, Liu S. Computational methods for detecting copy number variations in cancer genome using next generation sequencing: principles and challenges. Oncotarget. 2013;4:1868–81.

22. Gerstung M, Beisel C, Rechsteiner M, Wild P, Schraml P, Moch H, Beerenwinkel N. Reliable detection of subclonal single-nucleotide variants in tumour cell populations. Nat Commun. 2012;3:811.

23. Gerstung M, Papaemmanuil E, Campbell PJ. Subclonal variant calling with multiple samples and prior knowledge. Bioinformatics. 2014;30:1198–204.

24. Tanabe Y, Ichikawa H, Kohno T, Yoshida H, Kubo T, Kato M, Iwasa S, Ochiai A, Yamamoto N, Fujiwara Y, Tamura K. Comprehensive screening of target molecules by next-generation sequencing in patients with malignant solid tumors: guiding entry into phase I clinical trials. Mol Cancer. 2016;15:73.

25. Seki Y, Mizukami T, Kohno T. Molecular process producing oncogene fusion in lung cancer cells by illegitimate repair of DNA double-strand breaks. Biomol Ther. 2015;5:2464–76.

26. Mizukami T, Shiraishi K, Shimada Y, Ogiwara H, Tsuta K, Ichikawa H, Sakamoto H, Kato M, Shibata T, Nakano T, Kohno T. Molecular mechanisms underlying oncogenic RET fusion in lung adenocarcinoma. J Thorac Oncol. 2014;9:622–30.

27. Nakaoku T, Tsuta K, Ichikawa H, Shiraishi K, Sakamoto H, Enari M, Furuta K, Shimada Y, Ogiwara H, Watanabe S, et al. Druggable oncogene fusions in invasive mucinous lung adenocarcinoma. Clin Cancer Res. 2014;20:3087–93.

28. Kohno T, Ichikawa H, Totoki Y, Yasuda K, Hiramoto M, Nammo T, Sakamoto H, Tsuta K, Furuta K, Shimada Y, et al. KIF5B-RET fusions in lung adenocarcinoma. Nat Med. 2012;18:375–7.

29. Totoki Y, Tatsuno K, Yamamoto S, Arai Y, Hosoda F, Ishikawa S, Tsutsumi S, Sonoda K, Totsuka H, Shirakihara T, et al. High-resolution characterization of a hepatocellular carcinoma genome. Nat Genet. 2011;43:464–9.

30. Ji Y, Wu C, Liu P, Wang J, Coombes KR. Applications of beta-mixture models in bioinformatics. Bioinformatics. 2005;21:2118–22.

31. Biernacki C, Celeux G, Govaert G. Assessing a mixture model for clustering with the integrated completed likelihood. IEEE Trans Pattern Anal Mach Intell. 2000;22:719–25.

32. Wong SQ, Li J, Tan AY, Vedururu R, Pang JM, Do H, Ellul J, Doig K, Bell A, MacArthur GA, et al. Sequence artefacts in a prospective series of formalin-fixed tumours tested for mutations in hotspot regions by massively parallel sequencing. BMC Med Genet. 2014;7:23.

33. Robinson JT, Thorvaldsdottir H, Winckler W, Guttman M, Lander ES, Getz G, Mesirov JP. Integrative genomics viewer. Nat Biotechnol. 2011;29:24–6.

34. Li H, Durbin R. Fast and accurate long-read alignment with Burrows-Wheeler transform. Bioinformatics. 2010;26:589–95.

35. Kohno T, Nakaoku T, Tsuta K, Tsuchihara K, Matsumoto S, Yoh K, Goto K. Beyond ALK-RET, ROS1 and other oncogene fusions in lung cancer. Transl Lung Cancer Res. 2015;4:156–64.

36. Olshen AB, Venkatraman ES, Lucito R, Wigler M. Circular binary segmentation for the analysis of array-based DNA copy number data. Biostatistics. 2004;5:557–72.

37. Oh E, Choi YL, Kwon MJ, Kim RN, Kim YJ, Song JY, Jung KS, Shin YK. Comparison of accuracy of whole-exome sequencing with formalin-fixed paraffin-embedded and fresh frozen tissue samples. PLoS One. 2015;10: e0144162.

38. Wang M, Escudero-Ibarz L, Moody S, Zeng N, Clipson A, Huang Y, Xue X, Grigoropoulos NF, Barrans S, Worrillow L, et al. Somatic mutation screening using archival formalin-fixed, paraffin-embedded tissues by fluidigm multiplex PCR and Illumina sequencing. J Mol Diagn. 2015;17:521–32.

39. Kalatskaya I, Trinh QM, Spears M, McPherson JD, Bartlett JMS, Stein L. ISOWN: accurate somatic mutation identification in the absence of normal tissue controls. Genome Med. 2017;9:59.

40. Schweiger MR, Kerick M, Timmermann B, Albrecht MW, Borodina T, Parkhomchuk D, Zatloukal K, Lehrach H. Genome-wide massively parallel sequencing of formaldehyde fixed-paraffin embedded tumor tissues for copy-number- and mutation-analysis. PLoS One. 2009;4:e5548.

41. Scheinin I, Sie D, Bengtsson H, van de Wiel MA, Olshen AB, van Thuijl HF, van Essen HF, Eijk PP, Rustenburg F, Meijer GA, et al. DNA copy number analysis of fresh and formalin-fixed specimens by shallow whole-genome sequencing with identification and exclusion of problematic regions in the genome assembly. Genome Res. 2014;24:2022–32.

14

Exposure to the gut microbiota drives distinct methylome and transcriptome changes in intestinal epithelial cells during postnatal development

Wei-Hung Pan[1†], Felix Sommer[1,2†], Maren Falk-Paulsen[1], Thomas Ulas[3], Philipp Best[1], Antonella Fazio[1], Priyadarshini Kachroo[1], Anne Luzius[1], Marlene Jentzsch[1], Ateequr Rehman[1], Fabian Müller[4], Thomas Lengauer[4,5], Jörn Walter[6], Sven Künzel[7], John F. Baines[7,8], Stefan Schreiber[1,9], Andre Franke[1], Joachim L. Schultze[3,10], Fredrik Bäckhed[2,11] and Philip Rosenstiel[1*]

Abstract

Background: The interplay of epigenetic processes and the intestinal microbiota may play an important role in intestinal development and homeostasis. Previous studies have established that the microbiota regulates a large proportion of the intestinal epithelial transcriptome in the adult host, but microbial effects on DNA methylation and gene expression during early postnatal development are still poorly understood. Here, we sought to investigate the microbial effects on DNA methylation and the transcriptome of intestinal epithelial cells (IECs) during postnatal development.

Methods: We collected IECs from the small intestine of each of five 1-, 4- and 12 to 16-week-old mice representing the infant, juvenile, and adult states, raised either in the presence or absence of a microbiota. The DNA methylation profile was determined using reduced representation bisulfite sequencing (RRBS) and the epithelial transcriptome by RNA sequencing using paired samples from each individual mouse to analyze the link between microbiota, gene expression, and DNA methylation.

Results: We found that microbiota-dependent and -independent processes act together to shape the postnatal development of the transcriptome and DNA methylation signatures of IECs. The bacterial effect on the transcriptome increased over time, whereas most microbiota-dependent DNA methylation differences were detected already early after birth. Microbiota-responsive transcripts could be attributed to stage-specific cellular programs during postnatal development and regulated gene sets involved primarily immune pathways and metabolic processes. Integrated analysis of the methylome and transcriptome data identified 126 genomic loci at which coupled differential DNA methylation and RNA transcription were associated with the presence of intestinal microbiota. We validated a subset of differentially expressed and methylated genes in an independent mouse cohort, indicating the existence of microbiota-dependent "functional" methylation sites which may impact on long-term gene expression signatures in IECs.

Conclusions: Our study represents the first genome-wide analysis of microbiota-mediated effects on maturation of DNA methylation signatures and the transcriptional program of IECs after birth. It indicates that the gut microbiota dynamically modulates large portions of the epithelial transcriptome during postnatal development, but targets only a subset of microbially responsive genes through their DNA methylation status.

Keywords: Microbiota, Intestinal epithelial cell, Epigenetics, Methylation, Transcriptomics

* Correspondence: p.rosenstiel@mucosa.de
†Equal contributors
[1]Institute for Clinical Molecular Biology, University of Kiel,
Rosalind-Franklin-Straße 12, 24105 Kiel, Germany
Full list of author information is available at the end of the article

Background

A tremendously complex and dynamic union of microorganisms inhabits the mammalian gastrointestinal tract and contributes to several aspects of host physiology, including metabolism, maturation of the immune system, cellular homeostasis, and behavior [1–3]. However, the commensal microbial communities within the host also represent a danger due to their potential for infection and overgrowth. Thus, mechanisms are in place to assure a healthy beneficial coexistence. Intestinal epithelial cells (IECs) take a central role as they line the gastrointestinal mucosa and build a physicochemical and immunological barrier to restrain the microbiota and prevent invasion [4, 5]. Interactions between the microbiota and the host, especially IECs, have therefore been studied intensively in the past decade [6–11]. Previous studies have shown that under normal homeostatic conditions the gut microbiota regulates the expression of about 10% of host genes [6]. Several mechanisms have been implicated in how the gut microbiota can drive these global changes in the host transcriptome. Transcriptional regulators such as NFκB (nuclear factor kappa-light-chain-enhancer of activated B cells) or CEBPB (CCAAT/enhancer-binding protein beta) may be engaged by the microbiota to modulate the expression of specific target genes [6, 12]. Additionally, the microbiota have the potential to modulate host epigenetic mechanisms and thereby regulate transcription more globally [13–18]. The microbially produced short-chain fatty acids (SCFAs) butyrate and propionate are potent inhibitors of histone deacetylase (HDAC) enzymes [14] and therefore may promote heterochromatin formation and increase transcriptional activity. However, global changes in the accessible chromatin landscape by the gut microbiota were not detected in a previous study [12]. Additionally, the intestinal microbiota may modulate DNA methylation, since microbially produced folate is an essential methyl donor during DNA methylation [16].

DNA methyltransferases (DNMT) catalyze the transfer of the methylation group from methionine to cytosine if it is followed by a guanine (CpG). DNMT1 maintains the methylation pattern during DNA replication [19] whereas DNMT3a and DNMT3b perform de novo methylation [20]. DNA methylation occurs predominantly at a series of two or more CpGs [21–23]. DNA methylation is thought to inhibit gene transcription, but recent data indicate that the functional consequences may be more complex [24] and depend at least partially on the location of the methylated site. If 5-methylcytosine is situated in close vicinity to a transcription start site, transcription of the downstream gene is mainly blocked [25]. In contrast, methylation of CpGs in the gene body may rather influence transcript elongation or splicing [26]. DNA methylation plays a key role during development and cellular differentiation function [25, 27]. DNA methylation is mostly erased during zygote formation and reprogrammed during development [28].

Yu and colleagues have shown that during postnatal development both the epithelial transcriptome and the DNA methylation landscape undergo fundamental reshaping [29]. The early neonatal period is a critical phase not only for the development of the intestinal tract but also for the establishment of the microbiota and proper maturation of the immune system [30, 31]. A series of reports established the presence of a window of opportunity based on observations that lack of exposure to environmental microbes during early development may lead to immunological defects and autoimmune diseases later in life [32–37]. Notably, colonization at a later stage fails to normalize these immunological defects. This persistence of microbiota-dependent regulatory signatures points to microbial imprinting through epigenetic mechanisms (possibly DNA methylation) that are long lasting once they are established [2, 17]. However, whether microbial colonization early in life alters the DNA methylation pattern and alongside the epithelial transcriptome during postnatal development and maturation of the gut epithelium remains largely unknown. To address this issue, we collected IECs from the small intestine of 1-, 4- and 12 to 16-week-old mice, which were raised in either the presence or absence of a microbiota to represent the infant, juvenile, and adult states of the epithelium and the intestinal flora. We then measured the methylation variable positions using reduced representation bisulfite sequencing (RRBS) and analyzed the epithelial transcriptome by RNA sequencing (RNA-Seq) to investigate the association between gene expression, alternative splicing, and differential DNA methylation in IECs during postnatal ontogeny.

Methods

Mice

C57Bl6/N female littermate mice were maintained under standard specific pathogen-free or germ-free (GF) conditions in the laboratory for experimental biomedicine at University of Gothenburg as described previously [38]. Mice were kept under a 12-h light cycle and fed autoclaved chow diet *ad libitum* (Labdiet, St Louis, MO, USA). Mice were sacrificed at three different stages: 1, 4 and between 12 to 16 weeks of age with $n = 5$ animals for each of the groups. Mice were killed by cervical dislocation and the small intestine removed for isolation of IECs. All animal protocols were approved by the Gothenburg Animal Ethics Committee.

Isolation of IECs

IECs were isolated from small intestinal tissue using the Lamina Propria Dissociation Kit (Miltenyi BioTech, Bergisch Gladbach, Germany) according to the manufacturer's protocol. In brief, intestinal epithelial cells were isolated by disruption of the structural integrity of the epithelium using ethylenediaminetetraacetic acid (EDTA) and dithiothreitol (DTT). Purity of individual IEC fractions was analyzed by flow cytometry on a FACS Calibur flow cytometer (B&D, Heidelberg, Germany) with Cellquest analysis software from Becton Dickinson. We used the Anti-EpCam-PE (clone G8.8, Biolegend, San Diego, USA) antibody for analysis of IEC purity.

Transcriptional profiling by RNA sequencing

RNA was isolated from purified small intestinal IECs using the TRIZOL method. Briefly, 1 ml TRIzol was added to 50–75 mg pestle-homogenized tissue followed by vortexing, a 5-min incubation at room temperature, and addition of 200 μl chloroform. After mixing, further incubation at room temperature for 2–3 min and centrifugation (12.000 g) at 4 °C for 5 min, the clear supernatant was mixed with 500 μl isopropanol followed by incubation at room temperature for 10 min. After further centrifugation (12.000 g) at 4 °C for 10 min, the supernatant was discarded and the pellet washed with 1 ml cold 75% EtOH followed by vortexing and centrifugation (7.500 g, 4 °C, 5 min). The pellet was dried and dissolved in RNase-free water. RNA libraries were prepared using TruSeq v4 Kit (Illumina) according to the manufacturer's instructions. All samples were sequenced using an Illumina HiSeq 2000 sequencer (Illumina, San Diego,CA) with an average of 23 million paired-end reads (2 × 125 bp) at IKMB NGS core facilities. We used TopHat 2 [39] and Bowtie 2 [40] to align reads. Reads were mapped to the mouse genome (MGI assembly version 10) using TopHat 2. Average alignment rate for RNA-seq was 83.3% (73.3–89.9%, median = 85.7%) and the expression count was normalized by library size. Gene expression values of the transcripts were computed by HTSeq [41]. DEseq2 [42] was used to determine differentially expressed genes. Genes were considered as significant differentially expressed if the adjusted p value (Benjamini–Hochberg (BH) multiple test correction method) was less than 0.05. Gene expression differences were visualized using MA plot [43], a modification of a Bland–Altman plot for visual representation of genome-wide functional genomic data. M represents the log fold change for gene expression (y-axis) and A represents the mean normalized counts (x-axis). We've set the ceiling/floor to 2 on log fold change (y-axis) to achieve an optimal visualization. PCA was performed using plotpca in the R package DEseq2 and Euclidian distance was measured. Transcription factor binding site analysis was carried out using the Innate DB database [44] with implementation of the hypergeometric algorithm and the BH multiple test correction method (BH-corrected p value < 0.05). Only expressed transcription factors were considered for the analysis (raw read count > 3). Gene Ontology (GO) analysis was performed using the GOrilla (gene ontology enrichment analysis and visualization) tool [45]. GO terms with false discovery rate (FDR) < 0.05 were considered significantly altered. All

RNA-Seq data have been uploaded to the Gene Expression Omnibus (GEO) with accession number GEO:GSE94402.

Co-expression network analysis

For the establishment of a gene co-expression network, we built the union of differentially expressed genes comparing always the conventionally raised specific pathogen-free (CONV-R) and GF conditions at the same time point. Expression values of these genes over all 30 samples were used for the co-expression analysis using BioLayout Express 3D [46]. Applying a correlation cutoff of 0.8 resulted in a co-expression network with 970 nodes (genes) and 34,437 edges. The calculated gene–gene pairs and their Spearman correlation coefficients were imported into Cytoscape using organic layout for visualization. Subsequently, we mapped condition fold changes (based on the comparison of each condition with the mean of all conditions) individually for each condition onto the network, to identify condition-specific topological differences between the conditions in the co-expression network. Gene groups were assigned based on the temporal and microbiota-dependent expression changes with the following specific criteria: group 1, expressed high (Z-score > + 1 in condition gene expression value normalized by the mean condition value) in W1, low (condition Z-score < – 1) in W4 + W12/16, independent of GF/CONV-R; group 2, expressed high in W12 CONV-R but low in W12 GF, normal (condition Z-score – 1 to + 1) in W1 and W4 CONV-R, low in W4 GF; group 3, expressed high in W12 CONV-R but low in W12 GF, low in W1 + W4; group 4, expressed high in W12 CONV-R but low in W12 GF, low in W1 + W4; group 5, expressed high in W12 GF but low in W12 CONV-R, high in W4 GF, low in W1 GF, W1 CONV-R, and W4 CONV-R; group 6, expressed high in W12 GF but low in W12 CONV-R, high in W4 GF, low in W4 CONV-R, normal in W1 GF + CONV-R.

Transcript splicing analysis

Based on the updated genome annotation and our RNA-Seq data, we compared the alternative splicing events of each gene between CONV-R and GF in three stages. We used rMATS [47], which detects alternative splicing events such as skipped exons, alternative 5′ splice sites, alternative 3′ splice sites, mutually exclusive exons, and retained intron events. The events were identified as significantly different by choosing inclusion levels of |ΔPSI| ≥ 5% between CONV-R and GF at FDR q < 0.05.

Reduced representation bisulfite sequencing

DNA was isolated from purified IECs using a DNeasy Blood & Tissue Kit (Qiagen) according to the manufacturer's instructions. DNA libraries were sequenced at IKMB NGS core facilities using Illumina HiSeq 2500 sequencer (Illumina, San Diego, CA, USA) with an average of 127,000,000 single-end 50-bp reads. After removing adaptor sequences and low-quality tails, reads were mapped to the mouse genome (MGI version 10) using Bismark [48]. All CpG sites covered by less than five reads were removed along with SNPs specific to the C57BL/6 N strain (http://www.sanger.ac.uk/science/data/mouse-genomes-project). We used MethylKit [49] for gene category and CGI annotation and downloaded the gene information from Refseq. The average mapping efficiency of reduced representation bisulfite sequencing (RRBS) was 71.37% (63–78.28%, median = 70.73%). We used Dispersion shrinkage for sequencing data [50, 51] to identify differentially methylated loci based on a beta-binomial regression model with "arcsine" link function. Parameter estimation was based on transformed data with a generalized least square approach without relying on an iterative algorithm. One CONV-R W1 sample was excluded from the DNA methylation analysis due to failure of the bisulfite conversion. All RRBS data have been uploaded to GEO with accession number GEO:GSE94402.

Integrated analysis screening for differentially methylated and expressed genes

For integrated analysis of gene expression and DNA methylation, we applied a hierarchical testing approach [52] to detect DNA methylation sites around the differentially expressed gene. To that end, we identified all CpG sites 5 kb up- and downstream of the transcription start site of the microbially regulated genes. Second, we combined the neighborhood methylation positions to methylation regions (maximum distance 200 bp). Those regions, which contained less than 20% CpGs (BH-corrected p value < 0.05), were excluded and all retained regions were considered as differentially methylated regions. FDR correction was performed on all CpGs of the retained regions (BH-corrected p value < 0.05). The R code used for the integrated analysis is included in Additional file 1. The circular visualization plot was constructed using the R package *circlize* [53].

Functional network analysis for differentially methylated and expressed genes

To screen for functional networks among the differentially methylated and expressed genes (CONV-R versus GF) we employed the Functional Networks of Tissues in Mouse [54] prediction tool for mouse tissue-specific protein interactions, which integrates genomic data and prior knowledge of gene function. We used the small intestine tissue database and only kept edges with relationship confidence greater than 0.6.

Validation of identified microbiota-dependent genes and differentially methylated positions

To validate our findings in an independent set of animals, we isolated DNA and RNA from small intestinal epithelial scrapings of 4- and 12-week-old GF and CONV-R C57Bl6

mice (n = 10 per group) from the gnotobiotic animal facility of the Max Planck Institute for Evolutionary Biology in Plön, Germany. Among all of the genes with differential expression and methylation, we selected 3 out of 34 for W4 (Bcl3, Nfix, Cacnali) and 5 out of 79 for W12/16 (Rcbtb2, Mmp14, Itga5, Cd74, Pik3cd) based on the following criteria for the validation experiment: BH-corrected p value among the most significant; fold change among the most differential; validated qPCR primers available in either published studies or public databases.

For qPCR analysis, 1 μg of total RNA was reverse-transcribed to cDNA according to the manufacturer's instructions (MultiScribe Reverse Transcriptase; Applied Biosystems). qPCR was carried out using SYBR Select Master Mix (Applied Biosystems) according to the manufacturer's instructions. Primer sequences are given in Additional file 2. Reactions were carried out on the 7900HT Fast Real Time PCR System (Applied Biosystems). Expression levels were normalized to β-actin.

Region and base-specific methylation information was obtained via Bisulfite Amplicon Sequencing. This protocol involved bisulfite conversion of sample DNA (EpiTect Bisulfite Kit, QIAGEN) followed by PCR-amplification of target differentially methylated position (DMP)-containing regions (EpiMark Hot Start Taq, NEB). Primer pairs were designed using "MethPrimer" [55] and target specificity was evaluated using "BiSearch" [56]. PCR amplicons were normalized using SequalPrep plates (ThermoFisher), pooled sample-wise, and subjected to NGS library preparation (Nextera XT, Illumina) according to the manufacturer's instructions. Finally, the library pool was sequenced on a MiSeq platform (Illumina) with 150-bp, paired-end reads. Raw reads were trimmed for adapter and transposon sequences and only bases with a quality value below 30 were kept using Cutadapt 1.10. Reads were then mapped by Bismark 0.15.0 [48] with Bowtie 2.2.5 [40] to the mouse reference genome (mm10). Methylation ratios were extracted using Bismark and analyzed using R with the package bsseq [57].

Results

The gut microbiota and chronological age determine the epithelial transcriptome during postnatal development

To investigate potential effects of the gut microbiota and postnatal development on dynamic host epigenetic signatures and changes in the transcriptional profiles of the epithelial cells, we isolated DNA and RNA from IECs of conventionally raised and germ-free C57BL6 female mice (n = 5 per group) at three different stages during postnatal development—week 1, week 4, and week 12/16 (W1, W4, W12/16)—representative of the infant, juvenile, and adult states (Fig. 1a), respectively. RNA and DNA were isolated and subjected to RNA-Seq and RRBS to assess global mRNA expression and DNA methylation profiles,

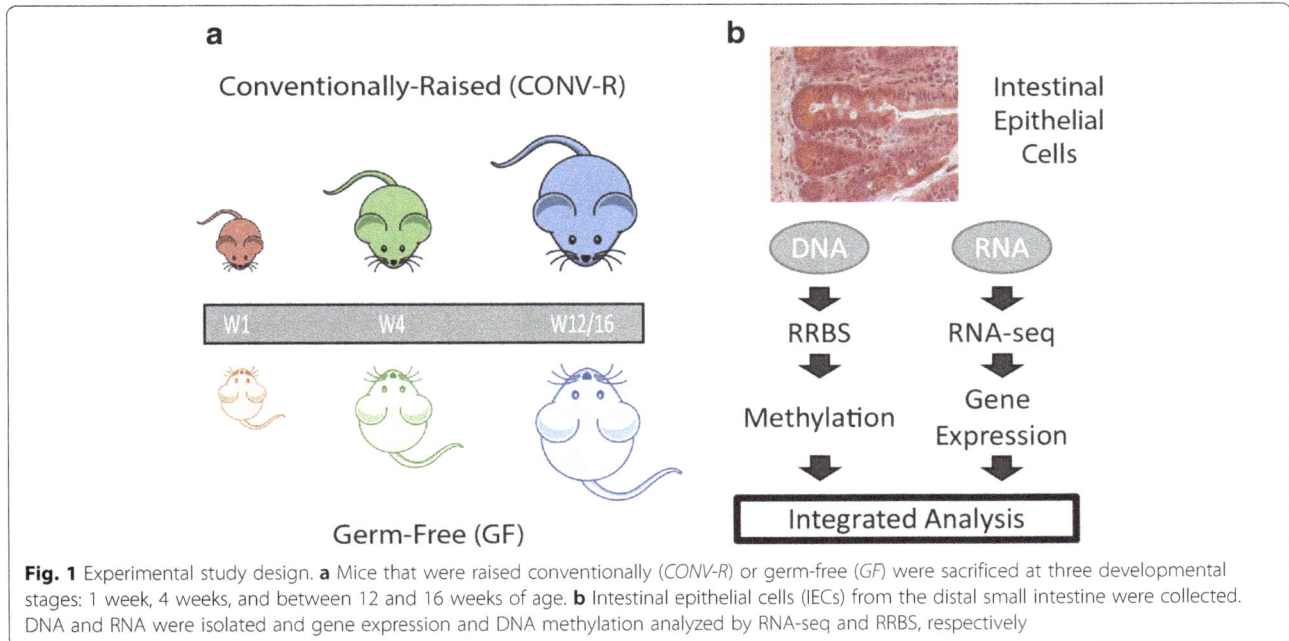

Fig. 1 Experimental study design. **a** Mice that were raised conventionally (*CONV-R*) or germ-free (*GF*) were sacrificed at three developmental stages: 1 week, 4 weeks, and between 12 and 16 weeks of age. **b** Intestinal epithelial cells (IECs) from the distal small intestine were collected. DNA and RNA were isolated and gene expression and DNA methylation analyzed by RNA-seq and RRBS, respectively

respectively (Fig. 1b). After quality control and data pre-processing, 21,619 gene transcripts and approximately 1.3 million methylation sites remained, which were employed in further downstream analyses.

First, we performed principal component analysis to visualize the global distribution of samples based on the expression data of the 21,619 transcripts. Samples were clustered according to both the developmental stage and microbial status (Fig. 2a). The first principal component explained 63% variation and separated samples from W1 and the other two stages, W4 and W12/16, indicating that gene expression changed dramatically during maturation of IECs, especially in the early postnatal period. The second principal component explained 8% of variation and separated W4 and W12/16 but also CONV-R and GF within a single developmental stage (Fig. 2a). Notably, the distance between CONV-R and GF samples increased along with time from W1 to W12/16. We detected 56 (0.3%) microbially regulated genes in W1 (differentially expressed in CONV-R vs GF comparison with BH-corrected p value < 0.05 and absolute fold change > 2), 614 (2.8%) in W4 and 1084 (5.0%) in W12/16 (Additional files 3 and 4). Moreover, the expression differences between CONV-R and GF (fold change) of the microbially regulated genes also increased with time (Additional files 3 and 5). Thus, ontogeny (developmental stage) and to a lesser extent bacterial status determine the epithelial transcriptional profile during postnatal development.

To gain insights into the biological functions of the microbially regulated genes during postnatal development, we employed Gene Ontology (GO) enrichment analysis on the differentially expressed genes in the three developmental stages. Supporting previous publications, enriched GO terms included mainly immune response-related or metabolic functions (Additional file 6).

We also tested whether postnatal and microbial status affected alternative splicing events. Overall, distribution of the splicing events did not differ significantly between CONV-R and GF mice or among the three developmental stages (Chi-squared test, p value = 0.99; Additional file 7). However, few distinct signatures were detectable that differentiated CONV-R from GF mice; for example, a higher number of microbiota-dependent intron retention events (2.3-fold higher, BH-corrected p value = 0.006, Chi-squared test with Yates continuity correction) in W1 compared to W4 or W12/16 (Additional files 7 and 8).

Next, we employed transcription factor binding site enrichment analysis among the promoters of microbially regulated genes to investigate the regulatory networks that underlie the microbiota-induced transcriptome alterations [58]. Interestingly, the transcriptional regulators most enriched among promoters of microbially regulated genes were unique to W1 whereas W4 and W12/16 shared several transcription factors (Fig. 2b). For example, in W1 the motif of the transcription factor XBP1, which functions in endoplasmic reticulum stress, cellular proliferation, and differentiation and protects from intestinal inflammation [59–61], was enriched in the promoters of genes upregulated by the microbiota. In W4 and W12/16 sites predicted to bind the transcription factor HIF1, which functions in mediating hypoxia effects and

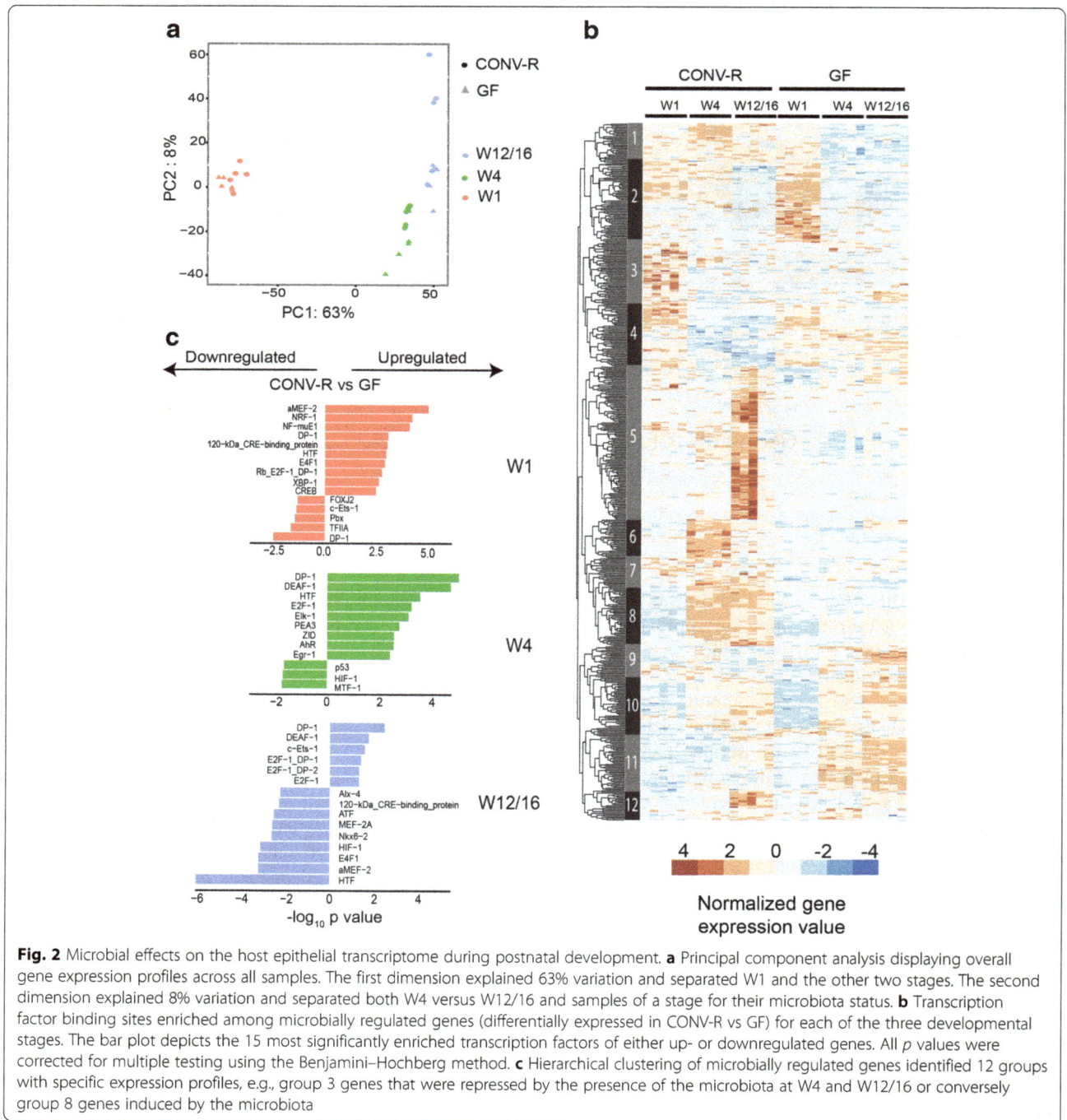

Fig. 2 Microbial effects on the host epithelial transcriptome during postnatal development. **a** Principal component analysis displaying overall gene expression profiles across all samples. The first dimension explained 63% variation and separated W1 and the other two stages. The second dimension explained 8% variation and separated both W4 versus W12/16 and samples of a stage for their microbiota status. **b** Transcription factor binding sites enriched among microbially regulated genes (differentially expressed in CONV-R vs GF) for each of the three developmental stages. The bar plot depicts the 15 most significantly enriched transcription factors of either up- or downregulated genes. All *p* values were corrected for multiple testing using the Benjamini–Hochberg method. **c** Hierarchical clustering of microbially regulated genes identified 12 groups with specific expression profiles, e.g., group 3 genes that were repressed by the presence of the microbiota at W4 and W12/16 or conversely group 8 genes induced by the microbiota

regulates metabolism and immune responses [62–64], were overrepresented among downregulated genes.

To identify co-regulated patterns of transcripts modulated by the microbiota we selected the 200 most significant genes regulated by microbial state at each of the three developmental stages, created the union of these genes (*n* = 547 genes), and performed hierarchical clustering analysis (depicted in the heatmap graph in Fig. 2c). A similar

analysis was performed based on the selection of developmentally regulated genes for the two bacterial conditions CONV-R and GF (*n* = 553 genes; Additional file 9). The analyses revealed both a microbial imprint (e.g., clusters 2, 3, 4, 8, 11 in Fig. 2c) as well as a developmental effect (e.g., clusters 8, 10 in Fig. 2c) irrespective of the presence of bacteria. However, while the impact of postnatal development stage is clearly detectable in the visualization of microbially regulated genes (Fig. 2c), the influence of the presence of microbiota is less pronounced in the signature of the developmentally regulated genes. These data therefore support the previous finding that endogenous ontogenetic programs have a larger impact on the epithelial transcriptome compared with environmental cues from the commensal microbiota. Cluster 8 contains microbially responsive genes that mainly have functions in immune responses and are induced by the microbiota and the effect increases during development (Fig. 2c). Notably, genes of this cluster include *Duox2* (dual oxidase 2), *Reg3g* (regenerating islet-derived protein 3 gamma), *Nos2* (inducible nitric oxide synthase), *Saa1* (serum amyloid A-1), and *Saa2*, which have been reported previously as microbially induced in IECs [6]. The clusters 3 and 4 contain genes such as *Sdr16c6* (short chain dehydrogenase/reductase family 16C, member 6) or *Fn3k* (fructosamine 3 kinase), which are associated with metabolic functions, and expression of these

genes increased specifically during W1 in colonized mice and then returned to basal level (Fig. 2c).

Next, we investigated the influence of the intestinal microbiota during postnatal development by co-expression network analysis [46, 65]. Co-expression network analysis builds on the hypothesis that genes with similar expression patterns are likely to have a functional relationship [66]. Following the procedure from Xue and colleagues [46], 970 co-expressed genes were selected based on a correlation cutoff of 0.8, normalized by their transcription level and tested for up- or downregulation compared to the average expression in the dataset (Additional file 4). Gene set enrichment analysis was used to identify the biological processes of individual time- and state-dependent co-expression subnetworks (Fig. 3, Additional file 10). At the W1 stage, we did not detect a prominent microbiota-dependent gene cluster (CONV-R and GF), but differential gene expression was exclusively time-dependent (W1 vs

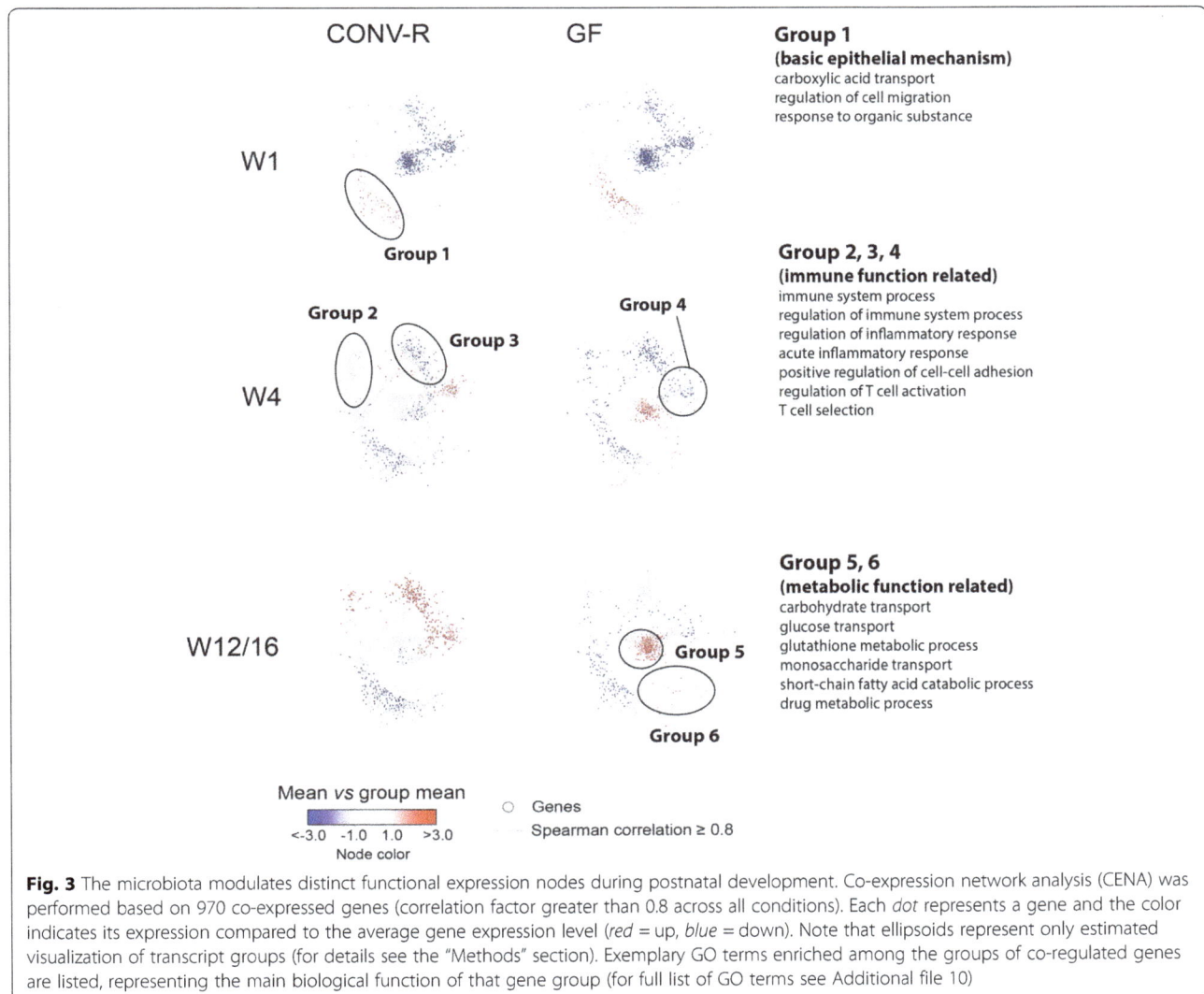

Fig. 3 The microbiota modulates distinct functional expression nodes during postnatal development. Co-expression network analysis (CENA) was performed based on 970 co-expressed genes (correlation factor greater than 0.8 across all conditions). Each *dot* represents a gene and the color indicates its expression compared to the average gene expression level (*red* = up, *blue* = down). Note that ellipsoids represent only estimated visualization of transcript groups (for details see the "Methods" section). Exemplary GO terms enriched among the groups of co-regulated genes are listed, representing the main biological function of that gene group (for full list of GO terms see Additional file 10)

W4 vs W12/16, group 1). Genes of this group 1 were involved in basic epithelial maintenance. At the later postnatal stages W4 and W12/16 two compensatory microbiota-dependent transcriptional responses were evident. Several genes involved in immune function (groups 2, 3, and 4)—for example, *Duox2* (dual oxidase 2), *Nod2* (nucleotide-binding oligomerization domain containing 2), *Fut2* (fucosyltransferase 2), *Pigr* (polymeric immunoglobulin receptor), *Nos2* (nitric oxide synthase 2), or *Reg3g* (Regenerating islet-derived protein 3-gamma), which are expressed by IECs—were upregulated in CONV-R compared to GF mice, whereas genes encoding metabolic functions (groups 5 and 6)—for example, *Ces1d* (carboxylesterase 1D), *Pnliprp2* (pancreatic lipase-related protein 2), and *Slc5a4b* (solute carrier family 5, neutral amino acid transporters system A, member 4b)—were downregulated in CONV-R mice.

Endogenous developmental programs as well as bacterial environmental cues affect the DNA methylation profile

To investigate how postnatal development and the microbial environment act on the DNA methylation pattern of IECs, we employed RRBS to determine the methylation level of isolated IECs from CONV-R and GF mice at W1, W4 and W12/16 (the identical samples used for transcriptome analysis). First, we examined the overall methylome pattern (1,296,536 CpG sites) by using multidimensional scaling analysis [67] instead of principal component analysis (PCA) due to data structure ("zero" inflation problem in RRBS as not all methylation sites can be detected in every sample regardless of sequencing depth). As for the transcriptome analysis, samples separated according to the developmental stage (Fig. 4a) and the methylation level increased with time (Additional file 11), indicating a

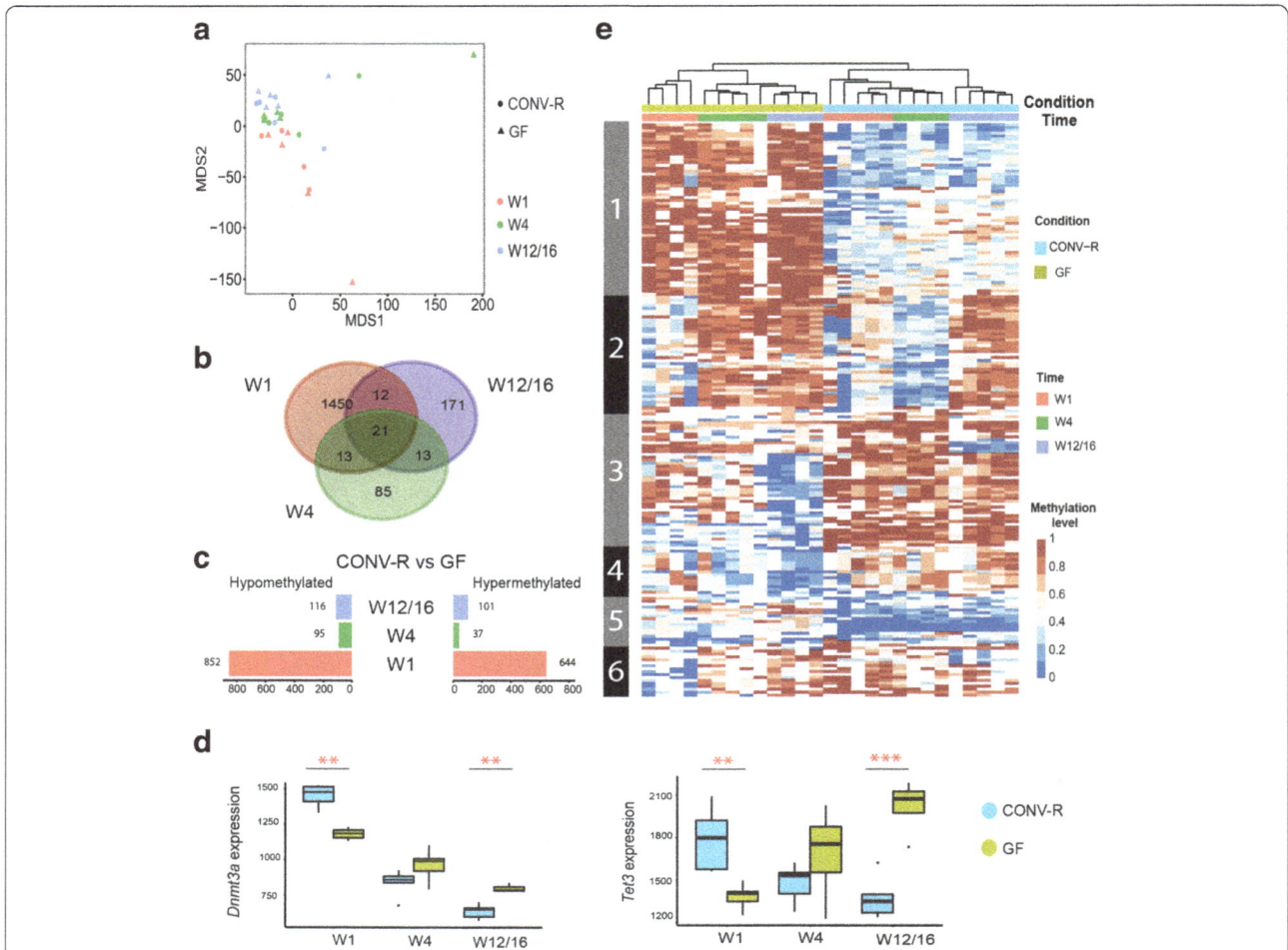

Fig. 4 Postnatal development and the microbiota affect the DNA methylation profile. **a** Multidimensional scaling analysis plot displaying the overall methylation profiles. **b** Venn plots showing the number of differentially methylated sites between CONV-R and GF at the three developmental stages. Note the high number of differentially methylated sites at W1. **c** Number of hypo- and hypomethylated sites among all DMPs (CONV-R vs GF) for each developmental stage. **d** Expression of *Dnmt3a* and *Tet3* genes, which function in de novo methylation and demethylation, respectively. **e** Hierarchical clustering of differentially methylated sites between CONV-R and GF in the three developmental stages. Each row indicates a CpG site and the color scale represents the methylation level

strong effect of postnatal developmental programs on DNA methylation. In contrast to transcriptional signatures, the global scaling analysis did not reveal a strong effect of the microbiota on the overall DNA methylation pattern. By individual comparison of the DNA methylome of CONV-R and GF at each time point, however, we were able to identify 1496, 132, and 217 DMPs (FDR < 0.05) in W1, W4, and W12/16, respectively (Fig. 4b). Interestingly, the number of DMPs at the earliest stage was about 10× higher compared to that of the later stages, indicating that the microbiota acted stronger on DNA methylation during W1 or that the microbial state already acts in utero. Detected DMPs were equally hypo- and hypermethylated (Fig. 4c). We classified the relative position of the variant sites according to their genomic location as exonic, intronic, intergenic, or promoter-associated DMPs. Notably, in W1 DMPs located in gene promoter regions were enriched (175 DMPs or 11. 7%) compared to W4 (one DMP or 0.8%) and W12/16 (15 DMPs or 6.9%) (Additional file 12). Given the enrichment of DMPs specifically during early development, we surveyed the expression of genes which are known to alter DNA methylation for microbial effects (Fig. 4d and Additional file 13). Expression of *Dnmt3a* and *Tet3* (Tet methylcytosine dioxygenase 3) were significantly altered by the microbiota in W1 and W12/16. DNMT3A is important for de novo methylation [68], whereas TET3 is essential for demethylation [69]. Similar to the approach of the transcriptome analysis, we ranked all DMPs based on their BH-corrected *p* value and chose the top 100 most significantly regulated DMPs from the microbiota-associated data set (Fig. 4e and Additional file 14) and from the developmental program (Additional file 15) for each time point to visualize differential methylation by hierarchical clustering. We chose a ranked approach and the top 100 to generate equal sample sizes for the analysis based on the total number of differentially methylated sites in the respective comparisons (minimum 132 for W4). For the microbiota-related DMPs, samples clustered according to microbial status and developmental stage (Fig. 4e) except for a few samples with several missing values only among these microbiota-related DMPs, which may be due to insufficient sequencing depth. However, these samples did contain data for many other of the almost 1.2 million CpG sites. As the samples overall met the quality criteria, they were not removed from the methylome analysis. For the top 100 developmentally related DMPs at each time point, samples clustered only by developmental stage but did not reveal a further stratification according to microbial status (Additional file 15).

Integrated analysis identifies a specific signature of loci with coupled DNA methylation and RNA transcription driven by the presence of microbiota

Next, we sought to identify microbiota-dependent DNA methylation changes linked to RNA expression differences.

We hypothesized that this mode of regulation may pinpoint important genes involved in epithelial–microbe interaction as it represents a potentially longer-term modulation of cellular programs. We employed a hierarchical testing approach [52] to identify interactions between the microbiota-dependent alterations in the transcriptome and DNA methylation signatures (Fig. 5a). To that end, we screened all differentially expressed genes (CONV-R vs GF) for DMPs within a 5-kb window up- and downstream. We identified 17, 34, and 79 microbially regulated genes both with altered expression and differentially methylated in W1, W4, and W12/16, respectively, and most (122 out of 126) were specific for the developmental stage (Additional files 16 and 17). Tracking both the transcriptome and DNA methylation in paired samples from individual mice throughout early postnatal development allowed us to identify specific changes in the DNA methylation signature that may underlie the microbiota-dependent transcriptome alterations. For example, expression of *Camk2b* (calcium/calmodulin-dependent protein kinase II), which is involved in calcium-dependent signaling [70], was only altered by the microbiota at W12/16 but not at the younger stages W1 or W4 (Fig. 5b). Interestingly, nearby CpG sites were not differentially methylated at W1, whereas in week W4 we detected three DMPs and another eight DMPs at W12/16 (Fig. 5b). Therefore, either the complete demethylation of all 11 DMPs or only the eight downstream DMPs may be required to mediate the microbial induction of *Camk2b* expression at W12/16. Similarly, *Mob3b* (MOB kinase activator 3B) and *Ube2a* (Ubiquitin conjugating enzyme E2 A) were differentially methylated and expressed only at W1 and W4, respectively, but not at any other developmental stage (Additional file 18). Of all 126 genes with differential expression and methylation 72 (57%) showed increased expression with reduced methylation or decreased expression with increased methylation, whereas 54 genes (43%) did not show a canonical association of expression and methylation shift, which is similar to previous studies [24]. Genome-wide mapping of the host–microbiota interactions for gene expression and DNA methylation during the three development stages revealed equal distribution among chromosomes (Fig. 5c). Among all genes that were differentially methylated and expressed depending on the microbiota, network analysis revealed an enrichment of genes involved in regulation of cellular proliferation and regeneration, such as *Pik3cd*, *Rb1*, *Grb10*, *Plagl1*, *Nfix*, and *Tab3*, or of genes functioning in immune responses, such as *Atp7a*, *Atf4*, and *Bcl3* (Fig. 6). For example, *Rb1* (retinoblastoma-associated protein) is a tumor suppressor inhibiting cell cycle progression, which may also recruit methylases [71]. *Rb1* expression was reduced in CONV-R mice, which is in line with an increased IEC proliferation in the presence of a microbiota [6, 9]. Similarly, *Bcl3* is a proto-oncogene promoting proliferation and also mediates immune tolerance by suppressing

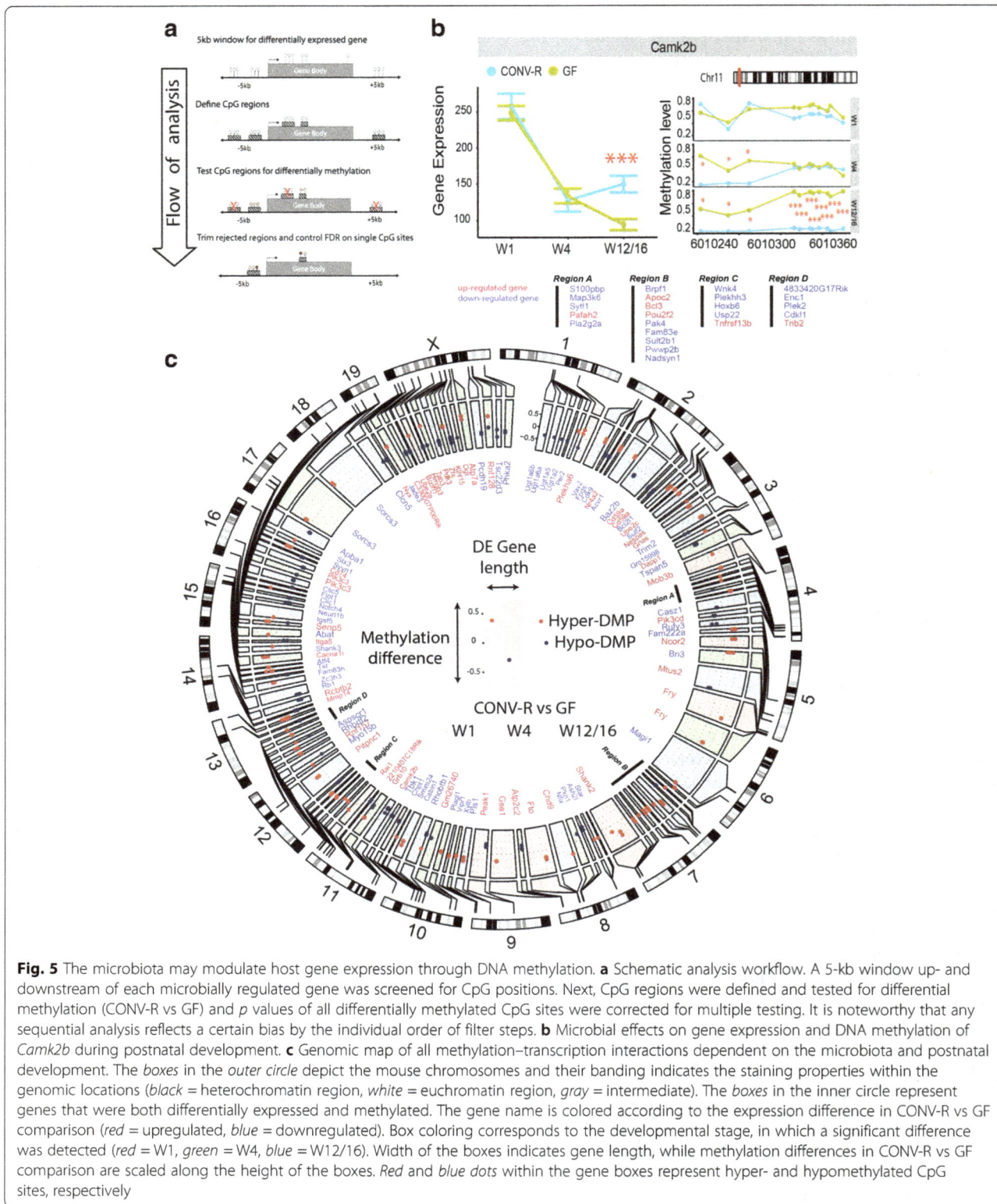

Fig. 5 The microbiota may modulate host gene expression through DNA methylation. **a** Schematic analysis workflow. A 5-kb window up- and downstream of each microbially regulated gene was screened for CpG positions. Next, CpG regions were defined and tested for differential methylation (CONV-R vs GF) and *p* values of all differentially methylated CpG sites were corrected for multiple testing. It is noteworthy that any sequential analysis reflects a certain bias by the individual order of filter steps. **b** Microbial effects on gene expression and DNA methylation of *Camk2b* during postnatal development. **c** Genomic map of all methylation–transcription interactions dependent on the microbiota and postnatal development. The *boxes* in the *outer circle* depict the mouse chromosomes and their banding indicates the staining properties within the genomic locations (*black* = heterochromatin region, *white* = euchromatin region, *gray* = intermediate). The *boxes* in the inner circle represent genes that were both differentially expressed and methylated. The gene name is colored according to the expression difference in CONV-R vs GF comparison (*red* = upregulated, *blue* = downregulated). Box coloring corresponds to the developmental stage, in which a significant difference was detected (*red* = W1, *green* = W4, *blue* = W12/16). Width of the boxes indicates gene length, while methylation differences in CONV-R vs GF comparison are scaled along the height of the boxes. *Red* and *blue dots* within the gene boxes represent hyper- and hypomethylated CpG sites, respectively

responses against microbial antigens [72]. In our analysis *Bcl3* was hypomethylated and expression increased in CONV-R mice, which is supported by a higher proliferative

capacity in the presence of a microbiota. Finally, as another example, *Plagl1* (pleiomorphic adenoma gene-like 1), which is another tumor suppressor inhibiting proliferation, was

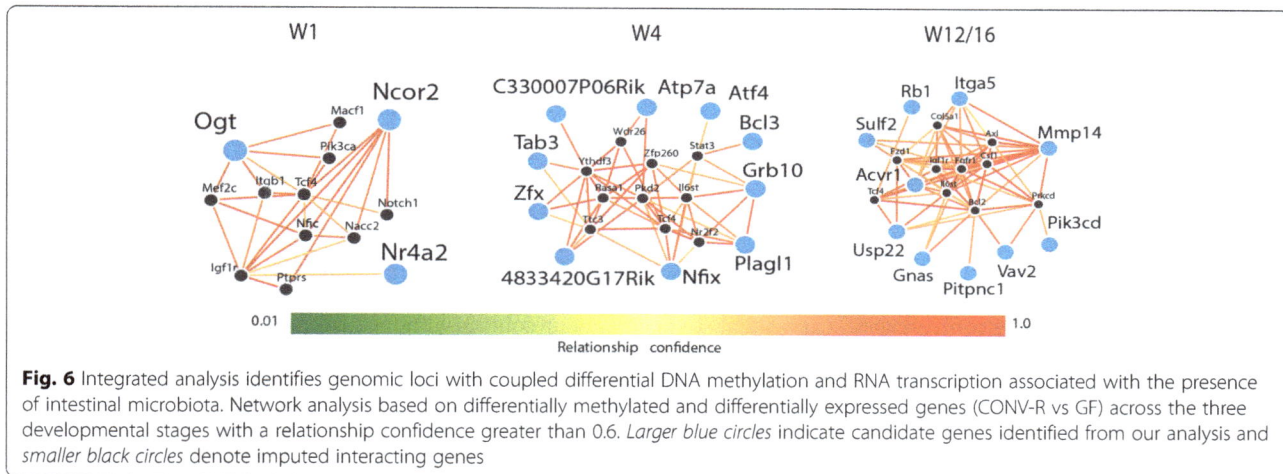

Fig. 6 Integrated analysis identifies genomic loci with coupled differential DNA methylation and RNA transcription associated with the presence of intestinal microbiota. Network analysis based on differentially methylated and differentially expressed genes (CONV-R vs GF) across the three developmental stages with a relationship confidence greater than 0.6. *Larger blue circles* indicate candidate genes identified from our analysis and *smaller black circles* denote imputed interacting genes

hypomethylated and had higher transcript levels in CONV-R mice, again supporting increased IEC proliferation in the presence of a microbiota.

To validate our findings, we selected a subset of the differentially expressed and methylated genes from our data and determined their expression and DNA methylation in an independent cohort of GF and CONV-R mice from another gnotobiotic animal facility. We harvested small intestinal epithelial tissue by scraping, isolated RNA and DNA as before, and performed qPCR analysis along with amplicon sequencing. For the eight tested genes (*Bcl3, Nfix, Cacna1i, Rcbtb2, Mmp14, Itga5, Cd74,* and *Pik3cd*) differential expression and methylation was reproduced for six genes in both cases (Additional file 19).

Discussion

We systematically investigated the regulatory effects of the microbiota on the transcriptome and the genome-wide DNA methylation status of IECs from the small intestine of infant, juvenile, and adult mice which were raised in either the presence or absence of a microbiota. This analysis revealed that both the IEC ontogeny and the microbiota affect the epithelial transcriptome signature along with the DNA methylation status and that the microbial effect increases during postnatal development. Furthermore, the microbial impact on the interplay of DNA methylation and the epithelial transcriptome were stage-specific as we detected almost no overlap between the genes that were regulated by the microbiota and also displayed an altered DNA methylation status for the three developmental stages. Our data provide groundwork to further dissect the endogenous developmental and microbial effects on the host's transcriptional and epigenetic program on a mechanistic level.

To fully understand the impact and role of the microbiota during adult development of IECs, it is required to assess the transcriptional and epigenetic changes over

time in both GF and CONV-R animals with a large enough size of biological replicates. While several studies have addressed selected aspects of the interplay of transcription, epigenetics, development, and microbiota [6–10, 12, 18, 29, 73, 74], an integrated genome-wide analysis of DNA methylation and transcriptional signatures in a single study using biological replicates and animals from different GF colonies has so far been lacking. In our current study, we therefore determined the epigenetic and transcriptional interactions between the gut microbiota and IECs using an integrated analysis of the methylome and transcriptome over time in both GF and CONV-R mice. The value of our experimental approach is demonstrated by the finding that although several previous studies established that the microbiota modulates the expression of more than 2000 genes in the intestinal epithelium [6, 9, 10], only a subset of these microbiota-responsive genes appear to be regulated by the epigenetic process of DNA methylation. Using our approach, we found that the microbiota seemed to inversely affect DNA methylation and gene expression throughout postnatal development. Whereas the number of differentially expressed (CONV-R vs GF) genes increased with postnatal development, the number of DMPs decreased from W1 to W12/16. The number of genes for which both transcription and DNA methylation are regulated by the microbiota (differentially expressed and DMPs within a 5-kb window) increased with time. Together these observations indicate that the microbial effect on modifying the epithelial DNA methylation and transcriptional status increased during maturation and postnatal development of the intestine. Notably, W1 samples differed substantially from W4 and W12/16 samples, indicating that further studies are required to describe the early dynamics from W1 to W4 in greater detail. However, the microbiota did not seem to engage DNA methylation to regulate transcriptional responses globally, but instead only seemed to target a specific subset of microbially responsive genes through their DNA methylation status. This unexpected finding is not caused by inherent differences in our and published datasets as, for example, our transcriptome sequencing data and the list of microbially regulated genes from the adult stage overlapped significantly with our previous data obtained from microarray analysis of laser-dissected ileal IECs [6]. Our observations are further supported by a study by Camp et al. which reported that the microbiota did not globally alter the chromatin architecture to drive gene expression, but only for specific genes [12]. Thus, host epigenetic mechanisms do not seem to be employed by the gut microbiota to drive transcriptional responses on a global scale.

Our study further validated that many developmentally regulated genes such as *Pigr*, which was reported to have increasing expression from infant to juvenile, or *Tet1*, having a decreasing expression from infant to juvenile [73], in addition also were differentially methylated and therefore appeared to be epigenetically regulated during postnatal development. Moreover, we could show that several of the genes which were previously reported as microbially regulated in the adult [6, 10] were also regulated transcriptionally during postnatal development. For example, the glycolysis regulator *Pfkfb3* (6-phosphofructo-2-kinase) was not only induced by the microbiota in the adult as reported [6, 10], but is already microbially regulated in the infant.

Surprisingly, we detected about ten times more DMPs in W1 compared to W4 or W12/16. Since methylation levels did not differ between the developmental stages, the increased number of DMPs in W1 did not seem to be simply due to higher overall methylation activity. Instead, the microbiota may differentially modulate de novo methylation and demethylation in the neonate mice. First, we detected generally higher levels of *Dnmt3a* during W1 compared to W4 or W12/16 and increased expression in CONV-R compared to GF mice. As DNMT3 mediates de novo methylation and parental imprinting [75], this temporal and microbiota-dependent expression pattern of *Dnmt3a* may therefore relate to the increased number of hypermethylated DMPs in the newborn mice. Conversely, *Tet3* expression was induced by the microbiota in W1 and since TET3 possesses hydroxymethylation activity [76, 77] and therefore mediates demethylation [69], the time- and microbiota-dependent expression pattern of *Tet3* may thus contribute to the increasing number of hypomethylated DMPs with increasing age. However, we can also not rule out a maternal imprinting effect, which may be dependent on the presence of microbiota in the mother before birth. Since the two groups of mice (CONV-R and GF) in the discovery cohort represent two separate colonies originating from different multiple mothers, we cannot exclude differential transgenerational inheritance of selected methylation marks (from the mother to the pups). In addition, as GF and CONV-R

mice have been maintained separately for several generations, genetic drift occurring in the two mouse colonies could theoretically contribute to the observed signatures, as genetic variants may have affected methylation sites. However, we validated a selection of identified differentially methylated and differentially expressed genes in an independent cohort of mice from another colony from a different gnotobiotic animal facility (Max-Planck Institute, Plön) using qPCR and targeted amplicon sequencing of the DMP loci. The validation of several candidate genes in an independent cohort—although of a smaller scale—corroborates the existence of microbiota-induced "functional" methylation sites, which may impact on long-term gene expression signatures in IECs.

Future studies are needed to functionally validate the involvement of methylation-modifying enzymes during early postnatal development and in relation to the microbiota. For example, tracking the changes in intestinal microbiota composition along with epithelial DNA methylation and transcriptome signatures of DNMT- or TET-deficient mice during postnatal development would be a promising approach. Together our data suggest that the microbiota seems to engage components of the DNA methylation machinery, which may at least partially translate into the observed epigenetic and transcriptional differences through postnatal development.

Conclusions
Postnatal development affects DNA methylation signatures and expression in intestinal epithelial cells, indicating that epigenetic processes contribute to developmental transitions largely driven by endogenous programs independent of microbial cues. However, our data also clearly show that the gut microbiota influences specific modules of the epithelial transcriptional network during postnatal development and targets only a subset of microbially responsive genes mainly functioning in IEC proliferation and immune responses through their DNA methylation status.

Additional files

Additional file 1: List of primers used for validation experiment (qPCR and amplicon sequencing). (XLSX 49 kb)

Additional file 2: R code used for the integrated analysis shown in Fig. 5a. (R 1 kb)

Additional file 3: Venn diagram of differentially expressed genes (CONV-R versus GF, adjusted *p* value < 0.05, fold change > 2) in the three developmental stages. (PDF 409 kb)

Additional file 4: Gene expression data of small intestinal epithelial cells from germ-free (GF) and conventionally raised (CONV-R) mice at the three developmental stages W1, W4, and W12/16 determined by RNA sequencing. (XLSX 9442 kb)

Additional file 5: MA transcriptome plot for CONV-R versus GF comparison. Every *dot* represents one transcript. The x-axis denotes the mean expression value and the y-axis denotes the log2 fold change of CONV-R versus GF. *Red dots* indicate statistically significant transcripts (CONV-R versus GF, adjusted *p* value < 0.05). The ceiling/floor of two on log2 fold change (y-axis) is set because of better visualization. (PDF 632 kb)

Additional file 6: Gene ontology (GO) analysis of the microbially regulated genes from each developmental stage. (XLSX 39 kb)

Additional file 7: Alternative splicing analysis. **a** Overview of the five categories of alternative splicing (skipped exon, alternative 5′ splice site, alternative 3′ splice site, mutually exclusive exons, and retained intron) as analyzed by the rMATS program. **b** Pie charts of the relative composition of alternative splicing events in each sample group. The relative composition patterns of alternative splicing do not differ significantly among the groups. **c** Count of significantly different (CONV-R versus GF, *p* < 0.05) alternative splicing events in the five categories for each developmental stage. The number of retained intron events in W1 was significantly higher than in the other stages. (PDF 529 kb)

Additional file 8: Alternative splicing events (total and only significant events in CONV-R versus GF) in the three developmental stages. (XLSX 9 kb)

Additional file 9: Heatmap of developmentally regulated genes (*n* = 553 genes). (PDF 818 kb)

Additional file 10: Gene ontology (GO) analysis of the co-expressed genes in different selected groups from Fig. 3. (XLSX 53 kb)

Additional file 11: Methylation levels across all samples (median ± standard deviation). (PDF 384 kb)

Additional file 12: Genomic location of DMPs (CONV-R versus GF) in the three developmental stages. (PDF 384 kb)

Additional file 13: Expression analysis of selected genes involved in DNA methylation: *Dnmt1* (DNA methyltransferase 1), *Dnmt3b* (DNA methyltransferase 3b), *Tet1* (Tet methylcytosine dioxygenase 1), *Tet2* (Tet methylcytosine dioxygenase 2), *Uhrf1* (Ubiquitin-like containing PHD and RING finger domains 1), *Uhrf2* (Ubiquitin-like containing PHD and RING finger domains 2), *Mbd2* (Methyl-CpG Binding Domain Protein 2), *Mbd3* (Methyl-CpG Binding Domain Protein 3), *Foxo3* (Forkhead box O3). (PDF 448 kb)

Additional file 14: Methylation levels of microbiota- (CONV-R versus GF) and development-dependent (W1 versus W4 versus W12/16) DMPs. Hierarchical clustering resulted in ten DMP groups. (XLSX 203 kb)

Additional file 15: Heatmap of methylation levels for developmentally related methylation sites. (PDF 658 kb)

Additional file 16: Venn diagram of differentially expressed genes (CONV-R versus GF) that also contain DMPs within a 5-kb window. (PDF 377 kb)

Additional file 17: List of differentially expressed genes (CONV-R versus GF) that also contain DMPs as depicted in Additional file 13. (XLSX 45 kb)

Additional file 18: Gene expression and DNA methylation levels of *Mob3b* (MOB kinase activator 3B) and *Ube2a* (Ubiquitin conjugating enzyme E2 A) genes and genomic loci in CONV-R and GF mice during postnatal development. (PDF 438 kb)

Additional file 19: Validation of a subset of differentially expressed and methylated genes. Small intestinal epithelial tissue was harvested by scraping from an independent cohort of GF and CONV-R mice from another gnotobiotic animal facility and both DNA and RNA were isolated for qPCR expression analysis and targeted methylation analysis using amplicon sequencing. *Asterisks* denote observations in the validation data that showed the same trend/direction as in the initial data, but were only very close to reaching the significance threshold after correction for multiple testing and therefore were considered as validation. (XLSX 48 kb)

Abbreviations

CONV-R: conventionally raised specific pathogen-free; CpG: DNA motif with cytosine followed by a guanine; DMP: differentially methylated position; DNMT: DNA methyltransferase; DTT: dithiothreitol; EDTA: ethylenediaminetetraacetic acid; FDR: false discovery rate; GF: germ-free; GO: Gene Ontology; HDAC: histone deacetylase; IEC: intestinal epithelial cell; MDS: multidimensional scaling; PCA: principal component analysis; RNA-Seq: RNA sequencing; RRBS: reduced representation bisulfite sequencing; SCFA: short-chain fatty acids; W1, W4, W12/16: 1, 4 or 12/16 week-old mice

Acknowledgements

We are indebted to Sabine Kock, Melanie Nebendahl, Carina Arvidsson, and the IKMB NGS team for excellent technical assistance. We thank Frauke Degenhardt and Dr. Anupam Sinha for helpful scientific discussions in gene expression analysis and methylation analysis.

Funding

This study was carried out as part of the Research Training Group "Genes, Environment and Inflammation", supported by the Deutsche Forschungsgemeinschaft (RTG 1743/1) and was further supported by the BMBF DEEP IHEC network grant (TP5.2, 2.3, 1.2, 3.1 and 3.3) and the DFG CRC1182, C2 and CRC877, B9 projects, as well as the Nucleotide Lab of the ExC 306 Inflammation at Interfaces. FB is Torsten Söderberg Professor in Medicine and recipient of an ERC Consolidator Grant (European Research Council, Consolidator grant 615362 - METABASE). JLS is a member of the ExC 1023 ImmunoSensation. This work was in part supported by DFG SFB 704 to JLS. The funding bodies had no part or influence on the design of the study and data collection, analysis, or interpretation.

Authors' contributions

FS, MFP, FB, and PR conceived the study. FS, MFP, AL, MJ, and PR performed the animal experiments and generated biological samples. WP, FS, MFP, TU, PB, and AF generated data. WP, FS, MFP, TU, PB, AF, JLS, FB, and PR analyzed the data. PK, AR, FM, TL, JW, SK, JFB, SS, and AF advised the various data analyses and contributed access to samples or infrastructure and techniques. WP, FS, MFP, and PR wrote the manuscript with input from all authors. All authors read and approved the final manuscript.

Authors' information

Not applicable

Competing interests

S.S. is a shareholder of CONARIS, has been a consultant to Allergosan, Danone, and Nestlé, and has received lectureship compensation from Allergosan. S.S. has lectured for Allergosan. F.B. is founder and owns equity in Metabogen AB. The remaining authors declare that they have no competing interests.

Author details

[1]Institute for Clinical Molecular Biology, University of Kiel, Rosalind-Franklin-Straße 12, 24105 Kiel, Germany. [2]The Wallenberg Laboratory, Department of Molecular and Clinical Medicine, University of Gothenburg, 41345 Gothenburg, Sweden. [3]Genomics and Immunoregulation, LIMES-Institute, University of Bonn, 53115 Bonn, Germany. [4]Max Planck Institute for Informatics, 66123 Saarbrücken, Germany. [5]Graduate School of Computer Science, Saarland University, 66123 Saarbrücken, Germany. [6]Department of Genetics, University of Saarland, 66123 Saarbrücken, Germany. [7]Institute for Experimental Medicine, Christian Albrechts University of Kiel, Kiel, Germany. [8]Max Planck Institute for Evolutionary Biology, Evolutionary Genomics, August-Thienemann-Str. 2, 24306 Plön, Germany. [9]Department of Internal Medicine I, University Hospital Schleswig Holstein, 24105 Kiel, Germany. [10]Platform for Single Cell Genomics and Epigenomics (PRECISE), German Center for Neurodegenerative Diseases

and the University of Bonn, Bonn, Germany. [11]Novo Nordisk Foundation Center for Basic Metabolic Research, Section for Metabolic Receptology and Enteroendocrinology, Faculty of Health Sciences, University of Copenhagen, 2200 Copenhagen, Denmark.

References

1. Hooper LV, Gordon JI, Venter JC, Savage DC, Brocks JJ, Logan GA, Buick R, Summons RE, Nelson KE, Paulsen IT, et al. Commensal host-bacterial relationships in the gut. Science (New York, NY). 2001;292:1115–8.
2. Sommer F, Backhed F. The gut microbiota - masters of host development and physiology. Nat Rev Microbiol. 2013;11:227–38.
3. Lozupone CA, Stombaugh JI, Gordon JI, Jansson JK, Knight R. Diversity, stability and resilience of the human gut microbiota. Nature. 2012;489:220–30.
4. Peterson LW, Artis D. Intestinal epithelial cells: regulators of barrier function and immune homeostasis. Nat Rev Immunol. 2014;14:141–53.
5. Rosenstiel P. Stories of love and hate: innate immunity and host-microbe crosstalk in the intestine. Curr Opin Gastroenterol. 2013;29:125–32.
6. Sommer F, Nookaew I, Sommer N, Fogelstrand P, Backhed F. Site-specific programming of the host epithelial transcriptome by the gut microbiota. Genome Biol. 2015;16:62.
7. El Aidy S, Derrien M, Merrifield CA, Levenez F, Dore J, Boekschoten MV, Dekker J, Holmes E, Zoetendal EG, van Baarlen P, et al. Gut bacteria-host metabolic interplay during conventionalisation of the mouse germfree colon. ISME J. 2013;7:743–55.
8. El Aidy S, Merrifield CA, Derrien M, van Baarlen P, Hooiveld G, Levenez F, Dore J, Dekker J, Holmes E, Claus SP, et al. The gut microbiota elicits a profound metabolic reorientation in the mouse jejunal mucosa during conventionalisation. Gut. 2013;62:1306–14.
9. El Aidy S, van Baarlen P, Derrien M, Lindenbergh-Kortleve DJ, Hooiveld G, Levenez F, Dore J, Dekker J, Samsom JN, Nieuwenhuis EE, Kleerebezem M. Temporal and spatial interplay of microbiota and intestinal mucosa drive establishment of immune homeostasis in conventionalized mice. Mucosal Immunol. 2012;5:567–79.
10. Larsson E, Tremaroli V, Lee YS, Koren O, Nookaew I, Fricker A, Nielsen J, Ley RE, Backhed F. Analysis of gut microbial regulation of host gene expression along the length of the gut and regulation of gut microbial ecology through MyD88. Gut. 2012;61:1124–31.
11. Gaboriau-Routhiau V, Rakotobe S, Lecuyer E, Mulder I, Lan A, Bridonneau C, Rochet V, Pisi A, De Paepe M, Brandi G, et al. The key role of segmented filamentous bacteria in the coordinated maturation of gut helper T cell responses. Immunity. 2009;31:677–89.
12. Camp JG, Frank CL, Lickwar CR, Guturu H, Rube T, Wenger AM, Chen J, Bejerano G, Crawford GE, Rawls JF. Microbiota modulate transcription in the intestinal epithelium without remodeling the accessible chromatin landscape. Genome Res. 2014;24:1504–16.
13. Alenghat T, Osborne LC, Saenz SA, Kobuley D, Ziegler CG, Mullican SE, Choi I, Grunberg S, Sinha R, Wynosky-Dolfi M, et al. Histone deacetylase 3 coordinates commensal-bacteria-dependent intestinal homeostasis. Nature. 2013;504(7478):153–7.
14. Arpaia N, Campbell C, Fan X, Dikiy S, van der Veeken J, Deroos P, Liu H, Cross JR, Pfeffer K, Coffer PJ, Rudensky AY. Metabolites produced by commensal bacteria promote peripheral regulatory T-cell generation. Nature. 2013;504(7480):451–5.
15. Kellermayer R, Dowd SE, Harris RA, Balasa A, Schaible TD, Wolcott RD, Tatevian N, Szigeti R, Li Z, Versalovic J, Smith CW. Colonic mucosal DNA methylation, immune response, and microbiome patterns in Toll-like receptor 2-knockout mice. FASEB J. 2011;25:1449–60.
16. Mischke M, Plosch T. More than just a gut instinct-the potential interplay between a baby's nutrition, its gut microbiome, and the epigenome. Am J Physiol Regul Integr Comp Physiol. 2013;304:R1065–9.
17. Celluzzi A, Masotti A. How our other genome controls our epi-genome. Trends Microbiol. 2016;24(10):777–87.
18. Krautkramer KA, Kreznar JH, Romano KA, Vivas EI, Barrett-Wilt GA, Rabaglia ME, Keller MP, Attie AD, Rey FE, Denu JM. Diet-Microbiota Interactions Mediate Global Epigenetic Programming in Multiple Host Tissues. Mol Cell. 2016;64:982–92.
19. Vertino PM, Sekowski JA, Coll JM, Applegreen N, Han S, Hickey RJ, Malkas LH. DNMT1 is a Component of a Multiprotein DNA Replication Complex. Cell Cycle. 2002;1:416–23.
20. Pradhan S, Esteve P-O. Mammalian DNA (cytosine-5) methyltransferases and their expression. Clin Immunol. 2003;109:6–16.
21. Goll MG, Bestor TH. Eukaryotic cytosine methyltransferases. Annu Rev Biochem. 2005;74:481–514.
22. Holliday R, Pugh J. DNA modification mechanisms and gene activity during development. Science. 1975;187:226–32.
23. Riggs AD. X inactivation, differentiation, and DNA methylation. Cytogenet Cell Genet. 1975;14:9–25.
24. Hasler R, Feng Z, Backdahl L, Spehlmann ME, Franke A, Teschendorff A, Rakyan VK, Down TA, Wilson GA, Feber A, et al. A functional methylome map of ulcerative colitis. Genome Res. 2012;22:2130–7.
25. Jones PA. Functions of DNA methylation: islands, start sites, gene bodies and beyond. Nat Rev Genet. 2012;13:484–92.
26. Yang X, Han H, De Carvalho DD, Lay FD, Jones PA, Liang G. Gene body methylation can alter gene expression and is a therapeutic target in cancer. Cancer Cell. 2014;26:577–90.
27. Lipka DB, Wang Q, Cabezas-Wallscheid N, Klimmeck D, Weichenhan D, Herrmann C, Lier A, Brocks D, Von Paleske L, Renders S, et al. Identification of dna methylation changes at cis-regulatory elements during early steps of hsc differentiation using tagmentation-based whole genome bisulfite sequencing. Cell Cycle. 2014;13:3476–87.
28. Lee HJ, Hore TA, Reik W. Reprogramming the methylome: erasing memory and creating diversity. Cell Stem Cell. 2014;14:710–9.
29. Yu D-H, Gadkari M, Zhou Q, Yu S, Gao N, Guan Y, Schady D, Roshan TN, Chen M-H, Laritsky E, et al. Postnatal epigenetic regulation of intestinal stem cells require DNA methylation and is guided by the microbiome. Genome Biol. 2015;16:211.
30. Van den Abbeele P, Van de Wiele T, Verstraete W, Possemiers S, Adlercreutz H, Akira S, Uematsu S, Takeuchi O, Alander M, Satokari R, et al. The host selects mucosal and luminal associations of coevolved gut microorganisms: a novel concept. FEMS Microbiol Rev. 2011;35:681–704.
31. Rodriguez JM, Murphy K, Stanton C, Ross RP, Kober OI, Juge N, Avershina E, Rudi K, Narbad A, Jenmalm MC, et al. The composition of the gut microbiota throughout life, with an emphasis on early life. Microb Ecol Health Dis. 2015;26:26050.
32. Gensollen T, Iyer SS, Kasper DL, Blumberg RS. How colonization by microbiota in early life shapes the immune system. Science. 2016;352:539–44.
33. Cahenzli J, Koller Y, Wyss M, Geuking MB, McCoy KD. Intestinal microbial diversity during early-life colonization shapes long-term IgE levels. Cell Host Microbe. 2013;14:559–70.
34. Olszak T, An D, Zeissig S, Vera MP, Richter J, Franke A, Glickman JN, Siebert R, Baron RM, Kasper DL, Blumberg RS. Microbial exposure during early life has persistent effects on natural killer T cell function. Science. 2012;336:489–93.
35. Gollwitzer ES, Saglani S, Trompette A, Yadava K, Sherburn R, McCoy KD, Nicod LP, Lloyd CM, Marsland BJ. Lung microbiota promotes tolerance to allergens in neonates via PD-L1. Nat Med. 2014;20:642–7.
36. Heijtz RD, Wang S, Anuar F, Qian Y, Bjorkholm B, Samuelsson A, Hibberd ML, Forssberg H, Pettersson S. Normal gut microbiota modulates brain development and behavior. Proc Natl Acad Sci U S A. 2011;108:3047–52.
37. Sudo N, Chida Y, Aiba Y, Sonoda J, Oyama N, Yu XN, Kubo C, Koga Y. Postnatal microbial colonization programs the hypothalamic-pituitary-adrenal system for stress response in mice. J Physiol. 2004;558:263–75.
38. Sommer F, Adam N, Johansson MEV, Xia L, Hansson GC, Bäckhed F. Altered mucus glycosylation in core 1 O-glycan-deficient mice affects microbiota composition and intestinal architecture. PLoS One. 2014;9:e85254.
39. Kim D, Pertea G, Trapnell C, Pimentel H, Kelley R, Salzberg SL, Mortazavi A, Williams B, McCue K, Schaeffer L, et al. TopHat2: accurate alignment of transcriptomes in the presence of insertions, deletions and gene fusions. Genome Biol. 2013;14:R36.
40. Langmead B, Salzberg SL. Fast gapped-read alignment with Bowtie 2. Nat Methods. 2012;9:357–9.
41. Anders S, Pyl PT, Huber W. HTSeq–a Python framework to work with high-throughput sequencing data. Bioinformatics. 2015;31:166–9.
42. Love MI, Huber W, Anders S. Moderated estimation of fold change and dispersion for RNA-seq data with DESeq2. Genome Biol. 2014;15:550.
43. Dudoit S, Yang YH, Callow MJ, Speed TP. Statistical methods for identifying genes with differential expression in replicated cDNA microarray experiments. Stat Sin. 2002;12:111–39.

44. Breuer K, Foroushani AK, Laird MR, Chen C, Sribnaia A, Lo R, Winsor GL, Hancock RE, Brinkman FS, Lynn DJ. InnateDB: systems biology of innate immunity and beyond–recent updates and continuing curation. Nucleic Acids Res. 2013;41:D1228–33.

45. Eden E, Navon R, Steinfeld I, Lipson D, Yakhini Z. GOrilla: a tool for discovery and visualization of enriched GO terms in ranked gene lists. BMC Bioinformatics. 2009;10:48.

46. Xue J, Schmidt SV, Sander J, Draffehn A, Krebs W, Quester I, De Nardo D, Gohel TD, Emde M, Schmidleithner L, et al. Transcriptome-based network analysis reveals a spectrum model of human macrophage activation. Immunity. 2014;40:274–88.

47. Shen S, Park JW, Lu ZX, Lin L, Henry MD, Wu YN, Zhou Q, Xing Y. rMATS: robust and flexible detection of differential alternative splicing from replicate RNA-Seq data. Proc Natl Acad Sci U S A. 2014;111:E5593–601.

48. Krueger F, Andrews SR. Bismark: a flexible aligner and methylation caller for Bisulfite-Seq applications. Bioinformatics (Oxford, England). 2011;27:1571–2.

49. Akalin A, Kormaksson M, Li S, Garrett-Bakelman FE, Figueroa ME, Melnick A, Mason CE, Deaton A, Bird A, Suzuki M, et al. methylKit: a comprehensive R package for the analysis of genome-wide DNA methylation profiles. Genome Biol. 2012;13:R87.

50. Park Y, Wu H. Differential methylation analysis for BS-seq data under general experimental design. Bioinformatics. 2016;32:1446–53.

51. Wu H, Xu T, Feng H, Chen L, Li B, Yao B, Qin Z, Jin P, Conneely KN. Detection of differentially methylated regions from whole-genome bisulfite sequencing data without replicates. Nucleic Acids Res. 2015;43:e141.

52. Hebestreit K, Dugas M, Klein HU. Detection of significantly differentially methylated regions in targeted bisulfite sequencing data. Bioinformatics. 2013;29:1647–53.

53. Gu Z, Gu L, Eils R, Schlesner M, Brors B. circlize Implements and enhances circular visualization in R. Bioinformatics. 2014;30:2811–2.

54. Goya J, Wong AK, Yao V, Krishnan A, Homilius M, Troyanskaya OG. FNTM: a server for predicting functional networks of tissues in mouse. Nucleic Acids Res. 2015;43:W182–7.

55. Li LC, Dahiya R. MethPrimer: designing primers for methylation PCRs. Bioinformatics. 2002;18:1427–31.

56. Tusnady GE, Simon I, Varadi A, Aranyi T. BiSearch: primer-design and search tool for PCR on bisulfite-treated genomes. Nucleic Acids Res. 2005;33:e9.

57. Hansen KD, Langmead B, Irizarry RA. BSmooth: from whole genome bisulfite sequencing reads to differentially methylated regions. Genome Biol. 2012;13:R83.

58. Hannenhalli S. Eukaryotic transcription factor binding sites–modeling and integrative search methods. Bioinformatics (Oxford, England). 2008;24:1325–31.

59. Kaser A, Lee AH, Franke A, Glickman JN, Zeissig S, Tilg H, Nieuwenhuis EE, Higgins DE, Schreiber S, Glimcher LH, Blumberg RS. XBP1 links ER stress to intestinal inflammation and confers genetic risk for human inflammatory bowel disease. Cell. 2008;134:743–56.

60. Hasegawa D, Calvo V, Avivar-Valderas A, Lade A, Chou H-I, Lee YA, Farias EF, Aguirre-Ghiso JA, Friedman SL. Epithelial Xbp1 is required for cellular proliferation and differentiation during mammary gland development. Mol Cell Biol. 2015;35:1543–56.

61. Adolph TE, Tomczak MF, Niederreiter L, Ko HJ, Bock J, Martinez-Naves E, Glickman JN, Tschurtschenthaler M, Hartwig J, Hosomi S, et al. Paneth cells as a site of origin for intestinal inflammation. Nature. 2013;503:272–6.

62. Glover LE, Colgan SP. Hypoxia and metabolic factors that influence inflammatory bowel disease pathogenesis. Gastroenterology. 2011;140:1748–55.

63. Benizri E, Ginouves A, Berra E. The magic of the hypoxia-signaling cascade. Cell Mol Life Sci. 2008;65:1133–49.

64. Formenti F, Constantin-Teodosiu D, Emmanuel Y, Cheeseman J, Dorrington KL, Edwards LM, Humphreys SM, Lappin TR, McMullin MF, McNamara CJ, et al. Regulation of human metabolism by hypoxia-inducible factor. Proc Natl Acad Sci U S A. 2010;107:12722–7.

65. Schmidt SV, Krebs W, Ulas T, Xue J, Bassler K, Gunther P, Hardt AL, Schultze H, Sander J, Klee K, et al. The transcriptional regulator network of human inflammatory macrophages is defined by open chromatin. Cell Res. 2016;26:151–70.

66. Lee HK, Hsu AK, Sajdak J, Qin J, Pavlidis P. Coexpression analysis of human genes across many microarray data sets. Genome Res. 2004;14:1085–94.

67. Legendre P, Legendre L. Numerical ecology. 3rd ed. Cambridge: Elsevier; 2012.

68. Fatemi M, Hermann A, Gowher H, Jeltsch A. Dnmt3a and Dnmt1 functionally cooperate during de novo methylation of DNA. Eur J Biochem. 2002;269:4981–4.

69. Shen L, Inoue A, He J, Liu Y, Lu F, Zhang Y. Tet3 and DNA Replication Mediate Demethylation of Both the Maternal and Paternal Genomes in Mouse Zygotes. Cell Stem Cell. 2014;15:459–70.

70. Yamauchi T. Neuronal Ca2+/calmodulin-dependent protein kinase II—discovery, progress in a quarter of a century, and perspective: implication for learning and memory. Biol Pharm Bull. 2005;28:1342–54.

71. Murphree AL, Benedict WF. Retinoblastoma: clues to human oncogenesis. Science. 1984;223:1028–33.

72. Muhlbauer M, Chilton PM, Mitchell TC, Jobin C. Impaired Bcl3 up-regulation leads to enhanced lipopolysaccharide-induced interleukin (IL)-23P19 gene expression in IL-10(−/−) mice. J Biol Chem. 2008;283:14182–9.

73. Kraiczy J, Nayak K, Ross A, Raine T, Mak TN, Gasparetto M, Cario E, Rakyan V, Heuschkel R, Zilbauer M. Assessing DNA methylation in the developing human intestinal epithelium: potential link to inflammatory bowel disease. Mucosal Immunol. 2016;9:647–58.

74. Rakoff-Nahoum S, Kong Y, Kleinstein SH, Subramanian S, Ahern PP, Gordon JI, Medzhitov R. Analysis of gene–environment interactions in postnatal development of the mammalian intestine. Proc Natl Acad Sci U S A. 2015;112:1929–36.

75. Okano M, Bell DW, Haber DA, Li E. DNA methyltransferases Dnmt3a and Dnmt3b are essential for de novo methylation and mammalian development. Cell. 1999;99:247–57.

76. He Y-F, Li B-Z, Li Z, Liu P, Wang Y, Tang Q, Ding J, Jia Y, Chen Z, Li L, et al. Tet-mediated formation of 5-carboxylcytosine and its excision by TDG in mammalian DNA. Science (New York, NY). 2011;333:1303–\.

77. Kang J, Kalantry S, Rao A. PGC7, H3K9me2 and Tet3: regulators of DNA methylation in zygotes. Cell Res. 2013;23:6–9.

15

Single-cell transcriptome analysis of lineage diversity in high-grade glioma

Jinzhou Yuan[1], Hanna Mendes Levitin[1], Veronique Frattini[2], Erin C. Bush[1,3], Deborah M. Boyett[4], Jorge Samanamud[4], Michele Ceccarelli[5], Athanassios Dovas[6], George Zanazzi[6], Peter Canoll[6], Jeffrey N. Bruce[4], Anna Lasorella[2,6,7], Antonio Iavarone[2,6,8] and Peter A. Sims[1,3,9*]

Abstract

Background: Despite extensive molecular characterization, we lack a comprehensive understanding of lineage identity, differentiation, and proliferation in high-grade gliomas (HGGs).

Methods: We sampled the cellular milieu of HGGs by profiling dissociated human surgical specimens with a high-density microwell system for massively parallel single-cell RNA-Seq. We analyzed the resulting profiles to identify subpopulations of both HGG and microenvironmental cells and applied graph-based methods to infer structural features of the malignantly transformed populations.

Results: While HGG cells can resemble glia or even immature neurons and form branched lineage structures, mesenchymal transformation results in unstructured populations. Glioma cells in a subset of mesenchymal tumors lose their neural lineage identity, express inflammatory genes, and co-exist with marked myeloid infiltration, reminiscent of molecular interactions between glioma and immune cells established in animal models. Additionally, we discovered a tight coupling between lineage resemblance and proliferation among malignantly transformed cells. Glioma cells that resemble oligodendrocyte progenitors, which proliferate in the brain, are often found in the cell cycle. Conversely, glioma cells that resemble astrocytes, neuroblasts, and oligodendrocytes, which are non-proliferative in the brain, are generally non-cycling in tumors.

Conclusions: These studies reveal a relationship between cellular identity and proliferation in HGG and distinct population structures that reflects the extent of neural and non-neural lineage resemblance among malignantly transformed cells.

Background

Gliomas are the most common malignant brain tumors in adults. High-grade gliomas (HGGs), which include grade III anaplastic astrocytomas and grade IV glioblastomas (GBMs), the deadliest form of brain tumor, are notoriously heterogeneous at the cellular level [1–5]. While it is well-established that transformed cells in HGG resemble glia [6, 7], the extent of neural lineage heterogeneity within individual tumors has not been thoroughly characterized. Furthermore, many studies have implied the existence of glioma stem cells—a rare subpopulation

that is capable of self-renewal and giving rise to the remaining glioma cells in the tumor [8]. Finally, the immune cells in the tumor microenvironment belong primarily to the myeloid lineage and drive tumor progression [9]. However, little is known about the diversity of immune populations that infiltrate HGGs and a potential role of immune cells for immunotherapeutic approaches in HGG remains elusive [10]. Therefore, questions about the nature and extent of interaction between transformed cells and the immune microenvironment in HGG persist despite extensive molecular profiling of bulk tumor specimens [3, 7, 11]. Single-cell RNA-Seq (scRNA-Seq) approaches are shedding light on immune cell diversity in healthy contexts [12], and marker discovery for brain resident and glioma-infiltrating immune populations is an area of active study [13, 14]. Pioneering work used scRNA-Seq to provide a snapshot of the formidable

* Correspondence: pas2182@cumc.columbia.edu
[1]Department of Systems Biology, Columbia University Medical Center, New York, NY 10032, USA
[3]Sulzberger Columbia Genome Center, Columbia University Medical Center, New York, NY 10032, USA
Full list of author information is available at the end of the article

heterogeneity characterizing human GBM [4, 15, 16]. However, these early studies employed relatively low-throughput scRNA-Seq analysis which lacked the resolution necessary to deconvolve the full complexity of tumor and immune cells within individual HGGs. Later single-cell studies in glioma focused on lower-grade gliomas and the effects of *IDH1* mutational status [15, 16]. Lower-grade gliomas are typically more diffuse, less proliferative, and associated with better survival compared to HGGs. Here, we use a new scalable scRNA-Seq method [17, 18] for massively parallel expression profiling of human HGG surgical specimens with single-cell resolution, focusing mainly on GBM. These data allow us to ask important questions such as What is the relationship between the neural lineage resemblance of HGG cells and their proliferative status? Are transformed HGG cells directly expressing the inflammatory signatures commonly associated with certain glioma subtypes or are these expression patterns restricted to tumor-associated immune cells? Is there patient-to-patient heterogeneity in the structures of HGG cell populations? We report the broad extent of neural and non-neural lineage resemblance among transformed glioma cells, a relationship between neural lineage identity and proliferation among transformed tumor cells, and new approaches to classifying HGGs based on population structure.

Methods

Procurement and dissociation of high-grade glioma tissue

Single-cell suspensions were obtained using excess material collected for clinical purposes from de-identified brain tumor specimens. Donors (patients diagnosed with HGG) were anonymous. Tissues were mechanically dissociated to single cells following a 30-min treatment with papain at 37 °C in Hank's balanced salt solution. After centrifugation at $100 \times g$, the cell pellet was re-suspended in Tris-buffered saline (TBS, pH 7.4) and red blood cells were lysed using ammonium chloride for 15 min at room temperature. Cells were washed in TBS, counted, and re-suspended in TBS at a concentration of 1 million cells per milliliter for immediate processing.

Massively parallel single-cell RNA-Seq

We used a previously reported, automated microwell array-based platform for pooled scRNA-Seq library construction and followed the procedures for device operation, library construction, and sequencing described by Yuan and Sims [18] with the following two modifications: (1) Live staining of single-cell suspensions was performed on ice for 15–30 min and (2) aliquots of amplified cDNA were pooled together before purification with Ampure XP beads (Beckman). Each device contained 150,000 microwells (50 μm diameter, 58 μm height) with center-to-center distance of 75 μm.

Low-pass whole genome sequencing

For each tumor, a 2–3-mm^3 piece was used for DNA extraction. Each section was re-suspended in 400 μL of DNA/RNA Lysis Buffer (Zymo) and homogenized with a Dounce homogenizer if necessary. DNA and RNA were then extracted for the tissue using the ZR-Duet Kit (Zymo) according to the manufacturer's instructions. DNA was quantified using the Qubit dsDNA High Sensitivity Kit (Thermo Fisher Scientific). Libraries for low-pass WGS were constructed using by in vitro transposition the Nextera XT kit (Illumina). DNA inputs for each sample were normalized to 1 ng and library preparation was performed according to the manufacturer's instructions, using unique i7 indices for each sample. Libraries from all eight tumors were pooled at equimolar concentrations, denatured, diluted, and sequenced on an Illumina NextSeq 500 using a 150-cycle High Output Kit (Illumina, 2 × 75 bp).

Whole genome sequencing analysis

Reads were aligned to the human genome (hg19) using bwa-mem, and coverage at each nucleotide position was quantified using bedtools after removing PCR duplicates with samtools. To generate the bulk WGS heatmaps in Fig. 1e, we computed the number of de-duplicated reads that aligned to each chromosome for each piece of tumor tissue and divided this by the number of de-duplicated reads that aligned to each chromosome for a diploid germline sample from one of the patients (pooled blood mononuclear cells) after normalizing both by total reads. We then normalized this ratio by the median ratio across all chromosomes and multiplied by two to estimate the average copy number of each chromosome.

Immunohistochemical analysis

Immunohistochemistry using standard immunoperoxidase staining was performed on formalin-fixed paraffin-embedded tissue sections (5 μm thick) from specimens of each of the tumor resections. Briefly, we used 3 × 3 min cycles of de-paraffinization in xylene, 2 × 1 min cycles of dehydration in 100% ethanol, 2 × 1 min cycles of dehydration in 95% ethanol, and a 1-min cycle of dehydration in 70% ethanol. Slides were then washed in water. We used 0.01 M citrate buffer (pH 6) for antigen retrieval in a microwaved pressure cooker for 20 min. We then washed the slides three times in phosphage-buffered saline (PBS) after cooling for 30 min. We quenched endogenous peroxidase in 3% hydrogen peroxide in PBS for 10 min, washed three times in PBS, and blocked with 10% goat serum for 25 min. We then incubated the slides with primary antibodies for 90 min at room temperature. We used the following primary antibodies: rabbit anti-CD163 (Abcam, ab182422, 1:50 dilution), rabbit anti-SOX2

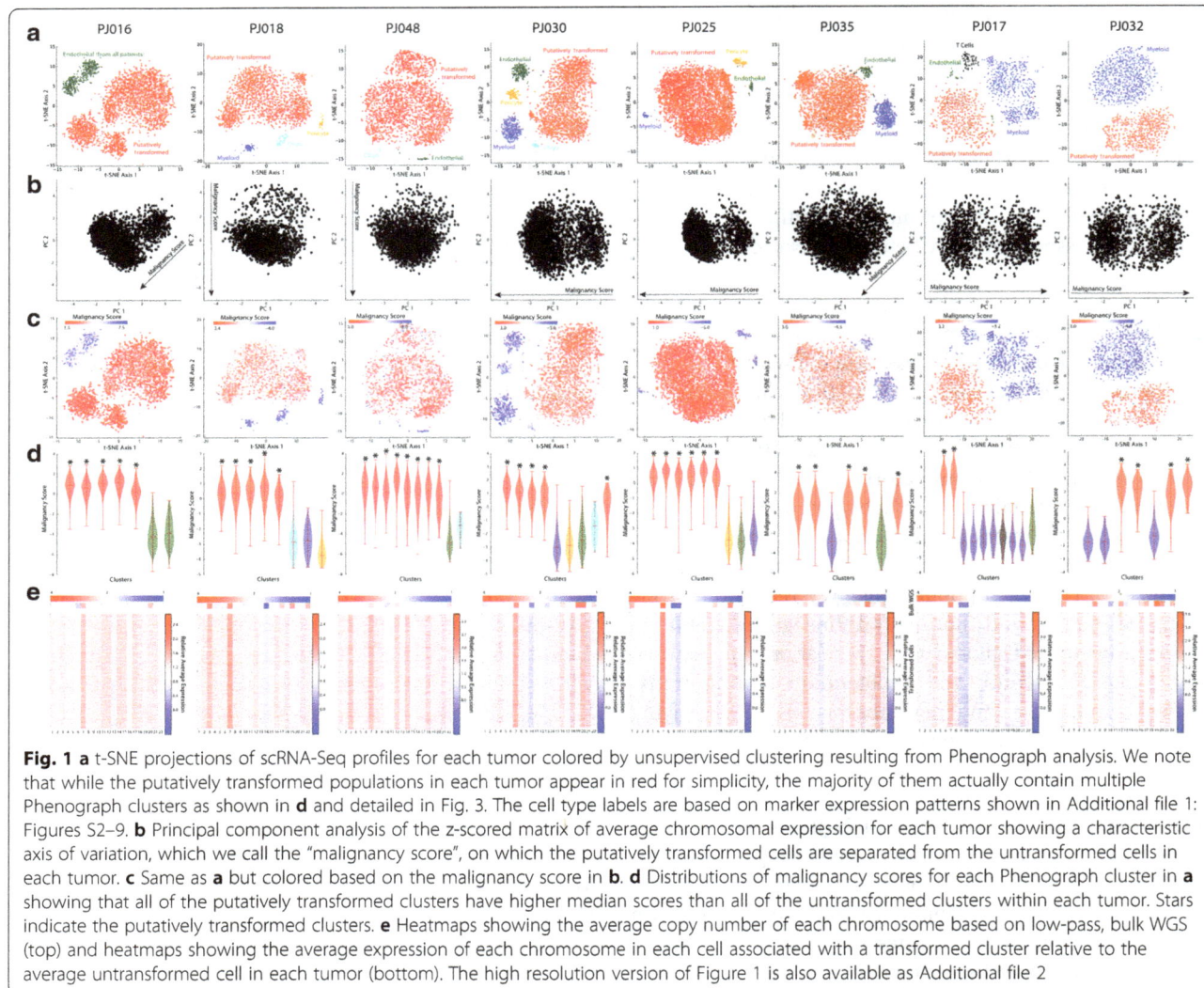

Fig. 1 a t-SNE projections of scRNA-Seq profiles for each tumor colored by unsupervised clustering resulting from Phenograph analysis. We note that while the putatively transformed populations in each tumor appear in red for simplicity, the majority of them actually contain multiple Phenograph clusters as shown in **d** and detailed in Fig. 3. The cell type labels are based on marker expression patterns shown in Additional file 1: Figures S2–9. **b** Principal component analysis of the z-scored matrix of average chromosomal expression for each tumor showing a characteristic axis of variation, which we call the "malignancy score", on which the putatively transformed cells are separated from the untransformed cells in each tumor. **c** Same as **a** but colored based on the malignancy score in **b**. **d** Distributions of malignancy scores for each Phenograph cluster in **a** showing that all of the putatively transformed clusters have higher median scores than all of the untransformed clusters within each tumor. Stars indicate the putatively transformed clusters. **e** Heatmaps showing the average copy number of each chromosome based on low-pass, bulk WGS (top) and heatmaps showing the average expression of each chromosome in each cell associated with a transformed cluster relative to the average untransformed cell in each tumor (bottom). The high resolution version of Figure 1 is also available as Additional file 2

(Abcam, ab92494, 1:100 dilution), rabbit anti-TMEM119 (Abcam, ab185333, 1:300 dilution). After washing three times in PBS, we incubated the slides with biotinylated goat anti-rabbit secondary antibody (Vector Laboratories, 1:200 dilution) for 30 min at room temperature, followed by additional PBS washing, 30-min incubation with ABC peroxidase reagent, development in DAB-peroxidase substrate solution (DAKO), and counter-staining in hematoxylin.

For the SOX2 validation cohort, tissue samples from 40 surgical resections of HGG (29 primary and 11 recurrent tumors) were fixed in 10% formalin and embedded in paraffin for immunohistochemical analysis. Five-micrometer sections were immunostained for SOX2 and counter-stained with hematoxylin. The slides were then scanned and digitized at 40× magnification on a Leica SCN400 system (Leica Biosystems). Total cell density and SOX2$^+$ nuclei were measured using a semi-automated cell-counting algorithm as

previously described [19]. Algorithm-derived cell counts were manually verified, and total cell density and SOX2 cell density were assessed for one representative high-power field from each sample. The labeling index was computed by dividing the total number of SOX2$^+$ cells by the total cell count for each high-power field.

Single-cell RNA-Seq alignment and data processing

As previously described, cell and molecular barcodes are contained in read 1 of our paired-end sequencing data, while all genomic information is contained in read 2 [18]. We trimmed read 2 to remove 3′ polyA tails (> 7 A's), and discarded fragments with fewer than 24 remaining nucleotides. Trimmed reads were aligned to GRCh38 (GENCODE v.24) using STAR v.2.5.0 with parameters "--sjdbOverhang 65 --twopassMode Basic --outSAMtype BAM Unsorted" [20]. Only reads with unique, strand-specific alignments to exons were kept for further analysis.

We extracted 12-nt cell barcodes (CBs) and 8-nt unique molecular identifiers (UMIs) from read 1. Degenerate CBs containing either 'N's or more than four consecutive 'G's were discarded. Synthesis errors, which can result in truncated 11-nt barcodes, were corrected similarly to a previously reported method [21]. Briefly, we identified all CBs with at least 20 apparent molecules and for which greater than 90% of UMI-terminal nucleotides were 'T'. These putative truncated CBs were corrected by removing their last nucleotide. This 12th nucleotide became the new first nucleotide of corresponding UMIs, which were also trimmed of their last ('T') base.

All reads with the same CB, UMI, and gene mapping were collapsed to represent a single molecule. To correct for sequencing errors in UMIs, we further collapsed UMIs that were within Hamming distance one of another UMI with the same barcode and gene. To correct for sequencing errors in cell barcodes, we then collapsed CBs that were within Hamming distance one of another barcode, had at least 20 unique UMI-gene pairs, and had at least 75% overlap of their UMI-gene pairs. Finally, we repeated UMI error correction and collapse using the error-corrected CBs. The remaining barcode-UMI-gene triplets were used to generate a digital gene expression matrix.

Filtering cell barcodes

We estimated the number of cell barcodes corresponding beads associated with cells in our microwell system using the cumulative histogram of reads associated with each barcode as described previously [22]. To avoid dead cells and library construction artifacts, we removed cell barcodes that failed to satisfy certain criteria. We removed all cells where > 10% of molecules aligned to genes expressed from the mitochondrial genome or where the ratio of molecules aligning to whole gene bodies (including introns) to molecules aligning exclusively to exons was > 1.5. These measures remove cells with compromised plasma membranes, which results in retention of mitochondrial or nuclear transcripts [23]. We also removed cells where the number of reads per molecule (indicative of amplification efficiency) or the number of molecules per gene deviated by more than 2.5 standard deviations from the mean for a given sample.

Unsupervised clustering, differential expression, and force-directed graphical analysis

To calculate k-nearest neighbor graphs, we computed a cell by cell Spearman's correlation matrix for each population and set $k = 20$. Spearman's correlation was calculated from a set of genes selected because they were detected in fewer cells than expected given their apparent expression level. For this step of our analysis only, molecular counts within each column of gene by cell expression matrices were normalized to sum to 1. Genes were then ordered by their mean normalized value in the population and placed into bins of 50 genes. A gene's detection frequency was calculated as fraction of cells in which at least one molecule of a gene was detected, and its score was defined as the maximum detection frequency in its bin minus its detection frequency. Genes with scores greater than 0.15 were considered markers and used to compute Spearman's correlation.

This k-nearest neighbors graph was used as input to Phenograph [24], a modularity-based clustering algorithm. The similarity matrix described above was converted to a distance matrix, and used as input to tSNE [25] for visualization. Differential expression analysis was conducted using a binomial test as previously described [21].

Force-directed graphs were generated from the k-nearest neighbor graphs described above using the *from_numpy_matrix*, *draw_networkx*, and *spring_layout* commands in the NetworkX v1.11 module for Python with default parameters.

Identification of transformed cells by single-cell analysis of copy number alterations

For unsupervised identification of transformed cells in our HGG data, we first converted the raw molecular counts for each cell to $\log_2$(counts per thousand molecules $+ 1$). We then discarded all genes that were expressed in fewer than 100 cells per tumor as well as the HLA genes on chromosome 6, which could manifest as copy number variants particularly in myeloid populations. Next, we computed the average of $\log_2$(counts per thousand molecules $+ 1$) across the genes on each somatic chromosome, resulting in an $N \times 22$ matrix, where N is the number of cells. Finally, we z-scored the resulting profile for each cell and computed the principal components (PCs) of the resulting z-matrix. For each tumor, either the first PC (PJ017, PJ025, PJ030, PJ032), second PC (PJ018, PJ048), or the sum of the first two PCs (PJ016, PJ035) yielded an axis along which the putatively transformed and untransformed cells identified by clustering were separated (Fig. 1b) as evidenced by the t-SNE projections in Fig. 1c in which the cells are colored based on their value along the appropriate axis. To compute the heatmaps of chromosomal gene expression in Fig. 1e, we took the average value of $\log_2$(counts per thousand molecules $+ 1$) for each chromosome in each transformed cell and divided by the average value of $\log_2$(counts per thousand molecules $+ 1$) for each chromosome averaged over all untransformed cells in a given tumor.

Subpopulation clustering with reference component analysis database

To identify cell types resembling the transformed subpopulations that we identified across our data set, we used the RNA-Seq databases curated for reference component analysis [26]. We first removed all transcriptomes of whole homogenized tissues (e.g., whole brain and whole blood) or that originated from cancers. We then computed Spearman's correlation coefficient between each cell type-specific transcriptome and the average expression profile of each transformed subpopulation across all eight tumors in our data set. All cell types with a below-median standard deviation were then removed to enrich for cell types with high variation across our data set, and the resulting correlation matrix was standardized and subjected to hierarchical clustering with a Euclidean distance metric using the *clustermap* function in the Seaborn Python module (Fig. 5a).

We have previously shown that molecular cross-contamination in our microfluidic system is ~ 1%. Such a cross-contamination rate slightly reduces the contrast in gene expression profiles between different cell subpopulations. However, it is unlikely that a gene would become highly differentially expressed in, and hence become a marker of, a population of cells due to cross-contamination. To address the possibility that the immune signature that is highly enriched in PJ017 and PJ032 arises from cross-contamination due to the high abundance of myeloid cells in these two tumors, we conducted an orthogonal and more direct analysis to determine whether or not glioma cells in PJ017 and PJ032 express higher levels of immune genes than other tumors. We first conducted a differential expression analysis between the combined transformed cells from PJ017/PJ032 and the remaining tumors along with parallel analyses comparing the transformed cells from PJ017 or PJ032 to their respective immune populations using the binomial test described above. We then selected all of the genes that were significantly more frequently detected in the PJ017/PJ032 transformed cells ($p < 0.01$ with fold-enrichment > 10) than other tumors and removed all genes that were more frequently detected in the immune cells in either tumor. Any remaining differentially expressed genes are more highly expressed in the transformed cells from PJ017/PJ032 and therefore cannot arise from molecular cross-contamination. Finally, we conducted a gene ontology analysis on the remaining differentially expressed genes that were either more frequently detected in PJ017/PJ032 (after filtering immune cell-specific genes) or in other tumors using Panther (www.pantherdb.org). Figure 5b shows the results for the lowest-level gene ontologies (top 15 biological process ontologies for each group) based on the Panther gene

ontology hierarchy (to avoid the use of extremely broad ontologies like "cell part").

Generation of myeloid signatures

To generate microglial- and macrophage-specific gene signatures for Additional file 1: Figure S17H, we started with the cell type-specific gene sets obtained from murine lineage-tracing studies (Additional file 1: Table S4 from Bowman et al.) [14], similar to previous analysis [27]. We then assembled all of the myeloid and non-myeloid cells in our data set and conducted a differential expression analysis using the binomial test described above to identify genes with at least fivefold specificity for the myeloid population and FDR < 0.01. We removed any genes from the Bowman et al. gene sets that did not intersect with this list to avoid inclusion of genes expressed in other cell types (particularly the transformed cells) to obtain the gene sets in Additional file 1: Table S4.

Results

Low-cost, scalable single-cell RNA-Seq of high-grade glioma surgical specimens

scRNA-Seq has emerged as a powerful approach to unbiased cellular and molecular profiling of complex tissues. Recent reports have highlighted its particular utility in solid tumors [4, 15, 16, 26, 28], where phenotypic alterations resulting from both malignant transformation and the tumor microenvironment may have great therapeutic or diagnostic significance, but are difficult to dissect from conventional bulk analysis. However, these studies employed relatively expensive and low-throughput technologies for scRNA-Seq, which complicate their sensitivity to small cellular subpopulations and ultimate routine deployment for clinical analysis. We recently reported a simple, microfluidic system for scRNA-Seq with a number of key advantages for profiling complex tissues including rapid cell loading, compatibility with live cell imaging, high-throughput (i.e., thousands of cells per sample), and low cost without requiring cell sorting [17, 18]. Here, we apply this system and demonstrate routine profiling of thousands of individual cells in parallel from HGG surgical specimens. Our data set includes ~ 24,000 scRNA-Seq profiles from eight patients and reveals new insights into the population structures of these extremely heterogeneous tumors, relationships between neural lineages and subpopulations of transformed cells, and the immune microenvironment.

We procure tissue from surgical resections and immediately subject it to mechanical and enzymatic dissociation to produce a single-cell suspension. These cells are rapidly loaded into a microfluidic device where they are captured in arrays of microwells (Additional file 1: Figure S1A), subjected to imaging-based quality control and automated cDNA barcoding for pooled scRNA-Seq. Importantly, we do not apply any cell sorting and attempt to randomly sample the cell suspension. Additional file 1: Table S1 and Figure S1B summarizes the data in terms of patient diagnosis and cell numbers, molecular, and gene detection rates, which are comparable to those obtained in previously reported, large-scale scRNA-Seq experiments in tissues [22, 29], and GBM subtype as determined by comparing the single-cell average profiles to bulk RNA-Seq from previously classified GBMs in TCGA [7].

Identification of malignantly transformed glioma cells with single-cell RNA-Seq

We used the Phenograph implementation of Louvain community detection [24], a commonly used method for unsupervised clustering of scRNA-Seq data [21, 30], to analyze the diversity of cell types in individual patients. Figure 1a shows t-distributed stochastic neighbor embedding (t-SNE) projections of the single-cell profiles in each patient colored based on the resulting Phenograph clusters. Differential expression analysis to identify genes specific to each cluster revealed discrete populations of endothelial cells, pericytes, T cells, myeloid cells, and oligodendrocytes (Fig. 1a and Additional file 1: Figures S2–9) as expected in HGGs. In addition, each tumor harbored a large, complex population of cells comprised of multiple clusters that were often contiguous in the corresponding t-SNE projection. These cells most commonly resembled glia, expressing markers of astrocytes like *GFAP*, *AQP4*, and *ALDOC* and oligodendrocyte progenitors like *OLIG1*, *OLIG2*, and *PDGFRA*. Because transformed glioma cells typically resemble glia at the level of gene expression, we considered these cells to be putatively transformed [6] and attempted to validate these candidate transformed cells by orthogonal means. Importantly, there is no known universal marker or set of markers that can be used for unambiguous sorting of transformed cells from glioma tissues [4]. Therefore, an analytical approach for distinguishing transformed and untransformed cells, which will inevitably be mixed in our scRNA-Seq data, is crucial.

Previous studies have shown that large copy number alterations and aneuploidies are readily detectable by scRNA-Seq of tumor tissues [4, 15, 16, 28]. We found that aneuploidies were evident in certain cellular populations based on the average expression of each chromosome in each cell. Principal component analysis (PCA) of the chromosomal expression matrix for each patient consistently revealed an axis of variation that separated the putatively transformed cells from those that expressed common markers of cells in the glioma microenvironment (Fig. 1b, c). We called this the malignancy score, which we found to be either the first PC, second

PC, or a linear combination thereof in each patient. Notably, we did not detect putatively untransformed cells in PJ016. ~ 90% of cells in each PJ016 cluster express *SOX2* (Additional file 1: Figure S10A), which is normally expressed in stem and precursor cells in the CNS and, as discussed below, is pervasively expressed in transformed HGG cells compared to the adult brain. To address this, we included the combined set of endothelial cells from all of the other tumors to enable comparative analysis. Importantly, each cluster of putatively transformed cells had a significantly higher median malignancy score than the microenvironmental cells in every patient (Fig. 1d). Finally, when we considered the relative expression of each chromosome for each putatively malignant cell compared to the average chromosomal expression of the microenvironmental cells in each patient, we observed clear evidence of aneuploidies that are common in HGG, such as amplification of chromosome 7 and loss of chromosome 10 (Fig. 1e). For further validation, we conducted low-coverage whole genome sequencing (WGS) of bulk tumor tissue from each patient and computed the average copy number of each chromosome by comparison to a diploid reference. We found that the copy number variants evident in bulk WGS were in good agreement with the most prominent alterations in our scRNA-Seq data (Fig. 1e). As expected, there are some exceptions likely due to the lack of resolution at the single-cell level and the potential for compensatory changes in gene expression. For example, there is an apparent loss of chromosome 13 in PJ016 that is distinctly less prominent in the bulk WGS. High-resolution analysis of the bulk WGS reveals that there is indeed loss of a large region of chromosome 13 (Additional file 1: Figure S11). While this analysis is not meant to enable quantitative assessment of copy number alterations, it gives us confidence that the putatively transformed populations of cells are indeed mutated.

SOX2 is pervasively expressed in high-grade glioma cells

There is currently no universal marker that can consistently and specifically label transformed cells across HGGs. While it is unlikely that such a marker exists, we sought to determine whether our scRNA-Seq profiles could reveal genes that are both highly specific to and pervasively expressed in transformed glioma cells in HGG tissue. Taking advantage of the results described above, we conducted a differential expression analysis between cells in all transformed and untransformed clusters across our data set. We then asked which genes were most frequently detected in the transformed population among those with at least eightfold higher expression ($p_{adj} < 0.01$) in transformed versus untransformed cells. Interestingly, we found that *SOX2*, a gene with a well-known and crucial role in stem cell biology that is commonly associated with glioma stem cells [31, 32], is the most frequently detected gene with at least eightfold specificity for the transformed cells (Fig. 2a). Indeed, previous studies have suggested that SOX2 protein is significantly more widely expressed in glioma tissue than in normal brain, with expression in the adult brain being typically restricted to ventricular stem cell niches [33, 34]. We found pervasive expression of *SOX2* across all eight patients profiled in this study (Additional file 1: Figure S10); *SOX2* is expressed by cells in every transformed cluster identified in these tumors. In fact, analysis of transcript drop-out in the transformed populations identified in these eight tumors suggests that the frequency with which we detect *SOX2* transcript likely underestimates its pervasiveness (Fig. 2b). This is unsurprising because we have limited sensitivity, and transcription factors like SOX2 tend to be lowly

expressed. To confirm these results, we carried out immunohistochemical (IHC) analysis of six of the eight tumors in our cohort and found widespread expression of SOX2 protein in every tumor (Fig. 2c). Notably, the fraction of SOX2$^+$ cells in the IHC specimens correlates strongly (r = 0.98, p = 0.001) with the fraction of transformed tumor cells inferred using our scRNA-Seq data and the analysis shown in Fig. 1 (Additional file 1: Figure S12).

To further validate this finding, we performed quantitative immunohistochemical analysis of SOX2 expression in a larger cohort of 40 surgical specimens from high-grade gliomas (Additional file 1: Figure S13). SOX2$^+$ cells were seen in all tumor samples, and the median labeling index of SOX2 in this cohort was 0.87 (Additional file 1: Figure S13A), suggesting that the vast majority of transformed HGG cells are SOX2$^+$. SOX2 staining varied across samples, with the highest density

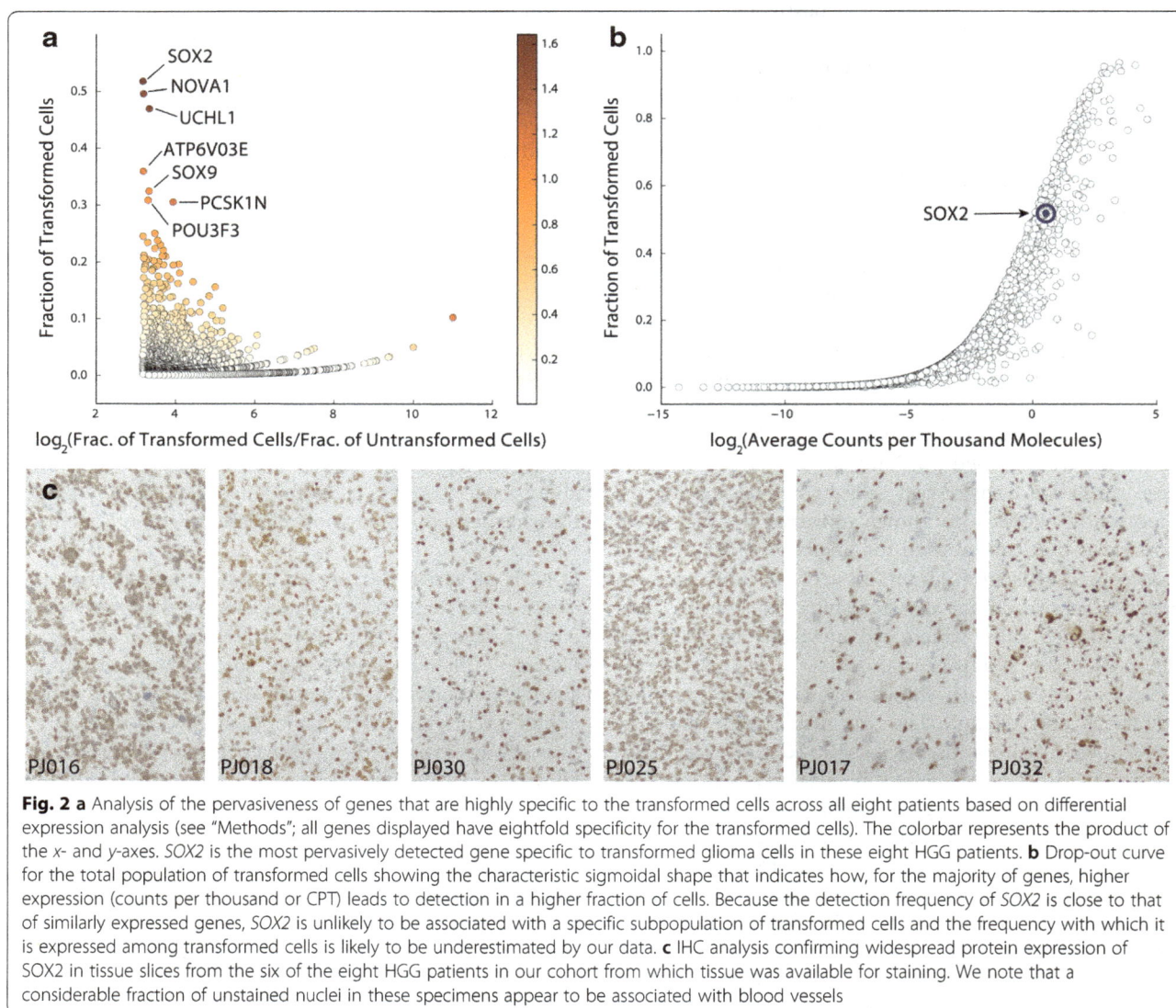

Fig. 2 a Analysis of the pervasiveness of genes that are highly specific to the transformed cells across all eight patients based on differential expression analysis (see "Methods"; all genes displayed have eightfold specificity for the transformed cells). The colorbar represents the product of the *x*- and *y*-axes. *SOX2* is the most pervasively detected gene specific to transformed glioma cells in these eight HGG patients. **b** Drop-out curve for the total population of transformed cells showing the characteristic sigmoidal shape that indicates how, for the majority of genes, higher expression (counts per thousand or CPT) leads to detection in a higher fraction of cells. Because the detection frequency of *SOX2* is close to that of similarly expressed genes, *SOX2* is unlikely to be associated with a specific subpopulation of transformed cells and the frequency with which it is expressed among transformed cells is likely to be underestimated by our data. **c** IHC analysis confirming widespread protein expression of SOX2 in tissue slices from the six of the eight HGG patients in our cohort from which tissue was available for staining. We note that a considerable fraction of unstained nuclei in these specimens appear to be associated with blood vessels

of SOX2⁺ cells seen in areas of highest cellularity (Additional file 1: Figure S13B, $r = 0.93$, $p = 10^{-18}$), which is also consistent with SOX2 expression in transformed HGG cells. Furthermore, regression analysis also showed a significant relationship between SOX2 labeling index and total cellularity (Additional file 1: Figure S13C, $r = 0.36$, $p = 0.02$). These results support the findings from scRNA-Seq analysis and suggest that SOX2 is a promising tumor cell marker for histopathological analysis of HGGs. In addition, we found no significant difference between primary and recurrent tumors in terms of SOX2 labeling index, suggesting that SOX2 is a useful marker of glioma cells in both pathological settings. While the pervasiveness of SOX2 is inconsistent with the idea that this protein marks a rare subpopulation of stem-like cells in HGG, the role of SOX2 in pluripotency implies that the majority of transformed glioma cells are in an immature and potentially plastic state.

Transformed cells resemble both glial and neuronal lineages in high-grade glioma

Previous studies of low-grade gliomas (LGGs) have used scRNA-Seq to draw comparisons between populations of glioma cells and certain neural lineages in the brain [15]. Subpopulations resembling oligodendrocyte progenitors (OPCs) and astrocytes were reported [15]. Bulk expression analysis of localized biopsies in HGG showed that different regions of the same tumor resembled disparate expression subtypes (e.g., proneural, classical, and mesenchymal) [2, 3] and subtype-specific differences in cellular composition and glial lineage resemblance [3]. Relatedly, scRNA-Seq of relatively small numbers of cells (tens per patient) in GBM found cellular subpopulations resembling different expression subtypes co-occurring in the same tumor [4]. These findings have implications for both cell-of-origin and the possibility that neurodevelopmental processes are occurring during glioma development and progression.

We sought to determine the extent to which subpopulations of transformed cells resemble neural lineages in HGGs subjected to large-scale scRNA-Seq. We performed unsupervised clustering of transformed glioma cells identified by the aneuploidy analysis described above and identified markers of the resulting subpopulations (Fig. 3a, see "Methods") [24]. The heatmaps in Fig. 3b show the expression of a subset of neural lineage markers found to associate specifically with certain subpopulations of transformed cells across our patients. As expected, we found that many of the commonly differentially expressed genes were markers of glial lineages including astrocytes (GFAP, AQP4, ALDOC) and OPCs (OLIG1, OLIG2, PDGFRA, DLL3). While multiple tumors contained cells that express genes associated with more mature oligodendrocytes, the tumor PJ018

contained a well-defined subpopulation that strongly resembled myelinating oligodendrocytes with specific expression of multiple myelin genes including MBP, MOG, and MAG. Hence, HGGs harbor cells that resemble a broad spectrum of glial developmental states and maturities. These findings are consistent with the well-established glial nature of these tumors and the numerous studies pointing to a glial cell-of-origin for gliomas [35–38]. Interestingly, in multiple patients, we also observed populations of transformed cells that closely resemble immature neurons or neuroblasts—progenitors that give rise to neurons (purple boxes, Fig. 3b). These cells express genes associated with neuroblasts like CD24 and STMN2 along with genes primarily expressed in the neuronal lineage in the brain, such as DCX [39, 40]. Interestingly, while we observe subpopulations that co-express these genes and have low expression of canonical glial markers (indicated by purple rectangles in Fig. 3b), we also find subpopulations with significant co-expression of neuroblast and OPC markers (e.g. OLIG2, PDGFRA), suggesting potential plasticity between these two cell types in HGG. PJ048 harbored a particularly well-defined population of immature neuronal cells, some of which even expressed markers of more mature neurons (Additional file 1: Figure S14). Taken together, our results indicate that the lineage resemblance of transformed glioma cells in HGG includes not only a diversity of glia, but even extends into the neuronal lineage.

Relationship between proliferation and lineage resemblance in high-grade glioma

Many studies have demonstrated the efficacy of scRNA-Seq for assessing the proliferative state of individual cells and even assigning cell cycle stage [4, 15, 22]. Recent scRNA-Seq experiments in LGGs showed that glioma cells with clear lineage resemblance to astrocytes and oligodendrocytes were generally non-proliferative, and cycling cells were largely restricted to a stem-like compartment [15]. Conversely, an earlier study of GBM with scRNA-Seq reported that the stem-like glioma signature was anti-correlated with expression of cell cycle control genes, suggesting that glioma stem cells are largely quiescent in GBM [4].

We used the expression of cell cycle control genes to assess active proliferation across the subpopulations we identified in transformed cells (Fig. 3b, Additional file 1: Table S2). Among transformed subpopulations with a clear neural lineage relationship, we never observed high expression of proliferation markers in those resembling astrocytes, myelinating oligodendrocytes, or neuroblast-like cells that lack co-expressed OPC markers. In contrast, a subset of OPC-like cells does express high levels of cell cycle control genes. These

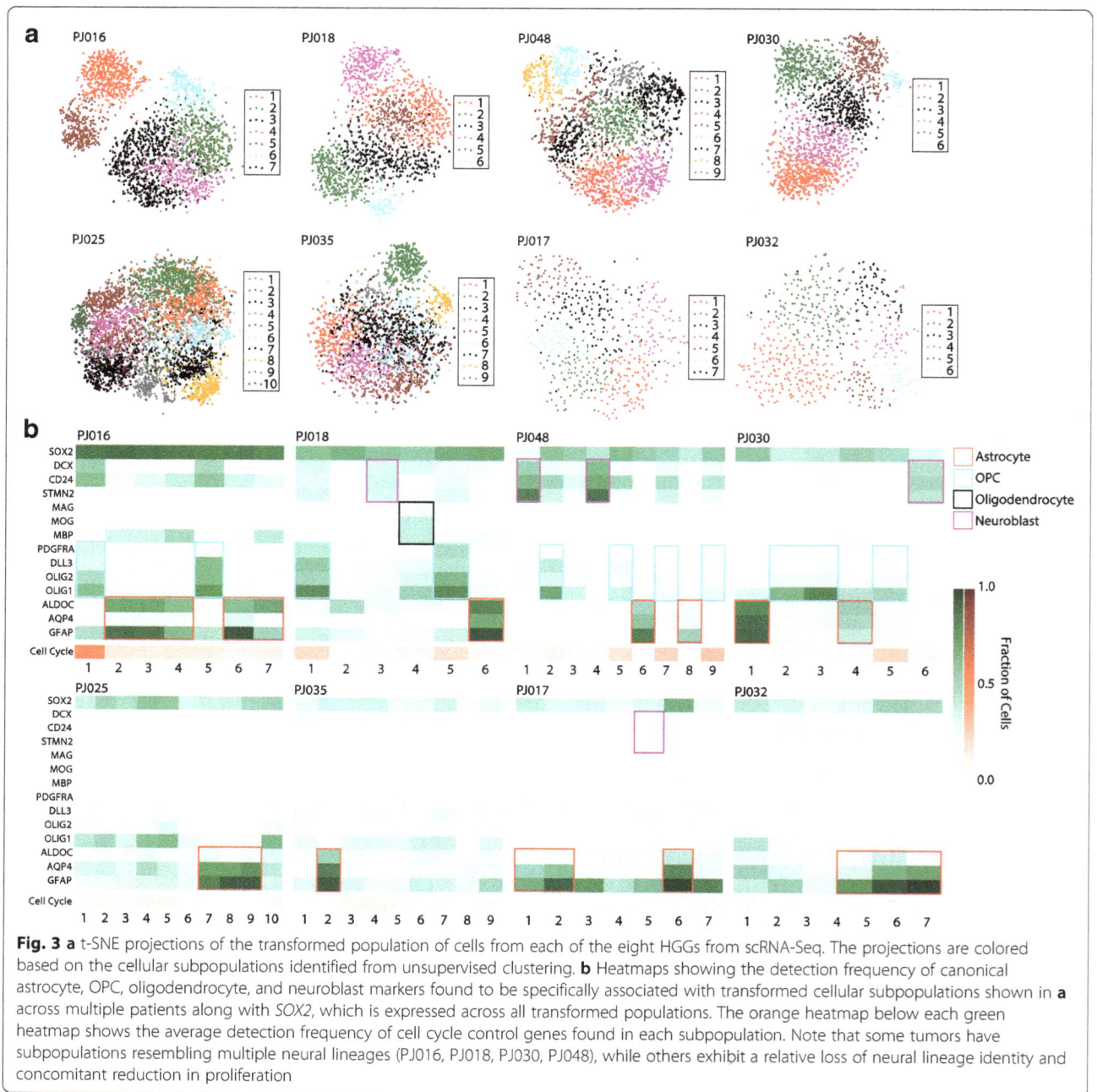

Fig. 3 a t-SNE projections of the transformed population of cells from each of the eight HGGs from scRNA-Seq. The projections are colored based on the cellular subpopulations identified from unsupervised clustering. **b** Heatmaps showing the detection frequency of canonical astrocyte, OPC, oligodendrocyte, and neuroblast markers found to be specifically associated with transformed cellular subpopulations shown in **a** across multiple patients along with *SOX2*, which is expressed across all transformed populations. The orange heatmap below each green heatmap shows the average detection frequency of cell cycle control genes found in each subpopulation. Note that some tumors have subpopulations resembling multiple neural lineages (PJ016, PJ018, PJ030, PJ048), while others exhibit a relative loss of neural lineage identity and concomitant reduction in proliferation

results are consistent with the behavior of these neural cell types in the adult brain, where OPCs are the predominant population of cycling cells and astrocytes, oligodendrocytes, and neuroblasts are generally not found in the cell cycle [41, 42].

Observation of distinct cellular population structures among transformed cells in high-grade glioma

Given the extent of neural lineage diversity represented in HGGs, we decided to investigate the underlying structure of the transformed population on an individual patient

basis. Recent reports describe analytical methods for identifying branching events and even pseudo-temporal ordering of scRNA-Seq profiles, particularly in the context of cellular differentiation [43–46]. Most of these approaches construct a graph from scRNA-Seq profiles in which each node represents a cell or group of cells and edges indicate similarity between nodes.

Our above analysis of cellular heterogeneity in HGG relies on the construction of a *k*-nearest neighbor graph from our scRNA-Seq profiles, which is then used for modularity clustering [24]. Therefore, to visualize the relationships between subpopulations, we plotted the k-nearest neighbor graph of the transformed cells from each patient as a force-directed graph in Fig. 4 (see "Methods"). This analysis revealed clear differences in the structures of these populations. In particular, the transformed cells in three of the tumors formed multi-branched structures (e.g., PJ016, PJ018, and PJ048), harbored cells resembling a diversity of neural lineages, and closely resembled the proneural subtype of GBM based on comparison of the single-cell average profiles of these tumors and classified bulk RNA-Seq data from TCGA [7]. A second set of three tumors resembled the classical subtype (PJ030, PJ025, and PJ035). PJ030 exhibited a branched structure with both OPC- and astrocyte-like branches and a small subpopulation of neuroblast-like cells, while PJ025 and PJ035 were less structured and less diverse in terms of neural lineage

resemblance. Finally, PJ017 and PJ032 exhibited relatively unstructured populations and closely resembled the Mesenchymal subtype. The number of cells sampled per tumor did not explain these structural differences (Additional file 1: Table S1). In most cases, cells at the termini of the branches resemble differentiated glia. For example, PJ016, PJ018, PJ030, and PJ048 each contain a branch that terminates in a subpopulation that resembles astrocytes (Fig. 4). PJ016 and PJ030 contain termini that resemble OPCs. The non-astrocyte branch of PJ018 strongly resembles oligodendrocyte differentiation. The terminus contains a subpopulation resembling an oligodendrocyte-like cell that expresses myelin genes and is adjacent to a subpopulation that expresses OPC markers (Fig. 4). At the branch point, PJ018 contains a lineage-ambiguous cell type with simultaneous expression of neuroblast and OPC markers, reminiscent of

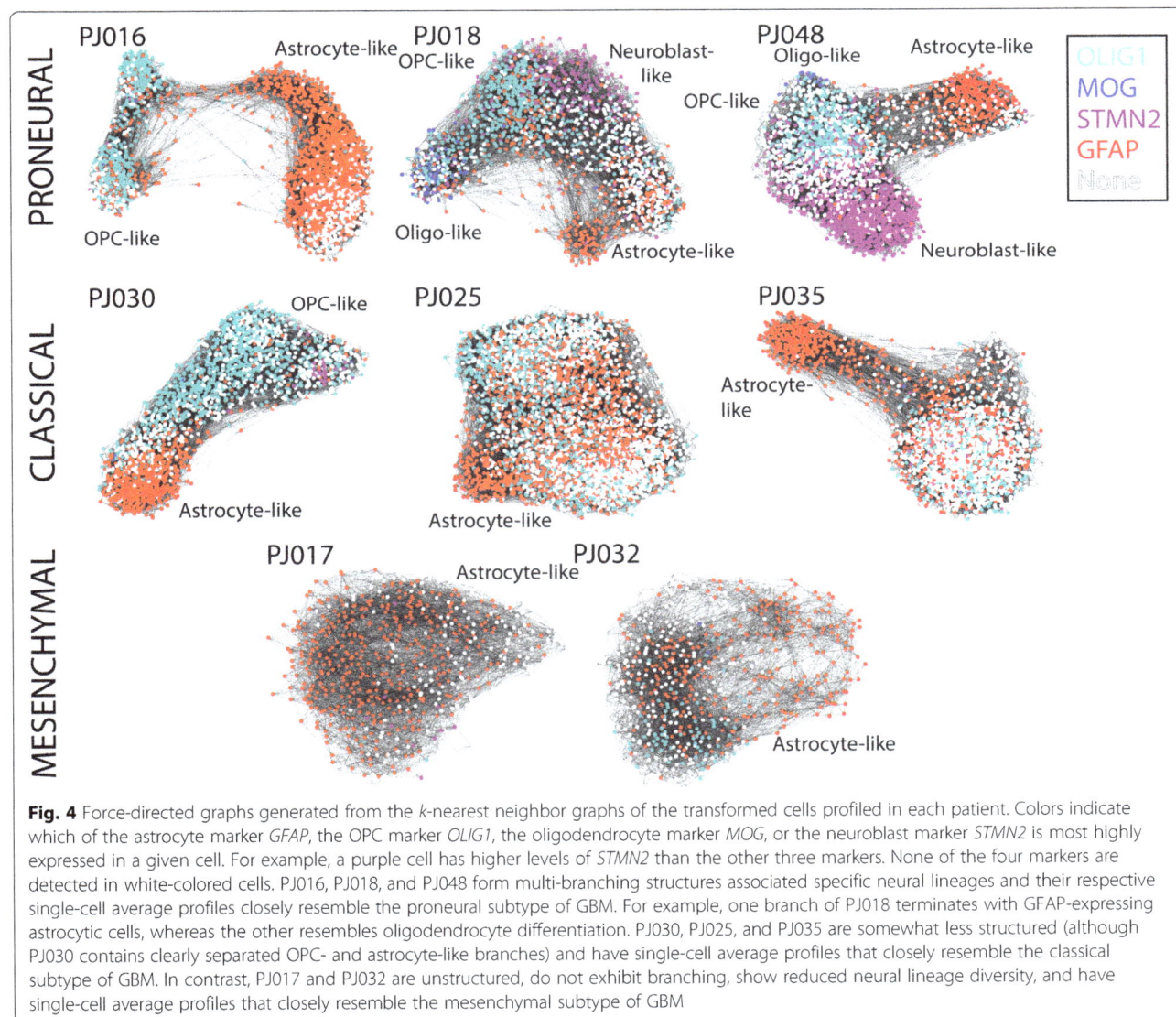

Fig. 4 Force-directed graphs generated from the k-nearest neighbor graphs of the transformed cells profiled in each patient. Colors indicate which of the astrocyte marker GFAP, the OPC marker OLIG1, the oligodendrocyte marker MOG, or the neuroblast marker STMN2 is most highly expressed in a given cell. For example, a purple cell has higher levels of STMN2 than the other three markers. None of the four markers are detected in white-colored cells. PJ016, PJ018, and PJ048 form multi-branching structures associated specific neural lineages and their respective single-cell average profiles closely resemble the proneural subtype of GBM. For example, one branch of PJ018 terminates with GFAP-expressing astrocytic cells, whereas the other resembles oligodendrocyte differentiation. PJ030, PJ025, and PJ035 are somewhat less structured (although PJ030 contains clearly separated OPC- and astrocyte-like branches) and have single-cell average profiles that closely resemble the classical subtype of GBM. In contrast, PJ017 and PJ032 are unstructured, do not exhibit branching, show reduced neural lineage diversity, and have single-cell average profiles that closely resemble the mesenchymal subtype of GBM

previous observations of multi-potent progenitors in the brain [47, 48]. PJ048 is particularly remarkable in that it harbors an astrocyte-like branch, an OPC-like branch terminating with a small population of myelin-expressing oligodendrocyte-like cells, and a large branch resembling neuroblasts or immature neurons (Additional file 1: Figure S14).

While the branching behavior represents neural lineage diversity and differentiation, the cellular states of the less structured tumors are less clear. The heatmaps in Fig. 3b show that four of the less structured tumors (PJ017, PJ025, PJ032, and PJ035) express relatively few neural lineage markers with the notable exception of astrocyte genes. We know from substantial prior work that glioma cells, and particularly GBM cells, are capable of differentiating along non-neural lineages. For example, some GBMs undergo mesenchymal transformation [49, 50].

To better understand these tumors, we sought to analyze their lineage resemblance across a large database of expression profiles representing cell types in many organs. We used a curated gene expression database to identify cell types that resemble the cellular subpopulations identified among the transformed glioma cells [26]. Figure 5a shows hierarchical clustering of correlation coefficients between the average profile of each transformed subpopulation in our data set and the cell type-specific expression profiles in the curated database. This analysis immediately reveals three clusters of cell type-specific expression profiles—one enriched in

embryonic stem and neural cells (neural/ESC), one enriched in immune cells (immune), and one enriched in mesenchymal and mesenchymal stem cells (mesenchymal/MSC)—along with three multi-tumor groups of transformed subpopulations. The first group of transformed cells (group I) is exclusively comprised of subpopulations from branched tumors PJ016, PJ030, and PJ048. Glioma cells in group I are correlated with the ESC/neural cluster, but bear the weakest resemblance to the MSC/mesenchymal and immune clusters. Group II contains clusters from all but one tumor (PJ032, a recurrent GBM) and is correlated with the neural/ESC signature, but unlike group I has some mesenchymal/MSC and immune character. Interestingly, group III is comprised of subpopulations from only two tumors, PJ017 and PJ032, which strongly resemble both the immune and MSC/mesenchymal clusters, but weakly resemble the ESC/neural cells.

The results in Fig. 5a are consistent with the notion that the tumors lacking clear neural lineage structure have undergone mesenchymal transformation. However, this analysis also highlights crucial distinctions among these tumors. First, as has been recognized from bulk expression analysis of GBM, mesenchymal gene expression is often accompanied by expression of inflammatory genes [3, 7]. However, the extent to which this inflammatory signature is expressed by transformed glioma cells has been difficult to discern from bulk analysis due to the presence of both transformed and untransformed cells. Here, we find that mesenchymally transformed

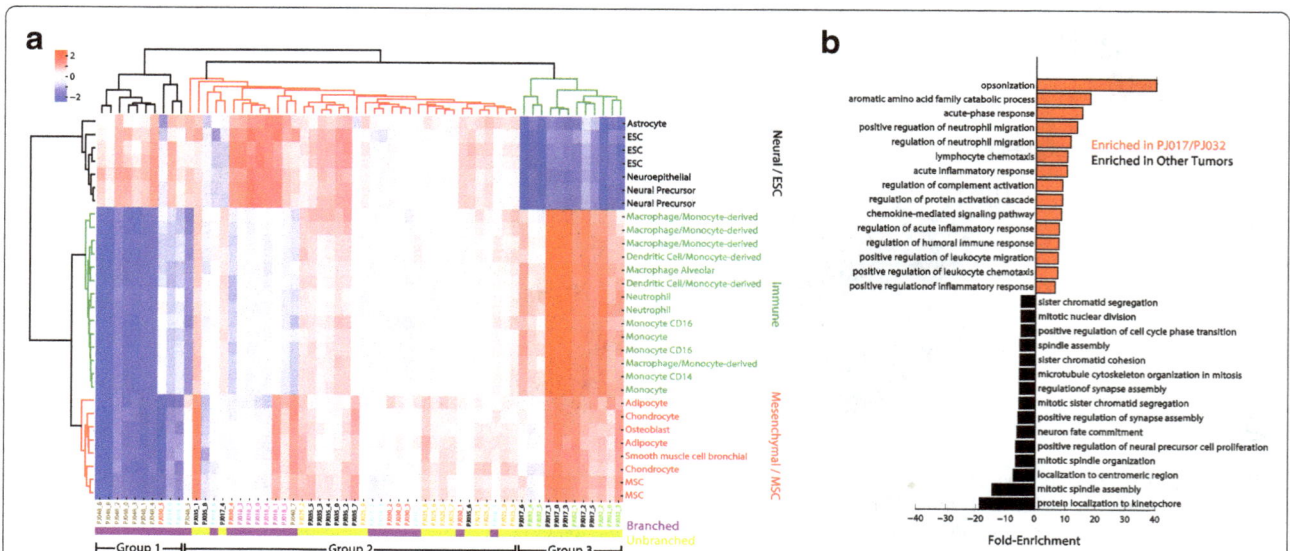

Fig. 5 a Hierarchical clustering of the correlation between each transformed subpopulation and a database of cell type-specific expression profiles with high variability across the data set. We find three cell type clusters referred to as Neural/ESC, Immune, and Mesenchymal/MSC which divide the tumor cell subpopulations into three major groups. **b** Gene ontology analysis of the differentially expressed genes between the group III tumors (PJ017/PJ032) and the remaining tumors (PJ016, PJ018, PJ025, PJ030, PJ035, PJ048) after removal of genes specific to the untransformed immune cells in PJ017 and PJ032. The group III tumors show a clear immunological gene signature that is specific to the transformed cells

glioma cells express many immune-related genes, but that there is also significant variability in the expression of these genes among subpopulations with mesenchymal gene expression (group II vs. group III). Second, the two tumors with high levels of inflammatory gene expression (PJ017 and PJ032 in group III) also bear the least resemblance to the neural/ESC clusters. Hence, expression of this mesenchymal-associated immune signature is accompanied by loss of neural lineage identity.

PJ017 and PJ032 are notable not just because of their unbranched structure, strong immunological gene expression, and loss of neural lineage identity, but also because they are the only two tumors in our data set where transformed glioma cells are in the minority of profiled cells. PJ017 is 48% myeloid cells, 5% T cells, and 45% transformed glioma cells; PJ032 is 57% myeloid cell and 43% transformed glioma cells based on scRNA-Seq. While the observation of extensive myeloid infiltration in tumors that express high levels of inflammatory markers is intriguing, it also raises the possibility that our observation arises from experimental cross-contamination either during mRNA capture or library construction. We compared the transformed cells in PJ017/PJ032 to the remaining tumors after stringent filtration of the differentially expressed genes to remove any genes that are more highly expressed in the myeloid compartment of these tumors and could result in cross-contamination (see "Methods"). Figure 5b shows that, despite our stringent filter, the transformed cells in PJ017/PJ032 express high levels of immune genes compared to the remaining tumors (Additional file 1: Table S3), thus indicating that tumor cells expressing an immune-like signature may recruit infiltration of myeloid cells. Interestingly, we were able to validate this finding in an independent patient cohort (Additional file 1: Figure S15) by re-analyzing an earlier, smaller-scale GBM data set from Patel et al. where one out of the five tumors profiled expressed this same signature at high levels among transformed cells [4].

We next asked if any of the genes in this signature have known receptor-ligand interactions with cognates expressed in the myeloid cells of these tumors. One interaction of potential therapeutic interest in glioma is the macrophage proliferation cytokine CSF1 and its cognate receptor CSF1R, which has been extensively validated in pre-clinical studies in glioma along with its potential therapeutic efficacy [51, 52]. Figure 6 shows that CSF1R is widely expressed in the myeloid populations in the seven tumors in which we detect myeloid cells. However, CSF1 is most highly expressed in the transformed glioma cells PJ017 and PJ032, the two tumors with the highest immune signature correlation in Fig. 5a and the highest proportion of tumor-associated myeloid cells. These results are consistent with a model

in which CSF1 secretion by glioma cells recruits CSF1R-expressing microglia or macrophages to the tumor microenvironment, as demonstrated previously in murine models [51, 52], and may point to a patient population that would be particularly susceptible to CSF1R blockade.

Previous studies have used scRNA-Seq to analyze the heterogeneity of tumor-associated myeloid cells in gliomas. One study focusing on IDH1 mutant gliomas found a continuous distribution of myeloid phenotypes ranging from more microglial on one extreme to more macrophage-like on the other [16]. In contrast, a recent study focusing on HGGs found a clear separation between cell of microglial origin and blood-derived macrophages [27]. We applied similar analytical methods in our patient cohort and found significant differences in myeloid phenotype dominated mainly by expression of pro-inflammatory cytokines and microglial versus macrophage lineage resemblance (Additional file 1: Figure S16–18).

Discussion

Large-scale scRNA-Seq has allowed us to dissect the lineage identity and proliferative status of malignant cells in HGG with unprecedented resolution. We find that only a subset of transformed cells resembles neural lineages and that there is significant inter-tumoral heterogeneity in the diversity of neural lineages represented among transformed cells. Furthermore, we find that neural lineage resemblance extends beyond glia. Subpopulations of transformed cells in multiple patients resemble neuroblasts or immature neurons. Moreover, we defined a molecular classification for HGGs based on population structure at the single-cell level that is closely related to the range of neural lineage resemblance among transformed cells in a tumor. Specifically, transformed populations with branched structures resemble a variety of neural lineages arranged similarly to normal neurodevelopment. These transformed populations appear to obey the same rules for proliferative potential as their corresponding neural lineages in the brain. Based on expression of cell cycle genes, the transformed cells resembling astrocytes, myelinating oligodendrocytes, and neuroblasts are generally not in the cell cycle, whereas those resembling OPCs are often found in a proliferative state. These observations are distinct from what has been reported previously in low-grade oligodendrogliomas, where a truncal, stem-like population was found to encompass the cycling cells in a tumor [15]. In HGG, we find that proliferative state is predominantly associated with cells expressing markers of OPC-like, glial progenitors.

A second group of tumors harbored transformed cells that either resemble astrocytes or exhibit a loss of neural lineage identity. The underlying subpopulations tend to

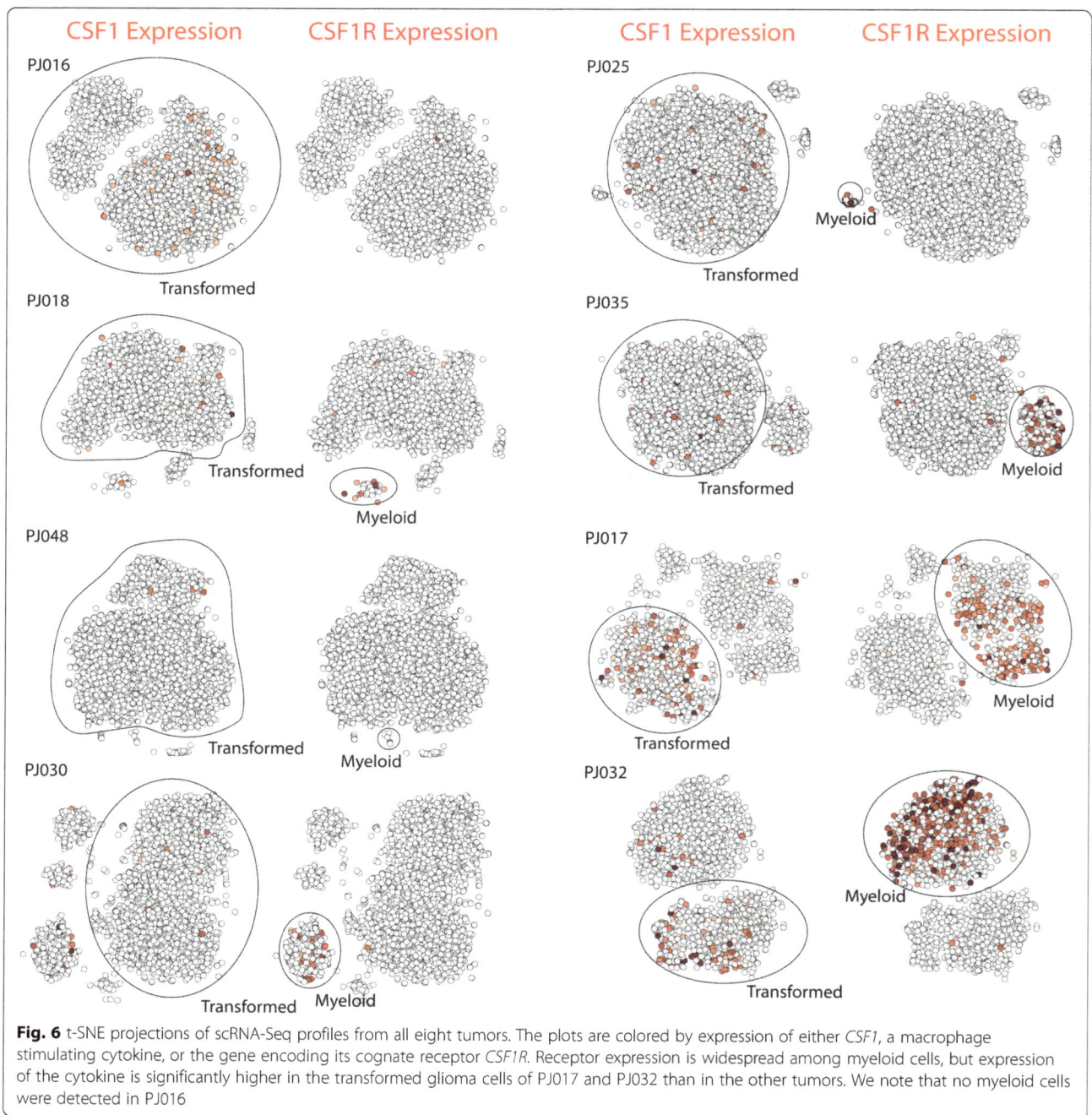

Fig. 6 t-SNE projections of scRNA-Seq profiles from all eight tumors. The plots are colored by expression of either *CSF1*, a macrophage stimulating cytokine, or the gene encoding its cognate receptor *CSF1R*. Receptor expression is widespread among myeloid cells, but expression of the cytokine is significantly higher in the transformed glioma cells of PJ017 and PJ032 than in the other tumors. We note that no myeloid cells were detected in PJ016

resemble mesenchymal and immune cell types and express low levels of proliferation markers. However, there is significant inter-tumoral heterogeneity among these HGGs, particularly with respect to immunological gene expression and corresponding myeloid infiltration. Mesenchymal gene expression in HGGs has long been associated with an inflammatory gene signature based on bulk analysis of tumor tissue [3, 7]. Indeed, previous studies have shown the essential role of inflammation-associated transcription factors such as

STAT3 and CEBPB in mesenchymal transformation [50]. Here, we define a mesenchymal-associated immunological signature expressed specifically by transformed glioma cells in a subset of patients. In addition, we find that these tumors express high levels of the macrophage recruitment factor gene *CSF1*, a cytokine whose cognate receptor *CSF1R* is widely expressed in myeloid cells across our patient cohort. One intriguing possibility is that CSF1 secretion by HGG cells is responsible for enhanced myeloid infiltration and that CSF1R blockade, which has been investigated as potential therapy for HGG [51, 52], would be particularly beneficial to this subset of patients.

Conclusions

The combined insights into both transformed population structure and microenvironment, even in the context of a modest cohort and a disease with extensive molecular characterization, highlight the utility of large-scale scRNA-Seq in complex tumors. We anticipate that the rapid, scalable, and inexpensive assessment of cellular composition, proliferative potential, tumor cell phenotype, and expression of therapeutic targets afforded by this approach will play a crucial role in molecular diagnosis and precision oncology for HGGs.

Acknowledgements
The authors thank the Molecular Pathology Core of the Herbert Irving Comprehensive Cancer Center and the Sulzberger Columbia Genome Center for technical assistance with immunohistochemistry and sequencing, respectively.

Funding
PAS is supported by NIH/NIBIB Grant K01EB016071, NIH/NCI Grant U54CA209997, and a Human Cell Atlas Pilot Project grant from the Chan-Zuckerberg Initiative. PAS, AI, and AL are supported by NIH/NCI Grant U54CA193313. PAS, PC, and JNB are supported by NIH/NINDS Grant R01NS103473.

Authors' contributions
JY conducted the scRNA-Seq experiments. JNB, JS, and PC procured the tissue. AL and VF prepared the tissue for scRNA-Seq. JY, HML, and PAS conducted the computational data processing and analysis with significant assistance and input from MC, AL, and AI. ECB conducted the DNA sequencing experiments. AD, GZ, DMB, and PC conducted the IHC analysis. All authors contributed to writing the paper. All authors read and approved the final manuscript.

Competing interests
Columbia University has filed patent applications based on the technology used in these studies with JY and PAS included as inventors. The remaining authors declare that they have no competing interests.

Author details
[1]Department of Systems Biology, Columbia University Medical Center, New York, NY 10032, USA. [2]Institute for Cancer Genetics, Herbert Irving Comprehensive Cancer Center, Columbia University Medical Center, New York, NY 10032, USA. [3]Sulzberger Columbia Genome Center, Columbia University Medical Center, New York, NY 10032, USA. [4]Department of Neurological Surgery, Columbia University Medical Center, New York, NY 10032, USA. [5]Department of Science and Technology, Università degli Studi del Sannio, 82100 Benevento, Italy. [6]Department of Pathology & Cell Biology, Columbia University Medical Center, New York, NY 10032, USA. [7]Department of Pediatrics, Columbia University Medical Center, New York, NY 10032, USA. [8]Department of Neurology, Columbia University Medical Center, New York, NY 10032, USA. [9]Department of Biochemistry & Molecular Biophysics, Columbia University Medical Center, New York, NY 10032, USA.

References
1. Huse JT, Holland EC. Targeting brain cancer: advances in the molecular pathology of malignant glioma and medulloblastoma. Nat Rev Cancer. 2010;10(5):319–31.
2. Sottoriva A, Spiteri I, Piccirillo SG, Touloumis A, Collins VP, Marioni JC, et al. Intratumor heterogeneity in human glioblastoma reflects cancer evolutionary dynamics. Proc Natl Acad Sci U S A. 2013;110(10):4009–14. https://doi.org/10.1073/pnas.1219747110.
3. Gill BJ, Pisapia DJ, Malone HR, Goldstein H, Lei L, Sonabend A, et al. MRI-localized biopsies reveal subtype-specific differences in molecular and cellular composition at the margins of glioblastoma. Proc Natl Acad Sci U S A. 2014;111(34):12550–5. https://doi.org/10.1073/pnas.1405839111.
4. Patel AP, Tirosh I, Trombetta JJ, Shalek AK, Gillespie SM, Wakimoto H, et al. Single-cell RNA-seq highlights intratumoral heterogeneity in primary glioblastoma. Science. 2014;344(6190):1396–401. https://doi.org/10.1126/science.1254257.
5. Szerlip NJ, Pedraza A, Chakravarty D, Azim M, McGuire J, Fang Y, et al. Intratumoral heterogeneity of receptor tyrosine kinases EGFR and PDGFRA amplification in glioblastoma defines subpopulations with distinct growth factor response. Proc Natl Acad Sci U S A. 2012;109(8):3041–6. https://doi.org/10.1073/pnas.1114033109.
6. Canoll P, Goldman JE. The interface between glial progenitors and gliomas. Acta Neuropathol. 2008;116(5):465–77. https://doi.org/10.1007/s00401-008-0432-9.
7. Verhaak RG, Hoadley KA, Purdom E, Wang V, Qi Y, Wilkerson MD, et al. Integrated genomic analysis identifies clinically relevant subtypes of glioblastoma characterized by abnormalities in PDGFRA, IDH1, EGFR, and NF1. Cancer Cell. 2010;17(1):98–110.
8. Lathia JD, Mack SC, Mulkearns-Hubert EE, Valentim CL, Rich JN. Cancer stem cells in glioblastoma. Genes Dev. 2015;29(12):1203–17. https://doi.org/10.1101/gad.261982.115.
9. Hambardzumyan D, Gutmann DH, Kettenmann H. The role of microglia and macrophages in glioma maintenance and progression. Nat Neurosci. 2016; 19(1):20–7. https://doi.org/10.1038/nn.4185.
10. Marsh JC, Goldfarb J, Shafman TD, Diaz AZ. Current status of immunotherapy and gene therapy for high-grade gliomas. Cancer Control. 2013;20(1):43–8.
11. Ceccarelli M, Barthel FP, Malta TM, Sabedot TS, Salama SR, Murray BA, et al. Molecular profiling reveals biologically discrete subsets and pathways of progression in diffuse glioma. Cell. 2016;164(3):550–63. https://doi.org/10.1016/j.cell.2015.12.028.
12. Villani AC, Satija R, Reynolds G, Sarkizova S, Shekhar K, Fletcher J, et al. Single-cell RNA-seq reveals new types of human blood dendritic cells, monocytes, and progenitors. Science. 2017;356(6335) https://doi.org/10.1126/science.aah4573.
13. Bennett ML, Bennett FC, Liddelow SA, Ajami B, Zamanian JL, Fernhoff NB, et al. New tools for studying microglia in the mouse and human CNS. Proc Natl Acad Sci U S A. 2016;113(12):E1738–46. https://doi.org/10.1073/pnas.1525528113.
14. Bowman RL, Klemm F, Akkari L, Pyonteck SM, Sevenich L, Quail DF, et al. Macrophage ontogeny underlies differences in tumor-specific education in brain malignancies. Cell Rep. 2016;17(9):2445–59. https://doi.org/10.1016/j.celrep.2016.10.052.

15. Tirosh I, Venteicher AS, Hebert C, Escalante LE, Patel AP, Yizhak K, et al. Single-cell RNA-seq supports a developmental hierarchy in human oligodendroglioma. Nature. 2016;539(7628):309–13. https://doi.org/10.1038/nature20123.

16. Venteicher AS, Tirosh I, Hebert C, Yizhak K, Neftel C, Filbin MG, et al. Decoupling genetics, lineages, and microenvironment in IDH-mutant gliomas by single-cell RNA-seq. Science. 2017;355(6332) https://doi.org/10.1126/science.aai8478.

17. Bose S, Wan Z, Carr A, Rizvi AH, Vieira G, Pe'er D, et al. Scalable microfluidics for single-cell RNA printing and sequencing. Genome Biol. 2015;16(1):120. https://doi.org/10.1186/s13059-015-0684-3.

18. Yuan J, Sims PA. An automated microwell platform for large-scale single cell RNA-Seq. Sci Rep. 2016;6:33883. https://doi.org/10.1038/srep33883.

19. Bowden SG, Gill BJA, Englander ZK, Horenstein CI, Zanazzi G, Chang PD, et al. Local glioma cells are associated with vascular dysregulation. AJNR Am J Neuroradiol. 2018; https://doi.org/10.3174/ajnr.A5526.

20. Dobin A, Davis CA, Schlesinger F, Drenkow J, Zaleski C, Jha S, et al. STAR: ultrafast universal RNA-seq aligner. Bioinformatics. 2013;29(1):15–21. https://doi.org/10.1093/bioinformatics/bts635.

21. Shekhar K, Lapan SW, Whitney IE, Tran NM, Macosko EZ, Kowalczyk M, et al. Comprehensive classification of retinal bipolar neurons by single-cell transcriptomics. Cell. 2016;166(5):1308–23 e30. https://doi.org/10.1016/j.cell.2016.07.054.

22. Macosko EZ, Basu A, Satija R, Nemesh J, Shekhar K, Goldman M, et al. Highly parallel genome-wide expression profiling of individual cells using nanoliter droplets. Cell. 2015;161(5):1202–14. https://doi.org/10.1016/j.cell.2015.05.002.

23. Ilicic T, Kim JK, Kolodziejczyk AA, Bagger FO, McCarthy DJ, Marioni JC, et al. Classification of low quality cells from single-cell RNA-seq data. Genome Biol. 2016;17:29. https://doi.org/10.1186/s13059-016-0888-1.

24. Levine JH, Simonds EF, Bendall SC, Davis KL, el AD A, Tadmor MD, et al. Data-driven phenotypic dissection of AML reveals progenitor-like cells that correlate with prognosis. Cell. 2015;162(1):184–97. https://doi.org/10.1016/j.cell.2015.05.047.

25. Van der Maaten L, Hinton G. Visualizing data using t-SNE. J Mach Learn Res. 2008;9(2579–2605):85.

26. Li H, Courtois ET, Sengupta D, Tan Y, Chen KH, Goh JJL, et al. Reference component analysis of single-cell transcriptomes elucidates cellular heterogeneity in human colorectal tumors. Nat Genet. 2017;49(5):708–18. https://doi.org/10.1038/ng.3818.

27. Muller S, Kohanbash G, Liu SJ, Alvarado B, Carrera D, Bhaduri A, et al. Single-cell profiling of human gliomas reveals macrophage ontogeny as a basis for regional differences in macrophage activation in the tumor microenvironment. Genome Biol. 2017;18(1):234. https://doi.org/10.1186/s13059-017-1362-4.

28. Tirosh I, Izar B, Prakadan SM, Wadsworth MH 2nd, Treacy D, Trombetta JJ, et al. Dissecting the multicellular ecosystem of metastatic melanoma by single-cell RNA-seq. Science. 2016;352(6282):189–96. https://doi.org/10.1126/science.aad0501.

29. Campbell JN, Macosko EZ, Fenselau H, Pers TH, Lyubetskaya A, Tenen D, et al. A molecular census of arcuate hypothalamus and median eminence cell types. Nat Neurosci. 2017;20(3):484–96. https://doi.org/10.1038/nn.4495.

30. Zheng GX, Terry JM, Belgrader P, Ryvkin P, Bent ZW, Wilson R, et al. Massively parallel digital transcriptional profiling of single cells. Nat Commun. 2017;8:14049. https://doi.org/10.1038/ncomms14049.

31. Suva ML, Rheinbay E, Gillespie SM, Patel AP, Wakimoto H, Rabkin SD, et al. Reconstructing and reprogramming the tumor-propagating potential of glioblastoma stem-like cells. Cell. 2014;157(3):580–94. https://doi.org/10.1016/j.cell.2014.02.030.

32. Gangemi RM, Griffero F, Marubbi D, Perera M, Capra MC, Malatesta P, et al. SOX2 silencing in glioblastoma tumor-initiating cells causes stop of proliferation and loss of tumorigenicity. Stem Cells. 2009;27(1):40–8. https://doi.org/10.1634/stemcells.2008-0493.

33. Annovazzi L, Mellai M, Caldera V, Valente G, Schiffer D. SOX2 expression and amplification in gliomas and glioma cell lines. Cancer Genomics Proteomics. 2011;8(3):139–47.

34. Schmitz M, Temme A, Senner V, Ebner R, Schwind S, Stevanovic S, et al. Identification of SOX2 as a novel glioma-associated antigen and potential target for T cell-based immunotherapy. Br J Cancer. 2007;96(8):1293–301. https://doi.org/10.1038/sj.bjc.6603696.

35. Assanah M, Lochhead R, Ogden A, Bruce J, Goldman J, Canoll P. Glial progenitors in adult white matter are driven to form malignant gliomas by platelet-derived growth factor-expressing retroviruses. J Neurosci. 2006;26(25):6781–90. https://doi.org/10.1523/jneurosci.0514-06.2006.

36. Liu C, Sage JC, Miller MR, Verhaak RG, Hippenmeyer S, Vogel H, et al. Mosaic analysis with double markers reveals tumor cell of origin in glioma. Cell. 2011;146(2):209–21. https://doi.org/10.1016/j.cell.2011.06.014.

37. Dai C, Celestino JC, Okada Y, Louis DN, Fuller GN, Holland EC. PDGF autocrine stimulation dedifferentiates cultured astrocytes and induces oligodendrogliomas and oligoastrocytomas from neural progenitors and astrocytes in vivo. Genes Dev. 2001;15(15):1913–25. https://doi.org/10.1101/gad.903001.

38. Lei L, Sonabend AM, Guarnieri P, Soderquist C, Ludwig T, Rosenfeld S, et al. Glioblastoma models reveal the connection between adult glial progenitors and the proneural phenotype. PLoS One. 2011;6(5):e20041.

39. Zhang Y, Chen K, Sloan SA, Bennett ML, Scholze AR, O'Keeffe S, et al. An RNA-sequencing transcriptome and splicing database of glia, neurons, and vascular cells of the cerebral cortex. J Neurosci. 2014;34(36):11929–47. https://doi.org/10.1523/jneurosci.1860-14.2014.

40. Pollen AA, Nowakowski TJ, Shuga J, Wang X, Leyrat AA, Lui JH, et al. Low-coverage single-cell mRNA sequencing reveals cellular heterogeneity and activated signaling pathways in developing cerebral cortex. Nat Biotechnol. 2014;32(10):1053–8. https://doi.org/10.1038/nbt.2967.

41. Rhee W, Ray S, Yokoo H, Hoane ME, Lee CC, Mikheev AM, et al. Quantitative analysis of mitotic Olig2 cells in adult human brain and gliomas: implications for glioma histogenesis and biology. Glia. 2009;57(5):510–23. https://doi.org/10.1002/glia.20780.

42. Dimou L, Gotz M. Glial cells as progenitors and stem cells: new roles in the healthy and diseased brain. Physiol Rev. 2014;94(3):709–37. https://doi.org/10.1152/physrev.00036.2013.

43. Trapnell C, Cacchiarelli D, Grimsby J, Pokharel P, Li S, Morse M, et al. The dynamics and regulators of cell fate decisions are revealed by pseudotemporal ordering of single cells. Nat Biotechnol. 2014;32(4):381–6. https://doi.org/10.1038/nbt.2859.

44. Setty M, Tadmor MD, Reich-Zeliger S, Angel O, Salame TM, Kathail P, et al. Wishbone identifies bifurcating developmental trajectories from single-cell data. Nat Biotechnol. 2016;34(6):637–45. https://doi.org/10.1038/nbt.3569.

45. Haghverdi L, Buettner F, Theis FJ. Diffusion maps for high-dimensional single-cell analysis of differentiation data. Bioinformatics. 2015;31(18):2989–98. https://doi.org/10.1093/bioinformatics/btv325.

46. Rizvi AH, Camara PG, Kandror EK, Roberts TJ, Schieren I, Maniatis T, et al. Single-cell topological RNA-seq analysis reveals insights into cellular differentiation and development. Nat Biotechnol. 2017;35(6):551–60. https://doi.org/10.1038/nbt.3854.

47. Belachew S, Chittajallu R, Aguirre AA, Yuan X, Kirby M, Anderson S, et al. Postnatal NG2 proteoglycan-expressing progenitor cells are intrinsically multipotent and generate functional neurons. J Cell Biol. 2003;161(1):169–86. https://doi.org/10.1083/jcb.200210110.

48. Clarke LE, Young KM, Hamilton NB, Li H, Richardson WD, Attwell D. Properties and fate of oligodendrocyte progenitor cells in the corpus callosum, motor cortex, and piriform cortex of the mouse. J Neurosci. 2012;32(24):8173–85. https://doi.org/10.1523/jneurosci.0928-12.2012.

49. Tso CL, Shintaku P, Chen J, Liu Q, Liu J, Chen Z, et al. Primary glioblastomas express mesenchymal stem-like properties. Mol Cancer Res. 2006;4(9):607–19.

50. Carro MS, Lim WK, Alvarez MJ, Bollo RJ, Zhao X, Snyder EY, et al. The transcriptional network for mesenchymal transformation of brain tumours. Nature. 2010;463(7279):318–25. https://doi.org/10.1038/nature08712.

51. Pyonteck SM, Akkari L, Schuhmacher AJ, Bowman RL, Sevenich L, Quail DF, et al. CSF-1R inhibition alters macrophage polarization and blocks glioma progression. Nat Med. 2013;19(10):1264–72. https://doi.org/10.1038/nm.3337.

52. Quail DF, Bowman RL, Akkari L, Quick ML, Schuhmacher AJ, Huse JT, et al. The tumor microenvironment underlies acquired resistance to CSF-1R inhibition in gliomas. Science. 2016;352(6288):aad3018. https://doi.org/10.1126/science.aad3018.

Permissions

All chapters in this book were first published in GM, by BioMed Central; hereby published with permission under the Creative Commons Attribution License or equivalent. Every chapter published in this book has been scrutinized by our experts. Their significance has been extensively debated. The topics covered herein carry significant findings which will fuel the growth of the discipline. They may even be implemented as practical applications or may be referred to as a beginning point for another development.

The contributors of this book come from diverse backgrounds, making this book a truly international effort. This book will bring forth new frontiers with its revolutionizing research information and detailed analysis of the nascent developments around the world.

We would like to thank all the contributing authors for lending their expertise to make the book truly unique. They have played a crucial role in the development of this book. Without their invaluable contributions this book wouldn't have been possible. They have made vital efforts to compile up to date information on the varied aspects of this subject to make this book a valuable addition to the collection of many professionals and students.

This book was conceptualized with the vision of imparting up-to-date information and advanced data in this field. To ensure the same, a matchless editorial board was set up. Every individual on the board went through rigorous rounds of assessment to prove their worth. After which they invested a large part of their time researching and compiling the most relevant data for our readers.

The editorial board has been involved in producing this book since its inception. They have spent rigorous hours researching and exploring the diverse topics which have resulted in the successful publishing of this book. They have passed on their knowledge of decades through this book. To expedite this challenging task, the publisher supported the team at every step. A small team of assistant editors was also appointed to further simplify the editing procedure and attain best results for the readers.

Apart from the editorial board, the designing team has also invested a significant amount of their time in understanding the subject and creating the most relevant covers. They scrutinized every image to scout for the most suitable representation of the subject and create an appropriate cover for the book.

The publishing team has been an ardent support to the editorial, designing and production team. Their endless efforts to recruit the best for this project, has resulted in the accomplishment of this book. They are a veteran in the field of academics and their pool of knowledge is as vast as their experience in printing. Their expertise and guidance has proved useful at every step. Their uncompromising quality standards have made this book an exceptional effort. Their encouragement from time to time has been an inspiration for everyone.

The publisher and the editorial board hope that this book will prove to be a valuable piece of knowledge for researchers, students, practitioners and scholars across the globe.

List of Contributors

Eilis Hannon
University of Exeter Medical School, University of Exeter, RILD Building, Level 4, Barrack Rd, Exeter EX2 5DW, UK

Diana Schendel
Department of Public Health, Aarhus University, Aarhus, Denmark

Christine Ladd-Acosta and Shan V. Andrews
Department of Epidemiology, Johns Hopkins Bloomberg School of Public Health, Baltimore, MD, USA
Wendy Klag Center for Autism and Developmental Disabilities, Johns Hopkins Bloomberg School of Public Health, Baltimore, MD, USA

Jakob Grove
Department of Biomedicine, Aarhus University, Aarhus, Denmark
iPSYCH, The Lundbeck Foundation Initiative for Integrative Psychiatric Research, Aarhus, Denmark
Centre for Integrative Sequencing, iSEQ, Aarhus University, Aarhus, Denmark
Bioinformatics Research Centre, Aarhus University, Aarhus, Denmark

Christine Søholm Hansen
iPSYCH, The Lundbeck Foundation Initiative for Integrative Psychiatric Research, Aarhus, Denmark
Center for Neonatal Screening, Department for Congenital Disorders, Statens Serum Institut, Copenhagen, Denmark
Institute of Biological Psychiatry, MHC Sct. Hans, Mental Health Services Copenhagen, Roskilde, Denmark

Ole Mors
iPSYCH, The Lundbeck Foundation Initiative for Integrative Psychiatric Research, Aarhus, Denmark
Psychosis Research Unit, Aarhus University Hospital, Risskov, Denmark

Mady Hornig
Center for Infection and Immunity, Columbia University Mailman School of Public Health, New York, USA
Department of Epidemiology, Columbia University Mailman School of Public Health, New York, USA

Preben Bo Mortensen
iPSYCH, The Lundbeck Foundation Initiative for Integrative Psychiatric Research, Aarhus, Denmark
Department of Clinical Medicine, Aarhus University; Aarhus University Hospital, Risskov, Denmark
National Centre for Register-Based Research, Aarhus University, Aarhus, Denmark
Centre for Integrated Register-based Research, Aarhus University, Aarhus, Denmark

M. Daniele Fallin
Wendy Klag Center for Autism and Developmental Disabilities, Johns Hopkins Bloomberg School of Public Health, Baltimore, MD, USA
Center for Infection and Immunity, Columbia University Mailman School of Public Health, New York, USA
Department of Psychiatry, Columbia University, New York, USA
Department of Mental Health, Johns Hopkins Bloomberg School of Public Health, Baltimore, MD, USA

Petar Scepanovic, Flavia Hodel, Christian W. Thorball and Nimisha Chaturvedi
School of Life Sciences, École Polytechnique Fédérale de Lausanne, Lausanne, Switzerland
Swiss Institute of Bioinformatics, Lausanne, Switzerland

Cécile Alanio and Darragh Duffy
Immunobiology of Dendritic Cell Unit, Institut Pasteur, Paris, France
Center for Translational Research, Institut Pasteur, Paris, France
Inserm U1223, Institut Pasteur, Paris, France

Jacques Fellay
School of Life Sciences, École Polytechnique Fédérale de Lausanne, Lausanne, Switzerland
Swiss Institute of Bioinformatics, Lausanne, Switzerland
Precision Medicine Unit, Lausanne University Hospital, Lausanne, Switzerland

Christian Hammer
School of Life Sciences, École Polytechnique Fédérale de Lausanne, Lausanne, Switzerland
Swiss Institute of Bioinformatics, Lausanne, Switzerland
Department of Cancer Immunology, Genentech, South San Francisco, CA, USA

Jacob Bergstedt
Department of Automatic Control, Lund University, Lund, Sweden

Etienne Patin and Lluis Quintana-Murci
Unit of Human Evolutionary Genetics, Department of Genomes and Genetics, Institut Pasteur, Paris, France
Centre National de la Recherche Scientifique, URA 3012, Paris, France
Center of Bioinformatics, Biostatistics and Integrative Biology, Institut Pasteur, 75015 Paris, France

Laurent Abel
Laboratory of Human Genetics of Infectious Diseases, Necker branch, Inserm U1163, Paris, France
Imagine Institute, Paris Descartes University, Paris, France
St Giles laboratory of Human Genetics of Infectious Diseases, Rockefeller Branch, The Rockefeller University, New York, NY, USA

João M. Alves and David Posada
Department of Biochemistry, Genetics and Immunology, University of Vigo, Vigo, Spain
Biomedical Research Center (CINBIO), University of Vigo, Vigo, Spain
Galicia Sur Health Research Institute, Vigo, Spain

Zeran Li, Jorge L. Del-Aguila, John Budde, Rita Martinez, Kathleen Black, Celeste M. Karch and Oscar Harari
Department of Psychiatry, Washington University School of Medicine, 660 S. Euclid Ave. B8134, St. Louis, MO 63110, USA

Joseph D. Dougherty
Department of Psychiatry, Washington University School of Medicine, 660 S. Euclid Ave. B8134, St. Louis, MO 63110, USA
Department of Genetics, Washington University School of Medicine, 660 S. Euclid Ave, St. Louis, MO 63110, USA

Umber Dube
Department of Psychiatry, Washington University School of Medicine, 660 S. Euclid Ave. B8134, St. Louis, MO 63110, USA
Medical Scientist Training Program, Washington University School of Medicine, 660 S. Euclid Ave, St. Louis, MO 63110, USA

Carlos Cruchaga
Department of Psychiatry, Washington University School of Medicine, 660 S. Euclid Ave. B8134, St. Louis, MO 63110, USA

Knight Alzheimer's Disease Research Center, Washington University School of Medicine, 660 S. Euclid Ave, St. Louis, MO 63110, USA
Hope Center for Neurological Disorders, Washington University School of Medicine, 660 S. Euclid Ave. B8111, St. Louis, MO 63110, USA

Qingli Xiao and Jin-Moo Lee
Department of Neurology, Washington University School of Medicine, 660 S. Euclid Ave, St. Louis, MO 63110, USA

Nigel J. Cairns
Department of Neurology, Washington University School of Medicine, 660 S. Euclid Ave, St. Louis, MO 63110, USA
Department of Pathology and Immunology, Washington University in St. Louis, School of Medicine, 510 S. Kingshighway, MC 8131, Saint Louis, MO 63110, USA
Knight Alzheimer's Disease Research Center, Washington University School of Medicine, 660 S. Euclid Ave, St. Louis, MO 63110, USA

John C. Morris and Randall J. Bateman
Department of Neurology, Washington University School of Medicine, 660 S. Euclid Ave, St. Louis, MO 63110, USA
Knight Alzheimer's Disease Research Center, Washington University School of Medicine, 660 S. Euclid Ave, St. Louis, MO 63110, USA
Hope Center for Neurological Disorders, Washington University School of Medicine, 660 S. Euclid Ave. B8111, St. Louis, MO 63110, USA

Carrie L. Welch, Philip M. Allen, Lijiang Ma and Usha Krishnan
Department of Pediatrics, Columbia University Medical Center, New York, NY, USA

Na Zhu and Jiayao Wang
Department of Pediatrics, Columbia University Medical Center, New York, NY, USA
Department of Systems Biology, Columbia University Medical Center, New York, NY, USA

Erika B. Rosenzweig
Department of Pediatrics, Columbia University Medical Center, New York, NY, USA
Department of Medicine, Columbia University Medical Center, New York, NY, USA

Yufeng Shen
Department of Systems Biology, Columbia University Medical Center, New York, NY, USA

Department of Biomedical Informatics, Columbia University, New York, NY, USA

Claudia Gonzaga-Jauregui, and Alejandra K. King, Jeffrey G. Reid, John D. Overton, Aris Baras and Frederick E. Dewey
Regeneron Genetics Center, Regeneron Pharmaceuticals, Tarrytown, New York, USA

D. Dunbar Ivy
Department of Pediatric Cardiology, Children's Hospital Colorado, Denver, CO, USA

Eric D. Austin and Rizwan Hamid
Department of Pediatrics, Vanderbilt University School of Medicine, Nashville, TN, USA

Michael W. Pauciulo and William C. Nichols
Division of Human Genetics, Cincinnati Children's Hospital Medical Center, Cincinnati, OH, USA
Department of Pediatrics, University of Cincinnati College of Medicine, Cincinnati, OH, USA

Katie A. Lutz
Division of Human Genetics, Cincinnati Children's Hospital Medical Center, Cincinnati, OH, USA

Wendy K. Chung
Department of Pediatrics, Columbia University Medical Center, New York, NY, USA
Department of Medicine, Columbia University Medical Center, New York, NY, USA
Herbert Irving Comprehensive Cancer Center, Columbia University Medical Center, New York, NY, USA
New York, USA

Michiko Sekiya, Yasufumi Sakakibara and Xiuming Quan
Department of Alzheimer's Disease Research, National Center for Geriatrics and Gerontology, 7-430 Moriokacho, Obu, Aichi 474-8511, Japan

Naoki Fujisaki and Koichi M. Iijima
Department of Alzheimer's Disease Research, National Center for Geriatrics and Gerontology, 7-430 Moriokacho, Obu, Aichi 474-8511, Japan
Department of Experimental Gerontology, Graduate School of Pharmaceutical Sciences, Nagoya City University, 3-1 Tanabe-dori, Mizuho-ku, Nagoya, Japan

Minghui Wang and Eric E. Schadt
Department of Genetics and Genomic Sciences, Icahn School of Medicine at Mount Sinai, 1470 Madison Avenue, Room 8-111, Box 1498, New York, NY 10029, USA

Icahn Institute of Genomics and Multiscale Biology, Icahn School of Medicine at Mount Sinai, One Gustave L. Levy Place, New York, NY, USA

Bin Zhang
Department of Genetics and Genomic Sciences, Icahn School of Medicine at Mount Sinai, 1470 Madison Avenue, Room 8-111, Box 1498, New York, NY 10029, USA
Icahn Institute of Genomics and Multiscale Biology, Icahn School of Medicine at Mount Sinai, One Gustave L. Levy Place, New York, NY, USA
Ronald M. Loeb Center for Alzheimer's Disease, Icahn School of Medicine at Mount Sinai, One Gustave L Levy Place, New York, NY, USA

Michelle E. Ehrlich
Department of Genetics and Genomic Sciences, Icahn School of Medicine at Mount Sinai, 1470 Madison Avenue, Room 8-111, Box 1498, New York, NY 10029, USA
Department of Neurology, Alzheimer's Disease Research Center, Icahn School of Medicine at Mount Sinai, New York, NY, USA
Department of Pediatrics, Icahn School of Medicine at Mount Sinai, New York, NY, USA

Sam Gandy
Department of Neurology, Alzheimer's Disease Research Center, Icahn School of Medicine at Mount Sinai, New York, NY, USA
Department of Psychiatry and Alzheimer's Disease Research Center, Icahn School of Medicine at Mount Sinai, New York, NY, USA
Center for NFL Neurological Care, Department of Neurology, New York, NY, USA
James J. Peters VA Medical Center, 130 West Kingsbridge Road, New York, NY, USA

Philip L. De Jager
Center for translational and Computational Neuroimmunology, Department of Neurology, The Neurological Institute of New York, Columbia University Medical Center, New York, NY, USA
Broad Institute, Cambridge, MA, USA

David A. Bennett
Rush Alzheimer's Disease Research Center and Department of Neurology, Rush University Medical Center, 1750 W. Congress Parkway, Chicago, IL 60612, USA

Kanae Ando
Department of Biological Sciences, Graduate School of Science and Engineering, Tokyo Metropolitan University, Tokyo, Japan

Alexandra R. Buckley
Biomedical Sciences Graduate Program, University of California San Diego, La Jolla, CA, USA
Human Biology Program, J. Craig Venter Institute, La Jolla, CA, USA

Trey Ideker and Hannah Carter
Division of Medical Genetics, Department of Medicine, University of California San Diego, La Jolla, CA, USA
Moores Cancer Center, University of California San Diego, La Jolla, CA, USA
Cancer Cell Map Initiative (CCMI), University of California San Diego, La Jolla, CA, USA

Nicholas J. Schork
Human Biology Program, J. Craig Venter Institute, La Jolla, CA, USA
Department of Quantitative Medicine and Systems Biology, The Translational Genomics Research Institute, Phoenix, AZ, USA
Departments of Family Medicine and Public Health and Psychiatry, University of California San Diego, La Jolla, CA, USA.

Olivier Harismendy
Moores Cancer Center, University of California San Diego, La Jolla, CA, USA
Division of Biomedical Informatics, Department of Medicine, University of California San Diego, La Jolla, CA, USA

Erika Bongen
Institute for Immunity, Transplantation and Infection, Stanford University School of Medicine, Stanford, CA 94305, USA
Program in Immunology, Stanford University School of Medicine, Stanford 94305, CA, USA

Francesco Vallania
Institute for Immunity, Transplantation and Infection, Stanford University School of Medicine, Stanford, CA 94305, USA
Department of Medicine, Division of Biomedical Informatics Research, Stanford University School of Medicine, Stanford, CA 94305, USA

Purvesh Khatri
Institute for Immunity, Transplantation and Infection, Stanford University School of Medicine, Stanford, CA 94305, USA
Program in Immunology, Stanford University School of Medicine, Stanford 94305, CA, USA
Department of Medicine, Division of Biomedical Informatics Research, Stanford University School of Medicine, Stanford, CA 94305, USA

Paul J. Utz
Institute for Immunity, Transplantation and Infection, Stanford University School of Medicine, Stanford, CA 94305, USA
Program in Immunology, Stanford University School of Medicine, Stanford 94305, CA, USA
Department of Medicine, Division of Immunology and Rheumatology, Stanford University School of Medicine, Stanford, CA 94305, USA

Margaret M. C. Lam, Kelly L. Wyres, Louise M. Judd and Ryan R. Wick
Department of Biochemistry and Molecular Biology, Bio21 Molecular Science and Biotechnology Institute, University of Melbourne, Parkville, Victoria 3010, Australia

Kathryn E. Holt
Department of Biochemistry and Molecular Biology, Bio21 Molecular Science and Biotechnology Institute, University of Melbourne, Parkville, Victoria 3010, Australia
London School of Hygiene and Tropical Medicine, London WC1E 7HT, UK

Sylvain Brisse
Biodiversity and Epidemiology of Bacterial Pathogens, Institut Pasteur, 75015 Paris, France

Adam Jenney
Department of Infectious Diseases and Microbiology Unit, The Alfred Hospital, Melbourne, Victoria 3004, Australia

Tianbao Li
College of Life Science, Jilin University, Changchun 130012, China
Department of Molecular Medicine, University of Texas Health, 8403 Floyd Curl, San Antonio, TX 78229, USA

Qi Liu and Victor X. Jin
Department of Molecular Medicine, University of Texas Health, 8403 Floyd Curl, San Antonio, TX 78229, USA

Nick Garza
Department of Molecular Medicine, University of Texas Health, 8403 Floyd Curl, San Antonio, TX 78229, USA
Department of Biomedical Engineering, Johns Hopkins University, Baltimore, MD 21218, USA

Steven Kornblau
Department of Leukemia, UT MD Anderson Cancer Center, Houston, TX 77030, USA

Amit A. Upadhyay, Amber N. Wolabaugh and Reem A. Dawoud
Division of Microbiology and Immunology, Yerkes National Primate Research Center, Atlanta, GA, USA

Steven E. Bosinger
Division of Microbiology and Immunology, Yerkes National Primate Research Center, Atlanta, GA, USA
Yerkes NHP Genomics Core Laboratory, Yerkes National Primate Research Center, 954 Gatewood Rd, Atlanta, GA 30329, USA
Department of Pathology and Laboratory Medicine, School of Medicine, Emory University, Atlanta, GA, USA

Robert C. Kauffman, Alice Cho and Jens Wrammert
Department of Pediatrics, School of Medicine, Emory University, Atlanta, GA, USA

Iñaki Sanz
Department of Pediatrics, School of Medicine, Emory University, Atlanta, GA, USA
Division of Rheumatology, School of Medicine, Emory University, Atlanta, GA, USA

F. Eun-Hyung Lee
Department of Pediatrics, School of Medicine, Emory University, Atlanta, GA, USA
Divisions of Pulmonary, Allergy and Critical Care Medicine, Emory University, Atlanta, GA, USA

Nirav B. Patel and Gregory K. Tharp
Yerkes NHP Genomics Core Laboratory, Yerkes National Primate Research Center, 954 Gatewood Rd, Atlanta, GA 30329, USA

Samantha M. Reiss and Colin Havenar-Daughton
Division of Vaccine Discovery, La Jolla Institute for Allergy and Immunology, La Jolla, CA, USA
Scripps Center for HIV/AIDS Vaccine Immunology and Immunogen Discovery (CHAVI-ID), La Jolla, CA, USA

Shane Crotty
Division of Vaccine Discovery, La Jolla Institute for Allergy and Immunology, La Jolla, CA, USA
Scripps Center for HIV/AIDS Vaccine Immunology and Immunogen Discovery (CHAVI-ID), La Jolla, CA, USA
Division of Infectious Diseases, Department of Medicine, University of California, San Diego, La Jolla, CA, USA

Bali Pulendran
Institute for Immunity, Transplantation and Infection, Stanford University School of Medicine, Stanford, CA, USA

Department of Pathology, Stanford University School of Medicine, Stanford, CA, USA
Department of Microbiology and Immunology, Stanford University School of Medicine, Stanford, CA, USA

Katherine Karakasis, Julia V. Burnier, Jeffery P. Bruce, Derek L. Clouthier, Arnavaz Danesh, Mark Dowar, Youstina Hanna, Tiantian Li, Lin Lu and Wei Xu
Princess Margaret Cancer Centre, University Health Network, 610 University Avenue, Toronto, Ontario M5G 2M9, Canada

S. Y. Cindy Yang and Rene Quevedo
Princess Margaret Cancer Centre, University Health Network, 610 University Avenue, Toronto, Ontario M5G 2M9, Canada
Department of Medical Biophysics, University of Toronto, Toronto, Ontario, Canada

Stephanie Lheureux and Amit M. Oza
Princess Margaret Cancer Centre, University Health Network, 610 University Avenue, Toronto, Ontario M5G 2M9, Canada
Department of Medicine, University of Toronto, Toronto, Canada

Pamela S. Ohashi
Princess Margaret Cancer Centre, University Health Network, 610 University Avenue, Toronto, Ontario M5G 2M9, Canada
Department of Medical Biophysics, University of Toronto, Toronto, Ontario, Canada
Department of Immunology, University of Toronto, Toronto, Canada

Trevor J. Pugh
Princess Margaret Cancer Centre, University Health Network, 610 University Avenue, Toronto, Ontario M5G 2M9, Canada
Department of Medical Biophysics, University of Toronto, Toronto, Ontario, Canada
Ontario Institute for Cancer Research, Toronto, Canada

Blaise A. Clarke and Patricia A. Shaw
Department of Laboratory Medicine and Pathobiology, University of Toronto, Toronto, Canada
Department of Pathology, University Health Network, Toronto, Canada

Mamoru Kato, Momoko Nagai, Asmaa Elzawahry, Eisaku Furukawa and Joe Miyamoto
Department of Bioinformatics, National Cancer Center Research Institute, Chuo-ku, Tokyo 104-0045, Japan

Hiromi Nakamura, Yasushi Totoki and Yasuhito Arai
Division of Cancer Genomics, National Cancer Center Research Institute, Chuo-ku, Tokyo 104-0045, Japan

Tatsuhiro Shibata
Division of Cancer Genomics, National Cancer Center Research Institute, Chuo-ku, Tokyo 104-0045, Japan
Laboratory of Molecular Medicine, Human Genome Center, The Institute of Medical Science, The University of Tokyo, Minato-ku, Tokyo 108-8639, Japan

Takashi Kubo and Hitoshi Ichikawa
Department of Clinical Genomics, National Cancer Center Research Institute, Chuo-ku, Tokyo 104-0045, Japan

Yuko Tanabe, Kenji Tamura and Noboru Yamamoto
Department of Experimental Therapeutics, National Cancer Center Hospital, Chuo-ku, Tokyo 104-0045, Japan

Hiromi Sakamoto and Teruhiko Yoshida
Division of Genetics, National Cancer Center Research Institute, Chuo-ku, Tokyo 104-0045, Japan

Shingo Matsumoto and Katsuya Tsuchihara
Division of Translational Genomics, Exploratory Oncology Research and Clinical Trial Center, National Cancer Center, Kashiwa, Chiba 277-8577, Japan

Kuniko Sunami and Takashi Kohno
Division of Genome Biology, National Cancer Center Research Institute, Chuo-ku, Tokyo 104-0045, Japan

Yutaka Suzuki
Department of Computational Biology and Medical Sciences, Graduate School of Frontier Sciences, The University of Tokyo, Kashiwa-shi, Chiba 277-8568, Japan

Wei-Hung Pan, Maren Falk-Paulsen, Philipp Best, Antonella Fazio, Priyadarshini Kachroo, Anne Luzius, Marlene Jentzsch, Ateequr Rehman, Andre Franke and Philip Rosenstiel
Institute for Clinical Molecular Biology, University of Kiel, Rosalind-Franklin-Straße 12, 24105 Kiel, Germany

Felix Sommer
Institute for Clinical Molecular Biology, University of Kiel, Rosalind-Franklin-Straße 12, 24105 Kiel, Germany
The Wallenberg Laboratory, Department of Molecular and Clinical Medicine, University of Gothenburg, 41345 Gothenburg, Sweden

Stefan Schreiber
Institute for Clinical Molecular Biology, University of Kiel, Rosalind-Franklin-Straße 12, 24105 Kiel, Germany

Department of Internal Medicine I, University Hospital Schleswig Holstein, 24105 Kiel, Germany

Fredrik Bäckhed
The Wallenberg Laboratory, Department of Molecular and Clinical Medicine, University of Gothenburg, 41345 Gothenburg, Sweden
Novo Nordisk Foundation Center for Basic Metabolic Research, Section for Metabolic Receptology and Enteroendocrinology, Faculty of Health Sciences, University of Copenhagen, 2200 Copenhagen, Denmark

Thomas Ulas
Genomics and Immunoregulation, LIMES-Institute, University of Bonn, 53115 Bonn, Germany

Joachim L. Schultze
Genomics and Immunoregulation, LIMES-Institute, University of Bonn, 53115 Bonn, Germany
Platform for Single Cell Genomics and Epigenomics (PRECISE), German Center for Neurodegenerative Diseases and the University of Bonn, Bonn, Germany

Fabian Müller
Max Planck Institute for Informatics, 66123 Saarbrücken, Germany

Thomas Lengauer
Max Planck Institute for Informatics, 66123 Saarbrücken, Germany
Graduate School of Computer Science, Saarland University, 66123 Saarbrücken, Germany

Jörn Walter
6Department of Genetics, University of Saarland, 66123 Saarbrücken, Germany

Sven Künzel
Institute for Experimental Medicine, Christian Albrechts University of Kiel, Kiel, Germany

John F. Baines
Institute for Experimental Medicine, Christian Albrechts University of Kiel, Kiel, Germany
Max Planck Institute for Evolutionary Biology, Evolutionary Genomics, August-Thienemann-Str. 2, 24306 Plön, Germany

Jinzhou Yuan and Hanna Mendes Levitin
Department of Systems Biology, Columbia University Medical Center, New York, NY 10032, USA

Erin C. Bush
Department of Systems Biology, Columbia University Medical Center, New York, NY 10032, USA
Sulzberger Columbia Genome Center, Columbia University Medical Center, New York, NY 10032, USA

Peter A. Sims
Department of Systems Biology, Columbia University
Medical Center, New York, NY 10032, USA
Sulzberger Columbia Genome Center, Columbia
University Medical Center, New York, NY 10032, USA
Department of Biochemistry and Molecular Biophysics,
Columbia University Medical Center, New York, NY
10032, USA

Veronique Frattini
Institute for Cancer Genetics, Herbert Irving
Comprehensive Cancer Center, Columbia University
Medical Center, New York, NY 10032, USA

Anna Lasorella
Institute for Cancer Genetics, Herbert Irving
Comprehensive Cancer Center, Columbia University
Medical Center, New York, NY 10032, USA
Department of Pathology and Cell Biology, Columbia
University Medical Center, New York, NY 10032, USA
Department of Pediatrics, Columbia University
Medical Center, New York, NY 10032, USA

Antonio Iavarone
Institute for Cancer Genetics, Herbert Irving
Comprehensive Cancer Center, Columbia University
Medical Center, New York, NY 10032, USA
Department of Pathology and Cell Biology, Columbia
University Medical Center, New York, NY 10032, USA
Department of Neurology, Columbia University
Medical Center, New York, NY 10032, USA

**Deborah M. Boyett, Jorge Samanamud and Jeffrey
N. Bruce**
Department of Neurological Surgery, Columbia
University Medical Center, New York, NY 10032, USA

Michele Ceccarelli
Department of Science and Technology, Università
degli Studi del Sannio, 82100 Benevento, Italy

Athanassios Dovas, George Zanazzi and Peter Canoll
Department of Pathology and Cell Biology, Columbia
University Medical Center, New York, NY 10032, USA

Index